FOOD HYGIENE, FOOD ADULTERATION, AND FOOD POISONING

Dr. Greeshma Sharma

ALLIED HEALTH PRESS

Food Hygiene, Food Adulteration, and Food Poisoning

Author: **Dr. Greeshma Sharma**

Allied Health Press
4164 Lakeshore Road
Burlington ON L7L 1A4
Canada
www.alliedhealthpress.com
Email: orders@arclereducation.com

ISBN: 978-1-77956-790-1

ABOUT THE AUTHOR

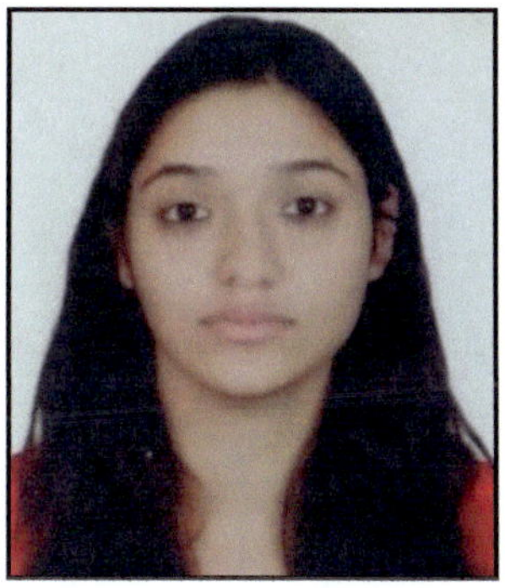

Dr. Greeshma Sharma, holds Ph.D. in Transfusion Medicine from PGIMER, Chandigarh, with a research focus on Neonatal Thrombocytopenia and Neonatal Alloimmune Thrombocytopenia (NAIT). She has completed her M.Sc. in Forensic Biotechnology from NFSU and a B.Sc. in Biological Sciences from Delhi University. She is currently working as a Project Research Scientist I under an ICMR-funded project on NAIT diagnosis and have previous experience as a Junior Research Fellow in DST-funded research. Some of her Publications include articles in Newborn Journal and Vox Sanguinis. She has qualified the UGC-NET (Forensic Science) and have received awards including the Harold Gunson Fellowship (ISBT 2020).

Brief Table of Contents

1. Introduction to Food Hygiene and Sanitation	1
2. Sources of Food Contamination	27
3. Personal Hygiene and Food Handler Responsibilities	55
4. Sanitation of Food Equipment and Premises	81
5. Safe Food Storage and Temperature Control	107
6. Common Foods and Adulteration	133
7. Detection of Adulterants	159
8. Consumer Awareness and Food Labeling	181
9. Understanding Food Poisoning	209
10. Bacterial and Viral Foodborne Illnesses	233
11. Poisoning from Chemicals and Natural Toxins	255
12. Food Allergies and Intolerances	273
13. Foodborne Outbreak Investigation	299
14. Emergency Food SafetyMeasures	325
15. Waste Management in Food Industry	353
Index	381

Detailed Table of Contents

List of Figures *xvii*
Preface *xxxiii*

CHAPTER 1

Introduction to Food Hygiene and Sanitation 1

Introduction **1**
1.1. Principles of Food Hygiene **4**
1.1.1. Personal Hygiene for Food Handlers 5
1.1.2. Cleanliness in Food Preparation Areas 5
1.1.3. Safe Food Storage Practices 5
1.1.4. Temperature Control in Food Safety 6
1.1.5. Cross-Contamination Prevention 6
1.1.6. Proper Cooking Techniques 7
1.1.8. Importance of Pest Control 7
1.1.9. Regular Cleaning and Sanitization Procedures 8
1.2. Foodborne Pathogens **8**
1.2.1. Common Types of Foodborne Pathogens 8
1.2.2. Symptoms of Foodborne Illnesses 9
1.2.3. Transmission Routes of Pathogens 9
1.2.4. High-Risk Foods for Contamination 10
1.2.5. Vulnerable Populations 10
1.2.6. Prevention Strategies for Pathogen Spread 11
1.2.7. Role of Laboratory Testing 11
1.3. Food Safety Regulations and Standards **12**
1.3.1. Overview of Food Safety Laws 12
1.3.2. Role of the FDA and USDA 12
1.3.3. Hazard Analysis Critical Control Point (HACCP) 13
1.3.4. International Food Safety Standards 13
1.3.5. Compliance and Enforcement Mechanisms 14
1.3.6. Certification Programs for Food Businesses 14
1.3.7. Impact of Non-Compliance 14
1.3.8. Consumer Awareness and Education 15
1.3.9. Future Trends in Food Safety Regulations 15
1.4. Best Practices in Food Hygiene **16**
1.4.1. Training Programs for Food Handlers 16
1.4.2. Implementation of Standard Operating Procedures 17
1.4.3. Importance of Regular Audits 17
1.4.4. Use of Technology in Food Safety 17
1.4.5. Community Involvement in Food Safety 18
1.4.6. Role of Food Safety Culture (FS-Culture) 18
1.4.7. Emergency Preparedness for Food Safety 18
1.4.8. Collaboration Between Stakeholders 19
1.4.9. Continuous Improvement in Food Hygiene Practices 19
Summary **21**
References **22**

CHAPTER 2

Sources of Food Contamination 27

Introduction **27**
2.1. Biological Contaminants **30**
2.1.1. Bacteria as a Source of Contamination 30

2.1.2. Viruses and Their Impact on Food Safety 31
2.1.3. Parasites in Food Products 31
2.1.4. Fungi and Mold Contamination 31
2.1.5. Sources of Biological Contaminants 32
2.1.6. Conditions that Promote Biological Growth 32
2.1.7. Symptoms of Foodborne Illnesses 33
2.1.8. Prevention Methods for Biological Contamination 33
2.2. Chemical Contaminants 34
2.2.1. Pesticides and Their Effects on Food 34
2.2.2. Heavy Metals in Food Sources 34
2.2.3. Food Additives and Preservatives 35
2.2.4. Industrial Chemicals and Their Risks 36
2.2.5. Natural Toxins in Food 36
2.2.6. Sources of Chemical Contamination 36
2.2.7. Regulations on Chemical Use in Food 37
2.2.8. Detection Methods for Chemical Contaminants 37
2.2.9. Long-Term Health Effects of Chemical Exposure 38
2.3. Physical Contaminants 38
2.3.1. Common Physical Contaminants in Food 38
2.3.2. Sources of Physical Contamination 39
2.3.3. Impact of Foreign Objects in Food 39
2.3.4. Prevention Strategies for Physical Contamination 40
2.3.5. Role of Food Processing in Contamination 40
2.3.6. Consumer Awareness and Reporting 41
2.3.7. Case Studies of Physical Contamination Incidents 41
2.3.8. Regulations Regarding Physical Contaminants 42
2.3.9. Importance of Quality Control in Food Production 42
2.4. Environmental Contaminants 42
2.4.1. Water Quality and Its Effect on Food 43
2.4.2. Soil Contamination and Agricultural Practices 43
2.4.3. Airborne Contaminants and Food Safety 44
2.4.4. Impact of Climate Change on Food Safety 45
2.4.5. Waste Management and Food Contamination 45
2.4.6. Role of Transportation in Contamination 45
2.4.7. Global Trade and Food Safety Risks 46
2.4.8. Community Practices Affecting Food Safety 46
2.4.9. Strategies for Reducing Environmental Contamination 46
Summary 49
References 50

CHAPTER 3

Personal Hygiene and Food Handler Responsibilities 55

Introduction 55
3.1. Importance of Personal Hygiene in Food Handling 58
3.1.1. Definition of Personal Hygiene in the Food Industry 58
3.1.2. Role of Personal Hygiene in Preventing Foodborne Illnesses 59
3.1.3. Common Pathogens Associated with Poor Hygiene 59
3.1.4. Legal Implications of Hygiene Violations 59
3.1.5. Consumer Expectations Regarding Hygiene 60
3.1.6. Cultural Differences in Hygiene Practices 60
3.1.7. Training and Education on Hygiene for Food Handlers 61
3.1.8. Best Practices for Maintaining Personal Hygiene 61
3.2. Key Personal Hygiene Practices for Food Handlers 61
3.2.1. Handwashing Techniques and Frequency 62
3.2.2. Use of Gloves and When to Change Them 62
3.2.3. Proper Grooming and Attire for Food Handlers 62
3.2.4. Importance of Nail Care and Jewelry Restrictions 63
3.2.5. Managing Personal Health and Illness 63
3.2.6. Avoiding Cross-contamination Through Hygiene 64
3.2.7. Safe Handling of Food and Utensils 64
3.2.8. Importance of Cleanliness in Food Preparation Areas 64
3.2.9. Regular Self-assessment of Hygiene Practices 65
3.3. Food Handler Responsibilities Beyond Personal Hygiene 65

3.3.1. Understanding Food Safety Regulations 66
3.3.2. Importance of Temperature Control in Food Storage 66
3.3.3. Safe Food Sourcing and Supplier Responsibilities 66
3.3.4. Importance of Cleanliness in Food Service Environments 67
3.3.5. Role of Food Handlers in Preventing Cross-Contamination 67
3.3.6. Reporting Illness and Symptoms to Management 68
3.3.7. Importance of Training and Certification 68
3.3.8. Collaboration with Health Inspectors 68
3.3.9. Continuous Improvement and Staying Updated on Best Practices 69
3.4. Consequences of Neglecting Personal Hygiene 69
3.4.1. Health Risks Associated with Poor Hygiene 69
3.4.2. Economic Impact on Food Businesses 70
3.4.3. Legal Repercussions for Food Handlers and Establishments 70
3.4.4. Loss of Consumer Trust and Brand Reputation 71
3.4.5. Impact on Employee Morale and Workplace Culture 71
3.4.6. Long-Term Effects on Public Health 71
3.4.7. Importance of Accountability in Food Handling 72
3.4.8. Strategies for Addressing Hygiene Failures 72
Summary 74
References 75

CHAPTER 4

Sanitation of Food Equipment and Premises 81

Introduction 81
4.1. Importance of Sanitation in Food Safety 84
4.1.1. Economic Consequences of Food Contamination 84
4.1.2. Consumer Trust and Business Reputation 85
4.1.3. Role of Sanitation in Food Quality 85
4.1.4. Connection Between Sanitation and Food Spoilage 85
4.1.5. Importance of Employee Training in Sanitation 86
4.1.6. Case Studies of Sanitation Failures 86
4.1.7. Best Practices for Maintaining Sanitation Standards 87
4.1.8. Future Trends in Food Safety and Sanitation 87
4.2. Sanitation Procedures for Food Equipment 87
4.2.1. Types of Food Equipment Requiring Sanitation 88
4.2.2. Cleaning vs. Sanitizing: Definitions and Differences 88
4.2.3. Recommended Cleaning Agents and Sanitizers 89
4.2.4. Proper Techniques for Cleaning Equipment 89
4.2.5. Frequency of Sanitation for Different Equipment 89
4.2.6. Importance of Equipment Maintenance 90
4.2.7. Role of Temperature in Sanitation Processes 90
4.2.8. Common Challenges in Equipment Sanitation 91
4.2.9. Innovations in Sanitation Technology for Food Equipment 91
4.3. Sanitation Practices for Food Premises 92
4.3.1. Importance of a Clean Food Preparation Area 92
4.3.2. Guidelines for Cleaning Floors and Surfaces 92
4.3.3. Waste Management and Its Role in Sanitation 93
4.3.4. Pest Control Measures in Food Premises 93
4.3.5. Importance of Handwashing Stations 93
4.3.6. Role of Personal Hygiene in Food Sanitation 94
4.3.7. Cleaning Schedules and Checklists 94
4.3.8. Training Staff on Premises Sanitation 95
4.3.9. Assessing the Effectiveness of Sanitation Practices 95
4.4. Regulatory Standards and Compliance 95
4.4.1. Overview of Food Safety Regulations 96
4.4.2. Role of the FDA and USDA in Sanitation 96
4.4.3. Local Health Department (LHDs) Regulations 97
4.4.4. Importance of Inspections and Audits 97
4.4.5. Consequences of Non-Compliance 97
4.4.6. Certification Programs for Food Handlers 98
4.4.7. Documentation and Record-Keeping Requirements 98
4.4.8. Role of Technology in Compliance Monitoring 99

4.4.9. Future Changes in Regulatory Standards 99
Summary **101**
References **102**

CHAPTER 5

Safe Food Storage and Temperature Control 107

Introduction **107**
5.1. Principles of Safe Food Storage **109**
5.1.1. Understanding Food Spoilage 109
5.1.2. Types of Food Storage Methods 110
5.1.3. Importance of Cleanliness in Storage Areas 110
5.1.4. Role of Packaging in Food Safety 111
5.1.5. FIFO (First In, First Out) Method 111
5.1.6. Temperature Zones for Food Storage 111
5.1.7. Importance of Labeling and Dating Food 112
5.1.8. Storage of Raw vs. Cooked Foods 112
5.1.9. Common Mistakes in Food Storage 112
5.2. Temperature Control Guidelines **113**
5.2.1. Recommended Temperature Ranges for Food Storage 113
5.2.2. Importance of Refrigeration 114
5.2.3. Freezing Food Safely 114
5.2.4. Temperature Monitoring Tools 114
5.2.5. Safe Thawing Methods 115
5.2.6. Cooking Temperatures for Different Foods 115
5.2.7. Effects of Temperature Abuse 115
5.2.8. Guidelines for Transporting Food 116
5.2.9. Role of Thermometers in Food Safety 116
5.3. Food Storage for Different Types of Food **117**
5.3.1. Meat and Poultry Storage Guidelines 117
5.3.2. Dairy Product Storage 117
5.3.3. Fruits and Vegetables Storage Tips 118
5.3.4. Grains and Dry Goods Storage 118
5.3.5. Canned and Preserved Foods 118
5.3.6. Leftovers and Reheating 119
5.3.7. Special Considerations for Allergens 119
5.3.8. Storage of Prepared Meals 120
5.3.9. Seasonal Food Storage Practices 120
5.4. Best Practices for Home and Commercial Storage **121**
5.4.1. Home Kitchen Organization 121
5.4.2. Commercial Kitchen Regulations 121
5.4.3. Employee Training on Food Safety 122
5.4.4. Use of Technology in Food Storage 122
5.4.5. Emergency Preparedness for Food Storage 123
5.4.6. Community Resources for Food Safety 123
5.4.7. Role of Government Regulations 123
5.4.8. Case Studies of Food Storage Failures 124
Summary **126**
References **127**

CHAPTER 6

Common Foods and Adulteration 133

Introduction **133**
6.1. Common Foods Prone to Adulteration **136**
6.1.1. Milk and Dairy Products 136
6.1.2. Grains and Cereals 137
6.1.3. Spices and Herbs 137
6.1.4. Oils and Fats 137
6.1.5. Fruits and Vegetables 138
6.1.6. Meat and Poultry 138
6.1.7. Fish and Seafood 138
6.1.8. Sugar and Sweeteners 139
6.1.9. Beverages 139
6.2. Methods of Adulteration **140**
6.2.1. Chemical Adulteration 140
6.2.2. Biological Adulteration 140
6.2.3. Physical Adulteration 141
6.2.4. Intentional vs. Unintentional Adulteration 141
6.2.5. Common Additives used in Adulteration 142
6.2.6. Techniques for Detecting Adulteration 142
6.2.7. Role of Technology in Adulteration 142
6.2.8. Case Studies of Notorious Adulteration Incidents 143
6.2.9. Consumer Awareness and Education 143
6.3. Health Implications of Food Adulteration **144**
6.3.1. Short-Term Health Effects 144

6.3.2. Long-Term Health Consequences 144
6.3.3. Vulnerable Populations at Risk 145
6.3.4. Allergic Reactions and Sensitivities 145
6.3.5. Impact on Nutritional Value 146
6.3.6. Psychological Effects of Food Safety Concerns 146
6.3.7. Role of Public Health Organizations 146
6.3.8. Case Studies of Health Crises Due to Adulteration 147
6.3.9. Preventive Measures for Consumers 147
6.4. Regulatory Measures and Consumer Protection 148
6.4.1. Overview of Food Safety Regulations 148
6.4.2. Role of Government Agencies 149
6.4.3. International Standards for Food Safety 149
6.4.4. Importance of Food Labeling 149
6.4.5. Consumer Rights and Advocacy 150
6.4.6. Challenges in Enforcement of Regulations 150
6.4.7. Role of NGOs in Food Safety 150
6.4.8. Innovations in Food Safety Practices 151
6.4.9. Future Directions for Food Safety Legislation 151
Summary 153
References 154

CHAPTER 7

Detection of Adulterants 159

Introduction 159
7.1. Methods of Detection 160
7.1.1. Sensory Evaluation Techniques 160
7.1.2. Chemical Tests for Adulterants 160
7.1.3. Spectroscopic Methods 161
7.1.4. Chromatographic Techniques 161
7.1.5. Microbiological Methods 161
7.1.6. Rapid Testing Kits 162
7.1.7. Advanced Technologies (e.g., DNA Barcoding) 162
7.1.8. Role of Food Laboratories 163
7.1.9. Limitations of Current Detection Methods 163
7.2. Current Laws and Regulations 164
7.2.1. Overview of National Laws on Adulteration 164
7.2.2. Role of the Food and Drug Administration (FDA) 165
7.2.3. State-Level Regulations and Enforcement 165
7.2.4. International Standards and Agreements 165
7.2.5. Penalties for Adulteration Violations 166
7.2.6. Recent Amendments to Existing Laws 166
7.2.7. Comparison of Laws Across Different Countries 166
7.2.8. Role of Consumer Protection Agencies 167
7.2.9. Challenges in Enforcing Adulteration Laws 167
7.3. Impact of Adulteration Laws on Society 168
7.3.1. Public Health Implications 168
7.3.2. Economic Consequences for Consumers 168
7.3.3. Impact on Food and Drug Industries 169
7.3.4. Consumer Trust and Confidence 169
7.3.5. Role of Advocacy Groups 170
7.3.6. Social Justice Issues Related to Adulteration 170
7.3.7. Global Implications of Local Laws 170
7.3.8. Trends in Consumer Behavior 171
7.3.9. Future Outlook on Adulteration Laws 171
Summary 174
References 175

CHAPTER 8

Consumer Awareness and Food Labeling 181

Introduction 181
8.1. The Importance of Food Labeling 185
8.1.1. Nutritional Information and Its Relevance 186
8.1.2. Ingredient Lists and Transparency 186
8.1.3. Allergen Information and Safety 186
8.1.4. Claims and Certifications (e.g., Organic, Non-GMO) 187
8.1.5. Serving Sizes and Portion Control 187
8.1.6. Date Labeling (e.g., Sell By, Use By) 187
8.1.7. Environmental Impact Labels 188
8.1.8. Ethical Considerations in Food Labeling 188
8.1.9. Consumer Trust and Brand Loyalty 189
8.2. Regulations Governing Food Labeling 189
8.2.1. Overview of the FDA and Its Role 190
8.2.2. Key Regulations (e.g., Nutrition Labeling and Education Act) 190

8.2.3. International Standards (e.g., Codex Alimentarius) 190
8.2.4. State vs. Federal Regulations 191
8.2.5. Enforcement and Compliance Issues 191
8.2.6. Labeling for Dietary Supplements 192
8.2.7. Misleading Labels and Consumer Protection 192
8.2.8. Recent Changes in Labeling Laws 193
8.2.9. Future Trends in Food Labeling Regulations 193
8.3. Consumer Behavior and Food Labeling 193
8.3.1. Factors Influencing Consumer Choices 194
8.3.2. The Role of Education in Consumer Awareness 194
8.3.3. Impact of Marketing on Food Labeling 194
8.3.4. Demographic Differences in Label Interpretation 195
8.3.5. The Influence of Social Media on Consumer Perceptions 195
8.3.6. Case Studies of Consumer Reactions to Labeling 196
8.3.7. The Role of Taste vs. Health in Purchasing Decisions 196
8.3.8. Consumer Advocacy Groups and Their Impact 197
8.3.9. Trends in Consumer Demand for Transparency 197
8.4. Challenges in Food Labeling 197
8.4.1. Complexity of Food Labeling Information 198
8.4.2. Misinterpretation of Labels by Consumers 198
8.4.3. The Issue of Food Fraud and Mislabeling 199
8.4.4. Balancing Information Overload and Simplicity 199
8.4.5. The Role of Technology in Labeling 199
8.4.6. Globalization and Labeling Challenges 200
8.4.7. Cultural Differences in Food Labeling 200
8.4.8. Economic Factors Affecting Labeling Practices 201
8.4.9. Future Challenges in Food Labeling 201
Summary 203
References 204

CHAPTER 9

Understanding Food Poisoning 209

Introduction 209
9.1. Causes of Food Poisoning 212
9.1.1. Bacterial Pathogens 212
9.1.2. Viral Pathogens 213
9.1.3. Parasitic Infections 213
9.1.4. Chemical Contaminants 214
9.1.5. Improper Food Handling 214
9.1.6. Cross-Contamination 214
9.1.7. Inadequate Cooking Temperatures 215
9.1.8. Food Storage Practices 215
9.1.9. Risk Factors in Food Production 215
9.2. Symptoms and Diagnosis 216
9.2.1. Common Symptoms of Food Poisoning 216
9.2.2. Duration of Symptoms 217
9.2.3. Variability of Symptoms by Pathogen 217
9.2.4. Diagnostic Methods Used 217
9.2.5. Importance of Medical History 218
9.2.6. Laboratory Tests for Pathogens 218
9.2.7. Differentiating Food Poisoning from Other Illnesses 219
9.2.8. When to Seek Medical Attention 219
9.2.9. Complications Arising from Food Poisoning 219
9.3. Treatment and Management 220
9.3.1. Home Remedies for Mild Cases 220
9.3.2. Importance of Hydration 221
9.3.3. Over-the-Counter Medications 221
9.3.4. Prescription Medications for Severe Cases 222
9.3.5. Role of Healthcare Providers 222
9.3.6. Monitoring for Complications 222
9.3.7. Dietary Recommendations During Recovery 223
9.3.8. Long-Term Effects of Severe Food Poisoning 223
9.3.9. Support Resources for Affected Individuals 223
Summary 226
References 227

CHAPTER 10

Bacterial and Viral Foodborne Illnesses 233

Introduction 233

10.1. Bacterial Foodborne Illnesses 234

10.1.1. Common Bacterial Pathogens (e.g., Salmonella, E. coli) 234

10.1.2. Mechanisms of Bacterial Infection 235

10.1.3. Symptoms of Bacterial Foodborne Illnesses 235

10.1.4. Transmission Routes of Bacterial Pathogens 236

10.1.5. Prevention Strategies for Bacterial Infections 236

10.1.6. Treatment Options for Bacterial Foodborne Illnesses 236

10.1.7. Role of Food Safety Regulations 237

10.1.8. Future Trends in Bacterial Foodborne Illness Research 237

10.2. Viral Foodborne Illnesses 238

10.2.1. Common Viral Pathogens (e.g., Norovirus, Hepatitis A) 238

10.2.2. Mechanisms of Viral Infection 238

10.2.3. Symptoms of Viral Foodborne Illnesses 239

10.2.4. Transmission Routes of Viral Pathogens 239

10.2.5. Prevention Strategies for Viral Infections 239

10.2.6. Treatment Options for Viral Foodborne Illnesses 240

10.2.7. Role of Food Safety Regulations 240

10.2.8. Future Trends in Viral Foodborne Illness Research 241

10.3. Comparison of Bacterial and Viral Foodborne Illnesses 241

10.3.1. Differences in Pathogen Structure and Function 241

10.3.2. Variations in Symptoms and Severity 242

10.3.3. Distinct Transmission Methods 242

10.3.4. Differences in Prevention Strategies 243

10.3.5. Treatment Approaches for Bacterial vs. Viral Infections 243

10.3.6. Public Health Responses to Outbreaks 244

10.3.7. Role of Education in Prevention 244

10.3.8. Future Research Directions in Foodborne Illnesses 244

10.4. Public Health and Food Safety Measures 245

10.4.1. Role of Government Agencies in Food Safety 245

10.4.2. Importance of Food Handling Practices 245

10.4.3. Education and Awareness Campaigns 246

10.4.4. Surveillance and Monitoring of Foodborne Illnesses 246

10.4.5. Role of Technology in Food Safety 247

10.4.6. International Collaboration on Food Safety 247

10.4.7. Impact of Foodborne Illness on Healthcare Systems 247

10.4.8. Community Involvement in Food Safety 248

10.4.9. Future Challenges in Public Health and Food Safety 248

Summary 250

References 251

CHAPTER 11

Poisoning from Chemicals and Natural Toxins 255

Introduction 255

11.1. Types of Chemicals Causing Food Poisoning 256

11.1.1. Pesticides and Herbicides 256

11.1.2. Heavy Metals (e.g., Lead, Mercury) 257

11.1.3. Food Additives and Preservatives 257

11.1.4. Industrial Chemicals (e.g., PCBs) 258

11.1.5. Contaminants from Packaging Materials 258

11.1.6. Chemical Residues in Processed Foods 259

11.1.7. Role of Food Processing in Chemical Exposure 259

11.1.8. Regulatory Standards for Chemical Use 259

11.2. Natural Toxins in Food 260

11.2.1. Mycotoxins From Mold 260

11.2.2. Plant Toxins (e.g., Solanine in Potatoes) 261

11.2.3. Marine Toxins (e.g., Ciguatera, Scombroid) 261

11.2.4. Bacterial Toxins (e.g., Botulinum Toxin) 261

11.2.5. Animal Toxins (e.g., Pufferfish Poison) 262

11.2.6. Fungal Toxins in Grains 262
11.2.7. Risk Factors for Natural Toxin Exposure 263
11.2.8. Identification and Testing of Natural Toxins 263
11.3. Prevention and Control Measures 263
11.3.1. Safe Food Handling Practices 264
11.3.2. Importance of Cooking Temperatures 264
11.3.3. Proper Food Storage Techniques 264
11.3.4. Role of Food Safety Education 265
11.3.5. Government Regulations and Inspections 265
11.3.6. Consumer Awareness and Labeling 266
11.3.7. Innovations in Food Safety Technology 266
11.3.8. Community Initiatives for Food Safety 267
11.3.9. Global Efforts to Combat Food Poisoning 267
Summary 269
References 270

CHAPTER 12

Food Allergies and Intolerances 273

Introduction 273
12.1. Types of Food Allergies 276
12.1.1. Common Food Allergens (e.g., Peanuts, Tree Nuts) 276
12.1.2. Less Common Food Allergens (e.g., Shellfish, Soy) 277
12.1.3. IgE-Mediated vs. Non-IgE-Mediated Allergies 277
12.1.4. Cross-Reactivity Among Allergens 278
12.1.5. Anaphylaxis and Its Implications 279
12.1.6. Diagnosis Methods for Food Allergies 279
12.1.7. Role of Genetic Factors in Food Allergies 279
12.1.8. Environmental Factors Contributing to Allergies 280
12.2. Types of Food Intolerances 280
12.2.1. Common Food Intolerances (e.g., Lactose, Gluten) 281
12.2.2. Symptoms of Food Intolerances 281
12.2.3. Mechanisms Behind Food Intolerances 282
12.2.4. Diagnosis Methods for Food Intolerances 282
12.2.5. Role of Gut Health in Food Intolerances 283
12.2.6. Impact of Food Intolerances on Nutrition 283
12.2.7. Psychological Effects of Food Intolerances 284
12.3. Management and Treatment 284
12.3.1. Avoidance Strategies for Allergens 284
12.3.2. Dietary Modifications for Intolerances 285
12.3.3. Use of Medications (e.g., Antihistamines, Epinephrine) 286
12.3.4. Importance of Reading Food Labels 286
12.3.5. Role of Allergists and Dietitians 286
12.3.6. Emergency Action Plans for Severe Reactions 287
12.3.7. Support Groups and Resources for Individuals 287
12.3.8. Education and Awareness Initiatives 288
12.4. Societal and Economic Impact 288
12.4.1. Economic Burden of Food Allergies and Intolerances 288
12.4.2. Impact on Food Industry and Labeling Practices 289
12.4.3. Social Implications for Affected Individuals 289
12.4.4. Public Health Policies Regarding Food Allergies 290
12.4.5. Role of Schools and Workplaces in Management 290
12.4.6. Cultural Attitudes Towards Food Allergies 290
12.4.7. Media Representation of Food Allergies 291
12.4.8. Advocacy and Legislation Efforts 291
12.4.9. Global Perspectives on Food Allergies and Intolerances 291
Summary 294
References 295

CHAPTER 13

Foodborne Outbreak Investigation 299

Introduction 299
13.1. Identifying Foodborne Outbreaks 301
13.1.1. Definition of an Outbreak 301
13.1.2. Symptoms and Signs of Foodborne Illnesses 302

13.1.3. Surveillance Systems for Detecting Outbreaks 302
13.1.4. Role of Healthcare Providers in Reporting 303
13.1.5. Importance of Epidemiological Data 303
13.1.6. Case Definitions and Criteria 304
13.1.7. Use of Laboratory Testing in Identification 304
13.1.8. Challenges in Outbreak Identification 305
13.1.9. Examples of Recent Outbreaks 305
13.2. Investigation Process 305
13.2.1. Initial Response to an Outbreak 306
13.2.2. Formation of an Investigation Team 306
13.2.3. Data Collection Methods 306
13.2.4. Interviews with Affected Individuals 307
13.2.5. Environmental Assessments 307
13.2.6. Laboratory Analysis of Food Samples 308
13.2.7. Timeline of the Investigation 308
13.2.8. Collaboration with Local Health Departments (LHDs) 309
13.2.9. Communication with the Public 309
13.3. Source Identification 309
13.3.1. Tracing the Food Supply Chain 310
13.3.2. Role of Traceback Investigations 310
13.3.3. Identifying Potential Sources of Contamination 310
13.3.4. Common Food Vehicles in Outbreaks 311
13.3.5. Environmental Factors Contributing to Outbreaks 312
13.3.6. Use of Technology in Source Identification 312
13.3.7. Challenges in Pinpointing Sources 312
13.3.8. Importance of Rapid Identification 313
13.4. Prevention and Control Measures 313
13.4.1. Public Health Recommendations 314
13.4.2. Role of Food Safety Regulations 314
13.4.3. Importance of Proper Food Handling 314
13.4.4. Education and Training for Food Industry Workers 315
13.4.5. Implementation of Hazard Analysis Critical Control Point (HACCP) 315
13.4.6. Role of Consumer Awareness 316
13.4.7. Strategies for Outbreak Prevention 316
13.4.8. Importance of Ongoing Research 316
Summary 319
References 320

CHAPTER 14

Emergency Food Safety Measures 325

Introduction 325
14.1. Types of Emergencies Affecting Food Safety 328
14.1.1. Natural Disasters (Hurricanes, Floods, Earthquakes) 328
14.1.2. Man-Made Disasters (Chemical Spills, Terrorist Attacks) 329
14.1.3. Public Health Emergencies (Pandemics, Outbreaks) 329
14.1.4. Power Outages and Their Impact on Food Storage 330
14.1.5. Transportation Disruptions Affecting Food Supply 330
14.1.6. Economic Crises Leading to Food Scarcity 330
14.1.7. Climate Change and Its Effects on Food Safety 331
14.1.8. Technological Failures in Food Production 331
14.1.9. Community-Level Emergencies and Their Implications 332
14.2. Key Emergency Food Safety Practices 332
14.2.1. Proper Food Storage Techniques During Emergencies 332
14.2.2. Safe Food Handling Practices 333
14.2.3. Importance of Food Temperature Control 333
14.2.4. Guidelines for Food Preservation Methods 334
14.2.5. Use of Safe Water Sources for Food Preparation 334
14.2.6. Emergency Food Supply Planning 334
14.2.7. Role of Food Safety Education and Training 335
14.2.8. Importance of Labeling and Tracking Food Supplies 335
14.2.9. Community Resources for Food Safety Information 336
14.3. Government and Organizational Roles in Food Safety 336
14.3.1. Federal Regulations and Guidelines for Food Safety 336
14.3.2. Role of Local Health Departments (LHDs) in Emergencies 337
14.3.3. Collaboration between Government and NGOs 337

14.3.4. Emergency Response Plans for Food Safety 338
14.3.5. Public Awareness Campaigns on Food Safety 338
14.3.6. Funding and Resources for Food Safety Initiatives 339
14.3.7. International Cooperation in Food Safety Measures 339
14.3.8. Case Studies of Successful Government Interventions 339
14.3.9. Challenges Faced by Organizations in Food Safety 340
14.4. Community Involvement and Education 340
14.4.1. Importance of Community Engagement in Food Safety 341
14.4.2. Training Programs for Local Volunteers 341
14.4.3. Role of Schools in Promoting Food Safety Education 342
14.4.4. Community Workshops on Emergency Preparedness 342
14.4.5. Building Local Food Safety Networks 342
14.4.6. Utilizing Social Media for Food Safety Awareness 343
14.4.7. Encouraging Local Food Production and Sustainability 343
14.4.8. Involving Local Businesses in Food Safety Initiatives 344
14.4.9. Evaluating Community Food Safety Programs 344
Summary 346
References 347

CHAPTER 15

Waste Management in Food Industry 353

Introduction 353
15.1. Types of Waste in the Food Industry 356
15.1.1. Organic Waste 357
15.1.2. Packaging Waste 357
15.1.3. Hazardous Waste 357
15.1.4. E-Waste From Food Processing Equipment 358
15.1.5. Wastewater and Its Treatment 358
15.1.6. By-Products From Food Processing 359
15.1.7. Spoilage and Unsold Inventory 359
15.1.8. Food Waste at the Consumer Level 360
15.2. Waste Management Strategies 360
15.2.1. Waste Reduction Techniques 360
15.2.2. Recycling and Composting Initiatives 361
15.2.3. Anaerobic Digestion for Organic Waste 361
15.2.4. Use of Food Waste as Compost 362
15.2.5. Technology in Waste Management 362
15.2.6. Employee Training and Awareness Programs 362
15.2.7. Sustainable Packaging Solutions 363
15.2.8. Collaboration with Waste Management Companies 363
15.3. Regulatory and Policy Framework 364
15.3.1. Overview of Local and National Regulations 364
15.3.2. International Guidelines on Food Waste 365
15.3.3. Role of Government in Waste Management 365
15.3.4. Incentives for Businesses to Reduce Waste 365
15.3.5. Penalties for Non-Compliance 366
15.3.6. Impact of Policies on Food Waste Reduction 366
15.3.7. Stakeholder Involvement in Policy-Making 367
15.3.8. Future Trends in Waste Management Legislation 367
15.3.9. Evaluation of Existing Policies and Their Effectiveness 367
15.4. Economic Impact of Food Waste 369
15.4.1. Cost Implications for Food Businesses 369
15.4.2. Economic Benefits of Waste Reduction 369
15.4.3. Impact on Food Prices 370
15.4.4. Job Creation in Waste Management Sectors 370
15.4.5. Investment in Sustainable Practices 370
15.4.6. Consumer Behavior and Its Economic Effects 371
15.4.7. Long-Term Financial Sustainability 371
15.4.8. Case Studies of Economic Success Through Waste Management 372
Summary 374
References 375

Index 381

LIST OF FIGURES

Figure 1.1. Food hygiene is an essential aspect of public health that encompasses practices aimed at ensuring the safety and quality of food from production to consumption

Figure 1.2. Wastewater irrigation

Figure 1.3. Government regulations play a pivotal role in safeguarding public health, especially within the domain of food hygiene and sanitation

Figure 1.4. Essential to ensuring public health, the objectives of food hygiene practices revolve around minimizing foodborne illnesses and safeguarding food quality throughout the supply chain

Figure 1.5: Personal hygiene for food handlers is a cornerstone of effective food safety practices, directly impacting the health of consumers and the integrity of food products

Figure 1.6. Proper storage techniques, such as keeping perishable items at appropriate temperatures, are crucial to reduce the risk of bacterial growth

Figure 1.7. Effective prevention of cross-contamination is pivotal in maintaining food hygiene and sanitation, particularly in environments where microbial contamination can lead to severe health risks

Figure 1.8. The quality of water utilized in food preparation directly impacts overall health and safety, particularly in developing regions where access to clean water is limited

Figure 1.9. Maintaining regular cleaning and sanitization procedures is crucial for ensuring food safety and hygiene within any food preparation environment

Figure 1.10. Campylobacter

Figure 1.11. The transmission routes of pathogens play a critical role in the dynamics of food hygiene and sanitation, particularly concerning zoonotic diseases

Figure 1.12. Understanding the unique challenges faced by vulnerable populations is essential in the context of food hygiene and sanitation

Figure 1.13. The role of laboratory testing in food hygiene and sanitation is paramount, as it acts as a crucial line of defense against zoonotic diseases and foodborne pathogens

Figure 1.14. The framework of food safety laws is essential for ensuring public health and maintaining the integrity of food systems worldwide

Figure 1.15. Hazard Analysis Critical Control Point (HACCP) serves as a pivotal framework in ensuring food safety within the realm of food hygiene and sanitation

Figure 1.16. Effective compliance and enforcement mechanisms are critical to maintaining food hygiene and sanitation standards, particularly in the face of evolving public health challenges

Figure 1.17. Non-compliance with food hygiene and sanitation standards has profound implications, particularly in the global marketplace, where food safety regulations are increasingly stringent

Figure 1.18. As global awareness of food safety escalates, future trends in regulations are poised to incorporate more comprehensive and interdisciplinary approaches

Figure 1.19. The implementation of effective training programs for food handlers is crucial in enhancing food hygiene and sanitation practices within the food industry

Figure 1.20. Regular audits are a critical component of maintaining high standards of food hygiene and sanitation within the food industry

Figure 1.21. Community involvement plays a critical role in enhancing food safety, as it fosters a collective responsibility towards maintaining hygiene and sanitation standards within local populations

Figure 1.22. Effective emergency preparedness for food safety is crucial in mitigating risks associated with foodborne illnesses, particularly during health crises such as pandemics

Figure 2.1. Food contamination is defined as the presence of harmful substances in food that can pose significant health risks to consumers

Figure 2.2. Contamination can broadly be classified into three main categories: biological, chemical, and physical

Figure 2.3. Foodborne illnesses continue to represent a significant public health challenge worldwide, with current statistics underscoring their impact

Figure 2.4. Bacterial pathogenicity

Figure 2.5. Parasites in food products

Figure 2.6. Fungi and mold contamination represent significant risks within the broader category of food contamination, primarily due to their ability to produce harmful mycotoxins such as aflatoxins

Figure 2.7. High moisture levels in food significantly increase the likelihood of microbial proliferation

Figure 2.8. Mycotoxins in food

Figure 2.9. Pesticides, widely utilized in agricultural practices, play a significant role in food production, but also contribute substantially to food contamination

Figure 2.10. Food additives and preservatives play a critical yet controversial role, often featuring prominently in discussions surrounding sources of food contamination

Figure 2.11. Natural toxins in food pose significant risks to human health and are an important aspect of food contamination

Figure 2.12. The regulation of chemical use in food is paramount to safeguarding public health and maintaining food safety

Figure 2.13. Microplastics, which infiltrate the food supply through various pathways, can carry hazardous chemicals that impact human health over time

Figure 2.14. Physical contaminants in food, ranging from foreign objects to naturally occurring materials, present significant risks to consumer safety and food quality

Figure 2.15. Contaminants such as pieces of glass, metal, plastic, or even natural elements like stones can lead to injuries, choking hazards, and more severe health complications

Figure 2.16. The role of food processing in contamination is a critical concern in understanding overall food safety

Figure 2.17. Salmonella in poultry and pesticides in tomatoes exemplify how such contamination can stem from inadequate handling or environmental factors, impacting consumer trust in food products

Figure 2.18. Quality control in food production is paramount for ensuring the safety and integrity of the food supply

Figure 2.19. The quality of water used in agricultural practices is profoundly linked to food safety and contamination, influencing not only crop yield but also the health of consumers

Figure 2.20. Airborne microorganisms, including various pathogens, can originate from food handlers, equipment, and even the surrounding environment, leading to the potential contamination of food products

Figure 2.21. Effective waste management practices play a crucial role in mitigating food contamination risks, particularly as societies increasingly rely on recycled materials for food packaging

Figure 2.22. The increasing globalization of trade significantly impacts food safety risks, presenting multifaceted challenges for contamination management

Figure 3.1. Personal hygiene encompasses a set of practices that individuals undertake to maintain health and prevent illness, particularly by limiting the spread of pathogens

Figure 3.2. Food handlers play a crucial role in ensuring food safety, which is essential for public health and well-being

Figure 3.3. Proper hygiene protocols serve as the frontline defense against foodborne illnesses, which continue to be a significant global health concern

Figure 3.4. In the food industry, personal hygiene refers to the practices and behaviors that food handlers must adhere to maintain the safety and quality of food products

Figure 3.5. Salmonella is a primary pathogen, responsible for numerous gastrointestinal disorders linked to the consumption of contaminated food products

Figure 3.6. Consumer expectations regarding hygiene in food handling have significantly evolved, particularly with the rise of online food delivery applications (OFD apps), which have transformed how consumers engage with food options

Figure 3.7. Effective training and education on hygiene for food handlers is paramount in safeguarding public health and ensuring food safety

Figure 3.8. Effective handwashing techniques and frequency are crucial components of personal hygiene for food handlers, significantly impacting food safety

Figure 3.9. Food handlers must maintain a clean and professional appearance, which begins with appropriate uniforms that are specifically designed to prevent contamination

Figure 3.10. Effective management of personal health and illness is crucial in ensuring the safety and well-being of food handlers, particularly in the context of public health

Figure 3.11. In the realm of personal hygiene and food handler responsibilities, the safe handling of food and utensils is paramount in preventing food-borne illnesses

Figure 3.12. Regular self-assessment of hygiene practices serves as a fundamental component in ensuring food safety and mitigating the risks associated with food-borne illnesses

Figure 3.13. Food safety regulations are crucial in protecting public health, particularly as foodborne illnesses continue to pose significant threats globally

Figure 3.14. Effective food safety practices begin at the source, where farmers must adhere to hygienic standards to mitigate risks associated with microbial and chemical contaminants

Figure 3.15. Food handlers play a critical role in preventing cross-contamination, a key factor in foodborne illness outbreaks

Figure 3.16. Effective training equips food handlers with the necessary knowledge and skills to recognize potential food safety hazards, implement best practices, and maintain cleanliness in food preparation environments

Figure 3.17. Continuous improvement and staying abreast of best practices are essential for ensuring food safety and protecting public health

Figure 3.18. The health risks associated with poor hygiene among food handlers are multifaceted and can lead to severe public health concerns

Figure 3.19. Violations can lead to severe penalties, including fines, loss of business licenses, and even criminal charges in cases of negligence that result in foodborne illnesses

Figure 3.20. Maintaining high standards of hygiene not only fosters a safer work environment but also enhances the overall well-being of employees

Figure 3.21. Food handlers play a critical role in preventing foodborne illnesses, yet research indicates that inadequate management practices often undermine this responsibility

Figure 4.1. Sanitation in food service encompasses the comprehensive practices and protocols that ensure food equipment and premises are maintained in a hygienic condition to prevent foodborne illnesses

Figure 4.2. *Listeria monocytogenes*, a pathogen known for forming resilient biofilms, which complicates effective sanitation protocols

Figure 4.3. Innovations such as integrated pest management (IPM) emphasized the selective application of insecticides as a cornerstone of food safety, enhancing traditional methods through new technologies

Figure 4.4. When foodborne illnesses occur, affected individuals burden healthcare resources, leading to increased medical expenses and loss of productivity due to missed workdays

Figure 4.5. Effective sanitation practices, particularly in food processing environments, are crucial for preventing contamination and the proliferation of harmful pathogens

Figure 4.6. Ensuring that employees are well-trained in sanitation practices is critical for maintaining the hygiene and safety of food equipment and premises

Figure 4.7. Regular and thorough cleaning schedules should be established, focusing on both surfaces and equipment that come into direct contact with food products

Figure 4.8. Equipment that requires thorough sanitation includes processing machinery, storage containers, utensils, and food preparation surfaces

Figure 4.9. Effective sanitation of food equipment and premises is paramount to ensuring food safety and preventing the spread of pathogens

Figure 4.10. Maintaining appropriate sanitation frequency for different food equipment is essential to ensure food safety and prevent contamination

Figure 4.11. Temperature plays a pivotal role in the sanitation processes of food equipment and premises, primarily through its influence on microbial survival and growth

Figure 4.12. Innovations such as automated cleaning systems, UV-C light sanitation methods, and smart sensors for real-time monitoring of hygienic conditions have significantly enhanced the efficiency and effectiveness of sanitation protocols

Figure 4.13. A sanitized environment minimizes the risk of foodborne illnesses, which are predominantly caused by harmful microorganisms that thrive in unsanitary conditions, particularly in meat, dairy, and egg products

Figure 4.14. Effective waste management is pivotal in ensuring proper sanitation within food equipment and premises, as it directly influences the prevention of contamination and the maintenance of hygiene standards

Figure 4.15. Handwashing stations play a pivotal role in ensuring the sanitation of food equipment and premises, particularly in environments where food safety is paramount

Figure 4.16. Effective cleaning schedules and checklists are vital components in the sanitation of food equipment and premises, as they ensure consistent adherence to hygiene protocols and the minimization of foodborne illnesses

Figure 4.17. The effectiveness of sanitation practices in the food industry is paramount to ensuring food safety and public health

Figure 4.18. Food safety regulations serve as a critical framework for ensuring the health and well-being of consumers in the food supply chain

Figure 4.19. Local health department regulations play a crucial role in ensuring the sanitation of food equipment and premises, which is pivotal for safeguarding public health

Figure 4.20. Non-compliance with sanitation standards in food equipment and premises can lead to severe consequences that undermine public health and safety

Figure 4.21. Effective documentation and record-keeping requirements play a crucial role in maintaining the sanitation of food equipment and premises

Figure 5.1. Food storage encompasses a fundamental practice aimed at preserving the quality and safety of perishable items, effectively preventing foodborne illnesses and spoilage

Figure 5.2. Effective temperature control is paramount in ensuring food safety and extending the shelf life of perishable items

Figure 5.3. Understanding food spoilage is essential for implementing effective safe food storage and temperature control practices

Figure 5.4. The significance of maintaining cleanliness in storage areas cannot be overstated, particularly within the framework of safe food storage and temperature control

Figure 5.5. The FIFO (First In, First Out) method is an essential practice in safe food storage and temperature control, particularly for perishable items

Figure 5.6. Effective food labeling and dating practices are vital components of safe food storage and temperature control, as they provide consumers with critical information regarding the freshness and safety of food products

Figure 5.7. Food storage often appears deceptively straightforward, yet numerous common mistakes can compromise both safety and quality

Figure 5.8. Effective food storage is crucial for maintaining food safety and preventing spoilage, with recommended temperature ranges playing a pivotal role in this process

Figure 5.9. The safe freezing of food is a critical aspect of food storage that helps maintain both quality and safety

Figure 5.10. Understanding safe thawing methods is essential for preventing foodborne illnesses and maintaining food quality during preparation

Figure 5.11. Temperature abuse, which occurs when food is stored outside the recommended temperature range, poses significant risks to food safety and public health

Figure 5.12. Thermometers play a crucial role in ensuring food safety, particularly in maintaining safe storage and temperature control

Figure 5.13. The safe storage of meat and poultry is paramount to preventing foodborne illness, and adhering to established guidelines is essential for maintaining food safety

Figure 5.14. Effective storage of fruits and vegetables is crucial for maintaining their freshness and preventing spoilage, ultimately contributing to safe food practices

Figure 5.15. Canned and preserved foods represent a crucial component of food safety and storage management, particularly as global trade increases the variety of products available

Figure 5.16. In the realm of safe food storage and temperature control, special considerations for allergens are paramount to ensure the health and safety of consumers

Figure 5.17. The concept of seasonal food storage practices plays a critical role within the framework of safe food storage and temperature control

Figure 5.18. Effective home kitchen organization is critical in ensuring safe food storage and maintaining appropriate temperature control, which are essential components in preventing foodborne illnesses

Figure 5.19. Effective employee training on food safety is paramount in ensuring that safe food storage and temperature control practices are consistently followed within food service establishments

Figure 5.20. The advancement of technology in food storage plays a critical role in enhancing food safety and extending shelf life

Figure 5.21. Effective community resources for food safety play a crucial role in ensuring safe food storage and temperature control practices, which are imperative for public health

Figure 6.1. Food adulteration refers to the intentional or unintentional alteration of food products, resulting in a lowered quality or safety standard

Figure 6.2. The significance of studying common foods extends beyond mere culinary interest; it encompasses critical health, economic, and social dimensions

Figure 6.3. The ramifications of food adulteration extend far beyond economic implications, significantly impacting public health and consumer safety

Figure 6.4. Milk and dairy products serve as staple components of many diets globally, not only for their nutritional value but also for their versatility in culinary applications

Figure 6.5. The integrity of spices and herbs has become a pressing concern in the context of food adulteration, particularly due to their significant economic value and widespread use in processed foods

Figure 6.6. The growing global trade in fruits and vegetables has significantly increased concerns about food adulteration and safety

Figure 6.7. The fish and seafood industry faces significant challenges related to adulteration and mislabeling, which undermine consumer trust and market integrity

Figure 6.8. Beverages represent a significant category within the food industry, often subject to adulteration that can compromise both quality and consumer trust

Figure 6.9. The practice of chemical adulteration poses significant challenges to food safety, often undermining the integrity of commonly consumed products

Figure 6.10. Physical adulteration presents a significant challenge within the broader issue of food safety, often compromising both the quality and integrity of commonly consumed products

Figure 6.11. The prevalence of food adulteration is often exacerbated by the use of common additives that serve to enhance the appearance, texture, or flavor of products without adding genuine nutritional value

Figure 6.12. Role of technology in adulteration

Figure 6.13. In an era marked by increasing concern over food safety and authenticity, consumer awareness and education play pivotal roles in combating food adulteration

Figure 6.14. The adulteration of common foods poses significant short-term health effects that can manifest rapidly and severely

Figure 6.15. The phenomenon of food adulteration poses significant risks to vulnerable populations, particularly those with limited access to safe and nutritious food sources

Figure 6.16. The adulteration of common foods significantly impacts their nutritional value, often diminishing the beneficial properties that consumers expect

Figure 6.17. Public health organizations play a crucial role in safeguarding the integrity of food supply chains, particularly in the context of common foods that may be subject to adulteration

Figure 6.18. Awareness of food origins, coupled with the ability to verify authenticity, empowers consumers to make informed choices about the products they purchase

Figure 6.19. In the realm of food safety, regulations serve as a critical framework aimed at safeguarding public health from the hazards associated with food adulteration

Figure 6.20. Understanding international standards for food safety is crucial in addressing the growing concerns related to food adulteration

Figure 6.21. The prevalence of food adulteration poses a significant threat to consumer rights, highlighting the urgent need for advocacy and awareness among the public

Figure 6.22. In the context of food safety, non-governmental organizations (NGOs) play a pivotal role by advocating for enhanced standards and promoting transparency throughout the food supply chain

Figure 7.1. The integration of sensory evaluation techniques serves as a crucial component in the detection of food adulterants, particularly in products like coffee, where visual inspection alone is insufficient due to the deceptive similarity in color and texture among adulterants

Figure 7.2. The application of spectroscopic methods has become increasingly vital in the detection of adulterants in food

Figure 7.3. Utilizing techniques such as culture-based assays, molecular methods, and rapid detection systems facilitates the identification of specific microbial contaminants that indicate adulteration

Figure 7.4. The effectiveness of DNA barcoding in food safety lies in its ability to authenticate raw materials and detect contaminants across various matrices

Figure 7.5. Conventional methods may struggle to detect low levels of adulterants that share similar properties with genuine products

Figure 7.6. Adulteration of food products remains a significant concern globally, necessitating stringent national laws and regulatory frameworks to safeguard public health

Figure 7.7. The role of state-level regulations and enforcement in the context of adulteration is crucial, as these local frameworks directly influence food safety and public health outcomes

Figure 7.8. Penalties for adulteration violations

Figure 7.9. Legal approaches shape the dynamics of food safety and adulteration across nations

Figure 7.10. The enforcement of adulteration laws faces numerous challenges that significantly affect public health and consumer safety

Figure 7.11. The implications of food and product adulteration on public health are profound, warranting immediate attention from policymakers and regulatory bodies

Figure 7.12. The intricate relationship between food safety regulations and the food and drug industries highlights the profound impact of adulteration laws on public health and economic stability

Figure 7.13. Advocacy groups play a pivotal role in shaping food safety regulations and combating the challenges posed by adulteration

Figure 7.14. The interplay between local laws and global implications becomes increasingly significant, particularly regarding food adulteration regulations

Figure 7.15. Policymakers are increasingly recognizing the importance of advanced technologies and data integration in combating food fraud

Figure 8.1. Consumer awareness is a critical component of an informed society, particularly in the context of food labeling

Figure 8.2. Nutritional Labeling Education Act (NLEA)

Figure 8.3. Informed choices significantly impact consumer behavior and preferences in the context of food labeling, highlighting the essential role of awareness in promoting sustainable consumption practices

Figure 8.4. Food labels serve not only as guides for nutritional value but also as instruments for promoting transparency in food production and safety standards

Figure 8.5. Understanding nutritional information is crucial for consumers aiming to make informed dietary choices, particularly in an age where food labeling regulations vary significantly

Figure 8.6. The increasing prevalence of food allergies necessitates robust allergen labeling to ensure consumer safety and awareness

Figure 8.7. The issue of serving sizes and portion control is critical in fostering consumer awareness and improving dietary choices

Figure 8.8. The phenomenon of environmental impact labels serves as a crucial intersection between consumer awareness and food labeling practices, thereby promoting sustainable consumption

Figure 8.9. In the contemporary marketplace, consumer trust and brand loyalty have emerged as critical components influencing purchasing behaviors, particularly concerning food products

Figure 8.10. The Food and Drug Administration (FDA) plays a pivotal role in regulating food safety, ensuring that consumers have access to products that meet strict health and safety standards

Figure 8.11. The establishment of international standards, such as those set by the Codex Alimentarius, plays a pivotal role in enhancing consumer awareness and guiding food labeling practices globally

Figure 8.12. Regulatory agencies like the Food and Drug Administration (FDA) have increasingly adopted punitive measures against non-compliance, but this shift has had mixed results

Figure 8.13. Misleading labels pose a significant challenge to consumer protection, particularly in an era where environmental claims and nutritional information are increasingly prominent in marketing strategies

Figure 8.14. As consumer awareness regarding health-related dietary choices continues to rise, future trends in food labeling regulations are likely to evolve significantly

Figure 8.15. Consumer choices are significantly shaped by a multitude of factors, including health consciousness, environmental awareness, and social influences

Figure 8.16. Retailers often adopt front-of-package (FOP) labels to enhance customer understanding and assist in food choice, responding both to market competition and regulatory pressures

Figure 8.17. Users often rely on social media to gather insights into product attributes, such as nutritional content and the authenticity of health claims, thus shaping their purchasing decisions

Figure 8.18. In consumer purchasing decisions, the interplay between taste and health considerations is increasingly pertinent, particularly in the context of food labeling

Figure 8.19. As consumers become more educated about the implications of their food choices, they actively seek clarity regarding sourcing, production methods, and ingredient origins

Figure 8.20. Despite the essential role that labels play in informing consumers about nutritional content and ingredients, many individuals struggle to decipher the complex language and varying formats employed

Figure 8.21. The prevalence of food fraud and mislabeling poses significant challenges to consumer safety and trust in the food supply

Figure 8.22. Innovations such as QR codes, augmented reality, and mobile applications now provide consumers with immediate access to detailed information about food products, including nutritional content, sourcing practices, and potential allergens

Figure 8.23. Cultural differences significantly influence the perceptions and effectiveness of food labeling, highlighting the need for tailored approaches in enhancing consumer awareness

Figure 9.1. Food poisoning is broadly defined as an illness resulting from the consumption of contaminated food or beverages, which can cause a range of symptoms including nausea, vomiting, diarrhea, and abdominal pain

Figure 9.2. The prevalence of food poisoning cases continues to be a significant public health concern, reflecting the complexities involved in food safety management

Figure 9.3. The impact of food poisoning on public health extends beyond immediate illness, highlighting systemic issues such as poverty and inadequate food safety protocols

Figure 9.4. *Clostridium perfringens*, recognized for its role in both foodborne and antibiotic-associated diarrheal diseases

Figure 9.5. Parasitic infections represent a significant, yet often underappreciated, portion of foodborne illnesses, contributing to the broader understanding of food poisoning

Figure 9.6. Improper food handling practices pose a significant threat to public health, particularly in settings where food is prepared for vulnerable populations, such as day care centers and restaurants

Figure 9.7. Inadequate cooking temperatures emerge as a critical factor in the prevalence of food poisoning, underscoring the importance of proper food handling practices

Figure 9.8. Food production is fraught with various risk factors that significantly influence food safety and contribute to the prevalence of food poisoning

Figure 9.9. The recognition of common symptoms associated with food poisoning is essential for prompt diagnosis and treatment, which can significantly mitigate illness severity

Figure 9.10. The variability of symptoms associated with food poisoning is significantly influenced by the specific pathogens involved, each of, which can elicit distinct clinical manifestations

Figure 9.11. An individual's medical history plays a crucial role in understanding food poisoning, as it provides significant insights into predispositions and potential vulnerabilities to various pathogens

Figure 9.12. Symptoms such as nausea, vomiting, diarrhea, and abdominal pain overlap significantly with conditions like viral gastroenteritis, pancreatitis, and even appendicitis, complicating clinical assessments

Figure 9.13. Many individuals experience severe long-term health effects, including the risk of neurodegenerative symptoms, which can arise from various pathogens and toxins found in contaminated food

Figure 9.14. Common approaches include hydration with clear fluids, ginger tea, and incorporating bland diets such as toast or rice to reduce gastrointestinal discomfort

Figure 9.15. The role of over-the-counter (OTC) medications in managing symptoms associated with food poisoning cannot be overstated, as these medications can offer relief from discomfort while the gastrointestinal system recovers

Figure 9.16. In the context of food poisoning, healthcare providers play an indispensable role in both the prevention and management of this public health concern

Figure 9.17. Recovery from food poisoning necessitates careful nutritional management to restore health and prevent further complications

Figure 10.1. The study of foodborne pathogens is vital for safeguarding public health and ensuring food security

Figure 10.2. Among the most prevalent bacterial pathogens associated with foodborne illnesses, Salmonella and *E. coli* are particularly noteworthy due to their significant public health impact

Figure 10.3. The symptoms of bacterial foodborne illnesses can vary widely, typically manifesting within hours to days after consumption of contaminated food

Figure 10.4. Effective prevention strategies for bacterial infections associated with foodborne illnesses are critical to safeguarding public health

Figure 10.5. The role of food safety regulations is crucial in mitigating the risk of bacterial and viral foodborne illnesses, as these laws are designed to ensure that food production, processing, and distribution adhere to stringent health standards

Figure 10.6. Norovirus, a leading cause of gastroenteritis, is notorious for its high contagion rates and can be transmitted through contaminated food, water, or direct contact with infected individuals

Figure 10.7. Common manifestations include gastrointestinal distress such as nausea, vomiting, diarrhea, and abdominal cramps, often accompanied by fever and malaise

Figure 10.8. Effective measures include the implementation of stringent food safety protocols, enhanced sanitation practices in food production and handling, and robust public education campaigns promoting awareness of viral transmission

Figure 10.9. Regulations ensure that food businesses adopt best practices to limit contamination, thereby protecting public health

Figure 10.10. Bacteria, as unicellular organisms, possess a rigid cell wall and replicate independently through binary fission, allowing rapid population increases in favorable environments

Figure 10.11. Understanding the distinct transmission methods of bacterial and viral foodborne illnesses is essential for effectively addressing food safety concerns

Figure 10.12. Bacterial infections are typically addressed with antibiotics, which target specific bacterial functions or structures, thereby halting their growth or killing them outright

Figure 10.13. An informed populace can significantly mitigate the impact of foodborne diseases, which are often exacerbated by poor hygiene and inadequate food handling procedures

Figure 10.14. The role of government agencies in food safety is pivotal in mitigating the incidence of bacterial and viral foodborne illnesses

Figure 10.15. Effective education and awareness campaigns are critical components in combating bacterial and viral foodborne illnesses

Figure 10.16. The role of technology in enhancing food safety is increasingly critical, particularly in mitigating the risks associated with bacterial and viral foodborne illnesses

Figure 10.17. The impact of foodborne illnesses on healthcare systems is profound, encompassing both direct and indirect consequences that strain resources and challenge public health initiatives

Figure 11.1. Understanding the nature of chemicals and natural toxins is vital for addressing food poisoning risks

Figure 11.2. The widespread use of pesticides and herbicides in modern agriculture plays a significant role in the incidence of food poisoning linked to chemical contaminants

Figure 11.3. As the demand for convenience and prolonged shelf-life in food products has surged, so too has the incorporation of various food additives and preservatives

Figure 11.4. Contaminants can leach from various packaging types, including plastic and cardboard, into food products, introducing harmful substances into the human diet

Figure 11.5. The role of food processing in chemical exposure is a critical factor in understanding the safety of our food supply

Figure 11.6. The presence of mycotoxins, toxic compounds produced by various molds, poses a significant risk in the realm of food safety, particularly concerning food poisoning caused by natural toxins

Figure 11.7. The phenomenon of marine toxins, particularly ciguatera and scombroid poisoning, exemplifies a critical aspect of foodborne illnesses stemming from natural toxins

Figure 11.8. The consumption of animal toxins, particularly pufferfish poison, raises significant public health concerns within the broader context of food poisoning from chemicals and natural toxins

Figure 11.9. Natural toxin exposure presents significant risk factors that can compromise food safety, particularly in agricultural practices

Figure 11.10. A critical aspect of mitigating food poisoning risks from chemicals and natural toxins is the implementation of safe food handling practices

Figure 11.11. Effective food storage practices not only slow down the proliferation of harmful microorganisms but also minimize the chances of chemical contamination from improperly stored items

Figure 11.12. Government regulations and inspections play a pivotal role in mitigating the risks associated with food poisoning from chemicals and natural toxins

Figure 11.13. As the prevalence of foodborne illnesses continues to impact public health, innovations in food safety technology have emerged as essential tools for mitigating risks associated with chemical and natural toxins

Figure 12.1. Food allergies are defined as adverse immune system reactions that occur when the body misidentifies certain proteins in food as harmful, prompting an immune response

Figure 12.2. The increasing prevalence of food allergies and intolerances has garnered significant attention from researchers and health professionals alike, revealing alarming trends, particularly among young populations

Figure 12.3. Food allergies and intolerances can significantly impact daily life and overall health, influencing not only dietary choices but also emotional well-being

Figure 12.4. Food allergies represent a significant public health concern, particularly among children, with common allergens including peanuts and tree nuts

Figure 12.5. The distinction between IgE-mediated and non-IgE-mediated allergies is crucial in understanding the complex nature of food allergies

Figure 12.6. Anaphylaxis, a severe and potentially life-threatening allergic reaction, often occurs in individuals with food allergies, highlighting the critical need for awareness and preparedness in managing such conditions

Figure 12.7. Multiple studies have indicated that a strong hereditary component exists in allergies, where children with a family history of atopy are at a heightened risk for food sensitivities

Figure 12.8. Lactose intolerance, caused by the insufficient production of lactase enzyme, leads to gastrointestinal distress upon the consumption of dairy products

Figure 12.9. Food intolerances are complex phenomena that involve various physiological mechanisms distinct from allergies, primarily concerning the digestive system's inability to process certain substances

Figure 12.10. The role of gut health in food intolerances has emerged as a critical area of research, given its implications for both prevalence and management

Figure 12.11. The psychological effects of food intolerances are increasingly recognized as significant, particularly among adolescents and young adults

Figure 12.12. The rising prevalence of food allergies has necessitated the development of effective avoidance strategies as a critical management approach for individuals at risk

Figure 12.13. Antihistamines are often utilized to mitigate mild allergic reactions, providing symptomatic relief from itching, hives, and other localized symptoms

Figure 12.14. The roles of allergists and dietitians are integral in managing food allergies and intolerances, as they provide specialized expertise essential for effective treatment and dietary planning

Figure 12.15. Navigating the challenges posed by food allergies and intolerances can be daunting, underscoring the importance of support groups and accessible resources for affected individuals

Figure 12.16. The economic burden of food allergies and intolerances is significant and multifaceted, affecting individuals and society at large

Figure 12.17. The social implications of food allergies and intolerances extend beyond mere dietary restrictions; they significantly impact the well-being of affected individuals

Figure 12.18. In managing food allergies and intolerances, both schools and workplaces play critical roles in fostering an environment conducive to safety and awareness

Figure 12.19. The media plays a pivotal role in shaping public perceptions of food allergies, often constructing narratives that reflect societal attitudes toward this emerging health concern

Figure 13.1. Foodborne outbreaks are defined as incidents in , which two or more individuals experience similar illnesses after consuming the same contaminated food or beverage

Figure 13.2. The role of government agencies in foodborne outbreak investigations is indispensable, as they are primarily responsible for safeguarding public health through effective surveillance and response mechanisms

Figure 13.3. The term outbreak in the context of foodborne illness refers to the occurrence of two or more cases of a similar illness resulting from the ingestion of a common food or drink

Figure 13.4. Surveillance systems play a crucial role in detecting foodborne outbreaks, facilitating rapid identification and response to potential health threats

Figure 13.5: Epidemiological data play a pivotal role in foodborne outbreak investigations, serving as a cornerstone for effective public health interventions

Figure 13.6. The use of laboratory testing in identification has become a cornerstone in managing foodborne outbreak investigations

Figure 13.7. Shiga toxin-producing *Escherichia coli* (STEC)

Figure 13.8. The initial response to a foodborne outbreak is crucial for mitigating public health risks and restoring consumer confidence

Figure 13.9. Effective data collection methods are essential in foodborne outbreak investigations, as they enable researchers to identify trends and sources of contamination

Figure 13.10. Environmental assessments play a crucial role in the investigation of foodborne outbreaks

Figure 13.11. The timeline of the investigation into foodborne outbreaks is critical for understanding the sequence of events leading to contamination and subsequent public health responses

Figure 13.12. Effective communication with the public plays a critical role in the management of foodborne outbreak investigations

Figure 13.13. In recent years, tracing the food supply chain has become a critical focus in the realm of foodborne outbreak investigation

Figure 13.14. Identifying potential sources of contamination is a critical component in the investigation of foodborne outbreaks, as demonstrated in recent epidemiological studies

Figure 13.15. Understanding the environmental factors contributing to foodborne outbreaks is crucial for mitigating public health risks

Figure 13.16. Identifying the sources of foodborne outbreaks presents significant challenges that complicate effective response and prevention efforts

Figure 13.17. Public health recommendations play a crucial role in mitigating the risks associated with foodborne outbreaks, as evidenced by various investigative studies that pinpoint the sources and necessary preventative measures

Figure 13.18. With foodborne pathogens such as Salmonella and *E. coli* posing significant health risks, understanding and implementing meticulous food safety practices is essential for both consumers and food industry professionals

Figure 13.19. The implementation of the Hazard Analysis Critical Control Point (HACCP) system represents a pivotal advancement in food safety management, particularly in the context of foodborne outbreak investigation

Figure 13.20. Effective strategies for outbreak prevention are integral to mitigating the public health risks associated with foodborne illnesses

Figure 14.1. Emergencies can disrupt food systems significantly, mandating robust food safety measures to mitigate health risks

Figure 14.2. Food safety is critically impacted by various emergencies that can arise from natural disasters, contamination, and bioterrorism threats

Figure 14.3. As emergencies such as natural disasters and disease outbreaks become increasingly prevalent, the integration of technology into food safety measures has emerged as a pivotal trend

Figure 14.4. Natural disasters, such as hurricanes, floods, and earthquakes, represent a significant challenge to food security, often leading to devastating consequences for vulnerable populations

Figure 14.5. The onset of public health emergencies, particularly pandemics such as COVID-19, profoundly impacts food safety measures worldwide

Figure 14.6. The intricate relationship between transportation disruptions and food supply chains has become especially pronounced in the context of recent global crises

Figure 14.7. The interplay between climate change and food safety presents significant challenges that necessitate urgent attention and action

Figure 14.8. Community-level emergencies, such as natural disasters or public health crises, significantly impact food safety and the availability of essential resources

Figure 14.9. During emergencies, proper food storage techniques are essential to ensure the safety and quality of food supplies

Figure 14.10. The significance of food temperature control cannot be overstated in the context of emergency food safety measures

Figure 14.11. Water contaminated with pathogens can lead to severe health risks, making it essential to source water from reliable and safe supplies such as treated municipal systems or bottled water

Figure 14.12. The role of food safety education and training is paramount in the framework of emergency food safety measures, as it equips individuals and organizations with critical knowledge and skills to mitigate risks associated with foodborne illnesses

Figure 14.13. Access to reliable community resources for food safety information is essential in ensuring public awareness and preparedness during emergencies

Figure 14.14. The Food Safety and Inspection Service (FSIS) and the Food and Drug Administration (FDA) establish standards that dictate how food should be produced, stored, and handled to minimize risks

Figure 14.15. Effective emergency food safety measures necessitate a robust collaboration between government agencies and non-governmental organizations (NGOs)

Figure 14.16. Public awareness campaigns on food safety play a vital role in promoting healthy practices and preventing foodborne illnesses, especially during emergencies

Figure 14.17. As global interconnectedness increases, foodborne risks transcend borders, making unilateral national measures insufficient to safeguard public health

Figure 14.18. Organizations involved in food safety encounter a myriad of challenges that complicate their efforts to guarantee public health

Figure 14.19. Community engagement in food safety is vital, particularly in emergency situations where swift communication and collective action can mitigate health risks

Figure 14.20. Schools play a pivotal role in promoting food safety education, serving as a foundation for instilling critical knowledge and practices in students from an early age

Figure 14.21. In the context of enhancing emergency food safety measures, building local food safety networks plays a critical role in effective risk management and response strategies

Figure 14.22. The promotion of local food production plays a critical role in enhancing sustainability, particularly in the context of emergency food safety measures

Figure 15.1. Waste management encompasses the collection, transportation, processing, and disposal of waste materials, aiming to mitigate their impact on the environment and public health

Figure 15.2. The food production sector generates a variety of waste types that significantly impact environmental sustainability

Figure 15.3. Food waste significantly contributes to environmental degradation, exacerbating climate change and resource depletion

Figure 15.4. Governments and organizations are implementing structured policies that not only address the efficient handling of food waste but also promote responsible practices throughout the food value chain

Figure 15.5. In the realm of waste management within the food industry, organic waste plays a crucial role that merits in-depth examination

Figure 15.6. Hazardous waste presents a significant challenge within the food industry, necessitating meticulous management to mitigate environmental and health risks

Figure 15.7. Effective wastewater management is crucial in the food industry, as this sector is a significant contributor to water pollution due to the high volume of organic waste generated during processing

Figure 15.8. The issue of spoilage and unsold inventory represents a significant challenge within the food industry, exacerbating the broader problem of food waste

Figure 15.9. In the food industry, effective waste reduction techniques are crucial for enhancing sustainability and operational efficiency

Figure 15.10. The adoption of anaerobic digestion as a method for managing organic waste within the food industry presents significant environmental and economic advantages

Figure 15.11. The integration of technology in waste management, particularly within the food industry, presents a transformative opportunity to address the pervasive issue of food waste

Figure 15.12. The integration of sustainable packaging solutions within the food industry is pivotal for enhancing waste management practices and minimizing environmental impact

Figure 15.13. Resource Conservation and Recovery Act (RCRA)

Figure 15.14. Effective waste management in the food industry hinges significantly on the role of government, which acts as a crucial regulatory body and facilitator for sustainable practices

Figure 15.15. The repercussions for failing to adhere to waste management regulations can vary significantly, ranging from monetary fines to more severe legal consequences, such as facility shutdowns

Figure 15.16. Effective stakeholder involvement in policy-making is essential for addressing the complex challenges posed by waste management in the food industry

Figure 15.17. Waste management policies within the food industry require rigorous evaluation to determine their effectiveness in mitigating food waste

Figure 15.18. Effective waste management in the food industry carries significant cost implications for businesses, influencing both operational efficiency and long-term profitability

Figure 15.19. Losses of food not only contribute to resource wastage but also inflate the costs associated with transportation and processing, which are passed on to consumers through higher retail prices

Figure 15.20. In the context of waste management in the food industry, investment in sustainable practices is increasingly recognized as a critical component for achieving both environmental and economic objectives

Figure 15.21. The integration of sustainable practices into waste management systems can streamline operations and reduce costs associated with waste disposal and resource consumption

PREFACE

Food safety and quality threats have been a core issue throughout human history; nowadays, in a condition of global interdependence, the consequences are greater than ever. Every day, consumers rely on vast supply chains across continents and climates to carry perishable commodities from farm producers to factories to local retail outlets. Along the way, there is the risk of contamination, spoilage, or intentional adulteration. When food commodities fail to meet minimum hygiene standards, either through the presence of pathogenic microorganisms, unsanitary handling, or contamination with toxic chemicals, the consequences can vary from slight discomfort to illness, chronic disease, or, in extreme cases, death. In addition to individual disease, foodborne disease outbreaks can strain public health systems, interfere with economic activity, and erode consumer confidence in producers and regulatory agencies.

No less disturbing is the practice of food adulteration, which consists of adding materials intentionally or inadvertently to enhance shelf life, alter appearance, or create perceived volume. While some adulterations are the result of a lack of knowledge or accidental contamination, others are driven by a desire for illicit profits and thus present hazards that the ordinary consumer may not easily discern. Added to these problematics are shifting patterns in food processing, a trend toward minimally processed and ready-to-eat (RTE) food, and the advent of direct-to-consumer sales that have completely reversed the paradigm of food safety roles. All segments of the supply chain, from the start of the harvest through to the position where a meal is served, must emulate strict standards of sanitation, good facility design, and vigilant monitoring to ensure safeguarding public health.

The book entitled *Food Hygiene, Food Adulteration, and Food Poisoning* has been authored as an encyclopedic handbook to be utilized by professionals, students, and stakeholders with mandates to ensure and promote safety in food systems. This book integrates key scientific principles, practical methods, and policy concerns to create an integrated reference that encourages theoretical understanding and practical application. Its audience will be exposed to evidence-based advice, authoritative procedures for the detection and control of common hazards, as well as analysis of emergent trends influencing regulatory regimes. By integrating perspectives from microbiology, chemistry, public health, and legal studies, this book aims to prepare its audience with the knowledge and skills required to uphold the integrity of the food supply.

Chapter 1 presents an overview of essential principles in food hygiene and sanitation, tracing the evolution of best practices and the rationale behind regulatory requirements. Chapter 2 focuses on identifying and characterizing the various sources of food contamination, from biological agents to physical debris, and examines the pathways through , which hazards can enter the food chain. Chapter 3 discusses personal hygiene and the duties of food handlers, emphasizing hand-washing techniques, health screening, and behavior that reduces risk in processing and preparation environments.

Chapter 4 examines the sanitation of food equipment and premises, offering detailed cleaning schedules, validation of cleaning methods, and design features that minimize harborage of pathogens. Chapter 5 explores safe food storage and temperature control, outlining the time-temperature relationships that govern microbial growth and the use of refrigeration, freezing, and hot-holding to preserve quality.

Chapter 6 addresses common foods prone to adulteration, from milk and spices to oils and grains, detailing the motivations behind adulteration and the implications for nutrition and safety. Chapter 7 provides techniques for detection of adulterants, covering chemical assays, spectroscopic methods, and rapid field tests that allow inspectors and industry personnel to verify authenticity. Chapter 8 considers consumer awareness and food labeling, analyzing how clear, accurate labels empower purchasers to make informed choices and how mislabeling can mislead or endanger vulnerable populations.

Chapter 9 introduces the clinical and epidemiological dimensions of food poisoning, defining symptoms, incubation periods, and the role of surveillance in detecting outbreaks. Chapter 10 delves into bacterial and viral foodborne illnesses, profiling key pathogens such as Salmonella, Listeria, norovirus, and Campylobacter, and describing prevention strategies from farm to fork. Chapter 11 examines poisoning from chemicals and natural toxins, including heavy metals, pesticide residues, mycotoxins, and plant or marine toxins, with guidance on risk assessment and mitigation.

Chapter 12 discusses food allergies and intolerances, elucidating immunological mechanisms, threshold levels, and the special labeling requirements that protect sensitive consumers. Chapter 13 outlines the process of foodborne outbreak investigation, from case definition and specimen collection to traceback procedures and assessment of control measures. Chapter 14 outlines emergency food safety measures, detailing contingency planning for natural disasters, supply disruptions, and large-scale contamination events. Finally, Chapter 15 addresses waste management in the food industry, describing systems for the disposal of organic refuse, treatment of wastewater, and recovery of by-products to reduce environmental impact and maintain hygiene standards.

This work is intended for food safety professionals, quality assurance managers, public health inspectors, regulatory authorities, academic researchers, and students in disciplines such as food science, nutrition, public health, and environmental health. It will also benefit industry stakeholders—ranging from farmers and processors to caterers and retailers—who seek to deepen their understanding of safe practices and compliance requirements. Providing clear explanations, practical tools, and up-to-date references, this book aims to support the efforts of everyone who contributes to the production, distribution, and consumption of safe, wholesome food. Through shared knowledge and consistent application of sound hygiene and quality principles, we can work together to reduce the burden of foodborne illness and ensure confidence in the meals that sustain us every day.

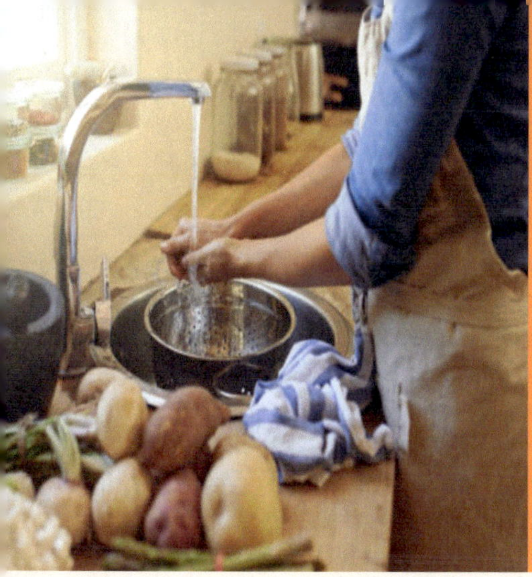

Chapter 1

INTRODUCTION TO FOOD HYGIENE AND SANITATION

Contents

Introduction....................1
1.1. Principles of Food Hygiene....................4
1.2. Foodborne Pathogens....................8
1.3. Food Safety Regulations and Standards....................12
1.4. Best Practices in Food Hygiene....................16
Summary....................21
References....................22

Introduction

Studying food sanitation and hygiene validates that, public health incorporates food safety. Any incident of food poisoning by a fast-food outlet validates that cleanliness is extremely critical. By studying, it is discovered that in developing nations such as Nigeria, a rise in food vendors is typically matched with a rise in cases of food poisoning that is related to poor sanitation levels and non-compliance with standards such as Hazard Analysis Critical Control Point (HACCP) (Usman, 2019). In the same way, in developed countries, pathogens such as Campylobacter, primarily attributed to the ingestion of undercooked chicken, put emphasis on adopting strong sanitation controls throughout the food chain (Vetchapitak & Misawa, 2019). All in all, these results show that good food hygiene is very important for both the well-being of the public and the quality of their meals.

Definition of Food Hygiene

Making sure food is safe and of good quality is a key part of public health, which includes steps from production to consumption. It requires understanding the steps of handling food, like storing it, preparing it, serving it and also knowing how to prevent contamination and diseases from food. Personal hygiene, cleanliness in the environment and proper use of equipment are all part of food hygiene, which helps reduce dangers to food safety. Consistent with the Intergovernmental Panel on Climate Changes report findings, a high association exists between food hygiene practices and sustainability, showing that default in this respect can aggravate public health issues and environmental problems (Calvin et al., 2023). Additionally, with the introduction of Industry 4.0 technologies, varied innovations are redesigning food hygiene practices, highlighting in particular the role of sustainable approaches to ensuring food safety (Bai et al., 2020) (Figure 1.1).

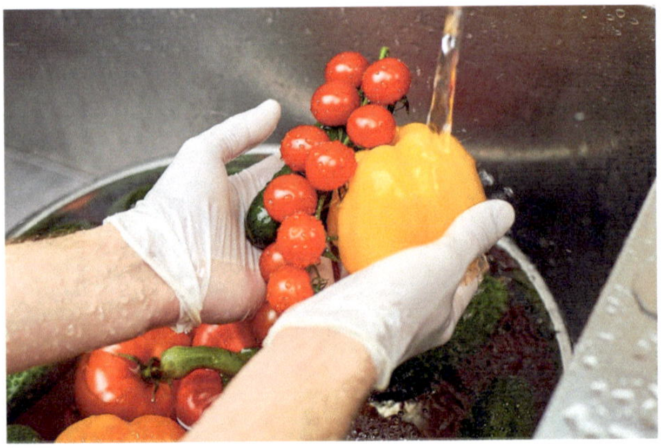

Figure 1.1. Food hygiene is an essential aspect of public health that encompasses practices aimed at ensuring the safety and quality of food from production to consumption.

Source: https://www.ficsi.in/blog/wp-content/uploads/2024/05/Blog-1-16.jpg.

Importance of Food Hygiene and Sanitation

The significance of keeping food hygienic and sanitary is very high, as it is the main way to prevent foodborne diseases and protect public health. If food is contaminated with pathogens, people may get sick, which weakens healthcare and reduces work productivity. When food preparation areas are clean, both hazards and consumer doubts about food safety are avoided. For instance, a recent advisory highlighted the need for more research in environmental health topics, especially in such regions as Malawi, to improve food hygiene practice gaps (Morse et al., 2010). In a similar way, USAID's Water and Development Strategy points out that having strong water management is necessary to support food hygiene programs. So, making sure food is clean and sanitary is necessary to protect health, people and the availability of safe food.

Historical Context of Food Safety

Food safety legislation shows how society responds to health emergencies and the increases in knowledge about what causes foodborne illnesses. After World War II, the partnership between the Food and Agriculture Organization (FAO) and the World Health Organization (WHO) established the International Codex Alimentarius in 1963, a turning point in uniforming food safety measures globally (Ramsingh, 2014). This partnership highlighted qualitative approaches' conflicts, specifically for combined food production systems, and WHOs preference for quantitative standards based on statistical comparisons of microbial quantities. A fundamental component of food safety has also included evaluating health threats related to agriculture, especially in developing nations where irrigation with wastewater creates formidable public health issues (Bahri et al., 2025). By studying these historical developments, it is clear that food safety frameworks have always evolved to meet new health challenges and the complexities of food manufacturing, highlighting their relevance in modern food sanitation and hygiene (Figure 1.2).

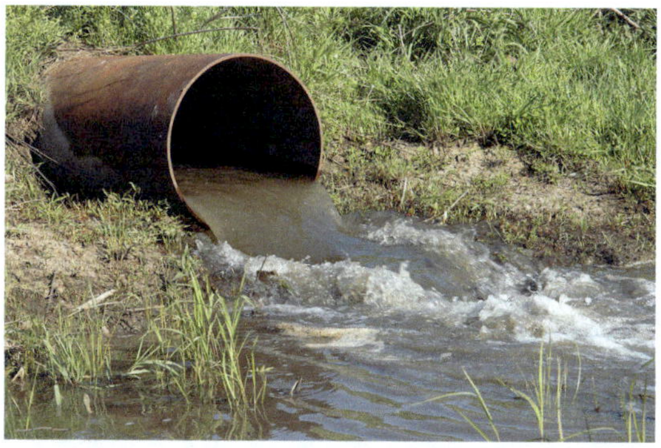

Figure 1.2. Wastewater irrigation.

Source: https://www.crawfordfund.org/wp-content/uploads/2015/11/1024px-Discharge_pipe.jpg.

Overview of Foodborne Illnesses

People often get sick from foodborne illness, which is usually caused by consuming contaminated food or handling it incorrectly. Because more people are eating fresh fruits and vegetables, which are generally healthy, there are now more outbreaks related to these foods. As per recent statistics, multistate outbreaks involving bacterial pathogens, most notably pathogenic *Escherichia coli*, *Listeria monocytogenes*, and *Salmonella enterica*, have increased, implicating different modes of contamination along the farm-to-fork supply chain (Carstens et al., 2019). Furthermore, viral foodborne diseases have become among the top priorities of food safety, highlighting the importance of effective control methods through the food chain (Bosch et al., 2018). Recognizing these factors is important for creating good food hygiene and sanitation habits, which will helps prevent risks and secure public health in a more complicated food system.

Role of Government Regulations

Government laws are very important for ensuring public health, mainly through their focus on food hygiene and sanitation. Agencies create regulating policies to ensure that food is produced and distributed under strict sanitary rules, which helps reduce foodborne illness outbreaks. Through regular updates to the rules, such as those in the agency's 2013–2018 Water and Development Strategy, governments can ensure that different ministries are working together to improve food safety. These rules make sure food handlers follow them and also help the public learn about hygiene standards. Additionally, in such settings as in Malawi, pointing out areas of environmental health research gaps, as well as suggesting implementable plans, highlights the importance of adaptive regulations that can deal with emerging food safety challenges (Morse et al., 2010). Eventually, effective government control is necessary to ensure a safe food supply, safeguard consumers, and improve health across the country (Figure 1.3).

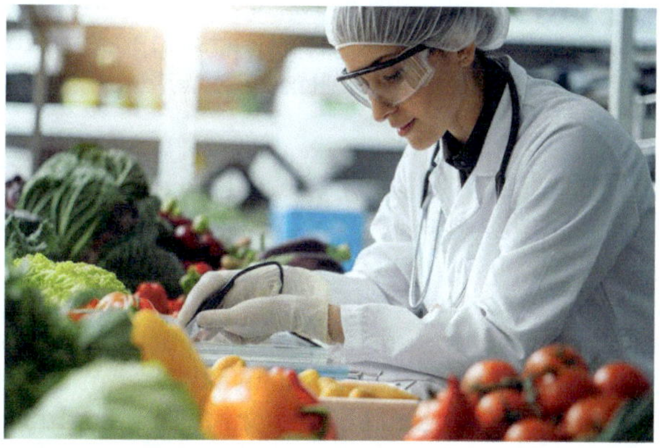

Figure 1.3. Government regulations play a pivotal role in safeguarding public health, especially within the domain of food hygiene and sanitation.

Source: https://www.foodinfotech.com/wp-content/uploads/2024/05/Safeguarding-Public-Health-Through-Modern-Food-Safety-Practices.jpg

Impact of Globalization on Food Safety

Because of globalization, food safety is affected by the changing food supply chains, which may bring more goods to people but also increase the risk of contamination. Because countries are more connected, foods are shipped more often, which makes making it difficult to regulate food hygiene issues. Because of cross-border trade, there needs to be strong rules in place to maintain hygiene throughout the supply chain. Also, tensions such as climate change and geopolitical inequalities aggravate weaknesses in existing food safety system weaknesses, as highlighted by emerging food and water security inequalities (United Nations System Standing Committee on Nutrition, 2020). The call for One Health response emphasizes the need for coordinated approaches aimed at addressing food security in environmental constraints of globalization to ensure that food safety interventions are comprehensive and sustainable (Angelos et al., 2017). In the end, dealing with these complexities is important for the safety of public health worldwide.

Objectives of Food Hygiene Practices

Maintaining public health depends on food hygiene, which focuses on stopping foodborne diseases and ensuring food quality from the start of production. By taking certain steps, these practices aim to prevent food from being contaminated at any point from being produced to being eaten. Teaching stakeholders about the value of hygiene is necessary, covering everything from how to handle food safely to what cross-contamination might be. Educational efforts are enriched by interdisciplinary strategies, as noted by the Western Institute for Food Safety and Security, , which calls for a One Health approach to food safety education, talking about interrelatedness between diverse disciplines and how they affect food security (Angelos et al., 2017). The US Agency for International Development's Water and Development Strategy also stresses that sustainability is important, since it helps ensure both safe food and the preservation of natural resources. Combined, these goals set a foundational structure for efficient food hygiene practices (Figure 1.4).

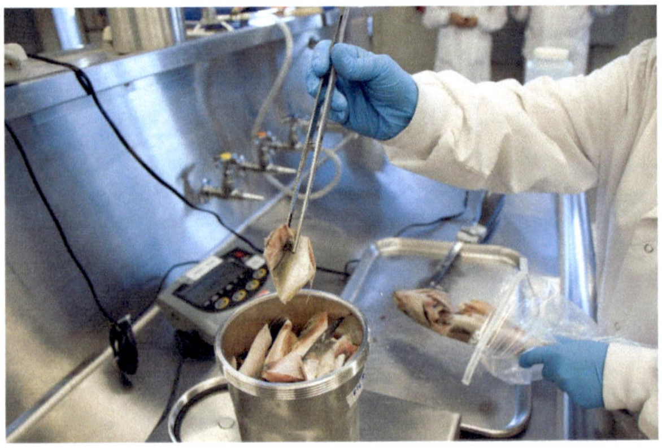

Figure 1.4. Essential to ensuring public health, the objectives of food hygiene practices revolve around minimizing foodborne illnesses and safeguarding food quality throughout the supply chain.

Source: https://upload.wikimedia.org/wikipedia/commons/1/11/Seafood-_FDA_Lab_2881_%284494783228%29.jpg.

1.1. Principles of Food Hygiene

One of the main parts of food safety is to strictly follow food hygiene rules to prevent foodborne diseases. Examples of these practices are washing your hands, cleaning the surfaces you use for food and cooking food at proper temperatures to kill bacteria. In addition, it is very important to be aware of cross-contamination to prevent pathogens from moving from food to food. Educating staff in these areas can make sure food service operations are clean and hygienic. The US Agency for International Development stresses sustainability and using lessons from the past in its Water and Development Strategy, showing that good hygiene should be part of all public health efforts. Developing useful advice regularly helps unite actions within the water sector, which is important for the main role of hygiene in keeping food safe.

1.1.1. Personal Hygiene for Food Handlers

Proper food safety depends on food handlers maintaining good personal hygiene, which contributes to consumer health and food quality. When food handlers keep high hygiene standards, the risk of foodborne diseases from pathogens is lowered. For example, research on the Hajj pilgrimage highlighted hygiene as a key concern, with evidence that non-adherence by food handlers negatively impacted food safety guidelines in pilgrim-serving kitchens (Asyary et al., 2024).

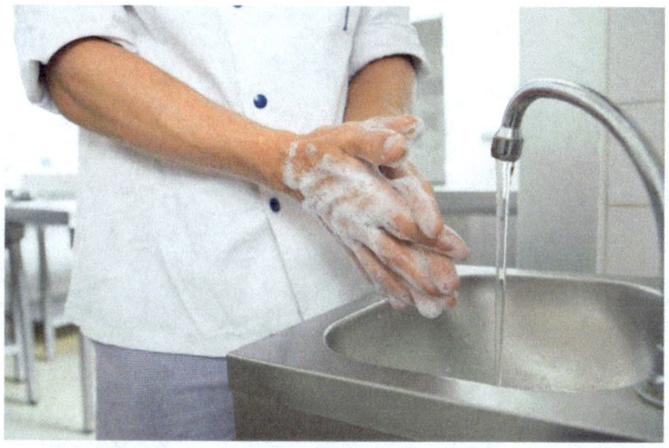

Figure 1.5. Personal hygiene for food handlers is a cornerstone of effective food safety practices, directly impacting the health of consumers and the integrity of food products.

Source: https://www.ficsi.in/blog/wp-content/uploads/2024/02/FICSI-Oct-4.jpg.

It is also very important to sanitize all the equipment and utensils used for preparing food. A study on the preparation of pastries has established the way in , which hygiene will directly impact food safety, consumer confidence, and product quality (Dianita et al., 2024). It is therefore crucial that food handlers adopt thorough personal hygiene measures such as extensive hand washing, correct clothing, and personal health care to facilitate a safe consuming experience (Figure 1.5).

1.1.2. Cleanliness in Food Preparation Areas

Keeping food preparation areas clean helps prevent food poisoning and many other diseases. A clean food preparation area is linked to both better food and better health. For example, a comprehensive approach in water, sanitation, and hygiene (WASH) has seen better food hygiene habits among households and has seen significant increases in the percentages of hygienically prepared food areas and safe food storage (Freeman et al., 2020). Further, research on street vendors indicates that although vendors tend to self-evaluate their sanitation procedures favorably, customers usually report inconsistency between these opinions and standards of hygiene in practice, especially in hand washing and food handling (Pula et al., 2019). For this reason, both homes and food businesses should keep cleanliness as their main goal to keep people safe and guarantee safe food.

1.1.3. Safe Food Storage Practices

When you store food properly, you are less likely to get sick and food stays clean. Storing perishable foods in a cold area stops bacteria from multiplying. For example, studies have uncovered that unsanitary food storage practices, including failing to manage cross-contamination and poorly designed cooling systems, can be major contributors to health hazards, especially in vulnerable groups like children (Dominguez-Salas et al., 2024). It must be imperative that water for food preparation and storing is highly sanitized. Research validates that treated water can even become contaminated if stored, hence causing serious public health concerns unless checked (Girmay et al., 2021). Thus, mandating rigorous safe storage practices not only ensures food integrity but also guarantees maximal possible sanitation regime efficiency, eventually contributing to improved community health (Figure 1.6).

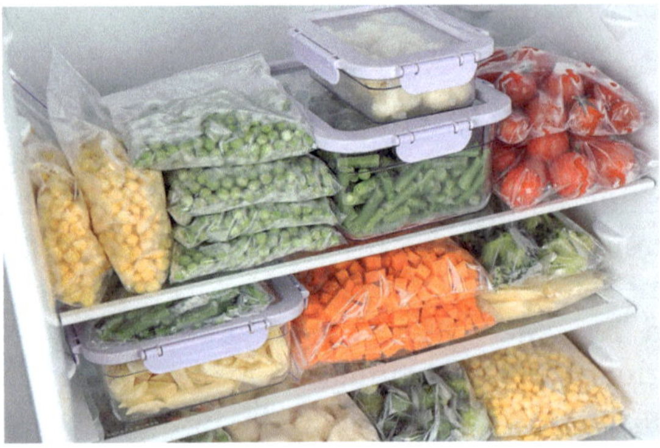

Figure 1.6. Proper storage techniques, such as keeping perishable items at appropriate temperatures, are crucial to reduce the risk of bacterial growth.

Source: https://cdn.cpdonline.co.uk/wp-content/uploads/2025/01/29145140/Food-Storage-Best-Practices-scaled.jpg.

1.1.4. Temperature Control in Food Safety

Proper temperature management is very important for food safety because failing to do so can cause dangerous pathogens to develop and threaten the public. Keeping temperatures at the right level helps stop bacteria from growing in meat, dairy, and cooked foods during storage, preparation and serving. Studies have shown an important correlation between knowledge of temperature control practices and application of Hazard Analysis Critical Control Point (HACCP) systems by the food industry, showing a lack of food hygiene procedures among different producers. Furthermore, research has proven that food and eating utensil sanitary handling, along with temperature control at service, has a great effect on the contamination risk, particularly by pathogens such as *E. coli* (Eryando et al., 2015). For this reason, more attention and efforts need to be given to training and supervision to promote food safety awareness, better hygiene and safeguard consumers.

1.1.5. Cross-Contamination Prevention

It is very important to stop cross-contamination to keep food safe and clean, especially in places where bacteria can be very harmful to health. Salmonella, *Escherichia coli* and Listeria can easily grow in places where food is not handled correctly, showing why we need strict food handling rules. Poor personal hygiene and a lack of knowledge regarding sanitation among food handlers significantly contribute to the spread of harmful microorganisms, as highlighted by the findings at Aji Santoso International Football Academy (ASIFA) (Fitriah et al., 2024).

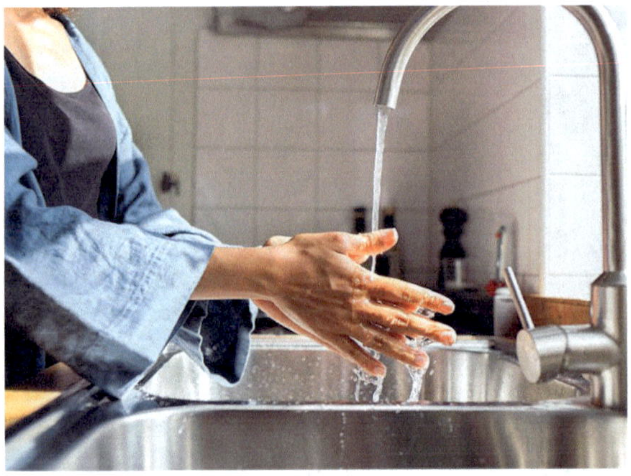

Figure 1.7. Effective prevention of cross-contamination is pivotal in maintaining food hygiene and sanitation, particularly in environments where microbial contamination can lead to severe health risks.

Source: https://media.post.rvohealth.io/wp-content/uploads/2020/01/washing-hands-kitchen-732x549-thumbnail.jpg.

Furthermore, awareness of the determinants that facilitate bacterial growth, represented by the acronym FATTOM (Food, Acid, Temperature,

Time, Oxygen, and Moisture), can mitigate risks of cross-contamination (Sunarti, 2024). Through effective training programs centered on hygiene and sanitation education, food handlers are able to contribute to minimizing cross-contamination and enhancing overall food safety (Figure 1.7).

1.1.6. Proper Cooking Techniques

Cooking is very important in food sanitation and hygiene because it helps ensure food is safe and of high quality. Good cooking skills make the food taste better and also act as a strong barriers against pathogens that can harm public health. For example, the right internal temperature (should be more than 70 degree Celsius) during cooking can kill dangerous bacteria such as *Salmonella* and *E. coli*, which are most often linked to raw animal foods (Abebe et al., 2020). Further, the application of good manufacturing practice (GMP) and normal food safety procedures can limit cross-contamination during food handling and cooking processes (Kumar et al., 2021). Sous-vide or high-heat cooking methods maintain the nutrition in food and also make it last longer, where science and cooking come together. So, it is very important to follow the correct steps when cooking to maintain food safety and hygiene.

1.1.7. Use of Safe Water and Raw Materials

It is very important to ensure that water and raw materials are safe for food hygiene and sanitation. Cooking with dirty water is very dangerous for health, mainly when clean water is not readily available. For instance, there is evidence that urbanization, particularly in Ghanaian urban areas, has the effect of increasing the demand for providing safe food since vendors on the streets do not have much access to hygienic conditions and clean water for food preparation (Johnson and Yawson, 2025). Enhanced management of resources and sanitation has been seen to enhance food safety and thereby guarantee public health. This emphasis on safety not only protects consumers but also promotes sustainable practice in the food sector, highlighting the necessity of the urgent need to prioritize safe water and raw materials for the topmost priority of food production and distribution systems (Figure 1.8).

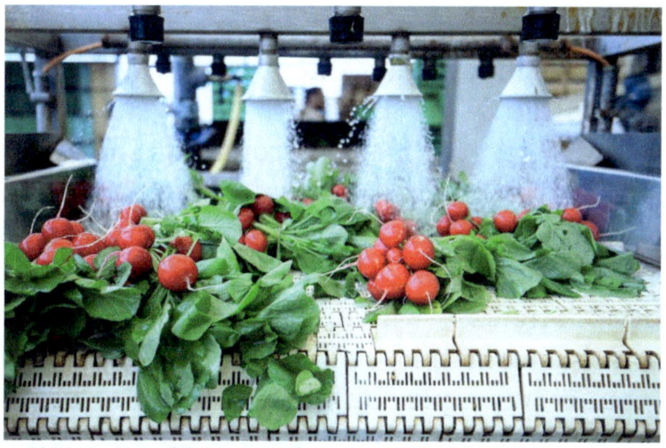

Figure 1.8. The quality of water utilized in food preparation directly impacts overall health and safety, particularly in developing regions where access to clean water is limited.

Source: https://nexteel.in/wp-content/uploads/2024/07/The-Impact-of-Water-Storage-on-Indias-Food-Supply-1024x683.jpg.

1.1.8. Importance of Pest Control

Because pests can cause major food safety problems, good food hygiene and sanitation rely on effective pest control. Food can become contaminated if it contains rodents or insects, which is very harmful to people. Food producers may lose money due to pests, since food that is not safe to eat is rarely sold, which can affect food security. Managing these problems requires you to learn about integrative pest management. This includes the assessment of environmental impacts on pest populations and the implementation of sustainable practices informed by innovative research (Angelos et al., 2017). For instance, in agricultural contexts, research has shown that inadequate sanitation practices in orchards can lead to persistent pest problems that necessitate the use of chemical controls to protect crops, underscoring the necessity for effective pest management programs throughout the food production process (Cooke et al., 2010).

1.1.9. Regular Cleaning and Sanitization Procedures

It is very important to keep up with cleaning and sanitizing, to maintain food safety and hygiene wherever food is prepared. They serve to decrease the chances of contamination and also ensure a healthy environment for all. Following a detailed cleaning routine removes food particles , which can invite pests and allow harmful microorganisms to grow. The impact of improper sanitation was underscored during the COVID-19 pandemic, as highlighted in Chamola et al. (2020), where inadequate hygiene contributed to widespread health crisis. Also, the link between cleanliness and fighting waterborne diseases highlights the need for a complete approach to hygiene. Effectively applying these regular cleaning and sanitization practices is essential for preventing foodborne illnesses and reinforcing public trust in food safety standards (Figure 1.9).

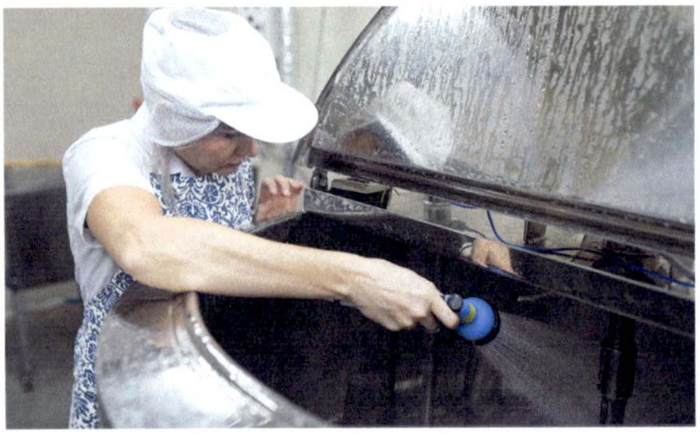

Figure 1.9. Maintaining regular cleaning and sanitization procedures is crucial for ensuring food safety and hygiene within any food preparation environment.

Source: https://www.foodengineeringmag.com/ext/resources/Issues/2020/01-January/GettyImages-1135928392.jpg?1577988061.

1.2. Foodborne Pathogens

People who are more likely to get sick, such as children, seniors and those with weak immune systems, may face serious problems because of foodborne diseases. Because patients in hospices may have weak immune systems, it is very important to keep their food safe and clean. Research has indicated outrageous levels of contamination, a study having identified that more than half of the food samples collected from vendors on campus were positive for *Escherichia coli*, indicating the direct correlation between improper sanitation and microbial food contamination (Eryando et al., 2015). Besides, HIV patients are also greatly susceptible to foodborne illness as their immune systems are compromised, signifying the utmost significance of adherence to good food hygiene procedures in healthcare facilities (Nkhebenyane et al., 2018). It is thus necessary to guarantee that the food handlers know the food safety rules so that foodborne pathogens do not multiply and the immunocompromised are not infected.

1.2.1. Common Types of Foodborne Pathogens

It is very important to know about common foodborne pathogens to protect the public from food safety and sanitation. Pathogens such as Salmonella, *E. coli*, and Campylobacter frequently emerge as primary agents of foodborne illnesses, with Salmonella accounting for a significant proportion of outbreaks globally, as reported by the European Food Safety Authority (EFSA) in 2006, which documented 5,719 incidents involving substantial hospitalization rates (Lee et al., 2009). Especially the O157:H7 strain of *E. coli* can be very dangerous if found in undercooked meat or infected produce. Furthermore, cross-contamination in food service environments significantly elevates the risk of pathogen transmission, as shown in studies indicating that food contact surfaces in child care centers often harbor high levels of microbiological contaminants (Cosby et al., 2005). These pathogens not only lead to severe gastrointestinal issues but also highlight the pressing need for stringent sanitation protocols in food handling practices to mitigate risks (Figure 1.10).

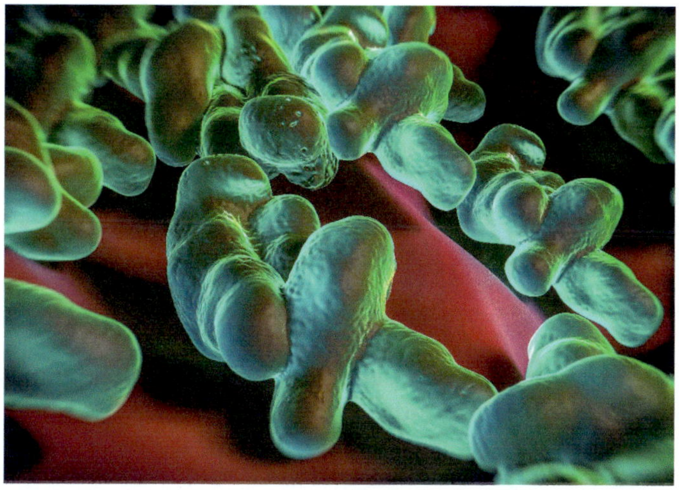

Figure 1.10. Campylobacter.

Source: https://www.biomerieux-industry.com/sites/default/files/2019-11/poultry-science-campylobacter-01.jpg.

1.2.2. Symptoms of Foodborne Illnesses

Foodborne illnesses might have various symptoms and can be very serious, which demonstrates the diversity among pathogens. Commonly associated gastrointestinal symptoms include nausea, vomiting, diarrhea, and abdominal cramps, which emerge due to infections caused by pathogenic bacteria such as Salmonella, *E. coli*, and Campylobacter found in contaminated animal products (Abebe et al., 2020). How fast the symptoms start is influenced by the type of infection and the health of the person and it can take from hours to several days. Additionally, certain zoonotic diseases, which are transmissible from animals to humans, may lead to more severe complications, highlighting the importance of recognizing early signs of foodborne illnesses (Rahman et al., 2020). To prevent these symptoms, we rely on proper food hygiene and sanitation, which help stop contamination and big outbreaks.

1.2.3. Transmission Routes of Pathogens

Many ways exist for pathogens to spread, which has a big impact on both food hygiene and the occurrence of zoonotic diseases. These diseases, which originate in animals and can be transmitted to humans, account for over 60% of human pathogens, highlighting the significance of understanding their pathways (Rahman et al., 2020). People usually get these illnesses by eating food that is contaminated, especially meat, dairy and eggs , which that can contain these bacterial pathogens. As bacteria like Salmonella species and *E. coli* proliferate in improperly handled or cooked food, they can lead to severe gastrointestinal illness and even complications such as hospitalization (Abebe et al., 2020). Thus, a comprehensive approach to food hygiene, encompassing GMP, sanitation, and effective monitoring systems, is essential for minimizing the transmission of pathogens and safeguarding public health (Figure 1.11).

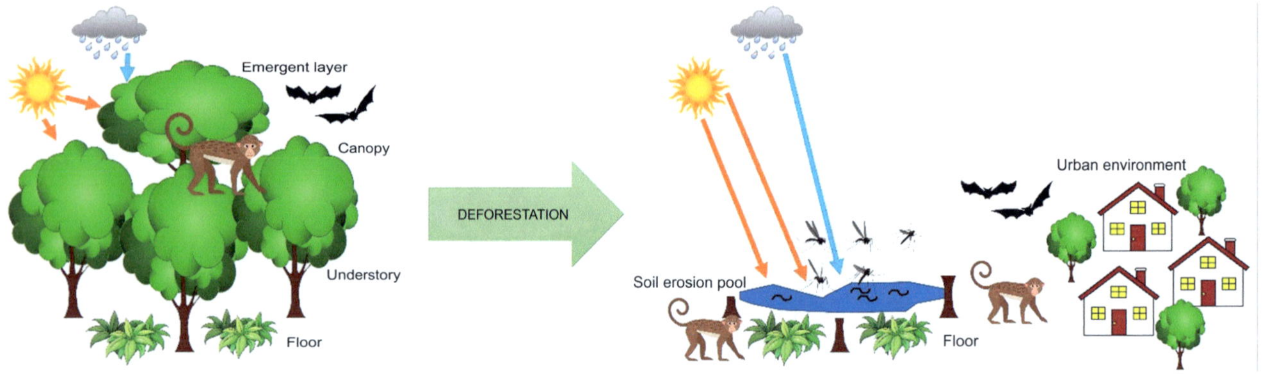

Figure 1.11. The transmission routes of pathogens play a critical role in the dynamics of food hygiene and sanitation, particularly concerning zoonotic diseases.

Source: Esposito MM, Turku S, Lehrfield L, Shoman A. The Impact of Human Activities on Zoonotic Infection Transmissions. *Animals.* 2023; 13(10):1646. https://doi.org/10.3390/ani13101646

1.2.4. High-Risk Foods for Contamination

It helps in food hygiene and sanitation to know the foods that are more likely to be contaminated to stop foodborne illnesses. Foods that are often implicated include raw meats, seafood, dairy products, and ready-to-eat (RTE) items such as salads and deli meats. Because moisture and food provide the right environment, pathogens can easily multiply. Mostly, serious problems from norovirus and Shigella spp. can occur when food is not handled or prepared correctly. Shigella, in particular, is known for its fecal-to-mouth transmission and is frequently associated with contaminated food and water, underscoring the importance of proper sanitation practices in the food industry (Simões et al., 2024). The complexities of food contamination highlight the need for stringent hygiene measures, as well as public awareness regarding the safe handling of potentially hazardous foods (Kaur et al., 2023).

1.2.5. Vulnerable Populations

Knowing about the special problems faced by vulnerable groups is very important in food hygiene and sanitation. Due to their financial and social challenges, such groups are more likely to suffer from foodborne diseases and lack access to clean water and sanitation. As highlighted in the Sustainable Development Goals, addressing the needs of the poor and vulnerable is crucial for fostering equitable service delivery and improving health outcomes (Kullman et al., 2017). Especially, poor WASH services add to existing health inequalities, since those who cannot use these services often suffer more illnesses and deaths. If policies focus on helping vulnerable groups, they can boost food safety and sanitation , which helps the community's health and reduces existing inequalities. Recognizing these dynamics is vital for effective advocacy and program implementation in food hygiene initiatives (Figure 1.12).

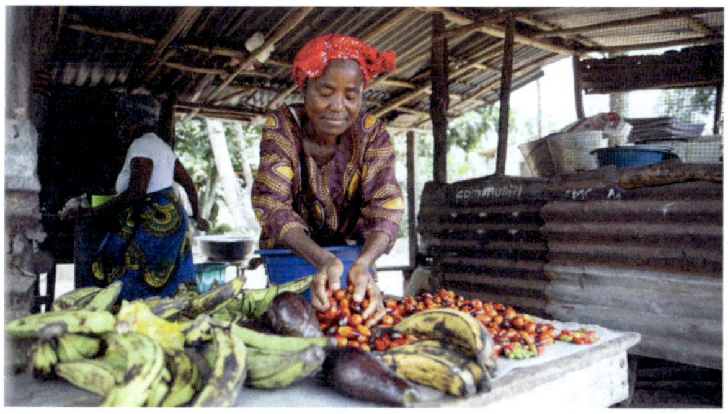

Figure 1.12. Understanding the unique challenges faced by vulnerable populations is essential in the context of food hygiene and sanitation.

Source: https://admin.concern.net/sites/default/files/styles/social_media/public/media/images/2025-03/concern-rs82217-liberia-food-security-agriculture.jpg?itok=8tNSXshz.

1.2.6. Prevention Strategies for Pathogen Spread

Education, good hygiene and understanding how different fields relate are important for stopping pathogens in food environments. The first thing to do in good food hygiene is to explain to food handlers why their actions matter for avoiding contamination. It shows people how to clean their hands and reminds them to prevent food from getting polluted and to store it properly. Educators and policymakers can benefit from frameworks such as those developed by the Western Institute for Food Safety and Security, which facilitate the integration of various disciplines within the food safety domain, thereby fostering a holistic approach to food hygiene (Angelos et al., 2017). Moreover, collaboration across sectors and research, as highlighted in the 2013 Annual Report, reinforces the necessity for continuous improvement and innovation in sanitation protocols (London School of Hygiene & Tropical Medicine, 2013). If we use different strategies, we can make it much less likely for pathogens to spread in food systems.

1.2.7. Role of Laboratory Testing

Laboratory testing plays a big role in food hygiene and sanitation because it helps to stop the spread of zoonotic diseases and foodborne pathogens. Testing food helps detect dangerous microorganisms and contaminants, which is important for public health.

For instance, zoonotic pathogen seroprevalence in pig herds was studied and found significant risks due to improper hygiene practices and eating contaminated pork products, leading to higher infection rates of, for instance, hepatitis E virus and *Trichinella spiralis* (Ito et al., 2016). HACCP is also used in the feed production industry , which demonstrates how important laboratory analysis is to feed safety. Compliance with HACCP procedures through monitoring and testing of foods is directly associated with a reduction in risks for Indonesian stock-feed production in the aspect of food safety. The incorporation of stringent laboratory testing constitutes an anticipatory approach towards the practice of food hygiene and sanitation, which indirectly results in healthier communities (Figure 1.13).

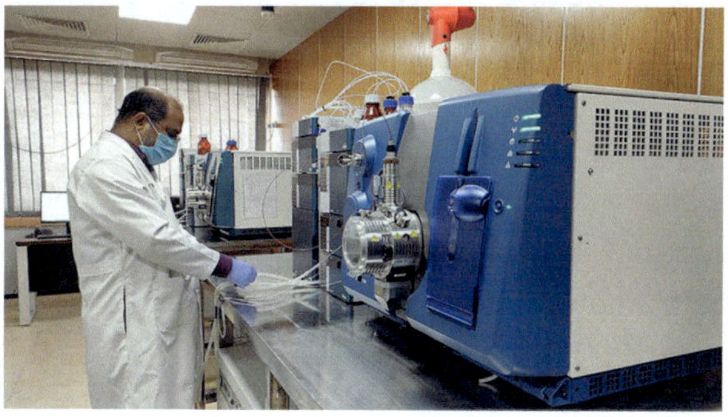

Figure 1.13. The role of laboratory testing in food hygiene and sanitation is paramount, as it acts as a crucial line of defense against zoonotic diseases and foodborne pathogens.

Source: https://www.iaea.org/sites/default/files/styles/full_page_width_landscape_16_9/public/labphoto-1.jpg?itok=YMM5He_R.

1.3. Food Safety Regulations and Standards

The foundation of effective food hygiene and sanitation is deeply rooted in robust food safety regulations and standards, which are essential in safeguarding public health. These regulations not only impose guidelines for food handling and preparation but also ensure compliance with environmental considerations, reflecting the interconnectedness of food safety and environmental health. For instance, initiatives developed from the One Health perspective emphasize the need for a multidisciplinary approach to food safety education, addressing how the effects of food production impact the environment and vice versa (Angelos et al., 2017). Furthermore, identifying gaps in research and prioritizing action plans are critical for improving environmental health sectors, which, in turn, enhances food safety protocols (Lungu et al., 2010). Such comprehensive frameworks ensure that food safety regulations are not merely reactive but are instead proactive in creating a sustainable and secure food supply that upholds both public health and environmental integrity.

1.3.1. Overview of Food Safety Laws

The safety of food and public health is secured by the framework of food safety laws in all places. Laws apply to all steps in food production, from farming to where it is sold and they also make safety rules for manufacturers, distributors and retailers. Food safety laws are handled by people such as food handlers and those who make the rules. Both must handle food safety hazards, and these are impacted by things like the environment and current social and political situations. Also, food safety laws are now being shaped by an emphasis on sustainability, as shown by the fact that food safety and SDGs are connected. This encapsulates the importance of comprehensive and adaptive food safety laws in promoting health and well-being in society, thereby addressing issues such as hunger and poverty (Jaffee et al., 2018; Novovesk et al., 2019) (Figure 1.14).

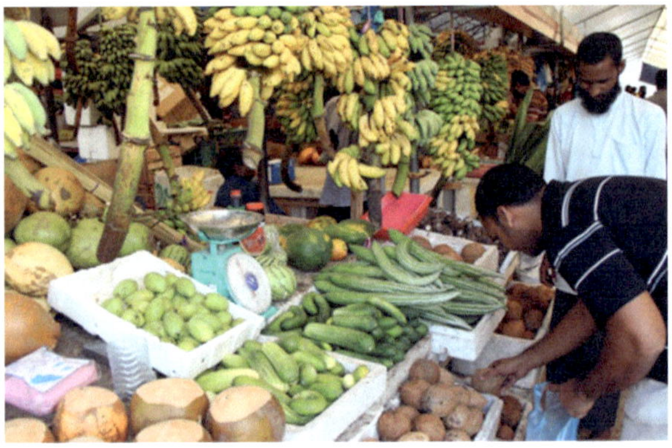

Figure 1.14. The framework of food safety laws is essential for ensuring public health and maintaining the integrity of food systems worldwide.

Source: https://cdn.who.int/media/images/default-source/imported/maldives-vegetables-market-healthy-dietaa6edaf996b74c81a254b79d79d140a8.tmb-479v.jpg?sfvrsn=97257d1f_25%20479w

1.3.2. Role of the FDA and USDA

The Food and Drug Administration (FDA) and the United States Department of Agriculture (USDA) play an important role in ensuring food sanitation and hygiene within the elaborate food system. With joint efforts, such agencies ensure the health of the public by offering regulations that guarantee foods are shielded from hazards related to the food and the environment. The FDA and USDA encourage people to adopt a whole-system approach to food safety that includes nutrition, environmental care, and the usual safety procedures. It is in accordance with growing recognition that food safety must guard against people becoming ill and also consider the way foods are prepared and disposed of.

By adopting this integrated perspective, such agencies facilitate more effective coordination of more efficient resource use and risk management in the food system, which ultimately results in enhancing the security and safety of the food supply (Angelos et al., 2017; Leib et al., 2019).

1.3.3. Hazard Analysis Critical Control Point (HACCP)

HACCP is a main guideline for maintaining food safety in food hygiene and sanitation. With HACCP, food producers can find and address risks, which helps them take steps to prevent health problems for people. A survey of Indonesian stock-feed producers found that most large companies (95%) and some medium-sized companies (65%) had adopted HACCP systems, suggesting that the framework is gaining popularity in the industry despite differences in how feed safety risks are seen by managers. Moreover, the integration of HACCP within a comprehensive One Health platform emphasizes the interconnectedness of food safety, public health, and environmental sustainability and therefore positions food safety education as an integral component for all stakeholders across all fields (Angelos et al., 2017). In addition to addressing short-term food safety concerns, thus, HACCP also supports the long-term security of the supply of food (Figure 1.15).

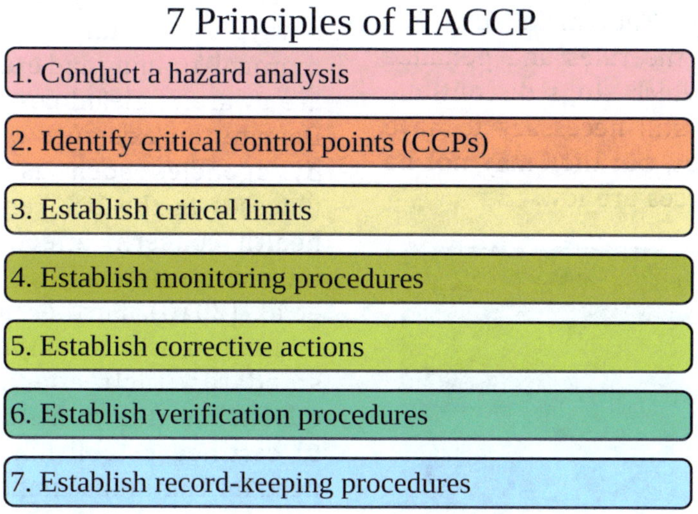

Figure 1.15. Hazard Analysis Critical Control Point (HACCP) serves as a pivotal framework in ensuring food safety within the realm of food hygiene and sanitation.

Source: By Surachit - Own work, CC BY-SA 4.0, https://commons.wikimedia.org/w/index.php?curid=123124814

1.3.4. International Food Safety Standards

The presence of International Food Safety Standards is very important for the safety and integrity of food systems everywhere. They offer a structure that helps countries make their food safety laws similar, which supports trade and keeps people healthy. When countries focus on better food hygiene, it is important to put such standards in place to reduce foodborne diseases and make consumers feel secure. For instance, educational initiatives that encompass a One Health perspective, which, , which considers the interconnectedness of human, animal, and environmental health, can further support these efforts; they encourage interdisciplinary approaches essential for comprehensive food safety curricula (Angelos et al., 2017). Moreover, addressing research gaps in environmental health, particularly in regions like Malawi, demonstrates the necessity of targeted action plans that align with international standards to promote effective food safety practices (Morse et al., 2010). Following these standards helps ensure that food is safe worldwide without using up too many natural resources.

1.3.5. Compliance and Enforcement Mechanisms

Good compliance and enforcement ensures food hygiene and sanitation, especially if public health problems change. They make sure that food industries follow the rules and penalize them if they do not, which stops discontinue any wrongdoing. It is still necessary to have inspections and licenses, but they may not be as helpful when resources are low.

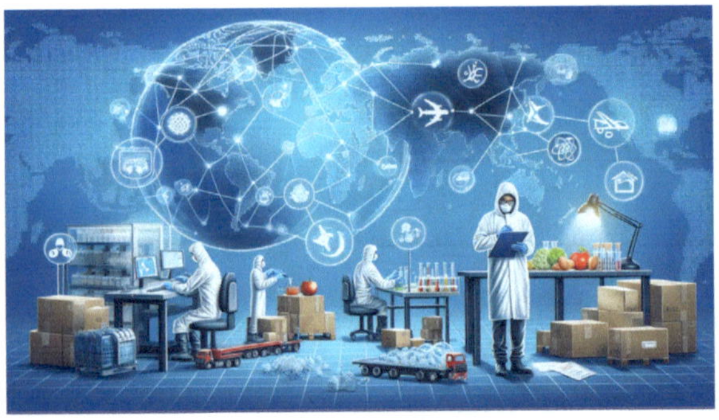

Figure 1.16. Effective compliance and enforcement mechanisms are critical to maintaining food hygiene and sanitation standards, particularly in the face of evolving public health challenges.

Source: https://sfkcorp.com/data/uploads/featured_image-43.webp.

Innovative approaches, such as public disclosure of non-compliance and escalating sanctions, can enhance adherence without significantly increasing administrative burdens (Gostin et al., 2010). Moreover, the development of universal human rights indicators related to water and sanitation can bolster accountability frameworks and improve enforcement through structured monitoring (Kim et al., 2015). As nations grapple with ensuring food safety, adapting these mechanisms to local contexts will be vital for their success, emphasizing that diligent oversight is essential for public health protection and consumer trust (Figure 1.16).

1.3.6. Certification Programs for Food Businesses

Food companies use certification programs to ensure their hygiene and food safety are always up to standard. Usually, they include thorough training and exams to prove employees are aware of cleanliness and how to stay safe. Despite the existence of stringent regulations by agencies such as the FDA, foodborne illnesses in the U.S. remain a pressing public health concern, affecting nearly 48 million individuals annually, as highlighted by Novak et al. (2016). Furthermore, while third-party audits can assess compliance with food safety standards, their effectiveness is sometimes questioned due to historical outbreaks linked to certified establishments, which raises the need for continuous improvement in food safety culture (FS-culture) and practices. Consequently, integrating comprehensive certification programs is crucial not only for compliance but also for fostering a proactive approach to food safety within food businesses, as suggested by Chapman et al. (2013).

1.3.7. Impact of Non-Compliance

Violating food hygiene and sanitation regulations can have serious implications, primarily due to the fact that food safety regulations are increasingly tightening in the international market. Due to such violations, nations stand to lose trade restrictions, as evidenced by the case of Kenyan fish exports to the EU that lost market access between 1997 and 2000 due to the failure to adhere to hygiene requirements. These measures pushed exporters to improve their hygiene controls with significant operational expenses, showing how compliance is not just a regulatory obstacle but a significant factor in market sustainability (Henson and Mitullah, 2025). Beyond this, good hygiene interventions, like encouraging hand-washing and enhancing water quality, have proven to effectively cut foodborne illnesses by half (Colford et al., 2004). Therefore, ensuring food safety compliance is not only necessary for public health but also the key to maintaining economic prosperity within food-exporting countries, highlighting the interdependence between hygiene culture and international trade patterns (Figure 1.17).

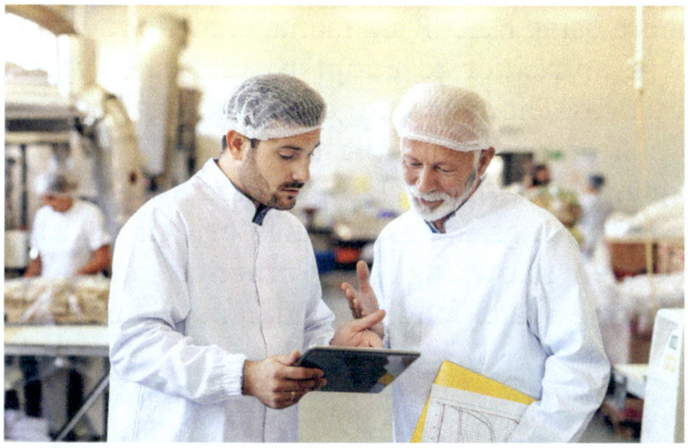

Figure 1.17. Non-compliance with food hygiene and sanitation standards has profound implications, particularly in the global marketplace, where food safety regulations are increasingly stringent.

Source: https://www.sesotec.com/sites/593fc2aac25e5b0640a20ff8/content_entry5996a921c25e5b2c7874b55f/5cecf9a6d1468d6425d9311d/files/audit-in-factory-food2-1000.jpg

1.3.8. Consumer Awareness and Education

For food hygiene and sanitation, educating consumers is very important for promoting safe food habits. If people understand the disadvantage of consuming dangers of fast food, it can strongly impact what they eat and how they eat it. As outlined in studies exploring the impact of *E. coli* outbreaks, consumers have shown a higher preference for establishments that prioritize hygienic practices and transparency regarding food handling (Ajekiigbe et al., 2025). Similarly, research on street food vendors demonstrates that even basic awareness of food safety can lead to better hygiene compliance, reducing the risk of contamination (Agrawal et al., 2025). Public health campaigns can encourage safety by teaching people and working with food service providers. In the end, increasing consumer knowledge about food hygiene helps prevent foodborne illnesses and supports the health of everyone.

1.3.9. Future Trends in Food Safety Regulations

Because food safety is gaining attention worldwide, future regulations are predicted to merge different areas of expertise. One notable shift is the integration of the One Health perspective, which recognizes the interconnectedness of human health, animal health, and environmental factors in food safety (Angelos et al., 2017). This way of thinking allows us to learn more about foodborne illness and back regulations that promote environmentally friendly farming. Furthermore, addressing the unique challenges in regions like Malawi exemplifies the urgent need for research-driven strategies that tackle food safety within the context of environmental health, underscoring the importance of targeted action plans (Morse et al., 2010). Ultimately, these evolving regulatory frameworks aim to strike a balance between safeguarding public health and preserving natural resources, reflecting a forward-looking approach that aligns with both societal needs and ecological realities (Figure 1.18).

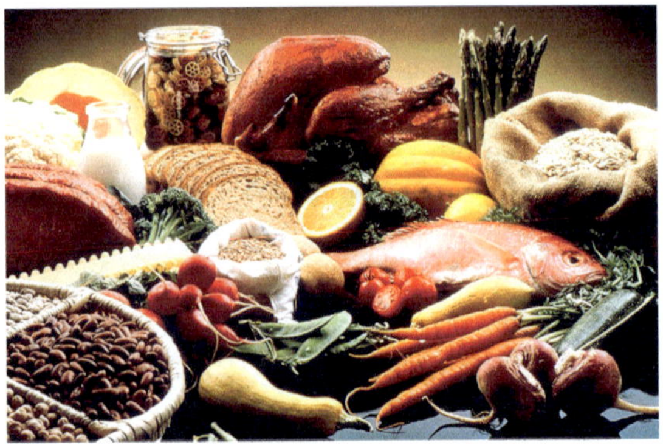

Figure 1.18. As global awareness of food safety escalates, future trends in regulations are poised to incorporate more comprehensive and interdisciplinary approaches.

Source: By Unknown author - This image was released by the National Cancer Institute, an agency part of the National Institutes of Health, with the ID 2397 (image) (next)., Public Domain, https://commons.wikimedia.org/w/index.php?curid=10531946

1.4. Best Practices in Food Hygiene

Ensuring food hygiene is very important for protecting the public's health and safety in the kitchen. There are many best practices designed to decrease the chance of foodborne illnesses. These steps are handwashing, putting food in the fridge promptly and using different utensils for raw and cooked foods. It is very important to train and educate food handlers, since not knowing the proper practices can cause serious health problems. The use of modern technology and new ideas can greatly boost how hygienic the environment is. For instance, industry advancements can optimize inventory management and improve monitoring systems, thereby reducing waste and promoting safer food handling operations (Bai et al., 2020). As demonstrated by recent studies, implementing robust hygiene protocols not only benefits consumer safety but also positively impacts public health by addressing the global challenge posed by antimicrobial resistance (Murray et al., 2022).

1.4.1. Training Programs for Food Handlers

Training food handlers effectively is very important for improving food hygiene and sanitation in the industry. Despite adequate knowledge and positive attitudes towards hygiene among food handlers, as observed in a psychiatric hospital study where 89% exhibited good knowledge and 84% a favorable attitude, there remains a significant gap in actual hygiene practices, with 38% demonstrating poor adherence to guidelines (Fitasari et al., 2021). In addition, the same issues are seen in other industries, for example, the feed industry, where using HACCP led managers who saw their work as riskier to adopt better feed hygiene practices. Therefore, targeted training programs, which address both the theoretical aspects of hygiene and practical applications within real-world settings, are essential in bridging the gap between knowledge and practice, ultimately fostering a safer food environment (Figure 1.19).

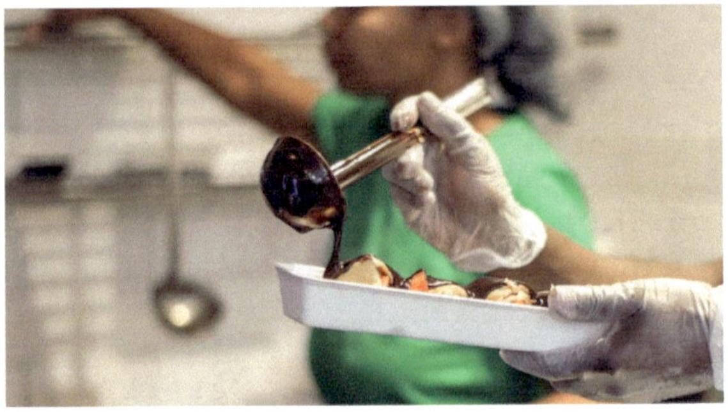

Figure 1.19. The implementation of effective training programs for food handlers is crucial in enhancing food hygiene and sanitation practices within the food industry.

Source: https://www.food-safety.com/ext/resources/eDigest/2022/man-and-woman-in-foodservice-kitchen-with-gloves-and-hairnets.png?1666745828.

1.4.2. Implementation of Standard Operating Procedures

Effective implementation of Standard Operating Procedures (SOPs) is crucial for maintaining food hygiene and sanitation within various food handling environments. SOPs help all employees know and follow safety measures , whichthat greatly lowers the risk of contamination. Consistently using these processes improves food safety and ensures the business follows regulations, which encourages accountability and quality among employees. Studies carried out recently point out that using HACCP in food production helps to boost hygiene standards. For example, HACCP systems were used differently by large and medium feed industries, which shows that one set of SOPs cannot cover all risks. Also, according to industry standards, it is important to keep evaluating and updating these SOPs to maintain improvement and adapt to new food safety issues.

1.4.3. Importance of Regular Audits

Maintaining good food hygiene and sanitation in the food industry depends a lot on regular audits. They are used to check if safety rules are being followed, find places where safety can be better and ensure hygiene is always maintained. During an audit, examining workflows, buildings and staff actions can help find risks, for example, unsafe food handling and inadequate cleaning. In addition, regular audits help create a sense of responsibility and encourage staff to keep improving, which improves how the company operates. The implementation of robust audit practices is vital in combating issues related to antimicrobial resistance, particularly in sectors like shrimp aquaculture, where unregulated antibiotic use poses significant public health threats (Thornber et al., 2019). Additionally, emphasizing gender considerations in decision-making processes surrounding food safety infrastructure can further empower women in the workforce and elevate overall food hygiene standards (OECD, 2021) (Figure 1.20).

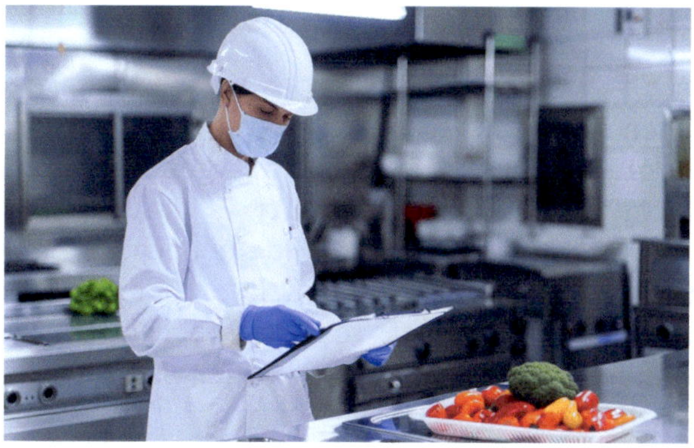

Figure 1.20. Regular audits are a critical component of maintaining high standards of food hygiene and sanitation within the food industry.

Source: https://www.capptions.com/_next/image?url=https%3A%2F%2Fcdn.sanity.io%2Fimages%2Fbs7uxmqc%2Fblog%2Fa117fd76d620ba73ab5663159adba7045768e4fa-1376x880.png&w=3840&q=75.

1.4.4. Use of Technology in Food Safety

Using technology in food safety has increased the cleanliness and safety in the food industry. Advanced tools such as blockchain, Internet of Things (IoT), and artificial intelligence (AI) enable real-time monitoring of food supply chains, ensuring traceability and transparency from farm to table. They can see potential risks, which makes it less likely that food will be contaminated or cause food poisoning. For example, if temperature changes are detected by sensors in storage, manufacturers are made aware of the problem early and this protects consumers. Food businesses can follow hygiene rules with the help of mobile apps, which give them training, reminders and checklists. Addressing research gaps in environmental health is crucial, particularly in regions like Malawi, which may lack sufficient technological resources (Morse et al., 2010). Using new science and technology, in the long run, makes food safer and more environmentally friendly.

1.4.5. Community Involvement in Food Safety

When communities join in, people are motivated to keep things clean, which is good for food safety. When the community is part of food safety, they feel more confident and active in food-related activities. Teaching people how to handle and cook food helps reduce the chances of contamination, which is good for public health.

Moreover, organizations such as Catholic Relief Services have demonstrated the effectiveness of integrating WASH practices into community-driven projects, which led to notable improvements in rural livelihoods (Emana et al., 2010). Similarly, assessments in various regions, including Malawi, highlight the necessity of addressing gaps in environmental health research to inform community-led action plans (Morse et al., 2010). Ultimately, the combined efforts of individuals and institutions are indispensable for creating safer food environments that benefit everyone (Figure 1.21).

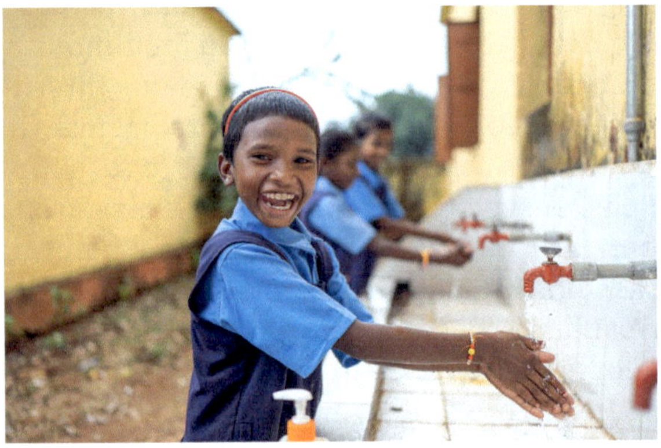

Figure 1.21. Community involvement plays a critical role in enhancing food safety, as it fosters a collective responsibility towards maintaining hygiene and sanitation standards within local populations.

Source: https://lindstrom-sites.s3.eu-north-1.amazonaws.com/wp-content/uploads/2023/12/UN0516991-1.jpg.

1.4.6. Role of Food Safety Culture (FS-Culture)

It is very important to understand FS-culture to ensure that food service environments keep proper hygiene and sanitation. FS-culture means the common beliefs, values and ways of doing things that guide employees in taking care of food safety. If a solid FS-culture is in place, employees are more likely to follow hygiene guidelines and take preventive actions , which can greatly decrease the number of foodborne illnesses. It has been found that companies with a solid FS-culture are more likely to follow food safety rules , which results in better public health. For instance, within the context of integrated programs such as Catholic Relief Services initiatives in Ethiopia, the emphasis on hygiene education and health promotion was critical in achieving sustainable improvements in community health and sanitation (Emana et al., 2010). Additionally, identifying and addressing gaps in food safety practices, like those noted in Malawi's environmental health assessments, can further refine strategies to cultivate a positive FS-culture (Morse et al., 2010).

1.4.7. Emergency Preparedness for Food Safety

Being well-prepared for emergencies in food safety is very important to prevent foodborne diseases, especially during pandemics. The complexity of zoonotic diseases, which account for over 60% of human pathogens, underscores the necessity for robust systems that can address these threats promptly and efficiently (Rahman et al., 2020). It requires being prepared by doing risk assessments, making plans and using One Health , which encourages the link between human, animal and environmental health. For instance, in Bangladesh, the government's initial lack of public health policies exacerbated challenges during the COVID-19 pandemic, revealing the importance of early groundwork and resource mobilization (Shammi et al.,

2020). By fostering coordinated efforts across various sectors, including food safety, health, and agriculture, communities can enhance resilience against potential crises, ensuring a safer food supply and minimizing health risks during emergencies (Figure 1.22).

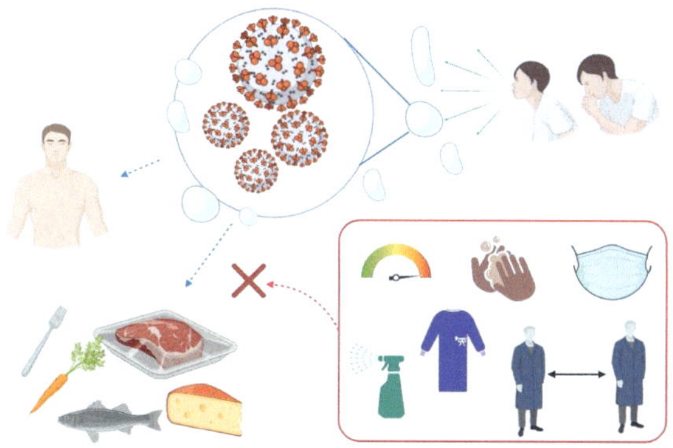

Figure 1.22. Effective emergency preparedness for food safety is crucial in mitigating risks associated with foodborne illnesses, particularly during health crises such as pandemics.

Source: Ceniti C, Tilocca B, Britti D, Santoro A, Costanzo N. Food Safety Concerns in "COVID-19 Era". *Microbiology Research*. 2021; 12(1):53-68. https://doi.org/10.3390/microbiolres12010006

1.4.8. Collaboration Between Stakeholders

Uniting various skills and resources by working together among stakeholders improves food hygiene and sanitation. Different stakeholders, including government agencies, non-governmental organizations (NGOs), and the private sector, play crucial roles in addressing food safety issues. For instance, a consultancy aimed at identifying research gaps in Malawi's environmental health sector emphasizes the importance of collaborative efforts in formulating research priorities and action plans to improve food hygiene standards (Morse et al., 2010). The concept is also shown in studies that point out how the use of primary healthcare, clean water, sanitation and nutrition in many countries helps solve difficult public health issues when stakeholders join forces. If they join forces, they might create programs that boost food safety, reduce the risk of diseases and protect public health.

1.4.9. Continuous Improvement in Food Hygiene Practices

Working to improve food hygiene at all times is important for improving health and food safety. This involves a systematic approach to evaluating and refining existing hygiene protocols, which is supported by research indicating that targeted promotional strategies can significantly influence sanitation behaviors, such as handwashing and safe food handling (Musekiwa et al., 2017). In addition, because food hygiene varies from place to place, policies should be able to change to meet local needs, as shown by studies on sanitation and hygiene improvements. By always evaluating and adjusting their practices, food businesses can satisfy rules and earn people's trust by always putting health and safety first. So, constant improvement is not only a requirement for procedures; it is also essential for the food industry to adapt to new health concerns.

A CLOSER LOOK

Hazard Analysis Critical Control Point (HACCP)

HACCP is designed to identify, look at and control any risks that could affect food safety during the entire production process. The purpose is to stop biological, chemical and physical hazards that might make food unsafe to eat. The HACCP system uses seven main principles , which are hazard analysis, identifying critical control points, setting critical limits, monitoring procedures, corrective actions, verification and documentation. HACCP is used in many places in the food industry to handle food safety problems before they happen. It supports both meeting regulations and encouraging buyers by always providing safe and high-quality food.

SUMMARY

Food needs to be clean and safe because it affects the health and safety of everyone. When good food handling practices are used, the risk of foodborne diseases is lowered and everyone in the community benefits. Since WASH relates to health, it is necessary to have high food hygiene standards. As seen in many studies, organizations like UNICEF realize key domains where WASH is crucial to affect health, such as nutrition and maternal health, highlighting the complexities between food safety and wider health programs (Mills et al., 2016). Because WASH impacts HIV/AIDS, we should make sure hygiene is included in public health efforts. For this reason, it is still necessary to back a unified way of ensuring food sanitation and hygiene to protect people from illnesses.

Examining food hygiene and sanitation makes it obvious that clean water and good sanitation are the main factors for public health. A thorough review indicates that the important interaction between water, sanitation, and nutrition is largely in reference to how enhanced WASH practices can prevent undernutrition, as described in the Bangladesh findings (Mahmud et al., 2016). Furthermore, the need for research specific to bridging gaps in the environmental health field is highlighted, especially in countries like Malawi, whose data can be used to guide strategic action plans to advance food safety and hygiene standards (Morse et al., 2010). So, this shows that better food hygiene and sanitation are needed to safeguard health and improve the nutrition of the community , which confirms the connection between hygiene and well-being.

KEY TERMS FROM THIS CHAPTER

- Advisory
- Association
- Campylobacter
- Climate change
- Consumer
- Contamination
- Cross-contamination
- Dangers
- Developing nations
- Assessment
- Bacteria
- Cleanliness
- Community health
- Consumption
- COVID-19 pandemic
- Dairy
- Deli meats
- World Health Organization (WHO)

REFERENCES

1. Abebe, E., Gugsa, G., & Ahmed, M. (2020). Review on major food-borne zoonotic bacterial pathogens. *Journal of Tropical Medicine, 2020*, Article 4674235. https://doi.org/10.1155/2020/4674235.
2. Agrawal, S., Vyas, M., Chauhan, T., & Patel, B. (2025). Street food safety: A study on hygiene practices and risk factors among vendors. *International Journal of Research Publication and Reviews*. https://www.semanticscholar.org/paper/69529e256227389d3d7f58bf2d641a62647cdccb (accessed on 29 May 2025).
3. Ajekiigbe, V., Ogieuhi, I., Anthony, C. S., Bakare, I. S., Anyacho, S., Ogunleke, P., Fatokun, D. I., et al. (2025). Consumer behavior and its role in *E. coli* outbreaks: The impact of fast-food preparation practices and hygiene awareness. *Tropical Medicine and Health, 53*. https://www.semanticscholar.org/paper/f0dcc4105d349fe365289c1ea7bc179c1d7d2a80 (accessed on 29 May 2025).
4. Angelos, J. A., Arens, A. L., Johnson, H. A., Cadriel, J. L., & Osburn, B. I. (2017). One Health in food safety and security education: Subject matter outline for a curricular framework. *One health (Amsterdam, Netherlands), 3*, 56–65. https://doi.org/10.1016/j.onehlt.2017.04.001
5. Asyary, A., Hayati, F., Memish, Z., et al. (2024). *Food Hygiene and Sanitation at the Jakarta Pondok Gede Hajj Embarkation Dormitory: Food Safety Efforts for the Hajj Pilgrims*. https://core.ac.uk/download/639388619.pdf (accessed on 29 May 2025).
6. Babcock, H. M., Garg, S., Kim, L., et al. (2017). *Preventing Respiratory Viral Transmission in Long-Term Care: Knowledge, Attitudes, And Practices of Healthcare Personnel*. https://core.ac.uk/download/212864305.pdf (accessed on 29 May 2025).
7. Bahri, A., Drechsel, P., Raschid-Sally, L., Redwood, L., et al. (2025). *Wastewater Irrigation and Health: Assessing and Mitigating Risk in Low-Income Countries*. https://core.ac.uk/download/pdf/6405282.pdf (accessed on 29 May 2025).
8. Bai, C., Dallasega, P., Orzes, G., & Sarkis, J. (2020). Industry 4.0 technologies assessment: A sustainability perspective. *International Journal of Production Economics, 229*, Article 107776. https://doi.org/10.1016/j.ijpe.2020.107776.
9. Ramsingh B. (2014). The emergence of international food safety standards and guidelines: understanding the current landscape through a historical approach. *Perspectives in public health, 134*(4), 206–215. https://doi.org/10.1177/1757913914536557 (accessed on 29 May 2025).
10. Bosch, A., Gkogka, E., Le Guyader, F. S., Loisy-Hamon, F., Lee, A., van Lieshout, L., Marthi, B., et al. (2018). Foodborne viruses: Detection, risk assessment, and control options in food processing. *International Journal of Food Microbiology, 285*, 110–128. https://doi.org/10.1016/j.ijfoodmicro.2018.06.001.
11. Broad Leib, E. M., & Pollans, M. J. (2019). *The New Food Safety*. https://core.ac.uk/download/231832064.pdf (accessed on 29 May 2025).
12. Calvin, K., Dasgupta, D., Krinner, G., Mukherji, A., Thorne, P., Trisos, C. H., Romero, J., et al. (2023). *Climate Change 2023: Synthesis Report. Contribution of Working Groups I, II and III to the Sixth Assessment Report of the Intergovernmental Panel on Climate Change* (H. Lee & J. Romero, Eds.). IPCC. https://doi.org/10.59327/ipcc/ar6-9789291691647.

13. Carstens, C. K., Salazar, J. K., & Darkoh, C. (2019). Multistate outbreaks of foodborne illness in the United States associated with fresh produce from 2010 to 2017. *Frontiers in Microbiology, 10*, Article 2667. https://doi.org/10.3389/fmicb.2019.02667.

14. Chamola, V., Hassija, V., Gupta, V., & Guizani, M. (2020). A comprehensive review of the COVID-19 pandemic and the role of IoT, drones, AI, blockchain, and 5G in managing its impact. *IEEE Access, 8*, 90225–90265. https://doi.org/10.1109/access.2020.2992341.

15. Chapman, B. J., Costa, R. E., Dodd, C., et al. (2013). *Audits and Inspections Are Never Enough: A Critique to Enhance Food Safety*. https://core.ac.uk/download/10653288.pdf (accessed on 29 May 2025).

16. Chinchilla Lee, A. C. (2009). *Assessment of Food Safety in Food Service Establishments*. https://core.ac.uk/download/543396598.pdf (accessed on 29 May 2025).

17. Colford, J. M., Jr., & Fewtrell, L. (2004). *Water, Sanitation and Hygiene: Interventions and Diarrhoea–A Systematic Review and Meta-Analysis*. https://core.ac.uk/download/71360183.pdf (accessed on 29 May 2025).

18. Cooke, L. R., Mac an tSaoir, S., & McCracken, A. R. (2010). *The Effects of Leaf Litter Treatments, Post-Harvest Urea and Omission of Early Season Fungicide Sprays on The Overwintering of Apple Scab on Bramley's Seedling Grown in A Maritime Environment*. https://core.ac.uk/download/45656428.pdf (accessed on 29 May 2025).

19. Cosby, C. M. (2005). *A Sanitation Assessment of Food Contact Surfaces in Child Care Centers Using Microbiological Analysis and Rapid Sanitation Assays*. https://core.ac.uk/download/268807029.pdf (accessed on 29 May 2025).

20. Dianita, I. A., Nurlena, N., & Sumarsih, U. (2024). *Evaluating Hygiene and Sanitation Practices in Pastry Equipment*. https://core.ac.uk/download/599141278.pdf (accessed on 29 May 2025).

21. Dominguez-Salas, P., Waddington, H., Grace, D., Bosire, C., Moodley, A., Kulkarni, B., Dasi, T., et al. (2024). Understanding the role of household hygiene practices and foodborne disease risks in child stunting: A UKRI GCRF Action Against Stunting Hub protocol paper. *BMJ Pediatrics Open, 8*. https://www.semanticscholar.org/paper/cbe56a6d09da0f10a7dd542240e7b213ead837fb (accessed on 29 May 2025).

22. Emana, B., Hebert, P. V., & Tessma, T. (2010). *Transforming Lives: An Evaluation of CRS Integrated Watershed Management Programs in Ethiopia*. https://core.ac.uk/download/71361177.pdf (accessed on 29 May 2025).

23. Eryando, T., Kusuma, A., Pratiwi, D., et al. (2015). *The Correlation Between Eating Utensils and Place of Sales in The Contamination of Escherichia Coli in Food Sold at Campus Food Stalls*. https://media.neliti.com/media/publications/150914-EN-the-correlation-between-eating-utensils.pdf (accessed on 29 May 2025).

24. Fitasari, R. P., Palupi, I. R., & Utami, F. A. (2021). *Knowledge, Attitude and Practice of Hygiene and Sanitation Among Food-Handlers in A Psychiatric Hospital in Indonesia: A Mixed Method Study*. https://core.ac.uk/download/386172170.pdf (accessed on 29 May 2025).

25. Fitriah, A. H., Heranisa, A., & Winarni, S. (2024). The evaluation of knowledge and behavior in hygiene sanitation of food handlers at Aji Santoso International Football Academy. *HEARTY*. https://www.semanticscholar.org/paper/918574b9e86ad3d0fc2317de275442cad183d7c6 (accessed on 29 May 2025).

26. Freeman, M., Ellis, A., Ogutu, E., Caruso, B., Linabarger, M., Micek, K., Muga, R., et al. (2020). Impact of a demand-side integrated WASH and nutrition community-based care group intervention on behavioural change: A randomised controlled trial in western Kenya. *BMJ Global Health, 5*. https://www.semanticscholar.org/paper/a129d7edff382caf1d612f58044571e9001e0bfa (accessed on 29 May 2025).

27. Girmay, A. M., Gari, S. R., Teklebirhan Gessew, G., & Tadesse Reta, M. (2021). Determinants of drinking-water quality and sanitary risk levels of water storages in food establishments of Addis Ababa, Ethiopia. *Journal of Water, Sanitation and Hygiene for Development*. https://www.semanticscholar.org/paper/518fd3cb4451e5457b1cefa3b50c53d35dc25ce6 (accessed on 29 May 2025).

28. Gostin, L. O., Gupta, M. D., Levin, M., et al. (2010). *Implementing Public Health Regulations in Developing Countries: Lessons from the OECD Countries*. https://core.ac.uk/download/70373906.pdf (accessed on 29 May 2025).

29. Habicht, J. P., Kim, S. S., Menon, P., et al. (2025). *How do Programs Work to Improve Child Nutrition? Program impact Pathways of Three Nongovernmental Organization Intervention Projects in The Peruvian Highlands*. https://core.ac.uk/download/pdf/6254914.pdf (accessed on 29 May 2025).

30. Heaviside, C., Lake, I., & Nichols, G. (2018). *Climate Change and Water-Related Infectious Diseases*. https://core.ac.uk/download/322490318.pdf (accessed on 29 May 2025).

31. Henson, S., & Mitullah, W. (2025). *Kenyan Exports of Nile Perch: The Impact of Food Safety Standards on An Export-Oriented Supply Chain*. https://core.ac.uk/download/pdf/6645136.pdf (accessed on 29 May 2025).

32. Ito, A., Steyer, A., van den Hurk, A. F., Willingham, A. L., Phongmany, A., Donnelly, B., Khamlome, B., et al. (2016). *Endemicity of Zoonotic Diseases in Pigs and Humans in Lowland and Upland Lao Pdr: Identification of Socio-Cultural Risk Factors*. https://core.ac.uk/download/45467782.pdf (accessed on 29 May 2025).

33. Jaffee, S., Henson, S., Unnevehr, L. J., Grace, D., & Cassou, E. (2018). *The Safe Food Imperative: Accelerating Progress in Low- And Middle-Income Countries*. World Bank. https://doi.org/10.1596/978-1-4648-1345-0.

34. Johnson, P. N. T., & Yawson, R. M. (2025). *Enhancing the Food Security of The Peri-Urban and Urban Poor Through Improvements to The Quality, Safety and Economics of Street-Vended Foods*. https://core.ac.uk/download/pdf/6618604.pdf (accessed on 29 May 2025).

35. Kaur, N., Satapathy, P., Neyazi, A., & Padhi, B. (2023). The outbreak of shigellosis in Sweden as a looming concern for public health: A correspondence. *Annals of Medicine and Surgery, 85*, 627–628. https://www.semanticscholar.org/paper/4a927af8979cbf9c79999aa2ac17f260b8c09649 (accessed on 29 May 2025).

36. Kim, Y., & Meier, B. M. (2015). *Human Rights Accountability Through Treaty Bodies: Examining Human Rights Treaty Monitoring for Water and Sanitation*. https://core.ac.uk/download/62570831.pdf (accessed on 29 May 2025).

37. Kullman, C., Skoufias, E., Andres, L. A., & Srivastava, V. (2017). *Reducing Inequalities in Water Supply, Sanitation, And Hygiene in The Era of The Sustainable Development Goals*. https://core.ac.uk/download/141922872.pdf (accessed on 29 May 2025).

38. Kumar, I., Rawat, J., Mohd, N., & Husain, S. (2021). Opportunities of artificial intelligence and machine learning in the food industry. *Journal of Food Quality, 2021*, 1–10. https://doi.org/10.1155/2021/4535567.

39. London School of Hygiene & Tropical Medicine. (2013). *Annual Report 2013*. https://core.ac.uk/download/19452766.pdf (accessed on 29 May 2025).

40. Morse, Tracy and Lungu, Kingsley and Taulo, Steven (2010) Gap Analysis of Environmental Health Research in Malawi : Report to the National Commission of Science and Technology. National Commission for Science and Technology (Malawi), Malawi.https://core.ac.uk/download/19610167.pdf (accessed on 29 May 2025).

41. Mahmud, I., & Mbuya, N. (2016). *Water, Sanitation, Hygiene, And Nutrition in Bangladesh: Can Building Toilets Affect Children's Growth?* https://core.ac.uk/download/75783689.pdf (accessed on 29 May 2025).

42. Mills, J. E., & Cumming, O. (2016). *The Impact of Water, Sanitation, And Hygiene on Key Health and Social Outcomes: Review of Evidence*. https://core.ac.uk/download/75761114.pdf (accessed on 29 May 2025).

43. Murray, C. J. L., Ikuta, K. S., Sharara, F., Swetschinski, L. R., Robles Aguilar, G., Gray, A. P., Han, C., et al. (2022). Global burden of bacterial antimicrobial resistance in 2019: A systematic analysis. *The Lancet, 399*, 629–655. https://doi.org/10.1016/s0140-6736(21)02724-0.

44. Musekiwa, A., Vande Veegaete, A., Avau, B., De Buck, E., Van Remoortel, H., Mosler, H. J., Hannes, K., et al. (2017). *Promoting Handwashing and Sanitation Behavior Change in Low- And Middle-Income Countries: A Mixed-Method Systematic Review*. https://core.ac.uk/download/141922886.pdf (accessed on 29 May 2025).

45. Nkhebenyane, J. S. (2018). *Food Hygiene Risks and Related Practices in Central South African HIV/Aids Hospices: A Qualitative Assessment* [Master's thesis, University of the Free State]. https://core.ac.uk/download/222968072.pdf (accessed on 29 May 2025).

46. Novak, A. C. (2016). *Increasing Food Safety Compliance with Online Resources* [Master's thesis, California State University, Northridge]. https://core.ac.uk/download/162578521.pdf (accessed on 29 May 2025).

47. Novoveská, L., Ross, M., Stanley, M. S., Pradelles, R., Wasiolek, V., & Sassi, J. F. (2019). Microalgal carotenoids: A review of production, current markets, regulations, and future direction. *Marine Drugs, 17*(11), 640. https://doi.org/10.3390/md17110640.

48. Olinto da Motta, S. P. (2016). *Consumer Behavior Concerning Food Safety in Brazil and New Zealand: Modelling Food Safety Risk in the Home* (Doctoral thesis, Massey University, Manawatu, New Zealand). https://core.ac.uk/download/148644581.pdf (accessed on 29 May 2025).

49. Organisation for Economic Co-operation and Development. (2021). *Women in Infrastructure* (Public Governance Policy Papers No. 10). https://doi.org/10.1787/9eab66a8-en.

50. Pula, J. J. I. B., & Pascual, M. P. (2019). Sanitation practices of street food vendors in Cabanatuan City. *International Journal of Advanced Engineering, Management and Science*. https://www.semanticscholar.org/paper/30c5b058b23bfc20e734b8d826acdf890699721d (accessed on 29 May 2025).

51. Rahman, M. T., Sobur, M. A., Islam, M. S., Ievy, S., Hossain, M. J., El Zowalaty, M. E., Rahman, A. T., et al. (2020). Zoonotic diseases: Etiology, impact, and control. *Microorganisms, 8*(9), 1405. https://doi.org/10.3390/microorganisms8091405.

52. Shammi, M., Bodrud-Doza, M., Islam, A. R. M. T., & Rahman, M. M. (2020). Strategic assessment of COVID-19 pandemic in Bangladesh: Comparative lockdown scenario analysis, public perception, and management for sustainability. *Environment, Development and Sustainability, 23*, 6148–6191. https://doi.org/10.1007/s10668-020-00867-y.

53. Simões, R. S. Q. (2024). Environmental virology linked to waterborne diseases and foodborne pathogens: Human and animal food viruses. *International Journal of Frontiers in Biology and Pharmacy Research.* https://www.semanticscholar.org/paper/fa69ce9c1ec7472adebffe2b0fa68320ed94141e (accessed on 29 May 2025).

54. Sunarti, L. S. (2024). Bacterial contamination in food: Sources, risks, and prevention strategies. *International Journal of Pathogen Research.* https://www.semanticscholar.org/paper/424b6e40290b771dbf75a50ca6bfbe9de762f0a6 (accessed on 29 May 2025).

55. Thornber, K., Verner–Jeffreys, D. W., Hinchliffe, S., Rahman, M. M., Bass, D., & Tyler, C. R. (2019). Evaluating antimicrobial resistance in the global shrimp industry. *Reviews in Aquaculture, 12*, 966–986. https://doi.org/10.1111/raq.12367.

56. United Nations System Standing Committee on Nutrition. (2020). *Water and Nutrition: Harmonizing Actions for the United Nations Decade of Action on Nutrition and the United Nations Water Action Decade.* https://core.ac.uk/download/288633623.pdf (accessed on 29 May 2025).

57. Usman, S. (2019). Evaluation of microbial load in fast food establishments in Kaduna Metropolis. *Community Medicine and Public Health Care.* https://www.semanticscholar.org/paper/3a09363422068d5444cce7b831c792dfaf16cc67 (accessed on 29 May 2025).

58. Vetchapitak, T., & Misawa, N. (2019). Current Status of *Campylobacter* Food Poisoning in Japan. *Food safety (Tokyo, Japan), 7*(3), 61–73. https://doi.org/10.14252/foodsafetyfscj.D-19-00001(accessed on 29 May 2025).

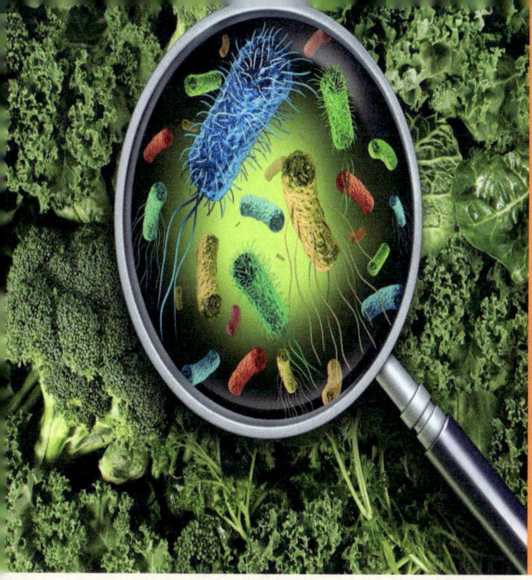

Chapter 2

SOURCES OF FOOD CONTAMINATION

Contents

Introduction 27
2.1. Biological Contaminants 30
2.2. Chemical Contaminants 34
2.3. Physical Contaminants 38
2.4. Environmental Contaminants 42
Summary 49
References 50

Introduction

Many different ways by which food gets contaminated today that can seriously endanger the health and safety of everyone. It is necessary to understand these sources to develop good ways to secure food and defend consumers. How food is made, the source of the ingredients and the methods used to grow it can all add contaminants. Since there is greater demand for organic food, extra care must be taken to ensure that organic food is safe, because quality matters a lot. Institutions such as the Western Institute for Food Safety and Security promote a multidisciplinary education approach to food safety, where the interrelated nature of various disciplines under the One Health umbrella is highlighted in order to address these issues comprehensively (Angelos et al., 2017). So, being aware of the different sources of food contamination helps us keep food safe and also supports environmental protection.

Definition of Food Contamination

Food contamination happens when dangerous substances are found in food , which can be very harmful to people who eat it. Such contaminants may be biological, chemical or physical and every type comes from different sources and affects food safety differently. When hygiene is poor during food preparation or storage, bacteria, viruses and parasites may increase in number, as pointed out in discussions about the food processing environment. If pesticides, additives or processing agents are used in excess, they can cause chemical contamination , which is dangerous for people. Also, during the manufacturing and handling of food, glass or metal pieces can end up in the product. The exhaustive knowledge of such forms of contamination supports the imperative of strict food safety procedures, such as the application of preventive steps, as noted in learning concepts for food safety and security (Angelos et al., 2017). Additionally, analyzing specific outbreaks, such as those linked to *Listeria monocytogenes* in frozen vegetables, illustrates the critical factors influencing contamination (EFSA BIOHAZ Panel (EFSA Panel on Biological Hazards), 2020) (Figure 2.1).

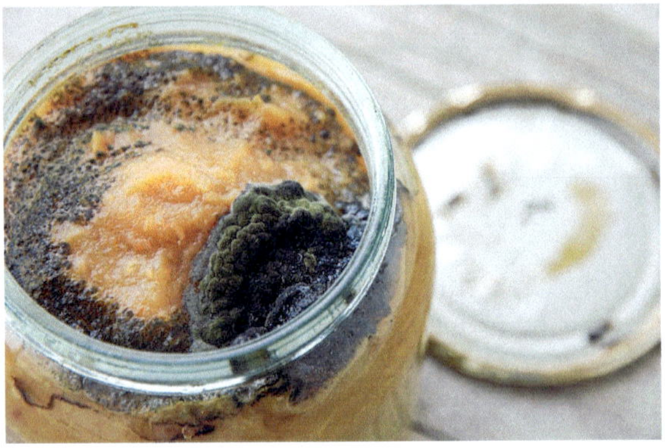

Figure 2.1. Food contamination is defined as the presence of harmful substances in food that can pose significant health risks to consumers.

Source: https://5845715.fs1.hubspotusercontent-na1.net/hub/5845715/hubfs/jam%20food%20contamination-1.jpg

Overview of Contamination Types

It is important to understand how food gets contaminated to ensure that food is safe and people remain healthy. Biological, chemical and physical are the key sources of contamination. Biological contaminants, in the form of mostly bacteria, viruses, and parasites, are very dangerous since they can cause foodborne diseases that require aggressive techniques like microbial source tracking (MST) to detect sources of fecal microbes in the food supply chain (Lihua et al., 2024).

Figure 2.2. Contamination can broadly be classified into three main categories: biological, chemical, and physical.

Source: By GNOME icon artists; Pbroks13 (talk) - Image:Gnome-applications-science.svg; Image:Gnome-appointment-soon.svg; Image:Gnome-dialog-warning.svg, CC BY-SA 4.0, https://commons.wikimedia.org/w/index.php?curid=4689247

Most frequently, the chemicals present in food obtained from farming or processing are pesticides, additives, and heavy metals. Small pieces of metal or glass can fall into the food by accident while manufacturing or packaging. The only way to properly solve these problems is to take a systems-based approach that is aware of the interplay between food safety and environmental concerns (as described by the Western Institute for Food Safety and Security, Angelos et al., 2017). This emphasizes the complex difficulties in keeping food supplies safe without sacrificing ecological integrity (Figure 2.2).

Historical Context of Food Contamination

The development of farming, industry and the world economy has made food contamination change over the years. Due to bacteria and fungi, early people had to handle the problem of food spoilage. Even so, when industrial farming started, more chemicals were needed , which boosted crop growth but made people worry about the safety of soil and water. Since cities were the main place people lived, food and waste were often close , which brought more heavy metals and pollutants and made it more difficult to keep food safe. Additionally, as identified in the recent discourse of sustainable water management, the union of man-made activities with natural processes requires interdisciplinary analysis for evaluation of the quality of water and contamination pathways (Akhtar et al., 2021). This path identifies the importance of continuous regulation and education in order to manage the historical effects of food contamination and the need to reshape these to respond to modern challenges within the global food system (Gann et al., 2019).

Current Statistics on Foodborne Illnesses

Foodborne illnesses are still a major public health problem globally, as current statistics prove. In 2022, the European Food Safety Authority found that campylobacteriosis and salmonellosis were the diseases reported most often in humans , which was similar to the pattern seen in previous years. Even though the food supply is stable, there has been a sharp increase in foodborne outbreaks and the number of deaths from these outbreaks hit a ten-year high, mainly because of infections from *L. monocytogenes* and *Salmonella*. Bacteria are responsible for approximately two-thirds of foodborne diseases (FBDs) globally, particularly affecting vulnerable populations in developing countries. Meat, dairy and eggs , which are major food products, are important for spreading these pathogens. These statistics highlight the urgent need for effective monitoring and preventive measures against food contamination (Figure 2.3).

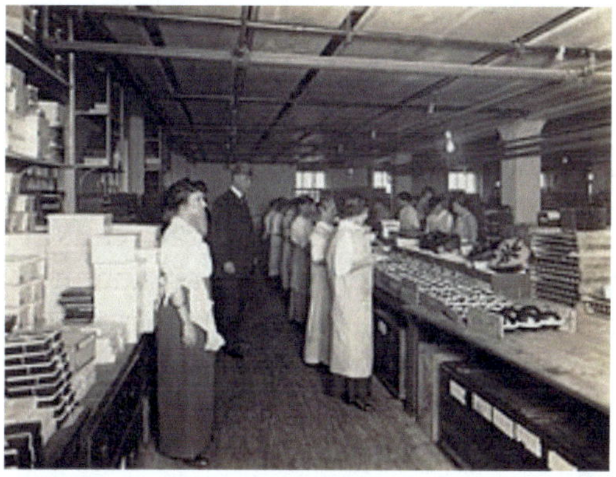

Figure 2.3. Foodborne illnesses continue to represent a significant public health challenge worldwide, with current statistics underscoring their impact.

Source: By The U.S. Food and Drug Administration - Inspecting a Candy Factory (FDA045), Public Domain, https://commons.wikimedia.org/w/index.php?curid=51272692

Relevance to Public Health

As food contamination can lead to injury among the more susceptible individuals, public health finds it extremely critical. As an example, the pathogen *Listeria monocytogenes*, associated with blanched frozen vegetables, has been found to lead to alarmingly higher probabilities of illness in elderly groups than in other food groups, which shows the need for strict food safety procedures in shielding the susceptible population (EFSA BIOHAZ Panel (EFSA Panel on Biological Hazards), 2020). Similarly, Shiga toxin-producing *Escherichia coli* (STEC) poses a critical concern, especially on dairy farms where environmental and husbandry practices can increase the rate of pathogen transmission. Research highlights that about 20% of young dairy calves carry STEC, thereby implicating livestock in the broader human health continuum (Browne, 2018). They prove that we need to keep checking food safety and have good strategies, since foodborne illnesses can affect everyone and the healthcare system.

2.1. Biological Contaminants

Among all the things that can cause food contamination, biological contaminants are a major problem because they can seriously harm people's health. The contaminants mentioned are bacteria, viruses, fungi and parasites that can come from soil, water and animal products. Eating food that is contaminated can result in foodborne illnesses and these illnesses may cause anything from stomach problems to infections throughout the body. According to food safety discussions, knowing how food is contaminated and taking steps to stop it is very important for public health. The need for rigorous hygiene standards during food processing and handling cannot be overstated, as emphasized in recent analyses of food safety practices (Abdurazakova et al., 2021) and the comprehensive review of microbial safety challenges (Heijden, 2019). In short, dealing with biological contaminants is necessary to uphold food safety and protect those who consume the food.

2.1.1. Bacteria as a Source of Contamination

Bacteria are a key reason for food contamination and this can be very harmful to people in many parts of the food supply chain.

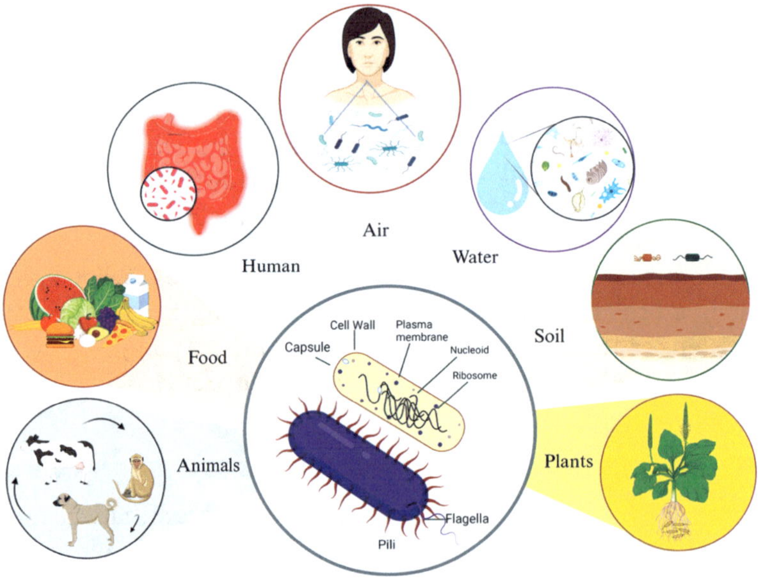

Figure 2.4. Bacterial pathogenicity.

Source: Soni J, Sinha S and Pandey R (2024) Understanding bacterial pathogenicity: a closer look at the journey of harmful microbes. Front. Microbiol. 15:1370818. doi: 10.3389/fmicb.2024.1370818

Because salmonella and similar pathogens can be found in plants and animals, there are many risks in food production and processing. For instance, Salmonella is particularly associated with pork, as evidenced by industry surveys indicating that effective management interventions are crucial during both the finishing and slaughtering stages to minimize contamination risks (Gaag et al., 2002). Because food is sent all over the world, it is difficult to maintain hygiene, so a small mistake can make a lot of people sick. As underscored by safety campaigns, ensuring food security and safety requires a comprehensive approach that addresses the intricate links between government regulations and societal engagement (Chattu et al., 2015). Thus, mitigating bacterial contamination is paramount to protecting consumer health across the food continuum (Figure 2.4).

2.1.2. Viruses and Their Impact on Food Safety

Even though viruses are not always acknowledged, they play a major part in making food unsafe. Such organisms can lead to foodborne illnesses and well-known examples like norovirus and hepatitis A are very dangerous through food. Food may become polluted at any point in its production, processing, handling or consumption , which is why good sanitation and hygiene are needed everywhere in the food industry. In particular, the potential for agroterrorism, which involves the deliberate introduction of plant pathogens to disrupt food security, highlights the vulnerability of agricultural systems to viral contamination (Forrest et al., 2020). The intricate relationship between human health and the safe production of food necessitates ongoing research into viral pathogens and comprehensive strategies for mitigation (Eijck et al., 2003). Taking care of these matters helps the food industry keep people safe and improve food safety.

2.1.3. Parasites in Food Products

Having parasites in food products is a major issue in food safety and this is influenced by different environmental and agricultural factors. Notably, *Toxoplasma gondii*, a zoonotic protozoan parasite, exemplifies this issue, as it disseminates through resilient oocysts that can infiltrate diverse food sources, including shellfish and fresh produce, thus magnifying the risk of human exposure (Bahia-Oliveira et al., 2019). Moreover, in organic agriculture, the increase in certain zoonotic diseases, including Toxoplasma, raises questions about the purported health advantages of organic products over conventional counterparts (Eijck et al., 2003). Occasionally, the way organic livestock is managed can accidentally create conditions that attract parasites , which makes it necessary to study these conditions and find better ways to control them. As such, addressing the role of parasites not only informs public health strategies but also guides agricultural practices aimed at reducing foodborne illnesses (Figure 2.5).

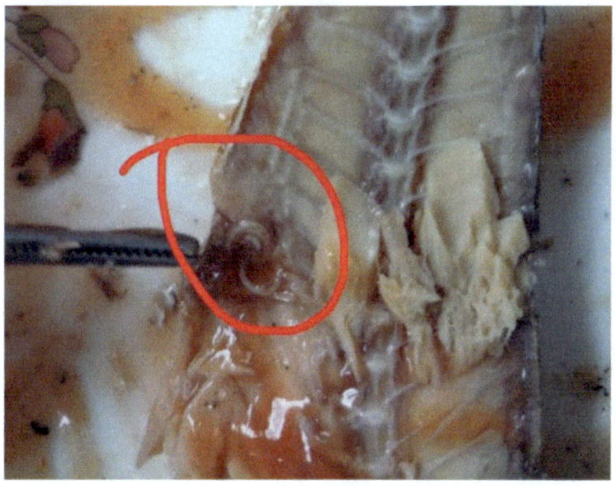

Figure 2.5. Parasites in food products.

Source: https://assets.nst.com.my/images/articles/02_sardin_ulat_1530458991.jpg.

2.1.4. Fungi and Mold Contamination

Aflatoxins , which are toxins, can be created by fungi and mold and these can contaminate food. Wheat , which is a staple in many places, is often linked to toxic chemicals. Research highlights that conditions conducive to fungal growth, such as humidity and temperature, often prevail in agricultural settings, particularly in areas like northern Iran, where environmental factors favor mold proliferation (Haji-Hoseeini et al., 2016). The effects of mold contamination can be significant, as indicated by results that a high proportion of local silos' wheat samples contained aflatoxins and therefore presented possible health hazards despite falling below acceptable levels (Audenaert et al., 2016). This implies that managing fungi and mold contamination by following proper storage and handling practices is important in maintaining food quality and health security (Figure 2.6).

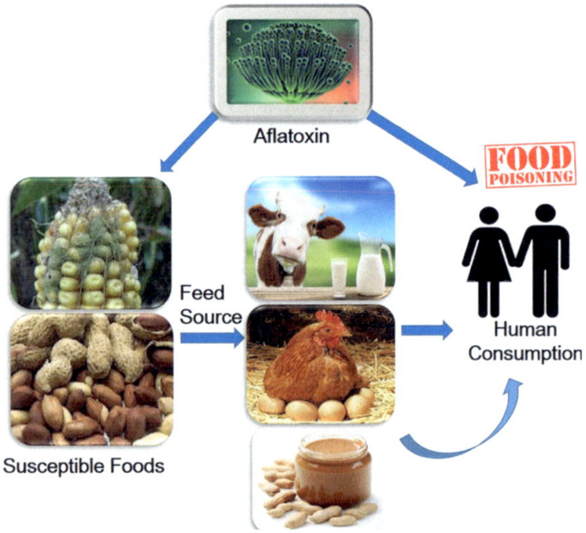

Figure 2.6. Fungi and mold contamination represent significant risks within the broader category of food contamination, primarily due to their ability to produce harmful mycotoxins such as aflatoxins.

Source: Kumar P, Mahato DK, Kamle M, Mohanta TK and Kang SG (2017) Aflatoxins: A Global Concern for Food Safety, Human Health and Their Management. Front. Microbiol. 7:2170. doi: 10.3389/fmicb.2016.02170

2.1.5. Sources of Biological Contaminants

Many factors in the environment and things people do can result in biological contaminants in food. One significant contributor is urban runoff, which can introduce harmful substances such as heavy metals and polycyclic aromatic hydrocarbons (PAHs) into water systems that support aquatic life crucial for human consumption. Urbanization alters natural watercourses, leading to sediment pollution that can decimate macroinvertebrate populations, thus destabilizing the food web and affecting the overall ecological health of these habitats (Beasley & Kneale, 2001). Additionally, studies within marine sanctuaries, such as Gray's Reef National Marine Sanctuary, have highlighted the relationship between contaminated sediments and the health of benthic organisms, which serve as vital links in the marine food chain (Balthis et al., 2004). So, it is necessary to understand these biological contaminants to ensure food safety and the health of the environment.

2.1.6. Conditions that Promote Biological Growth

Often, the environment helps microorganisms , which results in bacteria growing in food. Growth requires the proper temperature, water and nutrients and this can sometimes result in contamination. If the temperature is warm and food is very moist, bacteria and fungi can grow quickly , which increases the chance of microbial growth. Organisms that receive nutrient-rich food grow more quickly , which may cause an increase in food poisoning. The degradation of aquatic ecosystems, as noted in (Goethals et al., 2019), can exacerbate these issues, particularly in lakes and reservoirs where environmental quality is compromised by human activities. This is evident in studies on species like juvenile crayfish, which reveal that varying levels of environmental pollutants affect biological resilience and growth patterns, indicating how contamination can disrupt ecological balance and food safety (Alcorlo et al., 2019) (Figure 2.7).

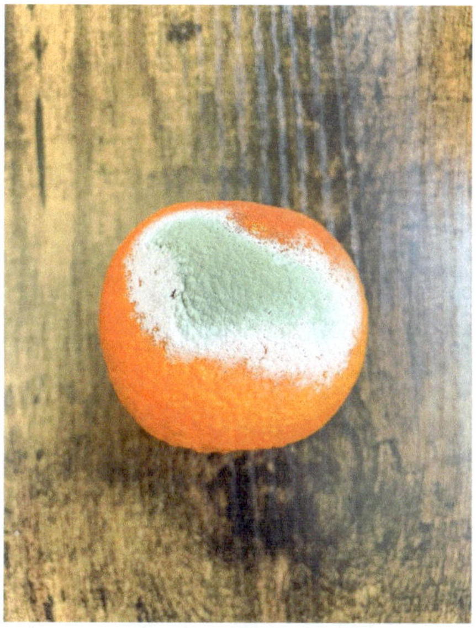

Figure 2.7. High moisture levels in food significantly increase the likelihood of microbial proliferation.

Source: https://nutritionmeetsfoodscience.com/wp-content/uploads/2022/08/img-10.jpg.

2.1.7. Symptoms of Foodborne Illnesses

What symptoms that appear from foodborne illnesses depend on the type of contaminant and the condition of the person. Most of the time, people experience nausea, vomiting, diarrhea, abdominal pain and fever and these usually start within a few hours or days after eating contaminated food. According to the CDC, pathogens like Salmonella and Listeria are frequently associated with specific foods, with Salmonella often linked to poultry and Listeria to deli meats, highlighting the importance of food source awareness in prevention efforts (Morris et al., 2011). Additionally, the economic burden stemming from these illnesses is substantial, as the costs related to medical treatment and productivity losses can outweigh the investments made in food safety systems such as HACCP (Gale & Buzby, 2025). If you are aware of these signs, you can get treated faster and it highlights the need for better food safety to avoid contamination.

2.1.8. Prevention Methods for Biological Contamination

Food production can be contaminated biologically , which is dangerous for health and food safety, so it is necessary to have effective ways to prevent it. A key technique is to reduce the risks caused by mycotoxins , which are toxins created by fungi. It is very important to take steps before and after harvesting to reduce mycotoxin growth in the field, but these actions alone may not be enough. The incorporation of sorbent materials in animal feed, for instance, has proven effective in adsorbing mycotoxins during digestion (Guyonvarc'h et al., 2011). Furthermore, the development of biological control mechanisms, such as utilizing beneficial microorganisms for pest management, can enhance grain storage cleanliness and efficacy (Anon, 2001). By integrating these multifaceted approaches, food producers can better safeguard their products from biological contamination and ensure safer consumption (Figure 2.8).

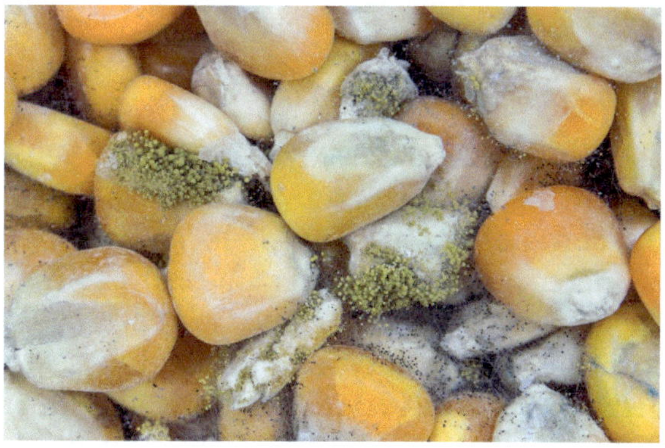

Figure 2.8. Mycotoxins in food.

Source: https://i0.wp.com/neosciencehub.com/wp-content/uploads/2024/01/Mycotoxins-blog-scaled-1.jpg.

2.2. Chemical Contaminants

Food safety can be endangered by chemical contaminants , which are most often introduced from the environment and the methods used to grow food. By accident, some of these substances, such as pesticides, veterinary drugs and industry chemicals, can get into the food supply. For instance, the Hazard Analysis by Critical Control Points (HACCP) approach emphasizes the need to identify and manage these chemical hazards, yet it has primarily focused on microbiological risks, resulting in insufficient attention to organic chemical contaminants within agriculture (Beck et al., 2003). Additionally, the rise of emerging organic groundwater contaminants (EGCs) has raised concerns about their prevalence and persistence in food systems. Compounds such as pharmaceuticals and pesticide metabolites, commonly detected in groundwater, can find their way into food products, heightening the risk of exposure to harmful substances (Crane et al., 2012). For this reason, proper monitoring and control are needed to limit the harm of chemical pollutants on both public health and food safety.

2.2.1. Pesticides and Their Effects on Food

Most of the pesticides used in farming are helpful for growing food, but they also cause a lot of food contamination. They help control pests and increase yields, but residues of pesticides are commonly found in food, which might be dangerous for people. Research indicates that levels of pesticide residues in organic products are consistently lower, approximately four to five times less than in conventionally produced items, which align with safer consumption practices (Brandt, 2007). Moreover, excessive pesticide application not only leads to food contamination but also threatens the integrity of environmental ecosystems, as pollutants can leach into water supplies, thereby impacting aquatic life and becoming further concentrated within the food chain (Hainzelin & Daviron, 2019). This dual impact underscores the need for stricter regulations and a move toward sustainable agricultural practices to mitigate health risks while maintaining food safety (Figure 2.9).

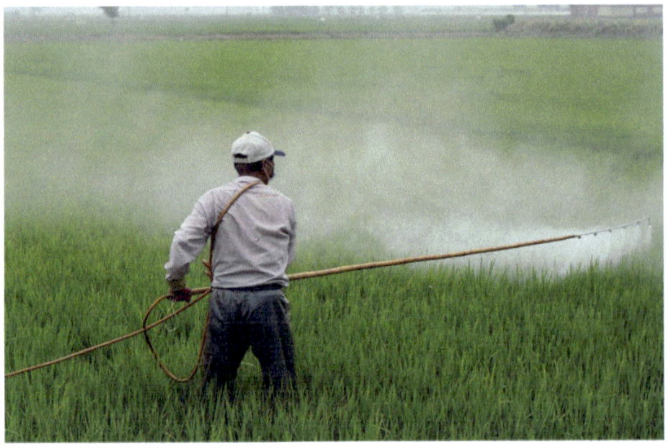

Figure 2.9. Pesticides, widely utilized in agricultural practices, play a significant role in food production but also contribute substantially to food contamination.

Source: https://earth.org/wp-content/uploads/2025/01/Copy-of-Untitled-683-x-1024-px-1-1.jpg.

2.2.2. Heavy Metals in Food Sources

Having heavy metals in food is very dangerous for health and remains a major issue in food safety discussions. Industry and farming are the main sources of heavy metals such as cadmium, lead and mercury , which can be found in the soil and water and then enter the food chain. Heavy metals in the soil can reduce crop yields and make food less safe , which makes sustainable farming more difficult. For instance, studies have shown that excessive heavy metal accumulation in aquaculture farm sediments can lead to potential risks that extend into the human food web, largely due to ineffective waste management and reliance on artificial feeds in commercial practices (Hossain et al., 2023). Furthermore, understanding the dynamics of soil heavy metal pollution is critical for developing strategies that can mitigate the uptake of these harmful substances by plants (Oyem & Oyem, 2024). It points out that several strategies are needed to deal with food safety problems from heavy metal contamination.

2.2.3. Food Additives and Preservatives

Food safety is a complicated topic and additives and preservatives are often important and controversial because they often come up in talks about food contamination. Even though they are used to improve taste, keep food fresh for longer and keep nutrients, their use causes many health concerns. The possibility of side effects, allergies and lasting health effects should never be ignored. For example, some artificial colors and flavors have been said to cause hyperactivity in children and other problems , which has led to their being watched more closely by regulators. Furthermore, the framework for assessing food quality and safety, particularly in the context of low-input processing, emphasizes the importance of transparent labeling and consumer education regarding these additives (Kretzschmar et al., 2005). As consumers increasingly prioritize organic and minimally processed foods, understanding the implications of these additives becomes essential for making informed dietary choices and mitigating the risks of contamination (Fernández Fernández et al., 2018) (Figure 2.10).

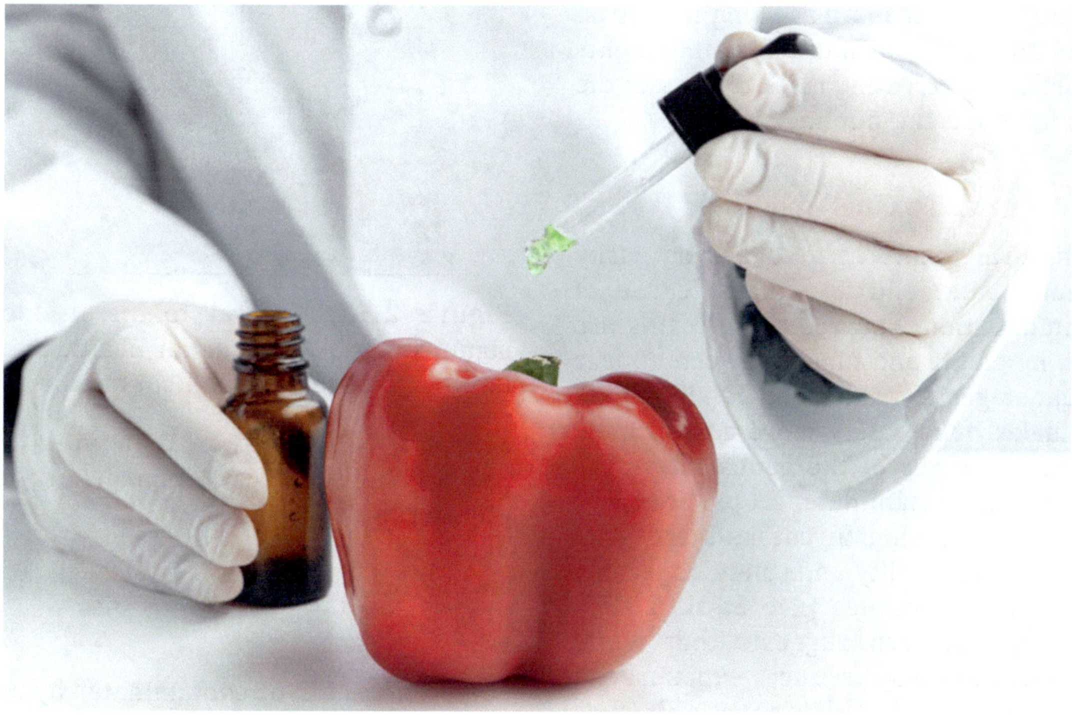

Figure 2.10. Food additives and preservatives play a critical yet controversial role, often featuring prominently in discussions surrounding sources of food contamination.

Source: https://foodnwellness.com/wp-content/uploads/2023/02/delicious-sweet-pepper-chemicals-1024x682.jpg

2.2.4. Industrial Chemicals and Their Risks

Industrial chemicals being used widely in farming and food processing cause concern about food safety. These chemicals , which are applied to control pests or help crops grow, might end up in the soil and water, then enter the food chain. Pollution of the soil by industry adds heavy metals and pesticides to farming , which reduces the fertility and variety of soil life. As highlighted in Koushal et al. (2025), the contamination of soil not only degrades its health but also poses substantial risks to human health through contaminated food sources. Moreover, metal contamination in water sources, often stemming from improper disposal of industrial waste, creates further risks as these metals bioaccumulate in aquatic organisms and eventually in human consumers (Gupta et al., 2025). This means that using industrial chemicals and their harmful effects highlights the importance of creating rules to protect the safety of food and the public.

2.2.5. Natural Toxins in Food

Having natural toxins in food is very risky for human health and is a major cause of food contamination. Because these toxins are produced by plants and fungi, they can appear at different stages of making and handling food , which makes food safety more complicated. For instance, species of the genus Alternaria are known to contaminate crops pre- and post-harvest, releasing mycotoxins that can compromise food quality and safety, especially in cereals and vegetables (Lee et al., 2015). Interestingly, research suggests that while organic farming may reduce exposure to synthetic pesticides, the levels of natural toxins in organic produce can be systematically higher, sometimes by 10 to 50 percent compared to conventional counterparts (Brandt, 2007). This highlights the complexity of food safety, where the presence of natural toxins necessitates careful monitoring to mitigate potential health risks, ensuring that food remains both safe and nutritious for consumers (Figure 2.11).

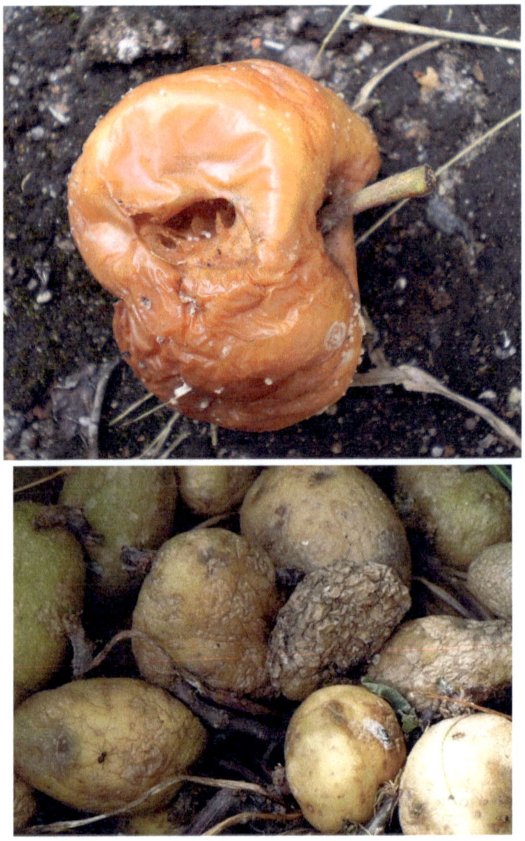

Figure 2.11. Natural toxins in food pose significant risks to human health and are an important aspect of food contamination.

Source: By Kulmalukko - Own work, CC BY-SA 3.0, https://commons.wikimedia.org/w/index.php?curid=8685553

2.2.6. Sources of Chemical Contamination

Food sources can be contaminated by chemicals , which is a major problem for public health, mainly because of farming, manufacturing and handling. Pesticides and herbicides used during crop cultivation can leave harmful residues that persist through to the final food product, leading to potential health risks (Olufemi et al., 2025).

Additionally, contaminated animal feed can introduce pathogens and mycotoxins into the food chain, notably in egg production systems, where organisms like Salmonella can proliferate and affect consumers (Olufemi et al., 2025).

These chemicals are dangerous to people and also lead to problems in the economy such as lower productivity and more food safety issues. Because food can be contaminated in many ways, it is necessary to have strong regulations and good monitoring in every stage of food production, processing and distribution. Therefore, dealing with chemical contamination is important for making sure food is safe and for safeguarding people's health from harmful exposures.

2.2.7. Regulations on Chemical Use in Food

It is very important to keep chemicals away from food to protect public health and food safety. Because of synthetic preservatives, food lasts longer without spoiling, but this has made some people concerned about their health, so they are encouraging the use of other types of preservatives.

Naturally occurring antimicrobials, such as nisin and essential oils, have emerged as safer options, but their regulatory status remains inadequately defined in many developing countries, complicating their widespread adoption (Afzaal et al., 2019). Furthermore, the integration of food safety education across disciplines, as highlighted by initiatives like the Western Institute for Food Safety and Security, underscores the necessity of a comprehensive framework that addresses chemical use while ensuring environmental sustainability (Angelos et al., 2017). In light of these factors, effective regulations are essential for balancing food preservation needs with consumer safety and ecological integrity (Figure 2.12).

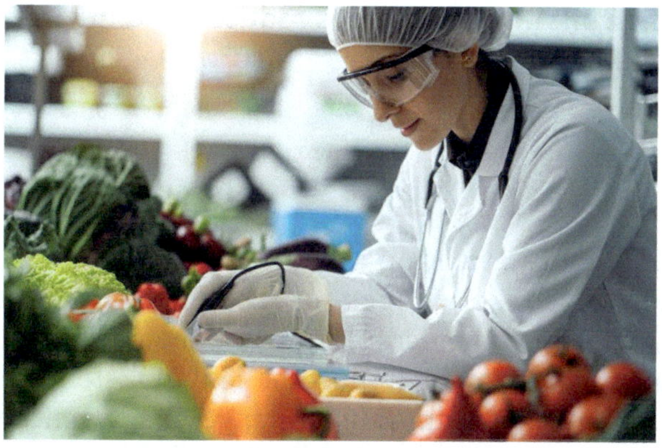

Figure 2.12. The regulation of chemical use in food is paramount to safeguarding public health and maintaining food safety.

Source: https://www.foodinfotech.com/wp-content/uploads/2024/05/Safeguarding-Public-Health-Through-Modern-Food-Safety-Practices.jpg.

2.2.8. Detection Methods for Chemical Contaminants

It is very important to detect chemical contaminants in food to protect the public , which means using different methods for various contaminants. Advanced analytical techniques such as gas chromatography-mass spectrometry (GC-MS) and liquid chromatography-tandem mass spectrometry (LC-MS/MS) are frequently employed to quantify trace levels of pesticides, pharmaceuticals, and other organic pollutants. They are useful because they are sensitive and specific , which helps detect new organic contaminants that might have been missed in the past. For instance, pesticides and their metabolites have been detected in groundwater sources, underscoring the complexities involved in safeguarding food supply chains (Crane et al., 2012). Furthermore, the establishment of baseline environmental conditions, as seen in studies of the Gray's Reef National Marine Sanctuary, facilitates the ongoing assessment of contaminant levels and their ecological impacts (Balthis et al., 2004). Using these methods to find contamination helps reduce the dangers of food being unsafe.

2.2.9. Long-Term Health Effects of Chemical Exposure

With more attention on food safety, the lasting health consequences of chemical contact, especially from microplastics and their additives, are becoming very important. Microplastics that enter our food can transfer dangerous chemicals to humans , which may cause health problems over the long term. Research indicates a strong correlation between prolonged exposure to these micro- and nano plastic particles and the development of several serious health conditions, including cancers and cardiovascular diseases (Chalannavar et al., 2025).

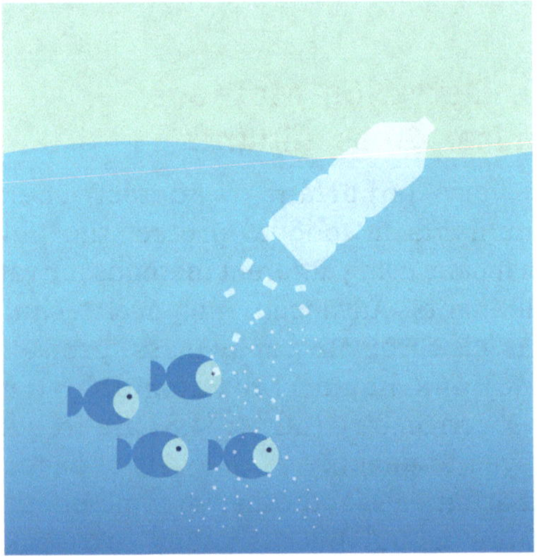

Figure 2.13. Microplastics, which infiltrate the food supply through various pathways, can carry hazardous chemicals that impact human health over time.

Source: By © European Union, 1998 – 2025, Attribution, https://commons.wikimedia.org/w/index.php?curid=116161052

Furthermore, these contaminants can disrupt not only individual health but also soil health and crop productivity, complicating food safety altogether (Boctor et al., 2025). It is very important to do more research on the long-term effects of chemical exposure, since not knowing enough about these risks can stop us from making good policies to handle plastic contamination in food. Such insights are essential to protect public health and ensure food safety in the face of increasing environmental challenges (Figure 2.13).

2.3. Physical Contaminants

The presence of soil, glass and plastic in food is a major problem for food safety. Food can be contaminated with these pollutants during farming and the processing of food. Notably, the intensification of agricultural production has led to soil degradation, resulting in higher rates of contamination from particulate matter, which directly impacts food quality and safety (Kopittke et al., 2019). Additionally, the proliferation of microplastics in marine environments raises concerns about seafood safety, as these small particles are ingested by fish and shellfish, ultimately affecting human health through consumption (Smith et al., 2018). Having physical contaminants in food can harm people's health and also lower consumer trust in the products. Since food systems are changing, handling physical contaminants is now crucial for both public health and sustainable farming.

2.3.1. Common Physical Contaminants in Food

When things that shouldn't be in food, such as foreign items or natural substances, are present, they can be unsafe for people and can reduce the quality of the food. Processing plants where cleanliness and equipment maintenance are ignored can cause hair, glass and metal to contaminate the food , which is why these are common contaminants. Food can sometimes contain natural materials like stones or insect parts , which may enter during harvesting and processing. The plastic pollution crisis also adds another layer of concern; microplastics can inadvertently infiltrate food through environmental pathways, potentially leading to ingestion by humans and wildlife alike (Rochman et al., 2019). Additionally, the presence of heavy metals in soil, water, and food can result from both natural occurrences and industrial activities, further complicating the contamination scenario (Ali et al., 2019). Consequently, understanding these physical contaminants is crucial for the development of effective prevention strategies and maintaining public health standards in the food supply chain (Figure 2.14).

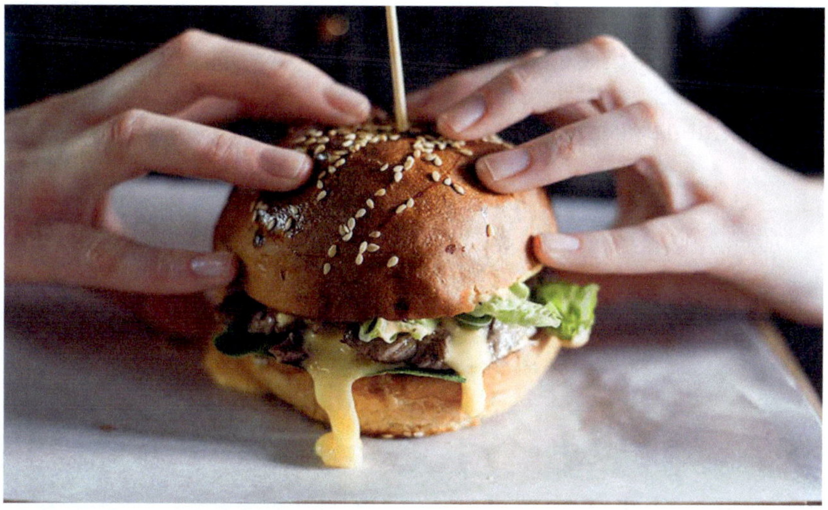

Figure 2.14. Physical contaminants in food, ranging from foreign objects to naturally occurring materials, present significant risks to consumer safety and food quality.

Source: https://www.food-safety.com/ext/resources/Images/2023/Apr_May/Testing-Img1-900.jpg?1681165578.

2.3.2. Sources of Physical Contamination

Any physical object that enters food during preparation or processing is called physical contamination and this is a major concern for both producers and consumers. Such contamination can come from worn-out machinery, bits of wood, plastic, metal and glass and also from environmental causes. Food can become contaminated by air pollutants such as suspended particles and products from burning , which settle on it during production. The impact of physical contamination extends beyond consumer safety, as it can result in serious financial repercussions, including costly product recalls and diminished brand loyalty (Crocco et al., 2019). To handle these risks, food manufacturers should always invest in advanced contamination detection systems and follow strict quality control standards, so that food products remain safe and intact throughout the supply chain.

2.3.3. Impact of Foreign Objects in Food

Having foreign objects in food can be very dangerous for health and cause serious worries about food safety. Having glass, metal, plastic or stones in food can cause injuries, choking and more serious health problems. The consequences go further than injuries; they can damage people's trust in the food industry , which may lead to reduced sales and legal problems. Also, not having enough controls during food processing and packaging leads to this, so stronger safety measures are needed. For example, research on food safety points out that having effective monitoring systems for contamination helps control these risks. Educational efforts that teach how to handle and process food properly may significantly cut down on foreign object contamination. Thus, addressing this challenge requires a multifaceted approach that prioritizes safety and consumer confidence (Figure 2.15).

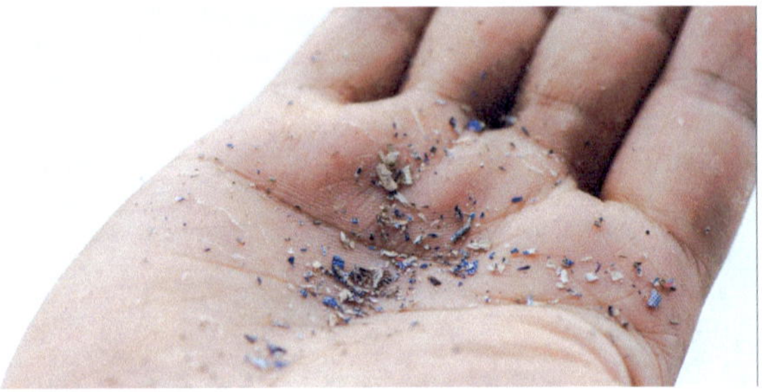

Figure 2.15. Contaminants such as pieces of glass, metal, plastic, or even natural elements like stones can lead to injuries, choking hazards, and more severe health complications.

Source: https://5845715.fs1.hubspotusercontent-na1.net/hub/5845715/hubfs/what%20is%20the%20best%20example%20of%20physical%20contamination.jpeg.

2.3.4. Prevention Strategies for Physical Contamination

Ensuring food is safe and of good quality requires using reliable strategies to avoid physical contamination in food production. Training should explain how to handle food and how to keep the workplace clean. It is also important to design facilities well so that hazards are avoided such as by making sure equipment and storage areas are always clean. Checking and maintaining the processing equipment can also stop foreign objects from entering the food supply. Moreover, educational curricula that encompass a range of disciplines related to food safety, as outlined by the Western Institute for Food Safety and Security, are essential for fostering an informed workforce capable of addressing these challenges effectively (Angelos et al., 2017). Thus, a multifaceted approach that emphasizes both training and environmental management is necessary to enhance food safety outcomes (Guyonvarc'h et al., 2011).

2.3.5. Role of Food Processing in Contamination

Food processing plays a major role in the risk of food contamination and is very important to consider when looking at food safety. During all the steps of food processing, from picking to packing, there are many chances for contaminants to get into the food.

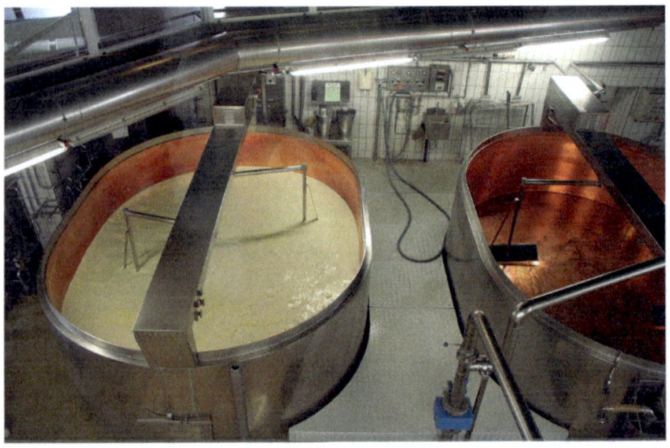

Figure 2.16. The role of food processing in contamination is a critical concern in understanding overall food safety.

Source: CC BY-SA 3.0, https://commons.wikimedia.org/w/index.php?curid=246468

When sanitation is poor, food is handled badly and the environment is not controlled, it can lead to the growth of dangerous microorganisms, for example Clostridium botulinum , which are very risky for consumers. Making honey , which is usually considered a natural food, can be quite difficult. Research indicates that contaminants can enter honey through various pathways, influenced by factors like plant origin and environmental conditions, causing significant economic losses in the industry due to contamination (Miglas, 2025). Furthermore, understanding these pathways is essential for developing educational frameworks for food safety and security, as emphasized by Angelos et al. (2017), which demand a multifaceted approach to mitigate the risks inherent in food processing (Figure 2.16).

2.3.6. Consumer Awareness and Reporting

Knowing and reporting about food safety issues is very important for avoiding the risks of food contamination, especially when it comes to pathogens such as *Listeria monocytogenes* in blanched frozen vegetables. The hygiene of raw materials, process water, and the food processing environment greatly influence the prevalence of such contaminants, necessitating rigorous consumer education about safe food practices and awareness of product labelling (EFSA BIOHAZ Panel (EFSA Panel on Biological Hazards), 2020). In addition, making sure people trust food safety is necessary, since how they perceive risk can greatly influence what they buy and eat. Research indicates that better understanding the intricate relationship between consumer trust and risk perception can lead to more effective policy initiatives that enhance communication about food safety issues (Lobb, 2025). Letting consumers know they can report anything suspicious in food safety can make the system stronger and better able to deal with contamination.

2.3.7. Case Studies of Physical Contamination Incidents

Reviewing case studies of physical contamination shows important details about the wider issues related to food safety. Both salmonella in poultry and pesticides in tomatoes show that inadequate handling or environmental reasons can lead to contamination , which can lower the trust people have in food products. It has been found that consumers consider food safety, especially for infants and as a result, they like to see safety labels and are ready to spend more for products they trust. Specifically, a study showed that 58% of respondents expressed a willingness to pay extra for safer milk, highlighting the economic implications of perceived risks (Meuwissen et al., 2025). Furthermore, analyses of malicious food contamination events from the past several decades underscore the varying motives and methods behind these incidents, revealing that opportunities for intervention are often tied to the accessibility of hazardous agents (France-Presse et al., 2016). Collectively, these case studies emphasize the necessity for enhanced safety measures within the food supply chain (Figure 2.17).

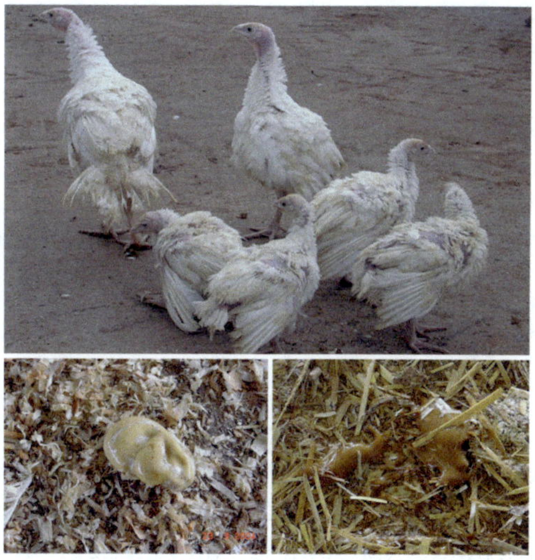

Figure 2.17. Salmonella in poultry and pesticides in tomatoes exemplify how such contamination can stem from inadequate handling or environmental factors, impacting consumer trust in food products.

Source: https://media.springernature.com/lw685/springer-static/image/chp%3A10.1007%2F978-3-031-63318-8_6/MediaObjects/446805_1_En_6_Fig3_HTML.png.

2.3.8. Regulations Regarding Physical Contaminants

The importance of rules about physical contaminants in food is very high, since they help protect people's health and the safety of what they eat. During the processing and distribution of food, unexpectedly, things like metal shards, glass pieces or plastic fragments can contaminate the food. Regulatory frameworks, often grounded in Hazard Analysis by Critical Control Points (HACCP), necessitate a systematic evaluation of potential hazards in food production. While HACCP primarily addresses microbiological risks, it is also crucial for identifying and controlling physical hazards, thereby enhancing the overall safety of food supplies (Beck et al., 2003). Furthermore, educational initiatives such as those outlined by the Western Institute for Food Safety and Security emphasize the importance of a One Health approach, integrating various disciplines to tackle food security challenges and mitigate risks associated with physical contaminants (Angelos et al., 2017). Following strong regulations and encouraging different experts to work together can help the food industry greatly lower the risks of physical contaminants.

2.3.9. Importance of Quality Control in Food Production

Checking food quality is very important to keep the food safe and reliable. Various sources can cause contaminants in food, such as environmental pollution and inadequate food processing. For instance, heavy metals such as lead and mercury, often originating from anthropogenic activities, can bioaccumulate in food products, posing significant health risks to consumers (Ali et al., 2019). Also, microbes can contaminate food if hygiene is poor or food is handled incorrectly, making it necessary to have strict quality control. Strict testing methods can spot and deal with these hazards, so public health is protected. Because the food industry is becoming more complex and demanding, quality control measures should focus on both safety and following health regulations. Ultimately, investing in comprehensive quality control programs is essential for preventing foodborne illnesses and ensuring consumer trust in food products (Bray et al., 2024) (Figure 2.18).

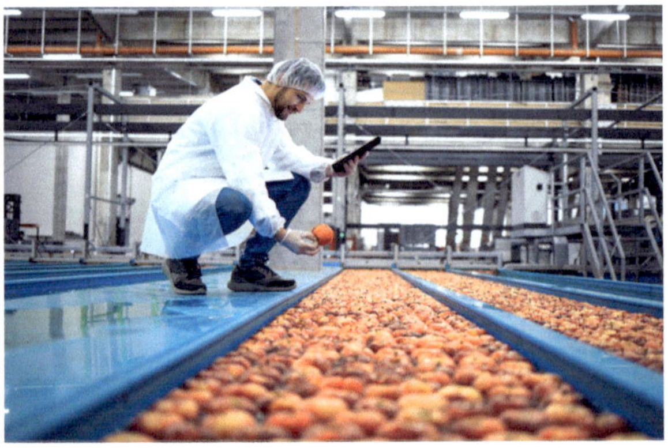

Figure 2.18. Quality control in food production is paramount for ensuring the safety and integrity of the food supply.

Source: https://www.ficsi.in/blog/wp-content/uploads/2023/09/blog1.jpg.

2.4. Environmental Contaminants

Environmental contaminants are very important in studying food contamination sources because they remain and build up in different environments. A recent study highlights the alarming presence of numerous halogenated organic compounds (HOCs) in marine mammals, specifically common bottlenose dolphins in the Southern California Bight, emphasizing that 86% of identified compounds are not currently monitored (Aluwihare et al., 2015). These compounds, including those related to dichlorodiphenyltrichloroethane (DDT), demonstrate how toxic substances can infiltrate food supplies, posing significant health risks to humans and wildlife alike. It is also emphasized by using a One Health approach , which shows that food safety, environmental problems and health are all connected. Such approaches guide curriculum development in food safety, emphasizing the need for comprehensive education about the effects of food production on the environment (Angelos et al., 2017). Looking after these environmental contaminants is necessary for both food safety and the environment.

2.4.1. Water Quality and Its Effect on Food

How safe food is and how much it is contaminated is strongly tied to the quality of water used in farming , which also affects the crops and the health of those who eat them. Water may contain pathogens, pesticides and heavy metals , which can cause food poisoning and health problems for people who consume it. For instance, improper water management can contribute to pathogen proliferation, thus posing a risk of zoonotic diseases as highlighted in the One Health perspective on food safety (Angelos et al., 2017). Fertilizers and pesticides can also end up in water , which can harm crops and cause food products to be unsafe. Organic farming practices tend to reduce the risk of such contamination by promoting sustainable water management and lower pesticide levels, ultimately fostering a safer food supply (Brandt, 2007). As water quality directly impacts food safety, maintaining and improving water standards is essential for safeguarding public health (Figure 2.19).

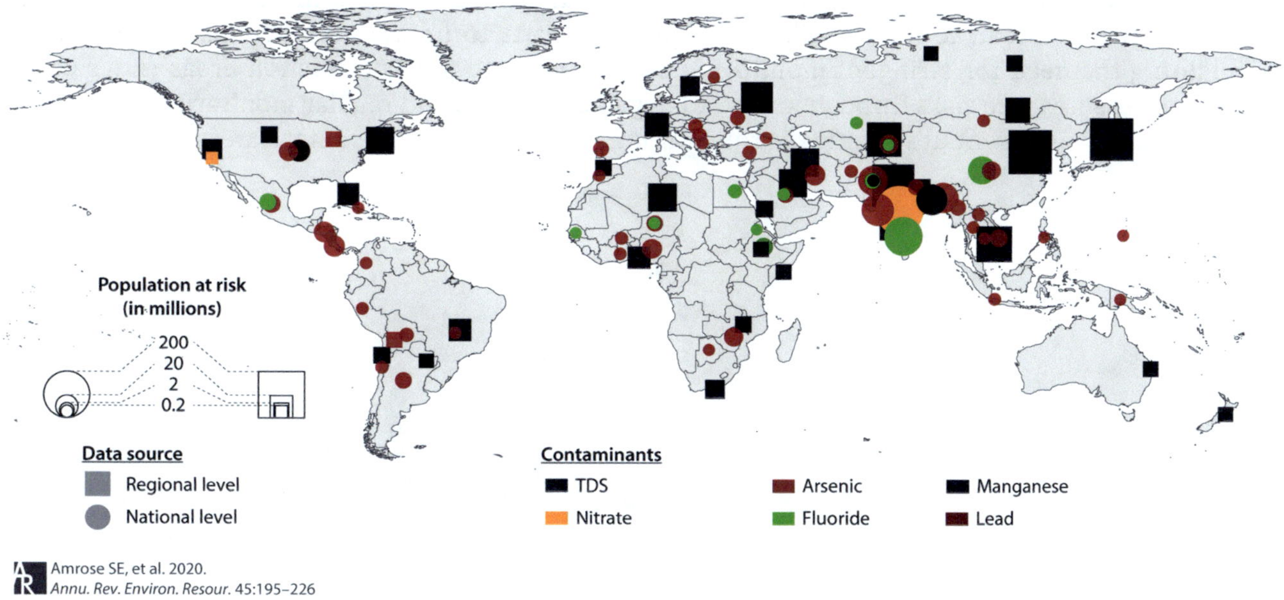

Figure 2.19. The quality of water used in agricultural practices is profoundly linked to food safety and contamination, influencing not only crop yield but also the health of consumers.

Source: By Susan E. Amrose,1 Katya Cherukumilli,2 and Natasha C. Wright3 - https://www.annualreviews.org/doi/full/10.1146/annurev-environ-012220-105152, CC BY 4.0, https://commons.wikimedia.org/w/index.php?curid=101285801

2.4.2. Soil Contamination and Agricultural Practices

Soil contamination and farming practices are very important in understanding how food can be contaminated. Using agrochemicals to increase farming output often causes soil pollution, mainly in places where development is slow. In Nigeria, for instance, studies have identified alarming levels of pesticides and heavy metals in agricultural soils, exceeding World Health Organization and Food and Agriculture Organization permissible limits, which profoundly affect food availability and safety (Vincent-Orugbo & Bemgba, 2025). Moreover, the rise of antibiotic-resistant bacteria and micro(nano)plastics in agricultural soils introduces new health risks, as these contaminants can enter the food chain through crops and livestock (Perković et al., 2022). As a result of such contamination, food is less nutritious and can cause serious health problems , which calls for quick changes in regulations and improved monitoring to preserve public health and support sustainable farming.

2.4.3. Airborne Contaminants and Food Safety

In food processing areas, the interaction between airborne contaminants and food safety is very important since microbes in the air can seriously affect both the quality of food and the health of the public. Microorganisms such as different pathogens can be airborne and come from food handlers, equipment or the environment , which may lead to food contamination. Studies have shown that bioaerosols can transport pathogenic microbes, which may compromise food safety and are linked to outbreaks of foodborne illnesses (Mokoena, 2013). Furthermore, in healthcare settings, airborne pathogens can also lead to food spoilage and pose a threat to immunocompromised individuals, highlighting the need for stringent monitoring of air quality in food production areas (Lues et al., 2014). Addressing these risks through improved hygiene practices and regular monitoring of airborne microorganisms is essential to mitigate contamination and ensure consumer safety (Figure 2.20).

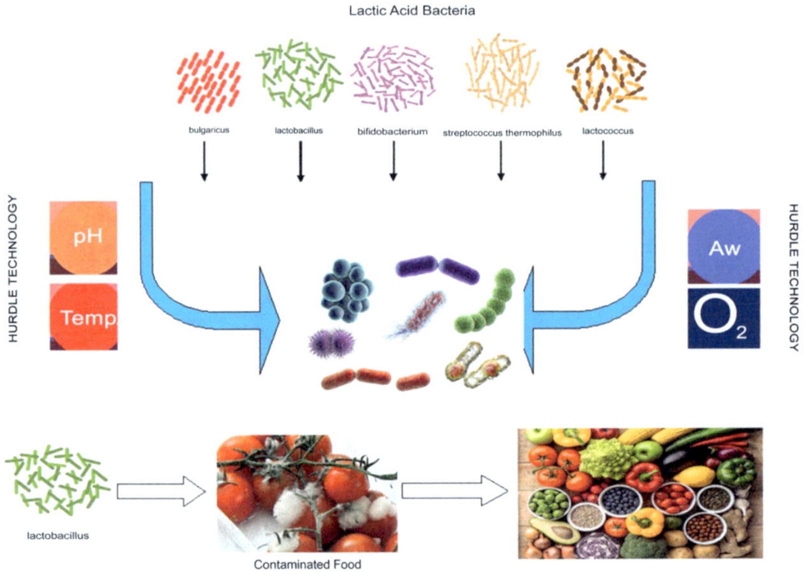

Figure 2.20. Airborne microorganisms, including various pathogens, can originate from food handlers, equipment, and even the surrounding environment, leading to the potential contamination of food products.

Source: Ibrahim SA, Ayivi RD, Zimmerman T, Siddiqui SA, Altemimi AB, Fidan H, Esatbeyoglu T, Bakhshayesh RV. Lactic Acid Bacteria as Antimicrobial Agents: Food Safety and Microbial Food Spoilage Prevention. *Foods*. 2021; 10(12):3131. https://doi.org/10.3390/foods10123131

2.4.4. Impact of Climate Change on Food Safety

It is becoming clear to people that climate change plays a big role in food contamination. When temperatures rise, there is more rain and severe weather happens, which helps pathogens and organisms that spoil food to grow in the food supply chain. For instance, pathogens such as Salmonella and *E. coli* thrive in warmer environments, potentially increasing the incidence of foodborne illnesses, as climate change disrupts traditional agricultural practices and food handling standards (Chattu et al., 2015). Additionally, climate change can also affect food security by limiting access to safe and nutritious food, addressing not just the health implications but also the socio-economic dimensions of food production (Angelos et al., 2017). Understanding these connections means we should design strategies that guarantee food safety and security as the climate changes , which requires quick education and policy changes in the food safety field.

2.4.5. Waste Management and Food Contamination

Practicing waste management well is important for preventing food from being contaminated, especially with the rise in recycled food packaging. Studies show that using recycled plastics for food packaging, as done in Bolivia, may introduce plasticizers and impurities from both fresh and used plastics. Moreover, inefficiencies in recycling processes can undermine the quality and safety of recycled PET, presenting significant health risks to consumers (Tejeda, 2024). Furthermore, addressing these contamination concerns involves not only improving waste collection and recycling systems but also enhancing consumer education regarding proper disposal and recycling practices (Angelos et al., 2017). For this reason, making sure there is a good waste management plan that focuses on new rules and educating the public is necessary to prevent food contamination and maintain a healthy circular economy. As food safety becomes increasingly intertwined with environmental practices, the need for effective waste management solutions cannot be overstated (Figure 2.21).

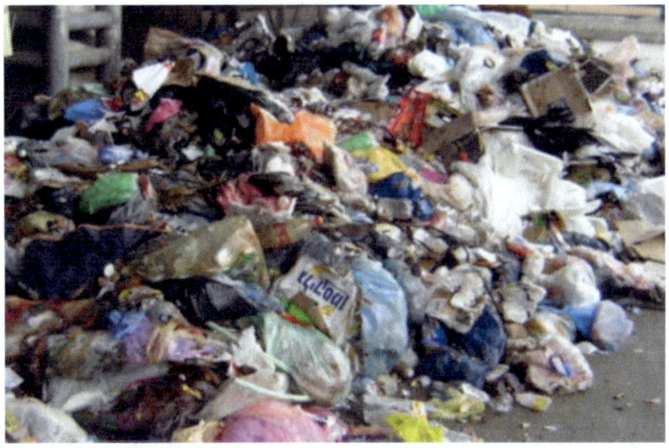

Figure 2.21. Effective waste management practices play a crucial role in mitigating food contamination risks, particularly as societies increasingly rely on recycled materials for food packaging.

Source: By Alex Marshall 2004, Clarke Energy Ltd - Originally uploaded to Wikipedia by Vortexrealm, here., CC BY-SA 2.5, https://commons.wikimedia.org/w/index.php?curid=2965770

2.4.6. Role of Transportation in Contamination

Food can be contaminated during transport , which affects its safety and quality from the farm to the consumer. When food is transported from one place to another, the risk of pathogens increasing becomes much higher. For instance, the transporting of poultry can lead to the spread of Campylobacter jejuni, a major pathogen associated with foodborne illness; colonized chickens can contaminate carcasses during processing, exacerbating the risk of transmission to humans (Haesebrouck et al., 2012). Similarly, in the pork supply chain, improper management during transportation can facilitate the spread of Salmonella, particularly when cross-contamination occurs during slaughter and distribution (Gaag et al., 2002). So, knowing how transportation affects food safety is necessary to locate possible sources of contamination and put in place proper measures to control the risks of foodborne pathogens. Concentrating on best practices in transportation can lead to better safety and health for people.

2.4.7. Global Trade and Food Safety Risks

Trade becoming more globalized has led to a rise in food safety risks , which brings many challenges for handling contamination. As people in different countries need more food, especially meat and fresh produce, the supply chains involved become more vulnerable to contamination , which might come from different sources such as the environment and how food is produced.

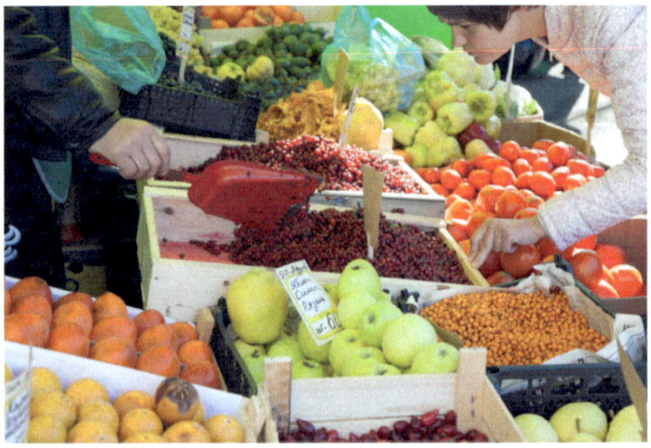

Figure 2.22. The increasing globalization of trade significantly impacts food safety risks, presenting multifaceted challenges for contamination management.

Source: https://cdn.who.int/media/images/default-source/impact-sheets/food-at-a-market.png?sfvrsn=360f608b_14.

The interrelations among disciplines outlined by the Western Institute for Food Safety and Security emphasize the necessity for a comprehensive educational framework addressing these risks within a One Health perspective (Angelos et al., 2017). Additionally, factors driving the surge in food-borne diseases include the anticipated doubling of global food demand and international trade, necessitating effective regulatory measures and innovation in food safety technologies to mitigate risks (Cole et al., 2010). Without coordinated efforts among governments and international organizations, the complexity of global trade could exacerbate food safety issues, undermining consumer confidence and public health (Figure 2.22).

2.4.8. Community Practices Affecting Food Safety

Community practices play a role in food safety and this is especially important now that farming and diets are becoming more complicated. When people understand food safety, they understand the links between food production, caring for nature and human health. Initiatives like the Western Institute for Food Safety and Security emphasize the importance of a One Health perspective, aiming to integrate diverse disciplines to create comprehensive food safety curricula that equip individuals with essential knowledge about sustainable practices (Angelos et al., 2017). Moreover, the consumer engagement with genetically modified organisms (GMOs) showcases a critical aspect of local discourse around food safety, reflecting community concerns about the socio-economic and ethical ramifications of such technologies (Mugwagwa et al., 2009). For this reason, people should be taught about food safety and discuss it to make sure their food is safe and less likely to be contaminated.

2.4.9. Strategies for Reducing Environmental Contamination

Looking after environmental contamination helps safeguard our food and improves public health. Effective strategies include the implementation of innovative agricultural practices aimed at mitigating the effects of heavy metals, such as root barrier formation and mycorrhizal symbiosis, which enhance plant resilience to contaminants (Vasilachi et al., 2023). It is also necessary to change to a green economy, mainly in places where industry often causes pollution. This transition necessitates identifying sources of contamination and understanding their impact on soil, groundwater, and crops (Economou-Eliopoulos et al., 2021). If we use metal-resistant crops and use sustainable soil methods, we can prevent metals from getting into our food. Many experts should collaborate to design solutions that lower pollution and keep future food safe.

A CLOSER LOOK

Organic Food

Organic food means food that is produced and processed without using synthetic fertilizers, pesticides, GMOs, antibiotics or growth hormones. Therefore, organic farming uses crop rotation, composting and natural ways to control pests to preserve the soil and the environment. Many people think that organic food is healthier and better for the environment since it cuts down on chemicals in food and lessens pollution in soil and water. A lot of people pick organic products because they think they are healthier, taste better and help protect the environment. Organic food certification rules may differ from country to country, but they usually demand that farmers strictly follow approved ways and are checked often for compliance.

SUMMARY

Learning the sources of food contamination helps us understand the environment and food safety. The findings underscore the significant impact of heavy metals, particularly as evidenced by their accumulation in bird eggs, which serves as a bioindicator of ecological conditions and pollution levels (Litvin et al., 2025). Furthermore, the contamination of agricultural soils with carcinogenic substances has been shown to pose serious risks to food production and public health, especially in the context of ongoing military conflicts (Chernychenko et al., 2024). Since there are many sources of contamination, it is necessary to closely watch and use preventive steps to limit harm to both nature and people. Therefore, dealing with food contamination and ensuring safety in agriculture requires working together in environmental sciences, public policy and with the community.

Finding out the causes of food contamination helps protect the public and guarantees there is enough safe food. Problems with the environment, how food is produced and water quality are all sources of contamination. For instance, the impact of water, sanitation, and hygiene (WASH) on nutrition has been thoroughly examined, highlighting the significant role that water quality plays in the contamination of food supplies and its subsequent effects on health outcomes (Mahmud et al., 2016). Additionally, research on marine environments, such as the studies conducted at the Gray's Reef National Marine Sanctuary, underscores how chemical contaminants in sediments can affect food sources, thus impacting the broader ecosystem and human food supplies (Balthis et al., 2004). It is important to handle both kinds of contamination properly to keep food safe and healthy , which means safety procedures should be used everywhere in the food process.

KEY TERMS FROM THIS CHAPTER

- Food products
- Foodborne diseases (FBDs)
- Fungi
- Habitats
- Heavy metals
- Industrial farming
- Listeria monocytogenes
- Manufacturing
- Food web
- Fungal growth
- Glass
- Health
- Hepatitis
- Juvenile crayfish
- Man-made activities

REFERENCES

1. Abdurazakova, K. N., Gitinova, P. S., & Abakarova, A. M. (2021). The modern state of the problem potential mutagenic and carcinogenic activity of food products. *Sanitarnyj Vrač (Sanitary Doctor)*. https://www.semanticscholar.org/paper/21b47a2186c8cac6595b5ad388dd2c6819425e50 (accessed on 29 May 2025).
2. Abebe, E., Gugsa, G., & Ahmed, M. (2020). Review on major food-borne zoonotic bacterial pathogens. *Journal of Tropical Medicine, 2020*, 1–19. https://doi.org/10.1155/2020/4674235.
3. Afzaal, M., Ahmad, A., Saeed, F., Tufail, M., et al. (2019). *Use of Natural Antimicrobial Agents: A Safe Preservation Approach*. https://core.ac.uk/download/322439164.pdf (accessed on 29 May 2025).
4. Agence France-Presse, Beilharz, N., Bianchin, R., Eckholm, E., Farwell, J., Felongco, G., et al. (2016). *Contextual Factors Among Indiscriminate or Larger Attacks on Food or Water Supplies, 1946–2015*. https://core.ac.uk/download/41993264.pdf (accessed on 29 May 2025).
5. Akhtar, N., Ishak, M. I. S., Bhawani, S. A., & Umar, K. (2021). Various natural and anthropogenic factors responsible for water quality degradation: A review. *Water, 13*(19), 2660. https://doi.org/10.3390/w13192660.
6. Alcorlo, P., Baltanás, A., & Lozano, I. (2019). *Heavy Metals Effects on Life Traits of Juveniles of Procambarus clarkii*. https://repositorio.uam.es/bitstream/10486/691062/1/heavy_alcorlo_aes_2019.pdf (accessed on 29 May 2025).
7. Ali, H., Khan, E., & Ilahi, I. (2019). Environmental chemistry and ecotoxicology of hazardous heavy metals: Environmental persistence, toxicity, and bioaccumulation. *Journal of Chemistry, 2019*, 1–14. https://doi.org/10.1155/2019/6730305.
8. Aluwihare, L. I., Chivers, S. J., Danil, K., Dodder, N. G., et al. (2015). *Nontargeted Biomonitoring of Halogenated Organic Compounds in Two Ecotypes of Bottlenose Dolphins (Tursiops truncatus) from the Southern California Bight*. https://core.ac.uk/download/323065203.pdf.
9. Angelos, J. A., Arens, A. L., Johnson, H. A., Cadriel, J. L., & Osburn, B. I. (2017). One Health in food safety and security education: Subject matter outline for a curricular framework. *One health (Amsterdam, Netherlands), 3*, 56–65. https://doi.org/10.1016/j.onehlt.2017.04.001Anon. (2001). *Integrated Grain Storage–Technology Transfer for Organic Farming*. https://core.ac.uk/download/10923913.pdf (accessed on 29 May 2025).
10. Audenaert, K., Croubels, S., & De Saeger, S. (2016). *Report from the 5th International Symposium on Mycotoxins and Toxigenic Moulds: Challenges and Perspectives (MYTOX) Held in Ghent, Belgium, May 2016*. https://core.ac.uk/download/74659735.pdf (accessed on 29 May 2025).
11. Bahia-Oliveira, L., de Wit, L. A., Dixon, B., Dumètre, A., et al. (2019). *Environmental Transmission of Toxoplasma gondii: Oocysts in Water, Soil and Food*. https://core.ac.uk/download/286729987.pdf (accessed on 29 May 2025).
12. Balthis, W. L., Bearden, D., Cooksey, C., Fulton, M. H., et al. (2004). *Soft-Bottom Benthic Assemblages and Levels of Contaminants in Sediments and Biota at Gray's Reef National Marine Sanctuary and Nearby Shelf Waters Off the Coast of Georgia (2000 and 2001)*. https://core.ac.uk/download/11017910.pdf (accessed on 29 May 2025).
13. Beasley, G. and Kneale, P. (2001) Macroinvertebrates, Heavy Metals and PAHs in Urban Watercourses. Working Paper. School of Geography , University of Leeds.Beck, A. J., Ferguson,

A., & Ropkins, K. (2003). *Development of Hazard Analysis and Critical Control Points (HACCP) Procedures to Control Organic Chemical Hazards in The Agricultural Production of Raw Food Commodities*. https://core.ac.uk/download/60392.pdf (accessed on 29 May 2025).

14. Boctor, J., Hoyle, F. C., Farag, M. A., Ebaid, M., Walsh, T., Whiteley, A. S., & Murphy, D. V. (2025). Microplastics and nano plastics: Fate, transport, and governance from agricultural soil to food webs and humans. *Environmental Sciences Europe*. https://www.semanticscholar.org/paper/86a93bc5bf07ecb4ffa613be778e0333c74e53fd (accessed on 29 May 2025).

15. Brandt, Dr Kirsten (2007) Organic Agriculture and Food Utilization. Paper at: Organic Agriculture and Food Security, FAO, Rome, 3-5 May. (accessed on 29 May 2025).

16. Bray, F., Laversanne, M., Sung, H., Ferlay, J., Siegel, R. L., Soerjomataram, I., & Jemal, A. (2024). Global cancer statistics 2022: GLOBOCAN estimates of incidence and mortality worldwide for 36 cancers in 185 countries. *CA: A Cancer Journal for Clinicians, 74*, 229–263. https://doi.org/10.3322/caac.21834.

17. Browne, A. S. (2018). *A Food Chain Approach to Control of Shiga Toxin-Producing Escherichia Coli In New Zealand: A Thesis Presented in Partial Fulfilment of The Requirements for The Degree of Doctor of Philosophy in Veterinary Science at Massey University, Palmerston North, New Zealand*. https://core.ac.uk/download/186668373.pdf (accessed on 29 May 2025).

18. Buzby, J. C., Crutchfield, S. R., Lin, C. T. J., Ollinger, M., et al. (2025). *Economic Assessment of Food Safety Regulations: The New Approach to Meat and Poultry Inspection*. https://core.ac.uk/download/pdf/6459734.pdf (accessed on 29 May 2025).

19. Chalannavar, R. K., Malabadi, R. B., Divakar, M. S., Swathi, Karamchand, K. S., Kamble, A. A., Kolkar, K. P., et al. (2025). Microplastic in food chain—Major health issues—An update. *World Journal of Advanced Research and Reviews*. https://www.semanticscholar.org/paper/72812af150d0852216911feb1615497bed750bf2 (accessed on 29 May 2025).

20. Chattu, V. K. (2015). *Food Safety as A Contributor to Food Security: Global Policy Concerns & Challenges*. https://core.ac.uk/download/348249090.pdf (accessed on 29 May 2025).

21. Chernychenko, I. O., Lytvychenko, O. M., Babii, V., Kondratenko, O. Ie., & Hlavachek, D. (2024). Soil contamination of agricultural territories of Ukraine with benz(a)pyrene in the pre-war period as a criteria of background pollution in the post-war period when determining the dangerous consequences of military actions. *Environment & Health*. https://www.semanticscholar.org/paper/35760721a2dcc13de1079dcf7d35f94f7686d916 (accessed on 29 May 2025).

22. Cole, M. B., Cook, P. E., Gorris, L. G. M., Quested, T., et al. (2010). *Trends in Technology, Trade and Consumption Likely to Impact on Microbial Food Safety*. https://core.ac.uk/download/pdf/29244276.pdf (accessed on 29 May 2025).

23. Crane, E., Hart, A., Lapworth, D., Stuart, M., et al. (2012). *Review of Risk from Potential Emerging Contaminants in UK Groundwater*. https://core.ac.uk/download/384302.pdf (accessed on 29 May 2025).

24. Crocco, L., Farina, L., Rivero Campos, F. J., Litman, A., Scapaticci, R., Tobon Vasquez, J. A., & Vipiana, F. (2019). *Microwave Imaging Technology for In-Line Food Contamination Monitoring*. https://core.ac.uk/download/524606956.pdf (accessed on 29 May 2025).

25. Hainzelin Etienne, Daviron Benoit. 2019. The effects of agriculture's environmental externalities on food systems. In : Food systems at risk. New trends and challenges. Dury Sandrine (ed.),

Bendjebbar Pauline (ed), Hainzelin Etienne (ed.), Giordano Thierry (ed.), Bricas Nicolas (ed.). Rome : CIRAD-FAO, pp. 63-66. ISBN 978-2-87614-751-5https://doi.org/10.19182/agritrop/00094. De Heijden, K. V. D. (2019). *International Food Safety Handbook*. https://www.semanticscholar.org/paper/debb460e257371bda64e5ce5f40266d96185a5ec (accessed on 29 May 2025).

26. Economou-Eliopoulos, M., & Megremi, I. (2021). Contamination of the soil–groundwater–crop system: Environmental risk and opportunities. *Minerals, 11*(7), 775. https://doi.org/10.3390/min11070775.

27. Eijck, I., Groot, M., Kasteel, D., Kijlstra, A., et al. (2003). *Analysis of Black Holes in Our Knowledge Concerning Animal Health in The Organic Food Production Chain*. https://core.ac.uk/download/10919416.pdf (accessed on 29 May 2025).

28. Fan, L., Wang, J., Ou, Z., Zhang, Y., Zhang, L., Liu, S., Zhou, Z., et al. (2024). *Research Progress on Microbial Source Tracking for Traceability of Pollution Sources in Food Chains*. https://core.ac.uk/download/615121087.pdf.

29. Fernández Fernández, J., Gutiérrez del Río Menéndez, I., & Lombó Brugos, F. (2018). *Plant Nutraceuticals as Antimicrobial Agents in Food Preservation: Terpenoids, Polyphenols and Thiols*. https://core.ac.uk/download/pdf/162571983.pdf (accessed on 29 May 2025).

30. Fomenko, O., Sagingalieva, A. G., Rudik, F., & Karpunina, L. V. (2024). Microbial safety issues in instant packaged meat and bone broths: Predicting the risks of occurrence. *Bulletin of the South Ural State University. Series Food and Biotechnology*. https://www.semanticscholar.org/paper/f6a6b38d54193a51e80d7707734ae039fc7509de (accessed on 29 May 2025).

31. Forrest, A. (2020). *The Growing Threat of Agroterrorism and Strategies for Agricultural Defense*. https://core.ac.uk/download/322850909.pdf (accessed on 29 May 2025).

32. Gaag, M. van der, & Huirne, R. B. M. (2002). *Elicitation of Expert Knowledge on Controlling Salmonella in The Pork Chain*. https://core.ac.uk/download/pdf/29298814.pdf (accessed on 29 May 2025).

33. Gann, G. D., McDonald, T., Walder, B., Aronson, J., Nelson, C. R., Jonson, J., Hallett, J. G., et al. (2019). International principles and standards for the practice of ecological restoration (2nd ed.). *Restoration Ecology, 27*. https://doi.org/10.1111/rec.13035.

34. Gao, S., Chen, Q., Chen, L., Cai, Y., Lin, D., Wang, L., Chen, M., et al. (2024). Analysis of foodborne outbreaks in Wenzhou City, China, 2012–2022. *Epidemiology and Infection, 152*. https://www.semanticscholar.org/paper/ba6b774ca926d22842f9ce5ea507f399750aa224 (accessed on 29 May 2025).

35. Goethals, P., & Ho, L. T. (2019). *Opportunities and Challenges for The Sustainability of Lakes and Reservoirs in Relation to The Sustainable Development Goals (SDGs)*. https://core.ac.uk/download/225020142.pdf (accessed on 29 May 2025).

36. Gupta, A., Gupta, R., & Sharma, R. K. (2025). Eriochrome Cyanine R immobilized Amberlite XAD-2 for efficient separation and preconcentration of Fe(III). *Current Analytical Chemistry*. https://www.semanticscholar.org/paper/1179d387b5eca98cb578d446f44ccfb455257557 (accessed on 29 May 2025).

37. Guyonvarc'h, A., Jard, G., Lebrihi, A., & Liboz, T. (2011). *Review of Mycotoxin Reduction in Food and Feed: From Prevention in The Field to Detoxification by Adsorption or Transformation*. https://core.ac.uk/download/12043388.pdf (accessed on 29 May 2025).

38. Haesebrouck, F., Hermans, D., Heyndrickx, M., & Martel, A. (2012). *Poultry as a Host for the Zoonotic Pathogen Campylobacter jejuni.* https://core.ac.uk/download/55843495.pdf (accessed on 29 May 2025).

39. Haji-Hoseeini, R., Joshaghani, H., Kohsar, F., & Namjoo, M. (2016). *Quantitative Determination of Aflatoxin by High Performance Liquid Chromatography in Wheat Silos in Golestan Province, North of Iran.* https://core.ac.uk/download/52205534.pdf (accessed on 29 May 2025).

40. Haynes, E., Bhagtani, D., Iese, V., Brown, C. R., Fesaitu, J., Hambleton, I., Badrie, N., et al. (2020). Food sources and dietary quality in Small Island Developing States: Development of methods and policy relevant novel survey data from the Pacific and Caribbean. *Nutrients, 12*, Article 1519. https://www.semanticscholar.org/paper/7b145421a077604d457c96d8095c98c7c697565f (accessed on 29 May 2025).

41. Hossain, M. B., Sultana, J., Pingki, F. H., Nur, A., Mia, M. S., Bakar, M. A., Yu, J., et al. (2023). Accumulation and contamination assessment of heavy metals in sediments of commercial aquaculture farms from a coastal area along the northern Bay of Bengal, *11*. https://www.semanticscholar.org/paper/fdc20c6bb37e8332f9dfca2ac62f016bade20ac1 (accessed on 29 May 2025).

42. Iqbal, J., Umair, M., Muhammad, R., Zafar, H., & Fatima, S. (2024). The food authority and its legal frameworks: An analysis in the context of Punjab, Pakistan. *The Critical Review of Social Sciences Studies.* https://www.semanticscholar.org/paper/847c995905a7c3d76770472b28418304d4b2a66c (accessed on 29 May 2025).

43. Kopittke, P. M., Menzies, N. W., Wang, P., McKenna, B. A., & Lombi, E. (2019). Soil and the intensification of agriculture for global food security. *Environment International, 132*, 105078. https://doi.org/10.1016/j.envint.2019.105078.

44. Koushal, S., Arya, D., Anbarasan, S., Haloi, D., Rashmi, M., Rahman, T., Singh, V., et al. (2025). Soil pollution: Sources, effects, and mitigation strategies. *Asian Journal of Soil Science and Plant Nutrition.* https://www.semanticscholar.org/paper/a4b45042ddfb55aab70b0c8949bfa02afa700908 (accessed on 29 May 2025).

45. Kretzschmar, U., & Schmid, O. (2005). Approaches used in organic and low input food processing–Impact on food quality and safety: Results of a Delphi survey from an expert consultation in 13 European countries. https://core.ac.uk/download/10923325.pdf (accessed on 29 May 2025).

46. Lee, H. B., Magan, N., & Patriarca, A. (2015). Alternaria in food: Ecophysiology, mycotoxin production and toxicology. https://core.ac.uk/download/74410111.pdf (accessed on 29 May 2025).

47. Litvin, L., & Chaplygina, A. (2025). Accumulation of heavy metals in bird's eggs in various transformed area Poltava Region (Ukraine). *Studia Biological.* https://www.semanticscholar.org/paper/5cf13eaf00e9af27d04b1045b8225bdc790c6c05 (accessed on 29 May 2025).

48. Lobb, A. E. (2025). A methodological review of the impacts of risk and trust on consumer behavior towards food safety. https://core.ac.uk/download/pdf/6459678.pdf (accessed on 29 May 2025).

49. Lues, R., Malebo, N., Setlhare, G., Shale, K., et al. (2014). Identification of airborne microbiota in selected areas in a health-care setting in South Africa. https://core.ac.uk/download/222967693.pdf (accessed on 29 May 2025).

50. Mahmud, I., & Mbuya, N. (2016). *Water, Sanitation, Hygiene, and Nutrition in Bangladesh: Can Building Toilets Affect Children's Growth?* https://core.ac.uk/download/75783689.pdf (accessed on 29 May 2025).

51. Meuwissen, M. P. M., Novoselova, T. A., Valeeva, N. I., van der Lans, I. A., et al. (2025). Consumers' perception of milk safety. https://core.ac.uk/download/pdf/6551237.pdf (accessed on 29 May 2025).

52. Miglas, H. (2025). Review on the hidden potential health risks of natural toxins in honey bees (*Apis mellifera*) "honey" in Tigray, Ethiopia. https://core.ac.uk/download/654538509.pdf (accessed on 29 May 2025).

53. Mokoena, K. K. (2013). Airborne microbiota and related environmental parameters associated with a typical dairy farm plant. https://core.ac.uk/download/222966349.pdf (accessed on 29 May 2025).

54. Morris, J. G., Jr., Batz, M. B., & Hoffmann, S. (2011). *Ranking the Risks: The 10 Pathogen-Food Combinations with the Greatest Burden on Public Health*. https://core.ac.uk/download/71358801.pdf (accessed on 29 May 2025).

55. Mugwagwa, J. T., & Rutivi, C. (2009). Socio-economic impact of GMOs on African consumers. https://core.ac.uk/download/81978.pdf (accessed on 29 May 2025).

56. Olufemi, O. I., Ayeni, O., & Olagoke-Komolafe, O. E. (2025). A systems dynamics model to mitigate the risk of contaminated feed in egg production systems in the USA. *International Journal of Research and Innovation in Social Science*. **https://dx.doi.org/10.47772/IJRISS.2025.9010144**(accessed on 29 May 2025).

57. Oyem, H. H., & Oyem, I. M. (2024). Safe utilization of heavy metals-polluted soils for healthy food production. *Nigerian Journal of Agriculture and Agricultural Technology*. https://www.semanticscholar.org/paper/d776c320c5191ff6142716b2cb556cd951c4317c (accessed on 29 May 2025).

58. Perković, S., Paul, C., Vasić, F., & Helming, K. (2022). Human health and soil health risks from heavy metals, micro(nano)plastics, and antibiotic-resistant bacteria in agricultural soils. *Agronomy*. https://www.semanticscholar.org/paper/19f7f1006df44b72ace8b26790ba11b284028503 (accessed on 29 May 2025).

59. Rochman, C. M., Brookson, C. B., Bikker, J., Djuric, N., Earn, A., Bucci, K., Athey, S. N., et al. (2019). Rethinking microplastics as a diverse contaminant suite. *Environmental Toxicology and Chemistry, 38*, 703–711. https://doi.org/10.1002/etc.4371.

60. Smith, M., Love, D. C., Rochman, C. M., & Neff, R. (2018). Microplastics in seafood and the implications for human health. *Current Environmental Health Reports, 5*, 375–386. https://doi.org/10.1007/s40572-018-0206-z.

61. Tejeda, Z. (2024). *Toxicity and Decision-Making in Circularity: Evaluation of The Environmental and Health Risks of Circular Economy Practices and Plastic Recycling in The Bolivian Beverage Industry* [Master's thesis or report, Institution if known]. https://core.ac.uk/download/631531507.pdf (accessed on 29 May 2025).

62. Vasilachi, I. C., Stoleru, V., & Gavrilescu, M. (2023). Analysis of heavy metal impacts on cereal crop growth and development in contaminated soils. *Agriculture, 13*, Article 1983. https://doi.org/10.3390/agriculture13101983.

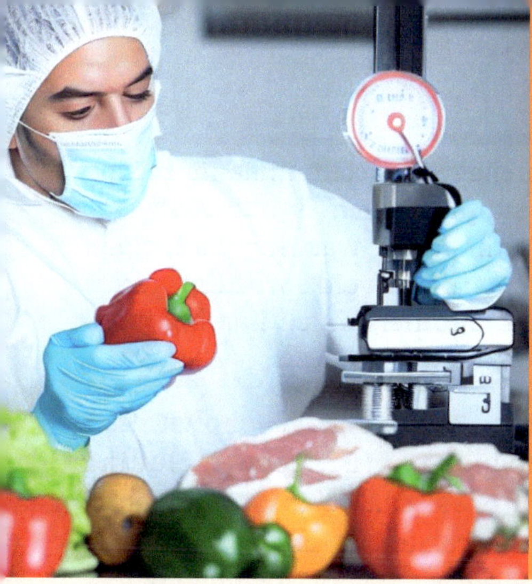

Chapter 3

PERSONAL HYGIENE AND FOOD HANDLER RESPONSIBILITIES

Contents

Introduction.......55
3.1. Importance of Personal Hygiene in Food Handling.......58
3.2. Key Personal Hygiene Practices for Food Handlers.......61
3.3. Food Handler Responsibilities Beyond Personal Hygiene.......65
3.4. Consequences of Neglecting Personal Hygiene.......69
Summary.......74
References.......75

Introduction

Maintaining personal cleanliness as a food handler is necessary to safeguard food safety and the well-being of everyone. Foodborne disease continues to be a top priority, costing millions each year, with an estimated almost 48 million incidents in the United States alone, a figure that demonstrates the need for proper training and management systems within the food service industry (Novak et al., 2016). In spite of regulations that have been put in place to enhance food safety practice, most outlets are still experiencing challenges regarding compliance, reinforcing the importance of both individual accountability and organizational culture that is based on a hygiene culture (Jackson, 2011). Therefore, food handlers need to be extra careful regarding hygiene in addition to code compliance. This chapter will explain the relationship between food handling and personal hygiene and will recommend effective training and management to avoid foodborne diseases.

Definition of Personal Hygiene

Personal hygiene is about taking care of yourself to avoid getting diseases. Regularly washing hands, bathing, brushing teeth and using clean clothes are important for food handlers to stop food contamination. A simple example is that failing to wash your hands properly can let bacteria get onto your food or surfaces. Additionally, healthcare professionals acknowledge that diseases such as hand eczema may hinder such practices, necessitating the preservation of healthy skin to ensure good hygiene (Thyssen et al., 2021). In the global perspective, access to clean water and soap is essential in realizing achieving the best personal hygiene, as it reflects considerable inequalities in practices among different socioeconomic backgrounds (Howard et al., 2020). Therefore, it is essential to understand personal hygiene not just for individual health but also for public health safety (Figure 3.1).

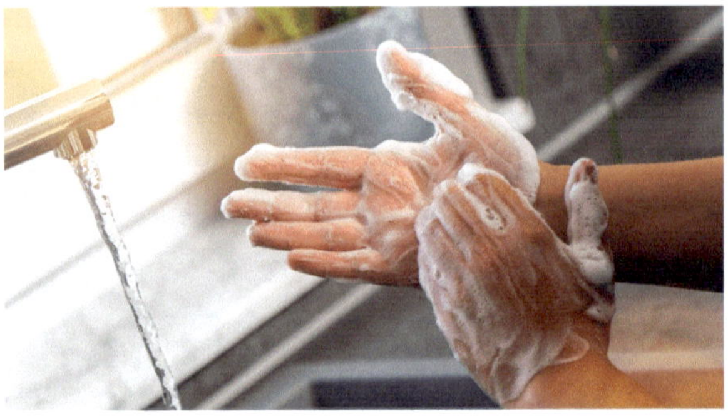

Figure 3.1. Personal hygiene encompasses a set of practices that individuals undertake to maintain health and prevent illness, particularly by limiting the spread of pathogens.

Source: https://plt4m.b-cdn.net/wp-content/uploads/2024/01/Hand-Washing-1.png.

Importance of Personal Hygiene in Food Handling

Since food safety and avoiding illness depend on it, personal hygiene is very important when working with food. Clean work areas by food handlers lowers the risk of contaminants getting into the food supply, which is necessary for everyone's health. Hand washing and clean clothes help kitchen staff avoid spreading germs from one food to another, which is a big issue in restaurants.

Furthermore, studies have shown that sustainable hygiene practices, including community awareness campaigns, significantly enhance behaviors related to safe food handling (Aregai et al., 2008). For this reason, food places begin to focus on keeping their places clean every day. Consequently, personal hygiene not only safeguards consumers but also enhances the reputation of food businesses, ultimately contributing to their long-term success in a highly competitive industry (Association, 2012).

Overview of Food Handler Responsibilities

Food handlers are important in making sure food is safe, which is necessary for the health and well-being of everyone. They are responsible for many tasks that stop foodborne illnesses , such as washing their hands, cleaning their work areas and storing food properly. It is especially important for handlers to know about microbial hazards and why good personal hygiene is necessary to avoid contamination. The effectiveness of their actions significantly influences food safety outcomes, as highlighted by the collaborative nature of food safety, which involves various stakeholders from farm to fork (Jaffee et al., 2018). Furthermore, food handlers must remain vigilant regarding potential chemical and environmental hazards, as neglecting these can lead to severe health consequences for consumers (Fung et al., 2018). Ultimately, the collective adherence to food safety protocols by handlers not only protects individual health but also supports broader public health initiatives aimed at reducing foodborne illnesses and ensuring safe consumption (Figure 3.2).

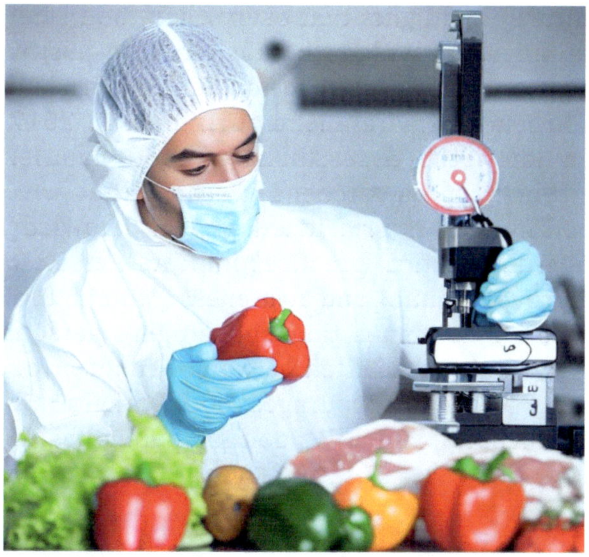

Figure 3.2. Food handlers play a crucial role in ensuring food safety, which is essential for public health and well-being.

Source: https://media.licdn.com/dms/image/v2/D4E12AQEPZKtgzTZu8A/article-cover_image-shrink_720_1280/article-cover_image-shrink_720_1280/0/1690893285673?e=2147483647&v=beta&t=8-2tjDNpqHJ69sjGpPn8EOrbOpczgUwKgGIObQMn-xE

Connection Between Hygiene and Food Safety

The connection between good hygiene and food safety is important to preventing foodborne illnesses , which strike millions of individuals in the United States annually. Practicing the rules of hygiene by food handlers is highly essential for consumer safety. Provided that you wash your hands frequently, use clean clothes and practice good hygiene rules when handling food, the possibility of contracting sickness from food is greatly reduced. As Food and Drug Administration (FDA) regulations have changed, they have also spurred increases in food safety compliance, but the existence of continued food safety infractions demonstrates the need for a continued focus on hygiene practices among food service workers. It is imperative that employers promote the conditions in , which proper hygiene is emphasized, as supported by studies that investigate obstacles to the practice of good food safety practices, showing a causal relationship between hygiene and overall food safety performance (Novak et al., 2016; Coyle et al., 2018).

Relevance to Public Health

It is very important and also complex how the personal hygiene of food handlers affects public health. Maintaining good hygiene is the main barrier to foodborne illnesses , which are still a major health problem for more than 600 million people around the world.

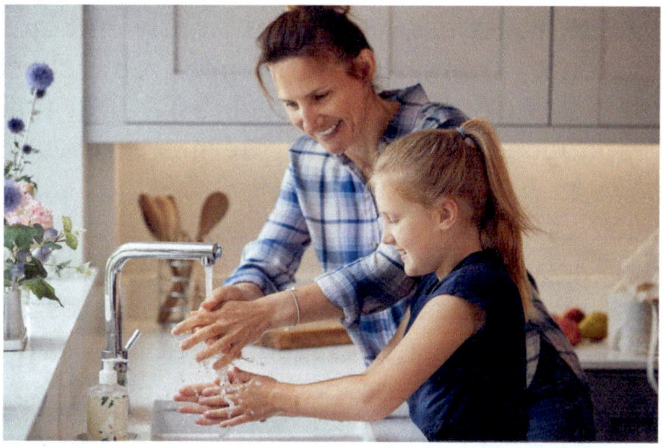

Figure 3.3. Proper hygiene protocols serve as the frontline defense against foodborne illnesses, which continue to be a significant global health concern.

Source: https://www.fsis.usda.gov/sites/default/files/2024-09/2024%20Handwashing.jpg.

As highlighted in the International Journal of Environmental Research and Public Health, foodborne diseases remain a pressing threat, necessitating robust strategies to mitigate their prevalence (Todd, 2020). This is particularly evident in regions , such as the Middle East and North Africa, where updated food laws and enhanced regulatory frameworks have emerged in response to this public health crisis (D-Klingbeil et al., 2019). The health and safety of food are largely dependent on food handlers following hygiene rules , which also affects the health of consumers. For this reason, improving how food handlers take care of themselves reduces illnesses and helps public health initiatives work better. (Figure 3.3).

Impact on Consumer Trust

Trust from customers is very important in the food industry, mainly when it comes to personal hygiene and how food is handled. When food handlers are very careful about hygiene, it gives consumers confidence in the safety and quality of their food. Evidence suggests that effective communication strategies, including transparent hygiene practices, can significantly enhance consumer trust and influence repurchase intentions in industries , such as frozen food (Prapdopo et al., 2024). Furthermore, research shows that personal encounters with food safety , such as dealing with food handlers, strongly affect how people view food safety. Notably, the presence of fundamental hygiene measures not only mitigates the risk of foodborne illnesses but also boosts customer confidence in food vendors, as demonstrated in research evaluating food handlers in Nnewi (Okwuanaso et al., 2024). Better hygiene helps create a good experience for consumers , which leads to more trust and loyalty in markets that care about health.

3.1. Importance of Personal Hygiene in Food Handling

Personal hygiene is very important in food handling since it helps prevent most foodborne illnesses. Rigorous cleanliness, including washing their hands often and wearing clean clothes, can help food handlers avoid contamination. A study focusing on food safety culture (FS-culture) highlights that even when food safety training is provided, the absence of a positive hygiene culture can lead to significant risks in food service environments (Griffith et al., 2017). Similarly, the assessment of food handlers within hospital kitchens revealed that while food hygiene is prioritized, gaps in knowledge regarding critical practices indicate a need for improved training and awareness (Mutalib et al., 2020). This means that encouraging personal hygiene in the kitchen helps ensure food safety and also encourages food workers to be responsible , which is good for public health.

3.1.1. Definition of Personal Hygiene in the Food Industry

Personal hygiene in the food industry means following certain actions and habits so that food products are safe and of good quality. Some of these activities are washing your hands, wearing clean clothes and covering any cuts or wounds properly.

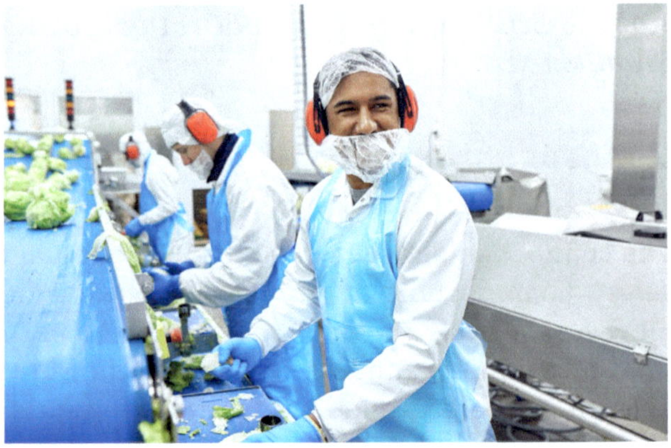

Figure 3.4. In the food industry, personal hygiene refers to the practices and behaviors that food handlers must adhere to in order to maintain the safety and quality of food products.

Source: https://lindstrom-sites.s3.eu-north-1.amazonaws.com/wp-content/uploads/sites/19/2024/01/012_Lindstrom_2016_hires_final.jpg.

High standards of personal hygiene are needed to prevent food contamination and to encourage a food safe culture in organizations, since the actions of food handlers play a big role in food safety. Failing to follow good personal hygiene can result in many health problems , which may also cause foodborne illnesses that can harm consumers and bring serious legal and financial consequences to food companies. The importance of cultivating a positive FS-culture, alongside formal policies and training, cannot be overstated, as it underpins the mechanisms that ensure food safety and public health (Griffith et al., 2017; Jaffee et al., 2018) (Figure 3.4).

3.1.2. Role of Personal Hygiene in Preventing Foodborne Illnesses

Looking after personal hygiene is necessary for food handlers to avoid foodborne illnesses. Even though it is very important that people know how to stay clean, the relationship between knowledge and prevention is not simple. For instance, a study conducted among street food handlers revealed that even though 70.65% had a moderate level of food hygiene knowledge, the correlation between this knowledge and their practices was weak, underscoring the necessity for effective training and enforcement of hygiene protocols (Dhudum & Bhosale, 2025). Additionally, traditional retail establishments have shown that over 95% of food handlers participated in hygiene training; however, many still failed to meet basic hygiene standards, such as providing hot water at handwashing stations (Oliveira et al., 2024). It shows that food handlers should learn about personal hygiene and that proper resources and systems should be available to support these practices , which benefits public health.

3.1.3. Common Pathogens Associated with Poor Hygiene

Incorrect handwashing when handling food can result in many common pathogens being spread , which is still a serious issue in food safety. A lot of gastrointestinal issues are caused by *Salmonella* , which can be found in contaminated food. *Salmonella* is a risky disease because it causes gastroenteritis and stomach cramps and this usually happens when food is not kept clean by handlers. In 2018, this pathogen was implicated in over half of foodborne illness outbreaks reported in the EU, emphasizing the critical role of food handlers in transmission dynamics (Ehuwa et al., 2021). In addition to this, the availability of certified food safety managers is not entirely sufficient in ensuring the prevention of food safety offenses, showing that ongoing training and good hygiene practices are necessary in order to prevent risks (Harris, 2015). Hence, recognizing such pathogens and following strict hygiene procedures are major responsibilities for food handlers (Figure 3.5).

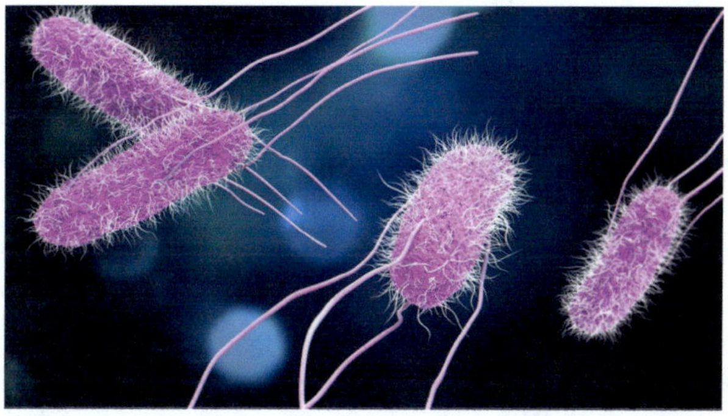

Figure 3.5. Salmonella is a primary pathogen, responsible for numerous gastrointestinal disorders linked to the consumption of contaminated food products.

Source: https://d2jx2rerrg6sh3.cloudfront.net/images/Article_Images/ImageForArticle_1970_1650606074420759.jpg.

3.1.4. Legal Implications of Hygiene Violations

If hygiene rules are ignored in food service, the public may get sick and it can be difficult for businesses to operate effectively. If food handlers do not wash their hands properly, there is a higher risk of foodborne illness , which could lead to problems with the law for companies. The obligation to maintain hygiene standards is codified in regulations like the Hazard Analysis Critical Control Point (HACCP) framework, which many jurisdictions have adopted to ensure safe food practices. Noncompliance can lead to fines, business shutdown, or criminal charges in extreme circumstances, as enumerated in reports outlining the relationship between managerial dedication and sanitary adherence (Jackson, 2011). Additionally, studies show that such businesses with bad hygiene have increased levels of infraction, further worsening their legal status and defiling their reputation (Clark et al., 2019). Therefore, employers and food handlers are obligated by law to practice good hygiene.

3.1.5. Consumer Expectations Regarding Hygiene

Consumer hygiene expectations in food handling have changed tremendously, especially with the emergence of online food delivery apps (OFD apps), which have revolutionized the way people interact with food choices. A study revealed that about 64% of the participants consumed OFD apps on a weekly basis, which indicated a rising reliance on digital means for making meal decisions (Osaili et al., 2023). There is a belief that fresh vegetables are a necessity for a healthy meal, and individuals are more focused on food safety and cleanliness. They indicate that individuals are more focused on hygiene during the preparation of food, as it is highly crucial to society now. In addition, the food choice implications of hygiene underscore the importance of stringent personal hygiene practices among food handlers since stakeholders need to work together to raise health standards to satisfy consumer demands and build confidence in food safety measures, both in terms of public health and consumer trust in the fast-evolving food environment (Awino et al., 2023) (Figure 3.6).

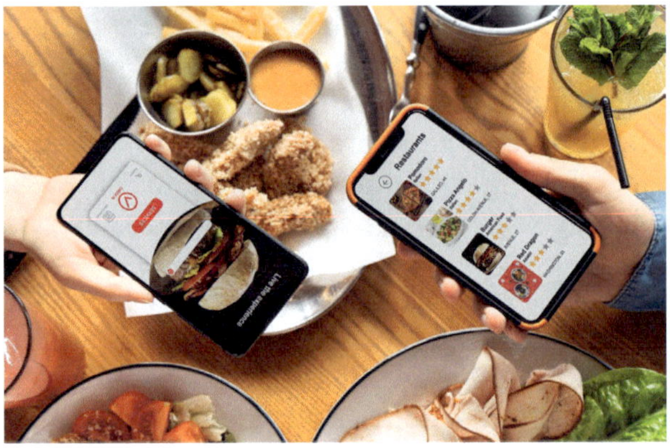

Figure 3.6. Consumer expectations regarding hygiene in food handling have significantly evolved, particularly with the rise of online food delivery applications (OFD apps), which have transformed how consumers engage with food options.

Source: https://ae.cms.pixbit.in/uploads/hands_holding_mobile_phones_with_food_delivery_app_screen_ebdf1cce59.jpg.

3.1.6. Cultural Differences in Hygiene Practices

How people from different cultures handle hygiene affects the tasks food handlers are responsible for. Different cultural traditions can impact how a person sees and handles personal hygiene , which then affects food safety. For some cultures, washing hands is tied to their religion, while others focus more on doing it quickly than on making sure it is very clean. When there is such a difference, food handling rules may not be followed as needed. A study revealed that only 2% of food handlers implemented fully compliant hand-hygiene practices, highlighting that prevalent knowledge alone does not ensure proper behavior (Evans & Redmond, 2019). Furthermore, the necessity of management support in enforcing effective food safety management systems becomes apparent, as workers often mirror the hygiene culture established by their supervisors (Jackson, 2011). Because of this, it is important to understand

and deal with cultural differences when setting up hygiene practices in food service.

3.1.7. Training and Education on Hygiene for Food Handlers

It is very important to train food handlers properly in hygiene to protect the public and make food safe. As foodborne illnesses rise, it is necessary for food handlers to understand how to be sanitary , such as by washing their hands and using protective gear. Training programs should be tailored to address common gaps in knowledge and practice, as evidenced by findings from studies , such as the one conducted in Jashore, where 72.5% of food vendors demonstrated good knowledge of food safety, yet only 0.5% exhibited good practices related to hygiene (Hossen et al., 2020). Moreover, continuous education is crucial as it must adapt to emerging challenges, such as skin disorders like hand eczema that affect food handlers, thereby requiring strategies for prevention and management (Thyssen et al., 2021). Ultimately, robust training initiatives can significantly enhance the overall hygiene practices among food handlers, contributing to safer food for consumers (Figure 3.7).

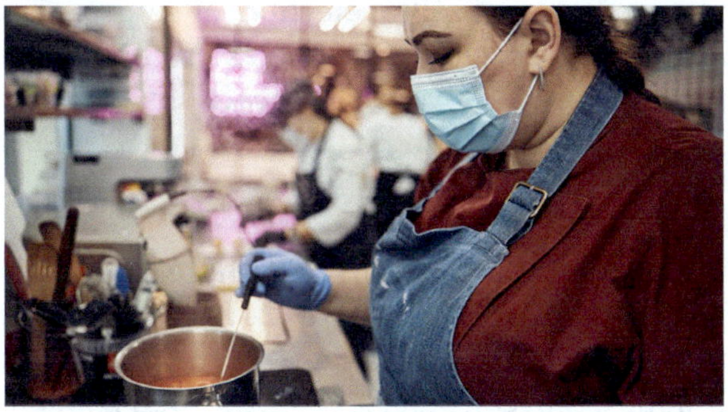

Figure 3.7. Effective training and education on hygiene for food handlers is paramount in safeguarding public health and ensuring food safety.

Source: https://firstaid4u.ca/wp-content/uploads/2024/08/Food-Handling.jpg.

3.1.8. Best Practices for Maintaining Personal Hygiene

Good personal hygiene is necessary for food handlers to stop foodborne illnesses and protect customers. Regularly wash your hands after handling raw food, after using the restroom and after touching your face or hair. Studies indicate that compliance with hand-hygiene protocols significantly mitigates risks associated with food preparation (Evans & Redmond, 2019). In addition, food handlers should learn that being clean, keeping their uniforms clean and not wearing jewelry that carries bacteria is very important. Implementation of robust food safety management systems, as highlighted in research, plays a crucial role in supporting hygienic practices within food service environments (Jackson, 2011). If hygiene is valued in the workplace, management can see a big improvement in food handlers' compliance. By always practicing good hygiene, a food service business helps protect the public and builds a reliable reputation.

3.2. Key Personal Hygiene Practices for Food Handlers

It is very important for food handlers to observe key personal hygiene habits to help prevent foodborne illnesses. Handwashing with soap and water after coming into contact with raw food, the restroom or anything that might be contaminated is the most important thing for good hygiene. As well as following proper hand hygiene, food handlers are supposed to keep their uniforms clean and put on gloves and hair restraints to minimize the chances of contamination. The significance of a positive FS-culture cannot be understated, as studies indicate that motivation and adherence to hygiene practices are often hindered by inadequate training and support systems within food service environments (Griffith et al., 2017). Furthermore, assessments of knowledge, attitude, and practice (KAP) highlight critical gaps in understanding temperature control, demonstrating the need for ongoing education to attain a prevailing FS-culture (Mutalib et al., 2020).

3.2.1. Handwashing Techniques and Frequency

Maintaining personal hygiene for food handlers requires them to wash their hands often and effectively , which is very important for food safety.

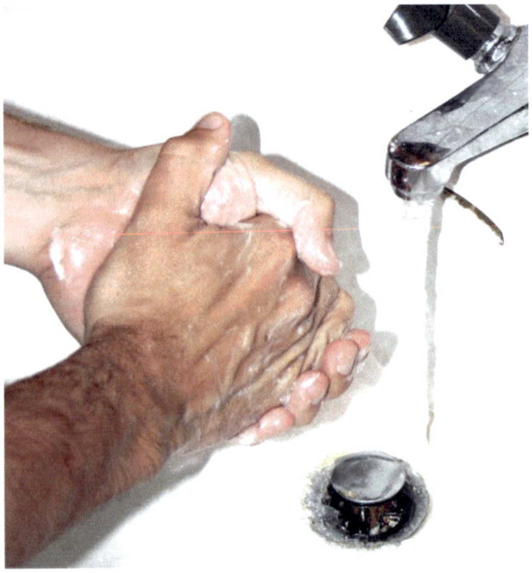

Figure 3.8. Effective handwashing techniques and frequency are crucial components of personal hygiene for food handlers, significantly impacting food safety.

Source: https://upload.wikimedia.org/wikipedia/commons/1/1b/OCD_handwash.jpg.

According to research, sub-optimal handwashing practices contribute to the transmission of foodborne illnesses, thereby posing a considerable public health risk (Clark et al., 2019). Warm water, enough soap and scrubbing all parts of the hands for at least 20 seconds are all important in critical hand hygiene. It is important to wash your hands more often , such as before starting to cook, after handling raw food and after using the restroom. Studies reveal that proper training and managerial commitment can greatly enhance compliance with handwashing protocols among food handlers (Gemeda et al., 2021). Lack of knowledge and bad attitudes about these practices are important reasons for food safety violations , which makes it necessary to keep educating staff and regularly inspect places where food is served. Hence, prioritizing effective handwashing strategies is essential for safeguarding public health (Figure 3.8).

3.2.2. Use of Gloves and When to Change Them

Gloves are used in food handling to keep hands clean and stop the spread of germs. Because food handlers handle many ingredients, the chance of spreading harmful pathogens rises, so it is important to change gloves often to prevent this. Gloves must be changed after touching raw products, after using the restroom and when they become dirty or torn, so that food stays safe to eat. Furthermore, the selection of appropriate glove materials is critical, as latex or vinyl gloves can sometimes provoke skin reactions, as noted in discussions surrounding hand eczema (Thyssen et al., 2021). Emphasizing proper glove usage is paramount; for example, when gloves are not changed frequently or correctly, there is potential for the transfer of bacteria, particularly when interacting with ready-to-eat (RTE) foods (Janik et al., 2023). Glove protocols motivate food handlers to act professionally and safely with food.

3.2.3. Proper Grooming and Attire for Food Handlers

In the food industry, how food handlers look and dress is very important for their personal hygiene and the safety of food and customers. Food handlers are expected to look professional and clean , which starts with wearing uniforms that help stop contamination. The materials used for these uniforms must be easy to clean and able to withstand tough cleaning to get rid of pathogens. Short nails are important in grooming, since bacteria on unkempt nails may be transferred to food. Loose strands of hair need to be held back so they do not get into food products, usually by wearing hairnets or caps. Such adherence to grooming standards not only fosters a safe food handling environment but also instills consumer confidence in the establishment (Missoula Vo Tech, 1973; Huot & Traiser, 2015) (Figure 3.9).

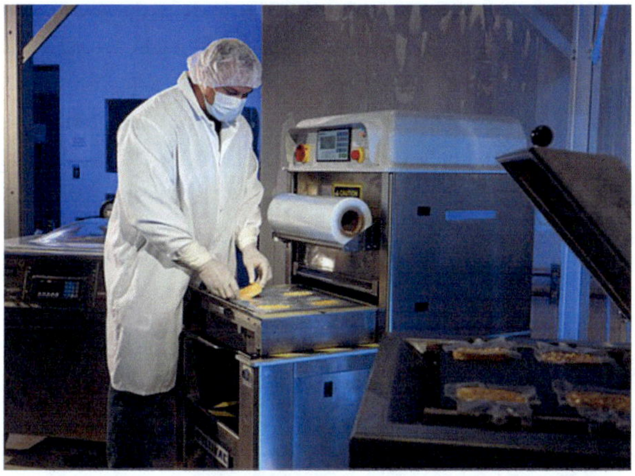

Figure 3.9. Food handlers must maintain a clean and professional appearance, which begins with appropriate uniforms that are specifically designed to prevent contamination.

Source: By Bill Stafford - https://www.nasa.gov/content/space-food-systems (direct link), Public Domain, https://commons.wikimedia.org/w/index.php?curid=93200006

3.2.4. Importance of Nail Care and Jewelry Restrictions

Personal hygiene for food handlers requires them to follow nail care and jewellery rules , which help keep food safe and healthy. When nails are properly cared for, they do not become a place for bacteria and other harmful germs to grow , which could contaminate food. Moreover, food handlers are generally advised to keep nails trimmed and clean, which not only promotes hygiene but also makes handwashing more effective (Rutherford et al., 2018).

Banning jewellery, such as rings and bracelets lowers the chance of spreading bacteria, since jewelry can hold germs and be hard to clean. A small mistake in these hygiene areas in food handling can cause the spread of infectious diseases, so sticking to these hygiene rules is very important for public health. So, it is very important to follow strict nail care and jewelry rules to maintain safety and quality in food service.

3.2.5. Managing Personal Health and Illness

It is very important to look after personal health and illness to ensure that food handlers in public health remain safe and healthy. Maintaining high hygiene standards can significantly prevent the transmission of zoonotic diseases, as over 60% of human pathogens originate from animal sources (Rahman et al., 2020).

Additionally, food handlers must be vigilant about environmental factors that may impact their health, as these can exacerbate conditions , such as asthma, which presents a unique challenge owing to its increasing prevalence in both children and adults (Dharmage et al., 2019). A full health plan , which includes health checkups, learning about health risks and proper food handling, can cut down on food contamination. Ultimately, the proactive management of personal health not only protects the food handler but also safeguards the health of consumers, fostering a safer food supply chain (Figure 3.10).

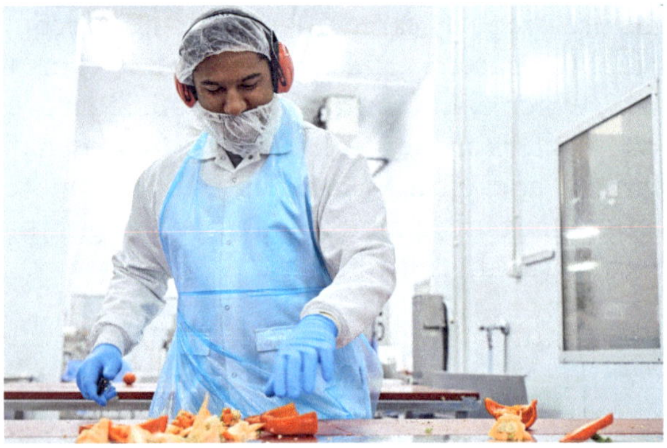

Figure 3.10. Effective management of personal health and illness is crucial in ensuring the safety and well-being of food handlers, particularly in the context of public health.

Source: https://lindstrom-sites.s3.eu-north-1.amazonaws.com/wp-content/uploads/sites/19/2024/06/012_Lindstrom_Set2_hires_final.jpg.

3.2.6. Avoiding Cross-contamination Through Hygiene

Not cross-contaminating food can prevent many foodborne illnesses and this is possible with good hygiene. Food handlers must know about hygiene and show hygienic behavior each day. According to studies, food handlers often understand how important good hygiene is, but it is still difficult for most to practice it on the job.

For instance, studies show a high level of awareness regarding cross-contamination and hygiene but identify gaps in consistent implementation due to socio-economic factors (Alter et al., 2016). Moreover, training in food safety has been associated with improved hygiene practices, underscoring its role in shaping food handling behaviors (Oumer, 2019). For this reason, we should keep teaching and supporting food handlers by finding solutions that suit them to avoid cross-contamination.

3.2.7. Safe Handling of Food and Utensils

Safe use of food and utensils is required in food handling to prevent foodborne illnesses from occurring. There has been evidence through research of a strong relationship between the attitudes of food service workers toward food safety and sanitation and overall hygiene procedures within food facilities, and this highlights the importance of proper training and following safety procedures (Lin et al., 2007). Additionally, lack of knowledge about handling foods can directly result in foodborne disease outbreaks, making a significant role of educational programs in public food facilities (Gemeda et al., 2021). Proper training and frequent checks on food safety enhance workers' skills , which reduce risks. Also, promoting a safety culture and individual responsibility among food handlers improves the standards of food preparation environments' safety, ensuring that the core principles of hygiene and safety are upheld at all times (Figure 3.11).

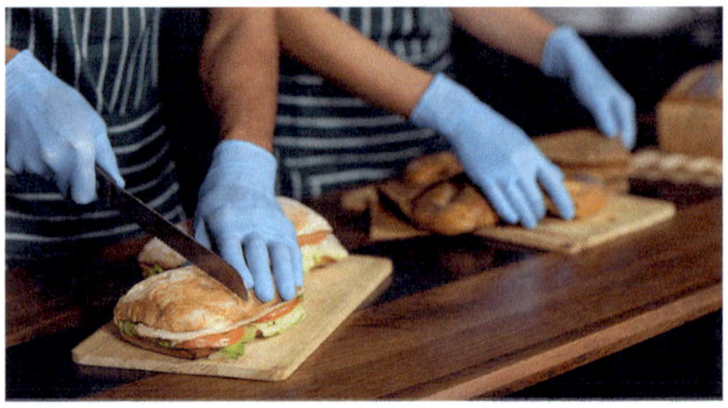

Figure 3.11. In the realm of personal hygiene and food handler responsibilities, the safe handling of food and utensils is paramount in preventing foodborne illnesses.

Source: https://www.i2comply.com/wp-content/uploads/2022/05/Article_Food_Header-1.png

3.2.8. Importance of Cleanliness in Food Preparation Areas

It is very important to clean food preparation areas to protect both food and the health of the public. If hygiene is ignored, the risk of food getting contaminated increases , which can cause foodborne diseases. This is particularly evident in environments , such as pastry production, where intricate tools and processes demand rigorous sanitation to prevent cross-contamination and uphold product quality, as outlined in the findings that highlight the relationship between good hygiene practices and culinary safety (Dianita et al., 2024). Furthermore, studies of food vendors emphasize the necessity for systematic hygiene training to mitigate health risks, underscoring the alarming microbial presence on popular street foods that frequently violates safety standards (Alindugan et al., 2024). If food preparation areas are clean, food handlers obey the rules, gain the confidence of customers and help ensure that food is safe for everyone.

3.2.9. Regular Self-assessment of Hygiene Practices

Often, considering your hygiene habits can help stop foodborne illnesses and ensure your food is safe to eat. Food handlers should often check their hygiene habits to confirm they are meeting all the required standards, especially those in HACCP. This reflective practice not only enhances personal accountability but also fosters a culture of safety within food service environments, where research has shown that traditional training alone does not guarantee proper implementation of food safety behaviors (Jackson, 2011). Furthermore, the critical observation of actual hygiene practices, rather than solely relying on self-reported data, highlights the need for frequent self-assessments, which have indicated alarming compliance failures in hand hygiene among food handlers (Evans & Redmond, 2019). By prioritizing regular self-assessment, food handlers can better align their practices with established safety standards, ultimately safeguarding public health (Figure 3.12).

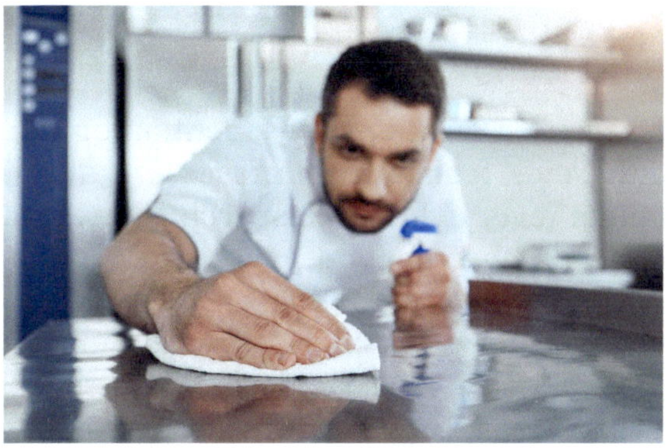

Figure 3.12. Regular self-assessment of hygiene practices serves as a fundamental component in ensuring food safety and mitigating the risks associated with food-borne illnesses.

Source: https://5845715.fs1.hubspotusercontent-na1.net/hub/5845715/hubfs/food%20hygiene%20rules.jpg.

3.3. Food Handler Responsibilities Beyond Personal Hygiene

Food handlers must do many important things, aside from keeping things clean, to prevent foodborne diseases. A good food safety plan includes learning the proper way to receive, store and rotate food. They ensure that a food safety plan is successful in keeping the company clean. Moreover, a positive FS-culture within an organization fosters an environment where food handlers are encouraged to prioritize safety and hygiene in all aspects of their work, as highlighted in recent research emphasizing the need for comprehensive FS-culture frameworks (Nyarugwe et al., 2020). Such frameworks not only enhance compliance with food safety regulations as outlined by industry standards (BC Cook Articulation Committee, 2015) but also promote a proactive mindset among employees, ultimately leading to improved food safety performance and reduced risk of contamination.

3.3.1. Understanding Food Safety Regulations

Food safety regulations are essential for public health since foodborne illnesses are a major problem everywhere. Research shows that a large number of food vendors understand food safety, but their actions and attitudes are not always as good. In Jashore, for instance, while 72.5% of food vendors exhibited solid awareness of essential safety measures, only a mere 0.5% demonstrated proper food handling practices, indicating a disconnection between knowledge and implementation (Hossen et al., 2020). It proves that training and strict use of hygiene rules are important for people who handle food. Additionally, the ongoing global struggle against foodborne diseases (FBDs) necessitates targeted public health strategies that promote comprehensive education on safe food handling practices (Todd, 2020). By addressing both knowledge and practical adherence to regulations, the food service industry can significantly reduce the risk of foodborne illnesses, thereby ensuring safer dining experiences for consumers (Figure 3.13).

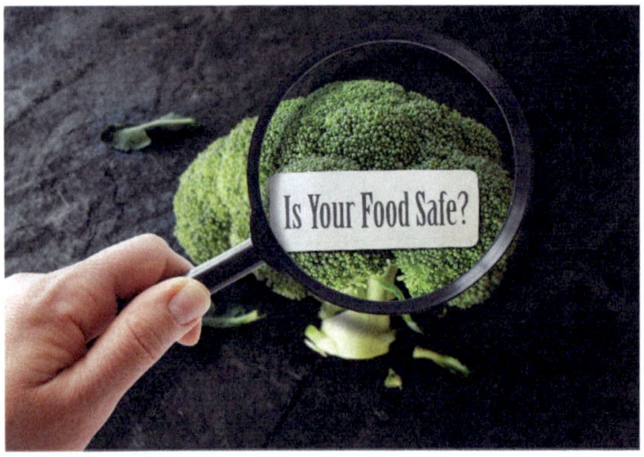

Figure 3.13. Food safety regulations are crucial in protecting public health, particularly as foodborne illnesses continue to pose significant threats globally.

Source: https://pnoe.com/wp-content/uploads/2024/06/iStock-822023804-scaled-1.jpg.

3.3.2. Importance of Temperature Control in Food Storage

It is very important to control the temperature in food storage, because wrong settings can quickly cause foodborne pathogens to grow. Strict rules for temperature are important because almost all open-air market stalls do not keep meat at the right temperature.

They raise the likelihood of food being contaminated and spoiled , which can endanger the public. If food handlers neglect temperature monitoring, the safety of the food supply is put at risk , which can result in outbreaks of foodborne illnesses that might have been avoided. Consequently, foodservice managers must instill a culture of awareness regarding temperature control among their staff, which is crucial for implementing safe food handling practices as noted in food safety management literature (Marule et al., 2024). Keeping the right temperatures helps ensure public health and also improves the image of food businesses.

3.3.3. Safe Food Sourcing and Supplier Responsibilities

It is not enough to only follow the regulations; everyone in the food supply chain must be actively involved in providing safe food. Farmers need to maintain high hygiene standards at the very beginning to protect against microbial and chemical contaminants in the food. Maintaining food safety during transportation and storage depends on the actions of food handlers and distributors. How people behave in the system plays a big role , which is why it's important to educate them about food safety dangers. Additionally, as highlighted by Jaffee et al. (2018), food safety not only safeguards public health but also impacts agricultural growth and market integration. Hence, government agencies must enforce stringent food safety laws to protect consumers, while suppliers and handlers must remain diligent and responsible stewards of food safety, as emphasized in the discussions surrounding (Fung et al., 2018) (Figure 3.14).

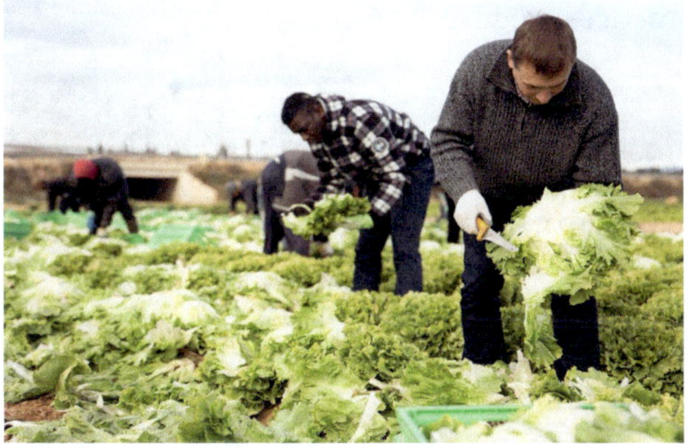

Figure 3.14. Effective food safety practices begin at the source, where farmers must adhere to hygienic standards to mitigate risks associated with microbial and chemical contaminants.

Source: https://cdn.wikifarmer.com/images/detailed/2024/04/Ensuring-Compliance-with-Food-Safety-Regulations-6-Tips-for-Farmers-and-Food-Processors.jpg.

3.3.4. Importance of Cleanliness in Food Service Environments

It is very important to keep food service areas clean to protect customers, since cleanliness affects both the food and public health. If sanitation is not good enough, it can cause foodborne illnesses , which can seriously harm consumers and harm the reputation of food businesses. According to recent studies, heightened awareness of hygiene practices has emerged due to the COVID-19 pandemic, prompting a reevaluation of cleanliness standards within the hospitality sector (Jiang et al., 2020). The pandemic has illuminated the need for rigorous sanitation protocols that align with evolving consumer expectations regarding health and safety (Wen et al., 2020). So, food handlers should always be clean and hygienic in the area where food is prepared, since these habits help prevent contamination and keep customers happy. Being very clean in food preparation makes the food safer and encourages customers to trust and stay loyal to the business.

3.3.5. Role of Food Handlers in Preventing Cross-Contamination

Food safety depends on food handlers preventing cross-contamination , which is the main cause of foodborne illness outbreaks. They have to use proper food preparation and make sure their personal hygiene is always very good. A study highlighted that misconceptions about food hygiene among food handlers can significantly contribute to contamination risk, underscoring the need for comprehensive training (Gemeda et al., 2021). Moreover, research indicates that while many food handlers possess basic knowledge of hygiene practices, gaps remain in their execution, particularly concerning handwashing procedures (Cheng et al., 2013). Since these differences exist, it may be hard to take enough preventive steps to stop dangerous pathogens from spreading. Therefore, it is imperative to emphasize continuous education for food handlers, ensuring they understand and implement best practices that mitigate cross-contamination, thus safeguarding public health through conscientious food handling (Figure 3.15).

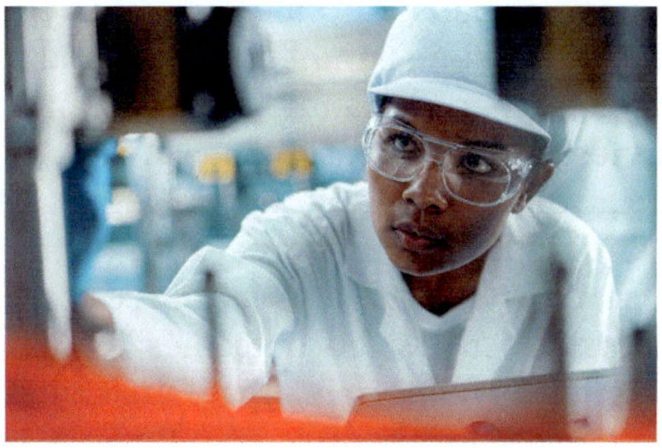

Figure 3.15. Food handlers play a critical role in preventing cross-contamination, a key factor in foodborne illness outbreaks.

Source: https://knowhow.distrelec.com/wp-content/uploads/2024/02/GettyImages-1656278047-min.jpg.

3.3.6. Reporting Illness and Symptoms to Management

Telling management about any illness or symptoms is very important for food handlers and helps ensure food safety in the kitchen. Food handlers should understand that any health problems that could affect food safety must be reported, because infections can quickly be transmitted to consumers through contaminated food. Research indicates that a culture of transparency, fostered by management, encourages employees to report their illnesses without fear of repercussion, thereby mitigating the risk of foodborne outbreaks (Jackson, 2011). Moreover, established protocols for illness reporting can enhance organizational food safety strategies, aligning with best practices in food management as indicated by studies assessing food safety knowledge and behavior among food handlers (Mutalib et al., 2020). In the end, having good reporting systems helps ensure public health and encourages food service workers to be more hygienic and careful.

3.3.7. Importance of Training and Certification

Being trained and having certificates is key in personal hygiene and food handling since it helps prevent people from eating unsafe foods. Training helps food handlers notice food safety issues, know how to handle them and maintain cleanliness in their areas. Being certified makes it official that a food handler is committed to following hygiene rules. Moreover, as highlighted by research, a well-trained workforce correlates with improved food safety outcomes; for instance, food handlers who participate in structured training programs exhibit significantly better hygiene practices than those without such credentials (Adane et al., 2018). Furthermore, adherence to rigorous food safety protocols supports broader agricultural and economic goals, as safe food systems are essential for sustainable development and consumer trust in food supply chains (Jaffee et al., 2018). Thus, prioritizing training and certification is fundamental to promoting safe food handling practices (Figure 3.16).

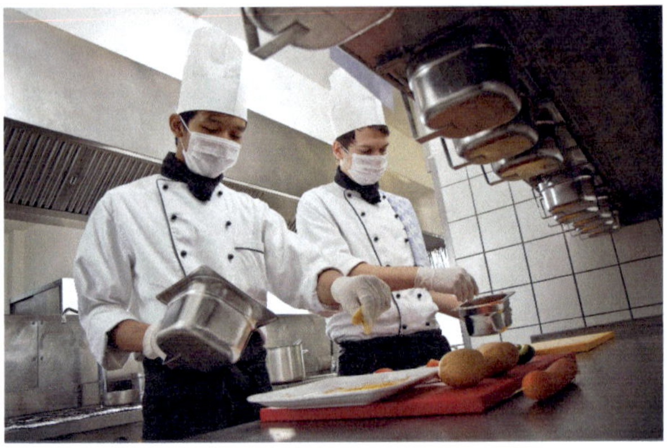

Figure 3.16. Effective training equips food handlers with the necessary knowledge and skills to recognize potential food safety hazards, implement best practices, and maintain cleanliness in food preparation environments.

Source: https://ugc.futurelearn.com/uploads/images/50/ab/50ab956f-2206-4be2-8f9f-241329b7dc30.jpg.

3.3.8. Collaboration with Health Inspectors

It is very important to work with health inspectors to ensure food safety in personal hygiene and food handling. Health inspectors connect the regulations to food establishments by offering tips on safe food handling and cleanliness. Their expertise is particularly significant in developing regions, where the informal food sector, , such as street food vendors, contributes greatly to the local economy yet often lacks rigorous safety protocols (Johnson and Yawson, 2025). By working closely with health inspectors, food handlers can receive tailored training that addresses specific challenges, , such as the prevalence of foodborne illnesses, which underscores the need for adherence to safety standards (Ber et al., 2015). When different agencies unite, everyone feels responsible and tries to improve , which means food handlers follow the rules and maintain good hygiene for all.

3.3.9. Continuous Improvement and Staying Updated on Best Practices

Being aware of new information and always trying to improve are important for both personal hygiene and food handling to maintain food safety and public health. A commitment to a proactive FS-culture can significantly bolster hygiene practices among food handlers, as evidenced by research highlighting the limitations of traditional food safety approaches in addressing persisting challenges within food companies (Nyarugwe et al., 2020). Moreover, studies conducted in Lebanon have shown that food handlers often exhibit gaps in knowledge regarding critical aspects of food safety, , such as safe food temperatures and cross-contamination prevention (Faour-Klingbeil et al., 2015). Hence, ongoing training and teamwork between public and private organizations can help build a workforce that knows how to maintain proper hygiene. This dedication not only enhances individual practices but also contributes to the overarching goal of sustained food safety in the industry (Figure 3.17).

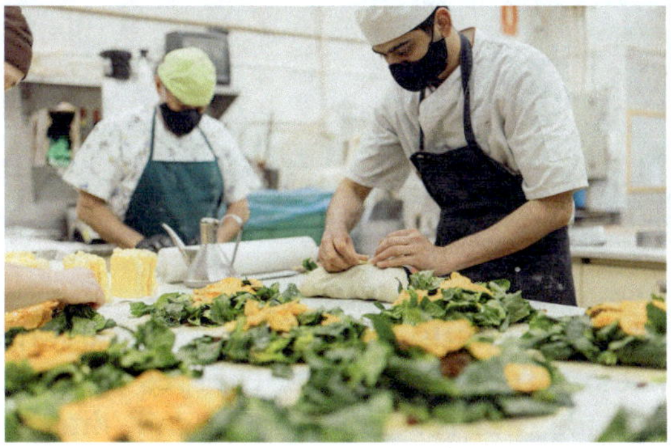

Figure 3.17. Continuous improvement and staying abreast of best practices are essential for ensuring food safety and protecting public health.

Source: https://www.ficsi.in/blog/wp-content/uploads/2024/03/Blog-4-1.jpg.

3.4. Consequences of Neglecting Personal Hygiene

If you do not follow proper hygiene when working with food, the results can be very serious for more than your own health. Lack of basic hygiene by food handlers unintentionally raises the chance of FBD for those who eat the food. Research indicates that food handlers often perceive themselves to be at a lower risk for causing FBD compared to their peers, a cognitive bias that can lead to unsafe practices in the kitchen (de Andrade et al., 2019). Additionally, the lack of adequate training in food safety further compounds this issue, as workers unaware of the critical nature of hygiene may not recognize potential risks associated with their actions (de Freitas et al., 2018). As a result, such negligence can make people sick and also reduce the trust they have in food service businesses. Fixing these issues in knowledge and practices is important for the safety of food and the health of consumers.

3.4.1. Health Risks Associated with Poor Hygiene

There are a lot of health issues that can arise if food handlers fail to practice good hygiene and the consequences can be highly detrimental to public health. Poor hygiene, like unclean hands and food not stored well, increases the chances of foodborne diseases. Most food handlers lack good training in food safety and therefore lack knowledge of key aspects of hygiene practices. For example, in most food handlers in a given study, the attitude towards food safety was positive, but observed practices were not sufficient, indicating a disconnect between knowledge and action (Jipiu, 2016). In addition, in another evaluation, low food safety practices among food handlers were found to be a direct consequence of poor knowledge and lack of supervision (Oumer, 2019). Therefore, hygiene must be addressed through thorough training and monitoring to reduce these health hazards and maintain the safety of food consumers (Figure 3.18).

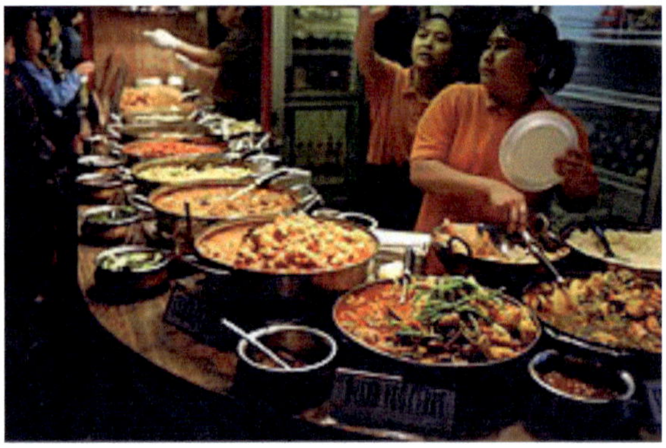

Figure 3.18. The health risks associated with poor hygiene among food handlers are multifaceted and can lead to severe public health concerns.

Source: By Karsten Seiferlin - https://www.flickr.com/photos/timecaptured/6182975764/, CC BY-SA 2.0, https://commons.wikimedia.org/w/index.php?curid=147925669

3.4.2. Economic Impact on Food Businesses

The way food businesses are affected economically depends on how well personal hygiene is followed and what food handlers do. A properly set up food safety management system , such as one based on HACCP, can prevent food-borne illnesses and strengthen a company's reputation in the market. As individuals become more concerned about food safety, companies that fail to be clean may lose a great deal of money since customers have less trust in such companies and the company might get into legal trouble. Literature emphasizes that successful employee training and management strategies strongly relate to food safety performance in food service facilities, indicating that how much effort is made in employee learning directly affects the economic sustainability of these operations (Jackson, 2011). In addition, adherence to changing regulations and consumer demands can prevent adverse economic consequences due to food safety violations (Tonder et al., 2004).

3.4.3. Legal Repercussions for Food Handlers and Establishments

Food premises and food handlers are legally liable for bad hygiene and non-compliance with food safety regulations , which serve to avoid such errors. When laws are violated, the penalties may be severe, including payment of fines, losing business rights and criminal prosecution if negligence leads to food poisoning. For example, unsanitary practices, for example, not cleaning utensils properly, can enhance the risk of contamination, as seen in the spread of foodborne pathogens , such as viruses from different studies (Cortés-Sánchez et al., 2022).

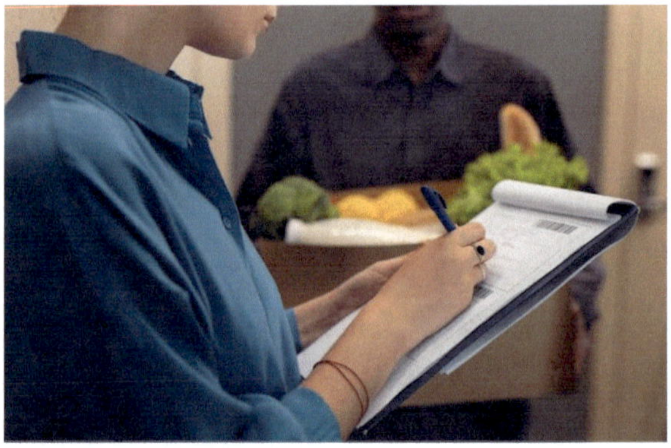

Figure 3.19. Violations can lead to severe penalties, including fines, loss of business licenses, and even criminal charges in cases of negligence that result in foodborne illnesses.

Source: https://metrobi.com/wp-content/uploads/2025/03/side-view-woman-receiving-groceries_23-2149722264.jpg.

When this negligence happens, it puts the public's health at risk along with the business's reputation, as trust is highly necessary for customer loyalty. Also, regulations are now enacting stricter sanitation standards, particularly in establishments where pastries and other high-risk foods are prepared. As underscored, improving equipment hygiene is critical to navigate the multifaceted environment of food safety measures and legal requirements for food handlers (Dianita et al., 2024) (Figure 3.19).

3.4.4. Loss of Consumer Trust and Brand Reputation

If people lose trust in a food industry brand because of hygiene or food handling, it can be very damaging for the business. Consumers rely on the perceived safety and quality of the food they purchase, often seeking assurance of "(cr)edibility," , which encompasses both credibility and edibility (Stearns, 2010). If foodborne illnesses happen because hygiene was not followed, the public's trust in the company quickly disappears , which can cause major issues for the brand and its ability to stay in business. This erosion is further compounded by the structural barriers in the food market that discourage accountability and transparency, which are essential for reinforcing consumer confidence (Stearns et al., 2010). Because food handlers are key to food safety, they must follow hygiene rules to ensure customers trust the business and its brand is protected , which makes proper training and supervision necessary.

3.4.5. Impact on Employee Morale and Workplace Culture

Maintaining good hygiene standards for personal use among food workers has a great impact on the workplace culture and atmosphere. Having stringent hygiene standards results in a safer working environment and also promotes the health of staff. If food handlers adhere to rigorous hygiene standards, it gives them a sense of pride and enables them to work professionally , which boosts employee engagement. When hygiene is prioritized in the workplace, absenteeism is reduced and job satisfaction increases, as employees feel valued and secure in their work. In addition, the establishment of a culture of hygiene supports other initiatives in sustainability and public health by incorporating shared organizational values that align with employees' own beliefs (Martín et al., 2022). This alignment can encourage employees to become more involved in their work, thereby generating a harmonious workplace culture based on collective responsibility and mutual respect (Martín et al., 2022) (Figure 3.20).

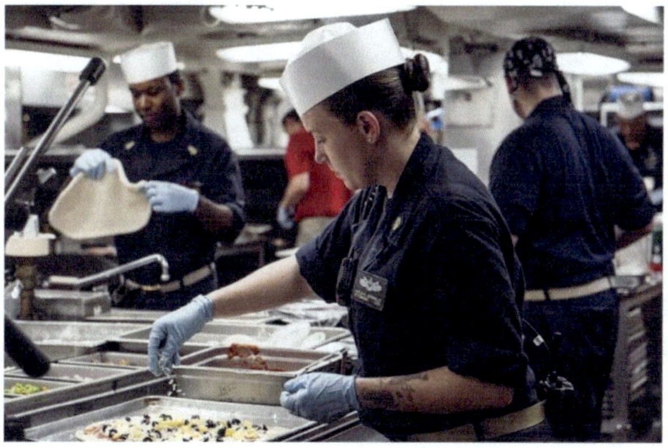

Figure 3.20. Maintaining high standards of hygiene not only fosters a safer work environment but also enhances the overall well-being of employees.

Source: https://easyfoodhandlers.com/wp-content/uploads/2024/04/SCR-20220517-tj-1024x686-1.jpeg

3.4.6. Long-Term Effects on Public Health

Personal hygiene and the actions of food handlers have a major and diverse impact on public health , which is reflected in the number of foodborne illnesses in the community. Insufficient hygiene in food preparation causes about 48 million cases of food poisoning in the U.S. each year, making it clear that food safety training and compliance are very important for food handlers. While regulatory measures from agencies , such as the FDA have contributed to a decline in confirmed outbreaks, ongoing food safety violations indicate a persistent risk that jeopardizes public health (Coyle et al., 2018). Therefore, enhancing food safety practices through targeted interventions, like those outlined in the Animal-Assisted Intervention for Healthcare Professionals program, becomes essential for both FS-culture and the well-being of food service employees (Coyle et al., 2018). Paying close attention to personal hygiene and food handling duties helps prevent diseases caused by contaminated food , which can reduce their occurrence over time.

3.4.7. Importance of Accountability in Food Handling

Having a culture where people are responsible for food handling is very important for keeping food safe and healthy for everyone. Although food handlers are important in stopping foodborne illnesses, studies reveal that poor management can make it harder for them to do their job well. Emphasizing accountability in a framework helps people see their duties and motivates them to follow the best standards for food safety. For instance, studies highlighting FS-culture in hospital kitchens reveal that while basic hygiene knowledge exists among staff, a lack of accountability can lead to lapses in crucial behaviors , such as timely temperature control (Mutalib et al., 2020). Furthermore, effective food safety management systems grounded in accountability have been shown to mitigate risks associated with foodborne pathogens, reinforcing the significance of management support and training in achieving compliance with safety standards (Jackson, 2011). Therefore, accountability is essential in cultivating responsible food handling practices that ultimately protect consumers (Figure 3.21).

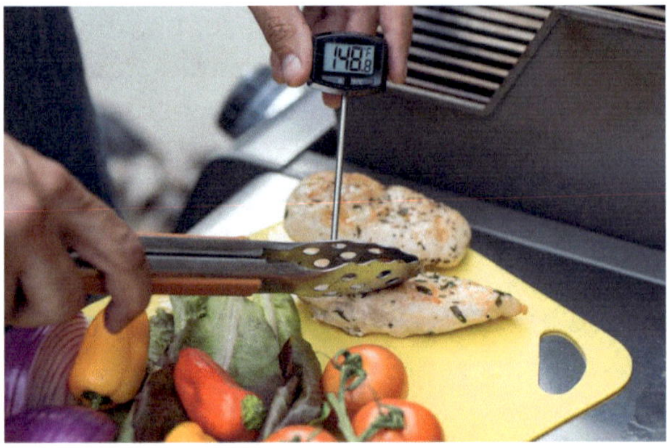

Figure 3.21. Food handlers play a critical role in preventing foodborne illnesses, yet research indicates that inadequate management practices often undermine this responsibility.

Source: https://www.ficsi.in/blog/wp-content/uploads/2024/02/FICSI-Aug-4.jpg.

3.4.8. Strategies for Addressing Hygiene Failures

It is very important to prevent hygiene failures when handling food to protect the public. It is necessary to use a combination of regular training, strict enforcement of hygiene rules and new technology. Training should focus on personal hygiene, especially by teaching how to wash hands and handle food safely. Regular checks and audits allow for spotting compliance issues , which motivates staff to follow best practices. Furthermore, the use of antimicrobial treatments and advanced monitoring systems can mitigate risks associated with bacterial contamination and multidrug-resistant organisms, as highlighted in recent studies (Uddin et al., 2021). It is also necessary to encourage food handlers to be responsible and keep improving, as this helps them see how important they are for food safety. By adopting these strategies, the food industry can effectively address hygiene failures and safeguard consumer health (Liu et al., 2020).

A CLOSER LOOK

Food-Borne Illnesses

Food-borne illnesses , which are the same as food poisoning, result from eating or drinking things that are contaminated. These illnesses are typically caused by harmful microorganisms , such as bacteria (e.g., Salmonella, E. coli, Listeria), viruses (e.g., Norovirus, Hepatitis A), parasites, or chemical substances. People may have nausea, vomit, get diarrhea, feel stomach pain, run a fever and feel tired. Some food-borne illnesses are not serious, but others can be very dangerous, mainly for young children, the elderly, pregnant women and people with weak immune systems. Food can be contaminated at any step in the process, from the farm to your plate, usually because of poor hygiene, wrong food handling, not cooking enough or unsafe storage. Food-borne illnesses can be prevented by handling food correctly, cooking it well, washing your hands often and sticking to food safety rules.

SUMMARY

Good personal hygiene helps food handlers ensure the safety of food in catering businesses. The increased trend of dining out has amplified the need for these stakeholders to adhere to stringent hygiene practices, as evidenced by the findings from focus group discussions , which revealed various barriers to compliance among food handlers, , such as a lack of time and entrenched traditional practices (Kumari et al., 2018). Caring about personal hygiene helps both with following the regulations and with keeping the community healthy. Ensuring safe food not only supports the well-being of consumers but also contributes to sustainable development, highlighting the interconnectedness of food safety, health, and economic growth (Jaffee et al., 2018). In this way, teaching food handlers about hygiene protects their health as well as the health of the community.

Being clean is important in food safety and public health since food handlers have to stop diseases that can be spread by food. Washing hands, keeping clean and using clean clothes and uniforms can stop the spread of dangerous bacteria and pathogens in food. Research shows that sanitation practice awareness plays a vital role in influencing personal behaviors, with the importance of having extensive food handler training programs to strengthen these notions (Aregai et al., 2008). In addition, personal hygiene not only maintains a food handling environment free of danger but also increases customers' confidence in food facilities, ultimately driving a healthier community (Fair Labor Association, 2012). Therefore, food handlers must be very careful about hygiene, because their actions can influence public health and the food chain. Stressing how important personal hygiene is for community health and well-being is very important.

KEY TERMS FROM THIS CHAPTER

- Organizational culture
- Personal hygiene
- Reliance
- Restroom
- Street food handlers
- Transmission
- Vinyl gloves
- Well-being
- Personal cleanliness
- Positive hygiene culture
- Responsible
- Soap
- Training
- Uniforms
- Washing hands
- Wounds

REFERENCES

1. Abdul Rashid, S., Abdul Mutalib, N. A., Ariffin, H. F., Mohd Izani, et al. (2020). *Knowledge, Attitude, And Practice on Food Safety Culture Among Kitchen Employees of Malaysian Government Hospitals*. https://core.ac.uk/download/324171185.pdf.
2. Adane, M., Teka, B., Gismu, Y., Halefom, G., & Ademe, M. (2018). Food hygiene and safety measures among food handlers in street food shops and food establishments of Dessie town, Ethiopia: A community-based cross-sectional study. *PLoS ONE, 13*, e0196919. https://doi.org/10.1371/journal.pone.0196919.
3. Alindugan, D. G., Castillo, P. B. D., De Sagun, L. M., et al. (2024). *Be Aware mga Suki: Practices of Food Safety and Appropriate Hygiene Among Sidewalk Vendors in Balayan, Batangas*. https://core.ac.uk/download/603657138.pdf (accessed on 29 May 2025).
4. Alter, T., Chaisowwong, W., Jenpanich, C., et al. (2016). *Assessment of Hygienic Practices Among Pig Slaughterhouses and Markets in Chiang Mai Province, Thailand*. https://core.ac.uk/download/132680354.pdf (accessed on 29 May 2025).
5. Aregai, B., & Dinku, S. (2008). *External Program Evaluation: Water, Sanitation and Hygiene (WASH) Program in Ethiopia*. https://core.ac.uk/download/71360955.pdf (accessed on 29 May 2025).
6. Awino, F. B., & Apitz, S. E. (2023). Solid waste management in the context of the waste hierarchy and circular economy frameworks: An international critical review. *Integrated Environmental Assessment and Management, 20*, 9–35. https://doi.org/10.1002/ieam.4774.
7. BC Cook Articulation Committee. (2015). *Food Safety, Sanitation, and Personal Hygiene*. Victoria, B.C.: BCcampus. Retrieved from https://opentextbc.ca/foodsafety/.(accessed on 29 May 2025).
8. Cheng, P. L., Ghazali, H., Mahyudin, N. A., & Soon, et al. (2013). *A Qualitative Study on Personal Hygiene Knowledge and Practices Among Food Handlers at Selected Primary Schools in Klang Valley area, Selangor, Malaysia*. https://core.ac.uk/download/153811705.pdf (accessed on 29 May 2025).
9. Clark, J. A. (2019). *Reducing the Risk: Psychological and Technological Approaches for Improving Handwashing Practices in The Foodservice Industry*. https://core.ac.uk/download/215464352.pdf.
10. Cortés-Sánchez, A. D. J. (2022). *About Food Safety, Viruses and Fish*. https://core.ac.uk/download/523087598.pdf (accessed on 29 May 2025).
11. Coyle, S., & Duggan, C. (2018). *Animal-Assisted Intervention for Healthcare Professionals: An Occupational Therapy Facilitated Program*. https://core.ac.uk/download/235073398.pdf.
12. Dharmage, S. C., Perret, J. L., & Ćustović, A. (2019). Epidemiology of asthma in children and adults. *Frontiers in Pediatrics, 7*, Article 246. https://doi.org/10.3389/fped.2019.00246.
13. Dhudum, B., & Bhosale, Y. (2025). Street Food Handlers' Knowledge and Hygiene Practices: A Descriptive Study. *Cureus, 17*(1), e77894. https://doi.org/10.7759/cureus.77894(accessed on 29 May 2025).
14. Dianita, I. A., Nurlena, N., & Sumarsih, U. (2024). *Evaluating Hygiene and Sanitation Practices in Pastry Equipment*. https://core.ac.uk/download/599141278.pdf.

15. Ehuwa, O., Jaiswal, A., & Jaiswal, S. (2021). *Salmonella, Food Safety and Food Handling Practices.* https://core.ac.uk/download/539113132.pdf (accessed on 29 May 2025).

16. Evans, E. W., & Redmond, E. C. (2019). Video observation of hand-hygiene compliance in a manufacturer of ready-to-eat pie and pastry products. *International journal of environmental health research, 29*(6), 593–606. https://doi.org/10.1080/09603123.2018.1558183(accessed on 29 May 2025).

17. Fair Labor Association. (2012). *Assessment Report 2012: Nike, USA AA0000000017.* https://core.ac.uk/download/33600680.pdf (accessed on 29 May 2025).

18. Faour-Klingbeil, D., & Todd, E. C. D. (2019). Prevention and control of foodborne diseases in Middle-East North African countries: Review of national control systems. *International Journal of Environmental Research and Public Health, 17*, 70. https://doi.org/10.3390/ijerph17010070.

19. Faour-Klingbeil, D., Kuri, V., & Todd, E. (2015). *Investigating a Link of Two Different Types of Food Business Management to The Food Safety Knowledge, Attitudes and Practices of Food Handlers in Beirut, Lebanon.* https://core.ac.uk/download/161938877.pdf.

20. Fung, F., Wang, H. S., & Menon, S. (2018). Food safety in the 21st century. *Biomedical Journal, 41*, 88–95. https://doi.org/10.1016/j.bj.2018.03.003.

21. Gemeda, A. A., Lemlem, G. A., Lemma, M. T., & Reta, M. A. (2021). *Food Handling Practices and Associated Factors Among Food Handlers Working in Public Food and Drink Service Establishments in Woldia Town, Northeast Ethiopia.* https://core.ac.uk/download/544239880.pdf (accessed on 29 May 2025).

22. Gomes de Freitas, R. S., da Cunha, D. T., & Stedefeldt, E. (2018). Food safety knowledge as gateway to cognitive illusions of food handlers and the different degrees of risk perception. *Food Research International, 116*, 126–134. https://doi.org/10.1016/j.foodres.2018.12.058.

23. Griffith, C. J., Jackson, L. M., & Lues, R. (2017). The food safety culture in a large South African food service complex. *British Food Journal, 119*, 729–743. https://doi.org/10.1108/bfj-11-2016-0533.

24. Griffith, C. J., Jackson, L. M., & Lues, R. (2017). The food safety culture in a large South African food service complex: Perspectives on a case study. https://core.ac.uk/download/222967850.pdf (accessed on 29 May 2025).

25. Harris, Jovan, "Risk Factors and Food-Borne Illness: An Analysis of Restaurant Violations in Georgia" (2015). *Walden Dissertations and Doctoral Studies.* 585. https://scholarworks.waldenu.edu/dissertations/585(accessed on 29 May 2025).

26. Hossen, M. T., Ferdaus, J., Hasan, M. M., Lina, N. N., Das, A. K., Barman, S. K., Paul, D. K., et al. (2020). Food safety knowledge, attitudes and practices of street food vendors in Jashore region, Bangladesh. *Food Science and Technology, 41*, 226–239. https://doi.org/10.1590/fst.13320.

27. Howard, G., Bartram, J., Brocklehurst, C., Colford, J. M., Costa, F., Cunliffe, D., Dreibelbis, R., et al. (2020). COVID-19: Urgent actions, critical reflections and future relevance of 'WaSH': Lessons for the current and future pandemics. *Journal of Water and Health, 18*, 613–630. https://doi.org/10.2166/wh.2020.162.

28. Huot, K. J., & Traiser, A. J. (2015). A protocol for animal assisted therapy in a Midwestern hospital. https://core.ac.uk/download/235073486.pdf (accessed on 29 May 2025).

29. Jackson, L. (2011). Food safety management and associated food handler behaviours in a prominent South African entertainment facility. Thesis (M. Tech. Environmental health) -- Central University of technology, Free State, 2011 (accessed on 29 May 2025).

30. Jaffee, S., Henson, S., Unnevehr, L. J., Grace, D., & Cassou, E. (2018). *The Safe Food Imperative: Accelerating Progress in Low- And Middle-Income Countries*. World Bank eBooks. https://doi.org/10.1596/978-1-4648-1345-0.

31. Jalaluddin, H., Karim, I. Q., Mohammad Nor, N., Senin, S., et al. (2020). Alternative sweetener from curculigo fruits. https://core.ac.uk/download/12007639.pdf (accessed on 29 May 2025).

32. Janik, E., Brancaleoni, R., Niemcewicz, M., Wojtas, W., Foco, M., Podogrocki, M., & Bijak, M. (2023). Healthcare waste—A serious problem for global health. *Healthcare, 11*, 242. https://doi.org/10.3390/healthcare11020242.

33. Jiang, Y., & Wen, J. (2020). Effects of COVID-19 on hotel marketing and management: A perspective article. *International Journal of Contemporary Hospitality Management, 32*, 2563–2573. https://doi.org/10.1108/ijchm-03-2020-0237.

34. Jipiu, L. B. (2016). Assessment of food safety knowledge, attitudes, practices, and training of food handlers in the context of HACCP guidelines in Malaysian public universities. https://core.ac.uk/download/89196997.pdf (accessed on 29 May 2025).

35. Johnson, P. N. T., & Yawson, R. M. (2025). Enhancing the food security of the peri-urban and urban poor through improvements to the quality, safety and economics of street-vended foods. https://core.ac.uk/download/pdf/6618604.pdf (accessed on 29 May 2025).

36. Kumari, V., & Kapur, D. (2018). Understanding barriers to compliance to food safety standards in the catering establishments using a qualitative research method: Focus group discussion. *International Journal of Scientific Research in Science and Technology*. https://doi.org/10.32628/ijsrst18401135.

37. Ogunjimi, B., Janzen Le Ber, M., (2015). Combating Food Borne Illnesses Through Safe Food Handling Practices in the United Nations/African Union Mission in Darfur (UNAMID), Sudan in: Speechley, M., & Terry, A.L. [eds] Western Public Health Casebook 2015. London, ON: Public Health Casebook Publishing. (accessed on 29 May 2025).

38. Levy de Andrade, M., Rocha Rodrigues, R., Antongiovanni, N., & da Cunha, D. T. (2019). Knowledge and risk perceptions of foodborne disease by consumers and food handlers at restaurants with different food safety profiles. *Food Research International, 121*, 845–853. https://doi.org/10.1016/j.foodres.2019.01.006.

39. Lin, S. C. (2007). Food facilities, food service workers and the flow of food: Food-borne illnesses in Taiwan's preschools. https://core.ac.uk/download/228459772.pdf (accessed on 29 May 2025).

40. Liu, Q., Luo, D., Haase, J. E., Guo, Q., Wang, X. Q., Liu, S., Xia, L., et al. (2020). The experiences of health-care providers during the COVID-19 crisis in China: A qualitative study. *The Lancet Global Health, 8*, e790–e798. https://doi.org/10.1016/s2214-109x(20)30204-7.

41. Martín, N., Mulligan, S., Shellard, I. J., & Hatton, P. V. (2022). Consensus on environmentally sustainable oral healthcare: A joint stakeholder statement. https://doi.org/10.22599/oralhealth.

42. Martín, N., Mulligan, S., Shellard, I. J., & Hatton, P. V. (2022). *Frame of Reference*. White Rose University Press eBooks. https://doi.org/10.22599/oralhealth.d.

43. Marule, N. L., du, G., & Marx-Pienaar, N. (2024). Gauteng's managers' implementation of food safety protocols and practices in their QSR environments. *Journal of Consumer Sciences*. https://www.semanticscholar.org/paper/506df82b5101cd300059e28908a5d233ff44c5d6 (accessed on 29 May 2025).

44. Missoula Vo Tech. (1973). *Missoula VoTech Course Catalog, 1973–1975*. https://core.ac.uk/download/289236229.pdf (accessed on 29 May 2025).

45. Nkhebenyane, J. S. (2018). Food hygiene risks and related practices in central South African HIV/AIDS hospices: A qualitative assessment. https://core.ac.uk/download/222968072.pdf (accessed on 29 May 2025).

46. Novak, A. C. (2016). Increasing food safety compliance with online resources. https://core.ac.uk/download/162578521.pdf (accessed on 29 May 2025).

47. Nyarugwe, S. P. (2020). *Influence of Food Safety Culture on Food Handler Behavior and Food Safety Performance of Food Processing Organizations* [Doctoral dissertation, Wageningen University]. CORE. https://core.ac.uk/download/pdf/287783995.pdf (accessed on 29 May 2025).

48. Okwuanaso, C., Onyemelukwe, N., & Ofodile, C. A. (2024). Food safety knowledge and hygiene practices among food handlers in Nnewi metropolis, southeast Nigeria. *African Journal of Clinical and Experimental Microbiology*. https://www.semanticscholar.org/paper/a56a934379d14561bdd5ae8e7511c7ae24620d2c (accessed on 29 May 2025).

49. Oliveira, I., Almeida, M., Gomes, J., & Henriques, A. R. (2024). Specific personal hygiene procedures and practices in food handlers—A cross-sectional study in butcher and fishmonger shops in Almada. *Hygiene*. https://www.semanticscholar.org/paper/a2fe172982acb009794627ce4dfccaafa10ad8fd (accessed on 29 May 2025).

50. Osaili, T. M., Al-Nabulsi, A. A., Taybeh, A. O., Ismail, L. C., & Saleh, S. T. (2023). Healthy food and determinants of food choice on online food delivery applications. *PLoS ONE, 18*, e0293004. https://doi.org/10.1371/journal.pone.0293004.

51. Oumer, A. (2019). *Determinants of Food Safety Practices Among Food Handlers in Selected Food Establishments* [Master's thesis, Addis Ababa University]. CORE. https://core.ac.uk/download/480549623.pdf (accessed on 29 May 2025).

52. Prapdopo, P., Melati, R., Nurhasanah, A., Away, J. L., & Kawuryan, R. (2024). Evaluating the role of integrated communication in enhancing brand awareness, trust, satisfaction, and repurchase intentions in Indonesia's frozen food industry. *Journal of Research in Business and Management*. https://www.semanticscholar.org/paper/21a8096a46d896baac98ce957fec8c9701b110c5 (accessed on 29 May 2025).

53. Rahman, M. T., Sobur, M. A., Islam, M. S., Ievy, S., Hossain, M. J., El Zowalaty, M. E., Rahman, A. T., et al. (2020). Zoonotic diseases: Etiology, impact, and control. *Microorganisms, 8*, 1405. https://doi.org/10.3390/microorganisms8091405.

54. Regina, G., Jing, L. S., & Hassan, Z. (2021). Food borne disease and the lifestyles of the students and food handlers in rural schools: A preliminary observation. https://core.ac.uk/download/480423510.pdf (accessed on 29 May 2025).

55. Rutherford, C. (2018). *Building Maintenance & Construction: Tools and Maintenance Tasks (Interactive)*. CORE. https://core.ac.uk/download/622362459.pdf (accessed on 29 May 2025).

56. Stearns, D. (2010). *On (cr)edibility: Why Food in The United States May Never Be Safe*. CORE. https://core.ac.uk/download/235982898.pdf (accessed on 29 May 2025).

57. Thyssen, J. P., Schuttelaar, M. L. A., Alfonso, J. H., Andersen, K. E., Angelova-Fischer, I., Arents, B. W. M., Bauer, A., et al. (2021). Guidelines for diagnosis, prevention, and treatment of hand eczema. *Contact Dermatitis, 86*, 357–378. https://doi.org/10.1111/cod.14035.

58. Todd, E. C. D. (2020). Food-borne disease prevention and risk assessment. *International Journal of Environmental Research and Public Health, 17*, 5129. https://doi.org/10.3390/ijerph17145129.

59. Uddin, T. M., Chakraborty, A., Khusro, A., Zidan, B. M. R. M., Mitra, S., Emran, T. B., Dhama, K., et al. (2021). Antibiotic resistance in microbes: History, mechanisms, therapeutic strategies and future prospects. *Journal of Infection and Public Health, 14*, 1750–1766. https://doi.org/10.1016/j.jiph.2021.10.020.

60. Van Tonder, I. (2004). *A Survey of Process Hygiene and Associated Food Handler Practices in A Retail Group in the Western Cape, South Africa* (Master's thesis, University of the Free State). CORE. https://core.ac.uk/download/222967214.pdf (accessed on 29 May 2025).

61. Wen, J., Kozak, M., Yang, S., & Liu, F. (2020). COVID-19: Potential effects on Chinese citizens' lifestyle and travel. *Tourism Review, 76*, 74–87. https://doi.org/10.1108/tr-03-2020-0110.

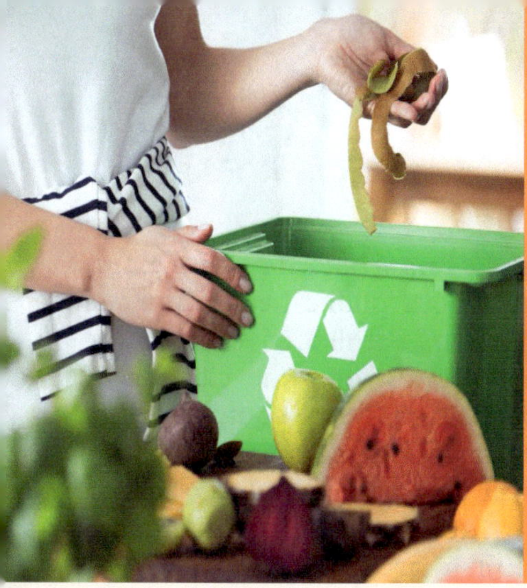

Chapter 4

SANITATION OF FOOD EQUIPMENT AND PREMISES

Contents

Introduction....81
4.1. Importance of Sanitation in Food Safety....84
4.2. Sanitation Procedures for Food Equipment....87
4.3. Sanitation Practices for Food Premises....92
4.4. Regulatory Standards and Compliance....95
Summary....101
References....102

Introduction

Food safety is improved by keeping food equipment and premises clean, which protects the health of people. Because the food industry is being watched more closely for hygiene, learning about how microbes contaminate food is now very important. Microorganisms that grow in biofilms are a major problem for keeping food areas clean. Biofilms consist of tightly bound microbial communities that can survive harsh cleaning conditions, leading to cross-contamination and spoilage, as highlighted in Carrascosa et al. (2021). Furthermore, the risk presented by emerging pathogens, such as the severe acute respiratory syndrome coronavirus 2 (SARS-CoV-2), emphasizes the need for robust sanitation protocols. With the pandemic underscoring the importance of effective food safety management systems like HACCP and GMP, maintaining sanitized environments from farm to fork has never been more crucial (Olaimat et al., 2020). So, putting more effort into sanitation helps stop foodborne illnesses and secures the health of everyone.

Definition of Sanitation in Food Service

Sanitation in food service includes all the necessary steps and rules to keep food equipment and the area clean, so food poisoning does not occur. The definition covers more than just keeping things clean by focusing on how to handle microbial risks, food leftovers and pollutants. Sanitation should include cleaning surfaces and utensils, using safe handling, storing food correctly and obeying the rules set for equipment and facilities. In addition, proper sanitation helps achieve the main goal of protecting public health by reducing the chances of contamination.

Current studies indicate significant gaps in research related to sanitation practices in various contexts, highlighting the need for targeted interventions to address these challenges and promote sustainable sanitation methods (Baquero et al., 2013; Morse et al., 2010). These factors are critical in reinforcing the importance of sanitation as a foundational element in the food service industry (Figure 4.1).

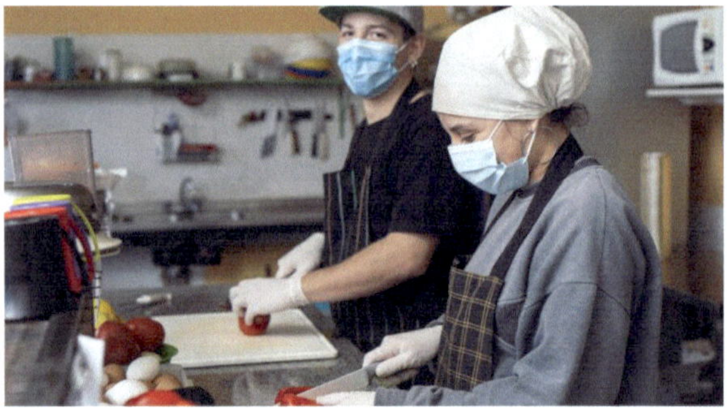

Figure 4.1. Sanitation in food service encompasses the comprehensive practices and protocols that ensure food equipment and premises are maintained in a hygienic condition to prevent foodborne illnesses.

Source: https://shapiroe.com/wp-content/uploads/2024/10/restaurant-food-safety-feature-image-770x428.jpg.

Importance of Sanitation in Food Safety

Sanitation is very important for food safety because it affects both public health and the quality of the food we eat. Effective sanitation practices encompass not only the cleanliness of food preparation areas and equipment but also involve the implementation of systematic approaches, such as Hazard Analysis Critical Control Point (HACCP) to identify potential risks and establish preventive measures. A study highlighted that while HACCP systems were adopted in 95% of large feed industries, a notable percentage of medium-sized operations lagged behind, indicating a crucial gap in food safety protocols (Sudibyo & Yulistia, 2011). Furthermore, robust legal frameworks and public health laws play an instrumental role in enforcing sanitation standards, thereby advancing the right to health and ensuring that all individuals have access to safe food (Cabrera et al., 2017). So, having a complete sanitation plan is necessary to prevent foodborne illnesses and protect the health of everyone.

Role of Sanitation in Preventing Contamination

It is very important to have good sanitation in food processing areas, especially to control biofilms. Such groups of microorganisms, protected by a strong layer, are very hard to remove from surfaces in food factories, even with traditional cleaning methods. A prime example is *Listeria monocytogenes*, a pathogen known for forming resilient biofilms, which complicates effective sanitation protocols (Mazaheri et al., 2021). Thus, creating specific disinfectants and thorough cleaning methods is necessary to stop biofilms from forming and to maintain cleanliness. Understanding the factors that contribute to biofilm development, such as surface material and environmental conditions, is essential for devising effective sanitation practices (Carrascosa et al., 2021).

By implementing rigorous sanitation measures tailored to the specific challenges posed by biofilms, food processing industries can significantly reduce the risk of contamination and enhance food safety (Figure 4.2).

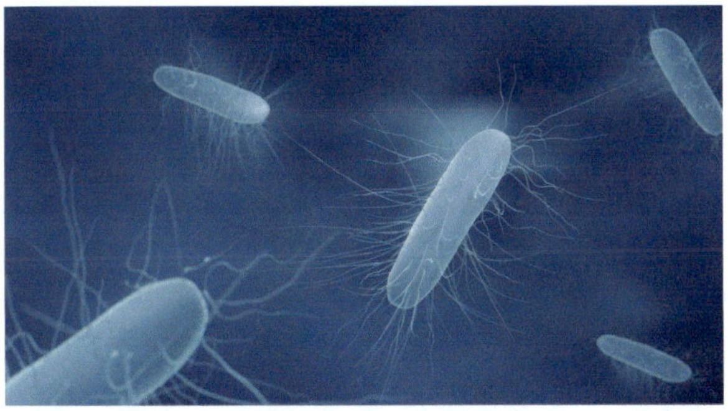

Figure 4.2. *Listeria monocytogenes*, a pathogen known for forming resilient biofilms, which complicates effective sanitation protocols.

Source: https://s7g10.scene7.com/is/image/biomerieux/Listeria-Image-1600x900?qlt=85&wid=480&ts=1719939286132&dpr=on,2.625

Legal Regulations Governing Food Sanitation

Rules for food sanitation in the law are important for public health by setting guidelines for food businesses. The laws help maintain cleanliness in food equipment and areas , which lowers the risk of food contamination and diseases. Effective public health laws are essential in creating an environment that supports the right to health, as evidenced in various successful case studies from around the world (Cabrera et al., 2017). Moreover, the comprehensive framework established by these regulations encompasses critical areas , such as cleanliness, proper waste disposal, and equipment maintenance, which are vital for the efficient functioning of food services (Fair Labor Association, 2006). Governments use these standards to ensure food is safe and to gain public trust in the food supply , which is good for the community's well-being.

Historical Context of Food Sanitation Practices

How food sanitation has changed over the years reflects the growth of public health and safety, resulting in better cleaning of food equipment and facilities. Local knowledge and customs were the main sources of food safety before the industrial era and there were few official rules. Because of the industrial revolution, food production and delivery increased , which pointed out the importance of proper sanitation to prevent foodborne illnesses. The early 20th century saw new knowledge about pathogens and hygiene , which led to better sanitation rules. Innovations , such as integrated pest management (IPM) emphasized the selective application of insecticides as a cornerstone of food safety, enhancing traditional methods through new technologies (Stejskal et al., 2021). Moreover, recognizing the socio-economic factors influencing health outcomes, as noted in the Nigerian context, underscores that equitable food sanitation practices must address not only technical measures but also broader societal issues (Abubakar et al., 2022) (Figure 4.3).

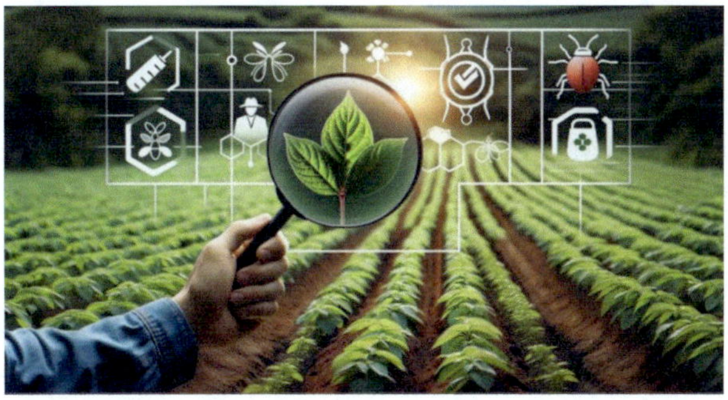

Figure 4.3. Innovations , such as integrated pest management (IPM) emphasized the selective application of insecticides as a cornerstone of food safety, enhancing traditional methods through new technologies.

Source: https://ardini.in/wp-content/uploads/2024/08/IPM-1024x553.png.

Scope of Sanitation in Food Equipment and Premises

Taking care of food equipment and premises is very important for food safety, as it involves many practices to avoid contamination. Sanitation practices help to keep food hygienic and also increase the quality of the food. When standard cleaning methods are used, food contact surfaces are clean and safe , which lessens the risk of foodborne illnesses. It has been found that using HACCP systems greatly affects the way food businesses handle sanitation. According to findings, 95% of large feed industries have implemented HACCP, highlighting the correlation between sanitation compliance and industry size, while only 65% of medium enterprises have followed suit (Sudibyo & Yulistia, 2011). Furthermore, a comprehensive understanding of potential critical control points can mitigate hazards effectively, ensuring safer food production in diverse settings, as demonstrated in various studies (Baquero et al., 2013).

4.1. Importance of Sanitation in Food Safety

Sanitation is very important in food safety because it helps protect us from foodborne diseases. When food is prepared in a clean environment, the chance of contamination is greatly decreased , which is good for public health. For instance, a study that analyzed ready-to-eat (RTE) foods demonstrated a concerning presence of Staphylococcus aureus, where findings indicated that 53% of the tested samples were contaminated. This points out that the cleanliness of food premises is important for the safety of the food made there. Although 92% of the surveyed food premises were classified as sanitary, the presence of *S. aureus* in cooked food highlights the potential hazards that persist, especially in establishments lacking rigorous sanitation standards (Wahab et al., 2016). Furthermore, assessing sanitation gaps can drive research priorities, as evidenced in Malawi's environmental health sector, ensuring that comprehensive action plans are developed to enhance food safety protocols (Morse et al., 2010).

4.1.1. Economic Consequences of Food Contamination

The results of food contamination can be seen right away in medical bills and later in problems for public health and the economy. If foodborne illnesses happen, people who are sick use more medical care , which increases costs and reduces their ability to work. If an outbreak occurs, it can lower consumer confidence , which leads to fewer sales for food businesses and suppliers and major financial losses along the supply chain.

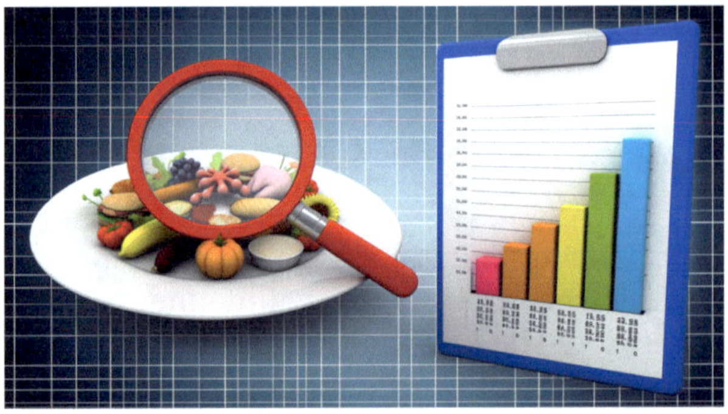

Figure 4.4. When foodborne illnesses occur, affected individuals burden healthcare resources, leading to increased medical expenses and loss of productivity due to missed workdays.

Source: https://media.licdn.com/dms/image/v2/D4D12AQG26jA0vWZgzg/article-cover_image-shrink_720_1280/article-cover_image-shrink_720_1280/0/1725278356033?e=2147483647&v=beta&t=GrSFcPRKNeGZck6-nql8mQanqPcFYTyAYY_NDQQWivY.

The role of zoonotic diseases, as noted in Rahman et al. (2020), exacerbates these concerns by highlighting the connection between animal health, food safety, and human disease transmission, thus necessitating robust sanitation practices. Additionally, water pollution contributes to food contamination risks, perpetuating a cycle of disease and economic strain, as indicated in Lin et al. (2022). Thus, effective sanitation of food equipment and premises emerges as a critical strategy not only for safeguarding health but also for mitigating extensive economic repercussions (Figure 4.4).

4.1.2. Consumer Trust and Business Reputation

Having trust from consumers and a good business reputation depends on how clean food equipment and premises are in the industry. If consumers think a business is very clean and follows strict sanitation rules, they are more likely to trust the food they serve. Having trust in a brand leads to more purchases and keeps customers loyal , which brings about more business and good references. Also, companies that handle sanitation well are usually regarded as more responsible and ethical , which helps improve their reputation. The main issue is putting proper sanitation measures in place while dealing with the difficulties of technology and running the business efficiently. For instance, as businesses explore automation and AI-driven analytics to maintain cleanliness, they must ensure that these technologies do not undermine consumer perceptions of safety and trustworthiness (Himeur et al., 2022; Giovanni, 2023). Taking action on sanitation helps build consumer trust and a good reputation for the business , which leads to lasting success.

4.1.3. Role of Sanitation in Food Quality

Sanitation is very important for food quality because it affects both safety and the health of those who eat it. Sanitation is very important in food processing to stop contamination and the spread of dangerous pathogens. According to recent studies, biofilms formed by microorganisms on food equipment can significantly compromise sanitation efforts; these resilient structures are notorious for their ability to withstand disinfectants, leading to potential outbreaks and food spoilage (Carrascosa et al., 2021). Moreover, inadequate sanitation practices contribute to broader public health challenges, as highlighted in discussions about Nigeria's health system, where significant food safety concerns intersect with poor sanitation infrastructure (Abubakar et al., 2022). By investing in robust sanitation protocols and regular cleaning regimens, the food industry can mitigate risks associated with foodborne illnesses, thereby enhancing overall food quality and ensuring the well-being of consumers (Figure 4.5).

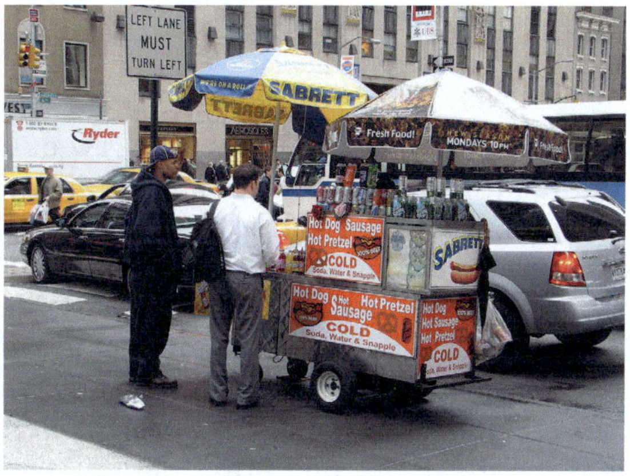

Figure 4.5. Effective sanitation practices, particularly in food processing environments, are crucial for preventing contamination and the proliferation of harmful pathogens.

Source: By hu:User:Totya - Own work, CC BY-SA 3.0, https://commons.wikimedia.org/w/index.php?curid=1561473

4.1.4. Connection Between Sanitation and Food Spoilage

It is important for food safety and quality in the food industry that sanitation and food spoilage are related. If sanitation is not done properly, it can allow microorganisms to multiply , which leads to food spoilage and both financial and health problems. Empirical evidence highlights that effective cleaning and sanitation measures not only reduce pathogenic viruses, , such as SARS-CoV-2, but also mitigate the growth of spoilage organisms that compromise food integrity, affirming the critical need for rigorous hygiene protocols (Ezzatpanah et al., 2022). Furthermore, the implementation of Environmental Monitoring Programs (EMPs) enables food producers to validate their cleaning efforts and adapt strategies against various microbial threats, including spoilage and hygiene indicators (Mota et al., 2022). Thus, strict sanitation is necessary to stop food from spoiling, guarantee its safety and keep products usable for as long as they are meant to be.

4.1.5. Importance of Employee Training in Sanitation

It is very important to train employees on sanitation to keep food equipment and the entire premises clean and safe. Good training programs help employees realize that sanitation is very important, so they can spot risks and clean properly. The training helps to prevent contamination and also encourages staff to be more careful and responsible, improving better management of the operation. Moreover, as illustrated by extensive research on workplace conditions, companies that prioritize sanitation training often experience lower rates of foodborne illnesses and comply better with regulatory standards, reflecting a commitment to both employee welfare and customer safety (Fair Labor Association, 2011). Additionally, a robust training program can empower staff to take ownership of sanitation processes, contributing to continuous improvement and adherence to best practices in food safety (Worker Rights Consortium, 2011). The importance of employee training in sanitation extends beyond compliance—it is an investment in the organization's integrity and reputation (Figure 4.6).

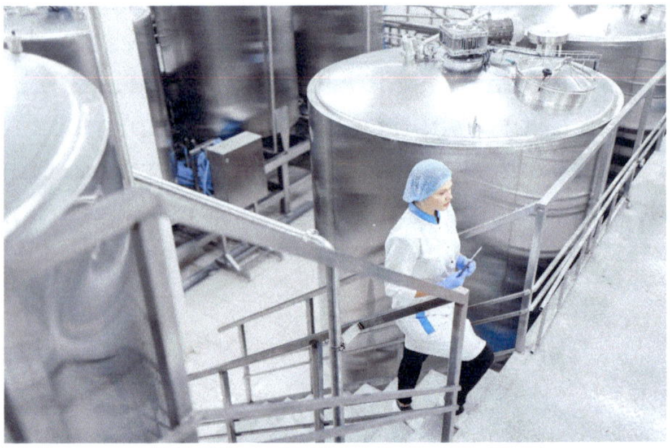

Figure 4.6. Ensuring that employees are well-trained in sanitation practices is critical for maintaining the hygiene and safety of food equipment and premises.

Source: https://d2evkimvhatqav.cloudfront.net/images/female_factory_tablet_164389055.jpg?v=1632174638.

4.1.6. Case Studies of Sanitation Failures

Sanitation problems seriously affect public health, especially in places where food is handled, as shown by a number of case studies about poor hygiene practices. A key example was when sanitation laws were not followed properly , which resulted in many people getting sick from food, proving how important effective laws are for health safety. The World Health Organization has emphasized that robust public health laws are essential in ensuring that fundamental functions, such as clean water and sanitation, are properly managed and regulated, which is crucial for food safety (Cabrera et al., 2017). In addition, new ways of handling sanitation can be profitable, as shown in a 2016 study by the Toilet Board Coalition , which looked at using sanitation resources in the circular economy and found that there are many unexplored opportunities to improve sanitation and meet market needs. Such information is necessary for improving sanitation in food areas.

4.1.7. Best Practices for Maintaining Sanitation Standards

Many important best practices arise in the effort to maintain high sanitation in food equipment and areas. A regular and effective cleaning plan should be set up, mainly for surfaces and equipment that are in touch with food items.

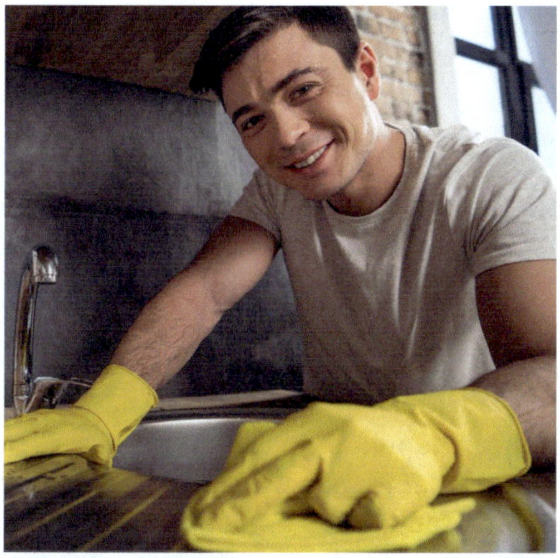

Figure 4.7. Regular and thorough cleaning schedules should be established, focusing on both surfaces and equipment that come into direct contact with food products.

Source: https://www.foodsafe.net.nz/wp-content/uploads/2021/09/A-food-handler-using-a-kitchen-cleaning-checklist-to-clean.jpg

Using the right cleaning products and making sure staff are trained to use them well can improve sanitation a lot. In addition, regular inspections and audits help find any possible contaminants and take care of them right away. HACCP helps food companies prevent food safety problems by focusing on prevention, rather than only reacting to them. Also, building a hygiene culture among staff, so that following sanitation rules is part of their daily tasks, helps to maintain these standards. Such comprehensive practices align with insights from industry reports, which highlight the intersection of labor rights and working conditions in achieving effective sanitation (Fair Labor Association, 2004) (Figure 4.7).

4.1.8. Future Trends in Food Safety and Sanitation

With changes in food safety and sanitation, more effort is being put into handling the challenges of microbial resistance and biofilm growth on equipment used for food. The advent of advanced technologies, including biofilm control strategies, is critical in managing persistent pathogens like *Listeria monocytogenes*, which thrive in food processing environments and resist conventional cleaning methods (Mazaheri et al., 2021). Future food sanitation will depend on having standardized rules that can be used in many areas and that are adjusted for different surfaces, types of products and the environment. Furthermore, integrating these sanitation efforts with broader public health initiatives, as highlighted in the context of Nigerian health outcomes, underscores the importance of sanitation in elevating overall population health (Abubakar et al., 2022). By using this approach, risks from foodborne illnesses will be reduced and a culture of safety and responsibility will grow within the industry.

4.2. Sanitation Procedures for Food Equipment

Using effective sanitation methods on food equipment helps prevent foodborne illnesses and keeps food service areas very clean. It is very important to clean everything regularly, inspect thoroughly and maintain all equipment, including mixers and slicers, to have an effective sanitation system. Implementation of systems like HACCP has been shown to significantly enhance food safety compliance, particularly within the feed industry, where the understanding of critical control points (CCPs) is crucial (Sudibyo & Yulistia, 2011). Since equipment can collect pathogens, using food-safe sanitizers and making sure everything is dried properly is very important. Furthermore, training staff on the significance of these procedures enhances overall safety awareness and operational efficiency, ultimately supporting public health objectives in food operations (Fair Labor Association, 2006). So, it is important to follow these strict sanitation rules to ensure food safety is maintained.

4.2.1. Types of Food Equipment Requiring Sanitation

Cleaning food equipment is very important for food safety and avoiding contamination in different parts of the food industry. You should clean processing machinery, storage containers, utensils and food preparation surfaces very well. These components are critical as they frequently come into contact with food products, making them susceptible to contamination by pathogens, particularly biofilms produced by microorganisms like *Listeria monocytogenes*, which may adhere firmly to surfaces and resist standard cleaning methods (Mazaheri et al., 2021).

Proper and frequent sanitation procedures are key to getting rid of biofilms and stop foodborne illnesses. Moreover, the specific sanitation methods should be tailored to the type of equipment and the nature of the food being processed, underlining the need for a multifaceted approach (Abubakar et al., 2022). Ultimately, ensuring the cleanliness of food equipment is vital not only for public health but also for ensuring the operational efficacy of food production systems (Figure 4.8).

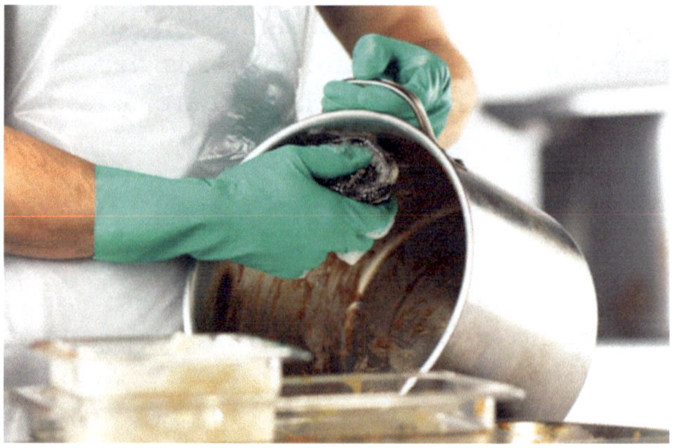

Figure 4.8. Equipment that requires thorough sanitation includes processing machinery, storage containers, utensils, and food preparation surfaces.

Source: https://foodhandler.com/webfoo/wp-content/uploads/2014/09/JS_Nitrile_Reusable-Gloves_Green-18-mil-Scouring_1212-03_01.jpg

4.2.2. Cleaning vs. Sanitizing: Definitions and Differences

Food safety depends on the difference between cleaning and sanitizing, which are both important for keeping food areas and equipment clean. To clean, you physically remove dirt, grease and food remains from surfaces along with using detergents, but to sanitize, you apply chemicals to lower the number of dangerous microorganisms. This difference is very important, especially in dairy facilities, since *Listeria monocytogenes* can easily survive in wet areas. Effective cleaning must precede sanitizing, as demonstrated in studies, the presence of organic matter, such as skim milk, can significantly diminish the effectiveness of sanitizers like peroxyacetic acid (PAA). Furthermore, regulations prohibit the sale of adulterated milk products, highlighting the importance of meticulous cleaning and sanitizing practices to ensure compliance and food safety (South Carolina Department of Health and Environmental Control, 2005).

4.2.3. Recommended Cleaning Agents and Sanitizers

Keeping food equipment and the premises clean is very important for food safety and to stop pathogens from spreading. Using detergents that clean away food and organic matter , which might contain harmful microorganisms, is advised. Once the first cleaning is done, chlorine compounds, quaternary ammonium compounds and hydrogen peroxide should be used to get pathogens down to a safe level. The efficacy of these agents is particularly critical in light of recent health concerns, like those raised during the COVID-19 pandemic, where heightened sanitation protocols became necessary to mitigate transmission risks (Chamola et al., 2020). Additionally, targeted strategies for controlling foodborne pathogens like *Listeria monocytogenes* emphasize not only the use of effective sanitizers but also the need for understanding specific food characteristics and environments that promote their survival (Buchanan et al., 2016). Implementing these recommended cleaning agents and sanitizers is essential for maintaining hygienic food preparation areas (Figure 4.9).

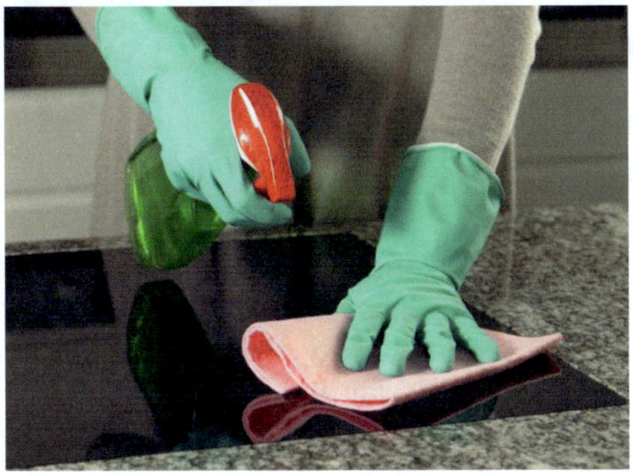

Figure 4.9. Effective sanitation of food equipment and premises is paramount to ensuring food safety and preventing the spread of pathogens.

Source: https://www.health.wa.gov.au/~/media/Corp/Images/Health-for/Food/Toolkit/images/cleaning.jpg.

4.2.4. Proper Techniques for Cleaning Equipment

Cleaning food equipment properly is necessary for food safety and to avoid contamination. A good way to clean is to pre-clean, wash, rinse and sanitize all the equipment. Removing residue and food at the start helps the other cleaning steps work much better. Using the correct cleaning agents and tools for different fabrics and kinds of dirt is very important to stop cross-contamination. Food service professionals should understand that different surfaces call for various methods and products, which helps maintain high sanitation standards everywhere. Furthermore, the incorporation of modern technologies, such as automated cleaning systems and IoT monitoring devices, enhances compliance with sanitation protocols, substantially reducing human error and improving operational efficiency (Bellini et al., 2022). Ultimately, adhering to established cleaning methodologies is vital to fostering public health and safeguarding the integrity of food supplies (Zandona et al., 2021).

4.2.5. Frequency of Sanitation for Different Equipment

Properly cleaning different food equipment frequently helps maintain food safety and avoid any contamination. Since different types of equipment, for example, slicers, mixers and food processors, are used differently, they need to be cleaned according to their own schedules and risk of bacteria. For example, equipment that comes into contact with raw foods should be cleaned after every use, but equipment for cooked foods needs to be cleaned less often, but still needs to be cleaned according to the rules. A strict cleaning schedule helps comply with regulations and improves how the food establishment works. Additionally, monitoring compliance is crucial; systems like Tracking Charts, as noted in the literature, provide transparency regarding sanitation practices and help identify areas for improvement (Fair Labor Association, 2008). Ultimately, understanding the specific sanitation needs of various kitchen equipment is critical to safeguarding public health and enhancing the overall efficacy of food safety protocols (Dutta et al., 2012) (Figure 4.10).

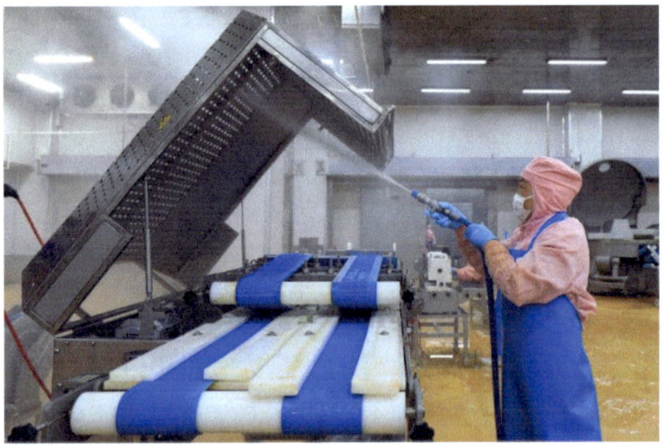

Figure 4.10. Maintaining appropriate sanitation frequency for different food equipment is essential to ensure food safety and prevent contamination.

Source: https://www.camcode.com/wp-content/uploads/2022/12/Food-Machinery-Cleaning.jpg.

4.2.6. Importance of Equipment Maintenance

Proper sanitation of food equipment and areas depends strongly on routine equipment maintenance. Looking after the equipment correctly helps keep it useful for a long time and also stops contamination and foodborne illness. If equipment is not maintained, it can allow harmful bacteria to grow , which can harm food safety and the health of the public. Moreover, carrying out maintenance activities, , such as equipment cleaning and inspection, can enhance the efficiency of the restaurant and avoid sudden breakdowns during peak usage in the restaurant. In addition, an analysis done to determine gaps in environmental health practices emphasizes the need for a systemic approach toward maintenance of equipment in food premises, which is vital in maintaining public health standards (Morse et al., 2010). Appropriate maintenance procedures, in turn, provide a more secure food handling environment, reflecting an interest in quality and cleanliness that is congruent with universal sanitation goals (Fair Labor Association, 2011).

4.2.7. Role of Temperature in Sanitation Processes

Temperature is very important in cleaning food equipment and areas, mainly because it affects the survival and growth of microbes. Effective sanitation relies on maintaining specific temperature thresholds during food processing, as evidenced in the production of pineapple juice, where temperatures must be carefully controlled to mitigate the growth of spoilage microorganisms like Saccharomyces cerevisiae (Ackah et al., 2014).

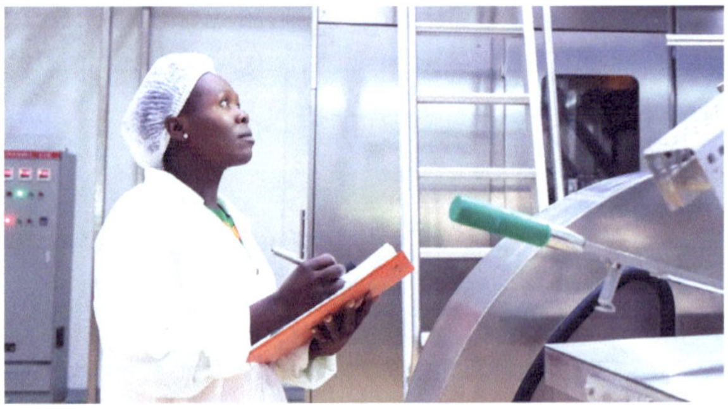

Figure 4.11. Temperature plays a pivotal role in the sanitation processes of food equipment and premises, primarily through its influence on microbial survival and growth.

Source: https://droppe-blog-media.s3.eu-north-1.amazonaws.com/Food_processing_1_970c03d7d2.webp.

Temperature control is also necessary in blanched frozen vegetable processing to stop *Listeria monocytogenes* from growing. The relationship between time and temperature (t/T) significantly impacts food safety during both processing and storage, where improper management can lead to severe health risks, particularly among vulnerable populations (FSA BIOHAZ Panel (EFSA Panel on Biological Hazards), 2020). Thus, incorporating stringent temperature protocols is essential for ensuring hygiene and prolonging the shelf life of food products, ultimately enhancing public health outcomes in food production environments (Figure 4.11).

4.2.8. Common Challenges in Equipment Sanitation

Proper cleaning of food equipment is often difficult, which can seriously affect public health. One big problem is that biofilms can remain on surfaces even after they have been cleaned and disinfected, so it becomes hard to maintain good sanitation. In addition, the use of stainless steel, plastic and wood in equipment means that cleaning must be done differently because each material absorbs and gets contaminated in its own way. Because there are no standard sanitation rules in food service industries, it is difficult to keep equipment clean, which can result in foodborne illnesses. Additionally, legal frameworks surrounding public health sanitation are often underutilized, which hinders the enforcement of rigorous cleaning standards and practices necessary for effective sanitation (Morse et al., 2010). Addressing these challenges is vital for ensuring safe food handling and compliance with health regulations (Cabrera et al., 2017).

4.2.9. Innovations in Sanitation Technology for Food Equipment

New technologies for cleaning food equipment have greatly improved how food safety is maintained in commercial kitchens and food processing areas. Automated cleaning, using UV-C light for disinfection and sensors that monitor cleanliness, have greatly improved how well sanitation is done. They help reduce mistakes by people and also make sure that health regulations are followed , which matters a lot now that foodborne illness outbreaks are on the rise. For instance, the application of HACCP regulations has shown that targeted inspections can yield higher compliance with sanitation standards, although the effects of HACCP on overall sanitation compliance remain complex, as indicated by investigations into FDA inspection practices (Alberini et al., 2025). Furthermore, the economic implications of these innovations underscore the need for strategic investments in sanitation technology to address both social and environmental needs, highlighting their potential as critical enablers in the food sector (Figure 4.12).

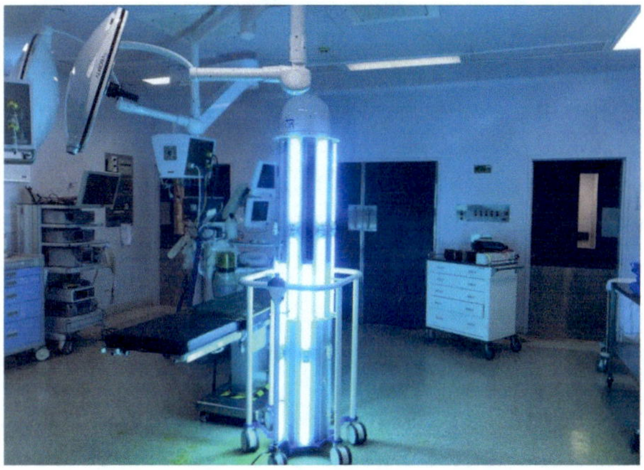

Figure 4.12. Innovations , such as automated cleaning systems, UV-C light sanitation methods, and smart sensors for real-time monitoring of hygienic conditions have significantly enhanced the efficiency and effectiveness of sanitation protocols.

Source: Browne K. Brought to Light: How Ultraviolet Disinfection Can Prevent the Nosocomial Transmission of COVID-19 and Other Infectious Diseases. *Applied Microbiology*. 2021; 1(3):537-556. https://doi.org/10.3390/applmicrobiol1030035

4.3. Sanitation Practices for Food Premises

Food premises need effective sanitation to protect both the food and the health of people. The use of protocols , such as HACCP is very important for finding and handling possible hazards in food processing. Research indicates that large feed industries show a higher degree of compliance with such systems, with 95% implementing HACCP, compared to only 65% in medium-sized operations, highlighting a significant variance in sanitation adherence across different business scales (Sudibyo & Yulistia, 2011). Also, the success of sanitation depends on both technical actions and the way management views and prioritizes food safety. Identifying research gaps within the environmental health sector can further refine sanitation practices and enhance compliance across all levels of food production (Morse et al., 2010). All these factors stress the role of good sanitation in ensuring food is safe and of good quality in any food business.

4.3.1. Importance of a Clean Food Preparation Area

It is very important to keep the food preparation area clean, since this helps keep food safe and protects the public. A sanitized environment minimizes the risk of foodborne illnesses, which are predominantly caused by harmful microorganisms that thrive in unsanitary conditions, particularly in meat, dairy, and egg products (Abebe et al., 2020). If food preparation areas are not clean, it can spread pathogens and cause gastrointestinal problems as well as other serious health issues. In addition, stricter food safety measures ensure that food is safe and make customers believe in the quality of the food served. Implementation of Good Manufacturing Practices (GMP) and compliance with HACCP standards are proven measures in ensuring cleanliness and the prevention of contamination (Chopra et al., 2020). Hence, a careful sanitation practice in food preparation environments must be pursued to ensure a safe food supply and the overall health of the community (Figure 4.13).

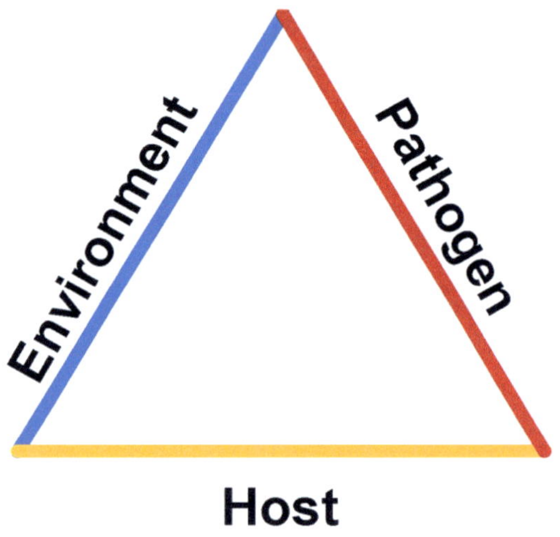

Figure 4.13. A sanitized environment minimizes the risk of foodborne illnesses, which are predominantly caused by harmful microorganisms that thrive in unsanitary conditions, particularly in meat, dairy, and egg products.

Source: Browne K. Brought to Light: How Ultraviolet Disinfection Can Prevent the Nosocomial Transmission of COVID-19 and Other Infectious Diseases. *Applied Microbiology*. 2021; 1(3):537-556. https://doi.org/10.3390/applmicrobiol1030035

4.3.2. Guidelines for Cleaning Floors and Surfaces

It is extremely crucial to thoroughly clean floors and surfaces in areas of food preparation to prevent illnesses and maintain cleanliness. Areas must have a standard procedure that entails cleaning and disinfecting. From research, visual inspections of cleanliness do not necessarily hold up against microbiological safety, highlighting the importance of rigorous cleaning processes to reduce chances of contamination, especially where there is a risk of cross-contamination, like kitchens and food preparation surfaces (Faour-Klingbeil et al., 2016). Additionally, businesses must ensure that cleaning supplies and methods align with GMP and Good Hygiene Practices (GHP) to meet regulatory standards (Laswai et al., 2013). Appropriate cleaning agents should be used, the manufacturer's directions for dilution and contact time should be followed and surfaces must be kept clean and tidy. Following these rules allows food service businesses to improve their hygiene and keep people safe.

4.3.3. Waste Management and Its Role in Sanitation

Good waste management is essential to cleanliness in food equipment and spaces, as it prevents contamination and ensures hygiene. Improper waste management can lead to more pathogenic microorganisms , which compromise food safety.

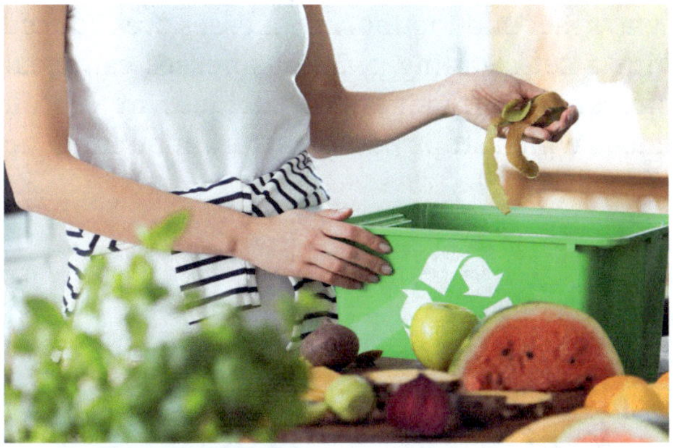

Figure 4.14. Effective waste management is pivotal in ensuring proper sanitation within food equipment and premises, as it directly influences the prevention of contamination and the maintenance of hygiene standards.

Source: https://evreka.co/wp-content/uploads/2021/01/woman-composting-organic-kitchen-waste-PGUM28D-1024x683.jpg

For example, biofilms with their reputation for disinfection resistance are known to develop on surfaces when organic waste lodges there, hence making it difficult to clean them and posing a high risk of foodborne disease (Carrascosa et al., 2021). In addition, it has been shown that creating efficient policies for waste management can considerably decrease the use of water and enhance hygiene standards, which is important in conditions where water shortage is an issue (Crouch et al., 2021). Thus, incorporating effective waste management systems not only helps in curbing environmental damage but also performs a crucial function of keeping food premises and equipment sanitary, ultimately protecting public health (Figure 4.14).

4.3.4. Pest Control Measures in Food Premises

Pest control is very important in food premises to ensure that food preparation and storage areas are safe and clean. They cover a variety of actions , such as checking the premises often, managing waste correctly and using IPM methods. Inspections done often help find pest problems early and strong waste management keeps pests away from food. Also, IPM works to stop pests in the long run by using biological, cultural and physical methods with pesticides , which helps reduce the risk of health problems from these chemicals. The integration of pest control measures must be complemented by robust sanitation protocols, as highlighted in recent research that emphasizes the importance of water, sanitation, and hygiene (WASH) in mitigating disease transmission in food settings (Howard et al., 2020). All of these approaches together support the maintenance of food safety in food businesses.

4.3.5. Importance of Handwashing Stations

Handwashing stations are very important for keeping food equipment and areas clean, mainly in places where food safety matters a lot.

They give food handlers a special area to stay clean , which greatly decreases the chances of contamination. The importance of these stations is underscored by findings from large-scale hygiene promotion campaigns, which highlight that effective handwashing practices are critical for achieving desired health outcomes (Coville et al., 2015). In addition, studies stress that both access to handwashing and changing people's habits are important for following handwashing guidelines. So, having handwashing stations alone is not enough; they should be well placed and encouraged so that food workers use them regularly. Such measures are essential in safeguarding public health and promoting overall sanitation in food-related settings (Figure 4.15).

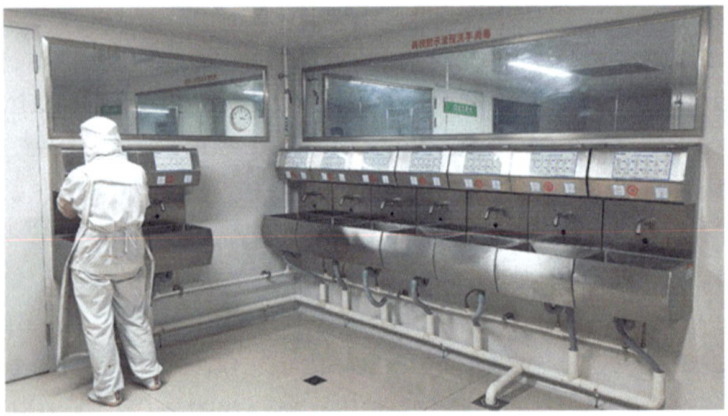

Figure 4.15. Handwashing stations play a pivotal role in ensuring the sanitation of food equipment and premises, particularly in environments where food safety is paramount.

Source: https://woneclean.com/wp-content/uploads/2024/12/%E5%B0%81%E9%9D%A2-4.png.

4.3.6. Role of Personal Hygiene in Food Sanitation

Looking after personal hygiene is very important for food sanitation and the health and safety of everyone. If food handlers do not wash their hands or keep themselves clean, they might transfer germs to the food preparation area , which can result in food illnesses. Many cases of cross-contamination happen when workers move from one task to another without cleaning their hands , which stresses the importance of strong personal hygiene rules in food service. Also, the study of government actions during the COVID-19 pandemic shows that hygiene is key to food safety, showing that society values health. The hospitality industry's alignment with sustainable practices, as documented in recent studies, reflects an awareness that personal hygiene not only safeguards customers but also enhances overall operational efficacy, thus reinforcing the importance of integrating effective hygiene management within the sanitation of food equipment and premises (E-Murage et al., 2022; Singh et al., 2024).

4.3.7. Cleaning Schedules and Checklists

For food equipment and premises to be kept clean, schedules and checklists are necessary since they guarantee that hygiene standards are always met and foodborne illnesses are reduced. With a set cleaning plan, businesses can clean different equipment and surfaces at certain times , which stops pathogens from building up.

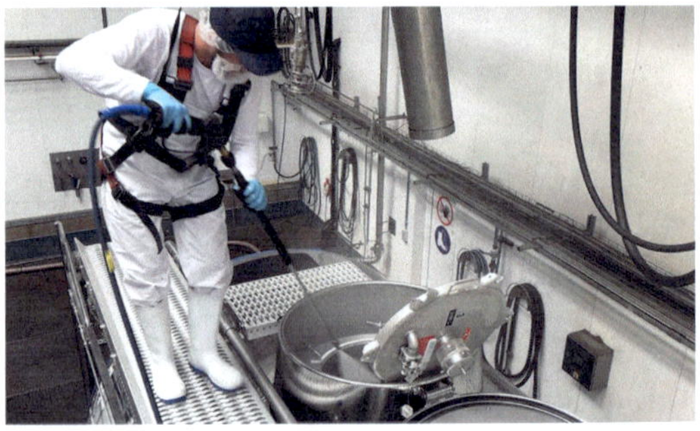

Figure 4.16. Effective cleaning schedules and checklists are vital components in the sanitation of food equipment and premises, as they ensure consistent adherence to hygiene protocols and the minimization of foodborne illnesses.

Source: https://www.food-safety.com/ext/resources/Images/2025/April/SC-0425-900-Img1.jpg?1745937291.

They not only improve how clean the area is but also help ensure food safety rules are met. For instance, a study highlighted that improving food safety knowledge and practices in restaurants is essential to mitigate bacterial hazards, including *Salmonella enterica* (Bolton et al., 2007). Also, in healthcare, guidelines encourage routine cleaning of the environment to emphasize the need for cleanliness in places that deal with food preparation. Consequently, the establishment and adherence to comprehensive cleaning schedules and checklists play an integral role in sustaining safe food environments and protecting public health (Figure 4.16)..

4.3.8. Training Staff on Premises Sanitation

It is very important to provide proper training on cleanliness for staff to keep food areas clean and avoid food poisoning. Training should cover the proper sanitation rules that are right for the facility, mainly in the food service industry. When employees are taught about the CCPs for sanitation, organizations help build a culture of safety and responsibility. Studies indicate a strong correlation between managerial awareness of hygiene practices and effective implementation of HACCP systems, highlighting the importance of thorough training (Sudibyo & Yulistia, 2011). Furthermore, comprehensive training not only reinforces compliance with health regulations but also enhances organizational resilience against potential sanitation failures (Fair Labor Association, 2006). Training staff on how to maintain cleanliness in the kitchen can result in much safer food for all and the continued success of the food business.

4.3.9. Assessing the Effectiveness of Sanitation Practices

It is very important for food safety and public health that sanitation practices in the food industry are effective. You should evaluate the ways these practices get rid of contaminants and in this case, biofilms are a main concern for food equipment and surfaces. Notably, *Listeria monocytogenes* thrives within biofilms and is notoriously difficult to eradicate due to its protective matrix, necessitating rigorous sanitation protocols tailored to specific environments and materials used in food processing (Mazaheri et al., 2021). Furthermore, Nigeria's public health system faces unique challenges, including inadequate sanitation and hygiene, exacerbated by socioeconomic disparities and insufficient resources (Abubakar et al., 2022). As a result, following good sanitation measures increases food safety and also helps with health issues related to nutrition and preventing diseases. Thus, a critical analysis of current sanitation strategies is essential for fostering a safer food environment (Figure 4.17).

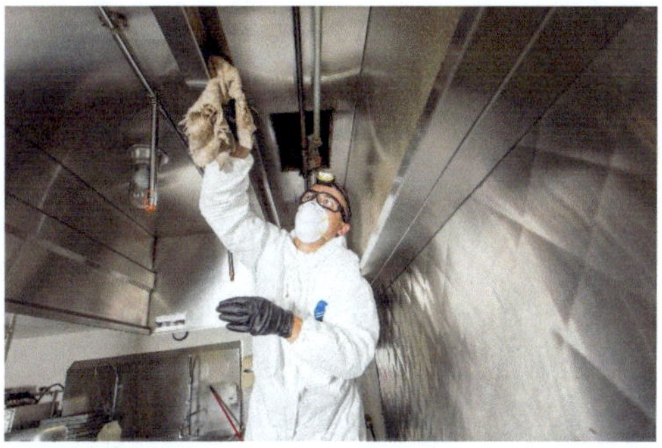

Figure 4.17. The effectiveness of sanitation practices in the food industry is paramount to ensuring food safety and public health.

Source: https://www.clearchoiceuk.com/wp-content/uploads/2022/12/10-Best-Practices-for-Cleaning-and-Sanitation-in-the-Food-Industry.jpg

4.4. Regulatory Standards and Compliance

Food safety is highly dependent on proper regulation and ensuring it is adhered to in ensuring food equipment and building cleanliness. Compliance with HACCP regulations requires rigorous inspection of facilities, ensuring sanitation requirements are upheld. Still, evidence indicates that the efficiency of such inspections can be derailed by an ineffectual targeted enforcement, seen in FDA practices where inspections were not concurrent with product risk or prior records of compliance, eventually influencing the compliance with sanitation standards (Alberini et al., 2025). In addition, the standards associated with organic and low-input foods add further complexity to compliance since processors have to deal with multiple quality parameters while balancing consumer safety requirements (Beck et al., 2006). Therefore, establishing specific guidelines for food processors becomes necessary in order to comply with regulations as well as make the whole food safety system more robust.

4.4.1. Overview of Food Safety Regulations

The safety of food regulations helps to ensure that people in the food supply chain are healthy. Effective laws are essential not only for safeguarding public health but also for advancing the right to health within communities, as highlighted by the collaborative efforts of organizations like the WHO and the International Development Law Organization (Cabrera et al., 2017). They cover different areas , such as food processing, sanitation and enforcing rules that prevent hazards, so that food equipment and premises are always safe. Moreover, regulations specifically target food processing procedures, offering guidance on the complex requirements in organic and low-input food sectors to enhance safety and quality (Beck et al., 2006). Ultimately, a robust regulatory environment is indispensable for fostering consumer confidence and promoting safe food practices across the industry (Figure 4.18).

Figure 4.18. Food safety regulations serve as a critical framework for ensuring the health and well-being of consumers in the food supply chain.

Source: https://www.ficsi.in/blog/wp-content/uploads/2023/09/blog21-1.jpg.

4.4.2. Role of the FDA and USDA in Sanitation

It all relies heavily upon the FDA and USDA to inspect for sanitation in premises and equipment for food. They employ strict guidelines and inspection techniques to ensure food-making facilities are safe and clean. The FDA is concerned with the general safety of the food supply, checking on sanitation procedures in all industries, whereas the USDA is particularly interested in meat, poultry, and egg products and implements HACCP plans to ensure sanitary conditions (Sant'Ana et al., 2023). In addition, their duties also involve the detection of emerging threats to food safety, as indicated by the systematic approach to emerging threats employed by the European Food Safety Authority (EFSA) that has impacted U.S. practice (Bottex et al., 2023). The FDA and USDA enhance sanitation by collaborating with industry players and utilizing scientific approaches , which safeguards consumers from contracting illnesses through food.

4.4.3. Local Health Department (LHDs) Regulations

Local health department (LHDs) regulations play a crucial role in ensuring the sanitation of food equipment and premises, which is pivotal for safeguarding public health. They set basic rules for cleanliness, sanitation and food safety , which help stop foodborne illnesses. As an illustration, they require routine checks of food service places to see if they are following sanitation rules and keeping equipment that touches food clean and well-maintained. Biofilms , which can protect pathogens from cleaning agents, show why strict rules are needed in the food industry. According to recent findings, biofilms can lead to significant food spoilage and equipment damage, necessitating a proactive approach to sanitation through the use of effective disinfectants (Carrascosa et al., 2021). Therefore, LHD regulations not only enforce compliance but also promote enhanced knowledge about the factors that contribute to food safety, ultimately leading to healthier communities (Abubakar et al., 2022) (Figure 4.19).

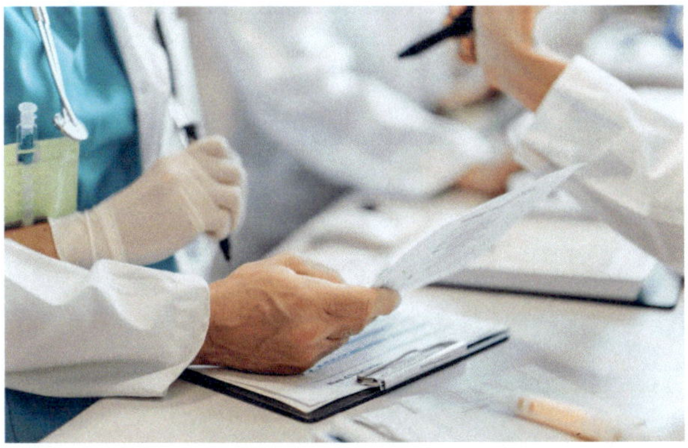

Figure 4.19. Local health department regulations play a crucial role in ensuring the sanitation of food equipment and premises, which is pivotal for safeguarding public health.

Source: https://www.capptions.com/_next/image?url=https%3A%2F%2Fcdn.sanity.io%2Fimages%2Fbs7uxmqc%2Fblog%2F1d1f0f6445ca6cbada2f1b795e28fd58efab5dee-1376x880.png&w=3840&q=75.

4.4.4. Importance of Inspections and Audits

It is very important to use inspections and audits to ensure that food equipment and premises are clean. They are important for discovering possible risks, checking that rules are met and raising the standard of food safety. Through routine audits, food processing plants can identify latent risks, including the accumulation of biofilms that are home to pathogens like *Listeria monocytogenes* that are resistant to traditional sanitizers (Mazaheri et al., 2021). In addition, as noted in current reviews of outdoor pig production, good biosecurity practices markedly decrease disease introduction and transmission risk, emphasizing the importance of inspections in dynamic agri-environments (Søren Nielsen et al., 2021). By keeping to rigorous auditing, food handlers are spurred on to abide by hygiene guidelines and continue improving that assists the trade in keeping up first-class hygiene standards.

4.4.5. Consequences of Non-Compliance

If food equipment and premises are not clean according to standards, it can seriously threaten the health and safety of the public. These issues go further than just foodborne illnesses , which can happen when food-contact surfaces are not kept clean and maintained. They can put customers' health at risk and harm the reputation of the establishments , which often leads to a drop in business and trust from customers. In addition, if operations do not comply, regulatory bodies may levy big fines or sanctions , which add to the financial problems of these businesses. When sanitation protocols are not followed, there is often more attention on the company and it may need to spend money to correct the issues. In considering the broader context, the consequences of non-compliance highlight a pressing need for stringent enforcement of hygiene regulations, as evidenced by labor market changes and working conditions described in the Fair Labor Association (2004, 2006), which reflect the interrelated nature of public health and workplace safety (Figure 4.20).

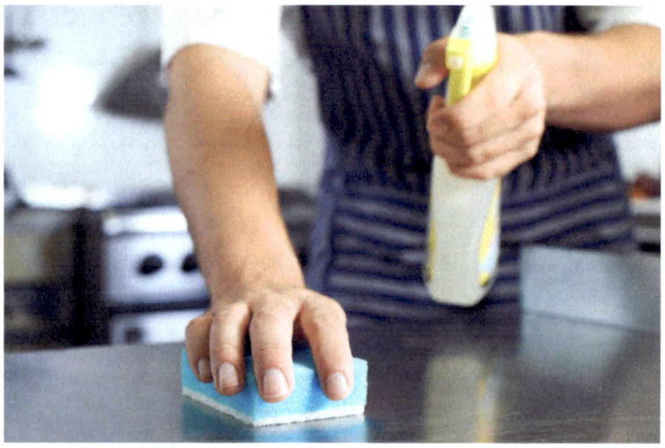

Figure 4.20. Non-compliance with sanitation standards in food equipment and premises can lead to severe consequences that undermine public health and safety.

Source: https://www.fooddocs.com/hs-fs/hubfs/chef%20sanitizing%20kitchen%20counter.jpg

4.4.6. Certification Programs for Food Handlers

Putting certification programs in place for food handlers is very important for boosting sanitation in food preparation areas. They give important instructions on safe food handling, covering the different risks that can happen during food production and service. When HACCP is used, food handlers can spot any biological, chemical or physical dangers that could endanger food safety. For instance, studies have demonstrated that training in HACCP principles significantly improves sanitation practices within food manufacturing facilities, as evidenced by research involving cake production processes in Dhaka, Bangladesh (Jubayer et al., 2022). Furthermore, certification programs also emphasize the importance of ongoing education in various food sectors, including meat supply chains, where inadequate training has been linked to poor hygiene practices and foodborne illness risks (Jeffer et al., 2021). In general, these programs help achieve the main goal of better public health by improving how food is handled.

4.4.7. Documentation and Record-Keeping Requirements

Keeping records and documentation is very important for keeping food equipment and areas clean. Good records allow companies to prove they are following food safety rules and sanitation standards. Regularly keeping logs of cleaning, equipment checks and employee training helps a business follow health rules and prevents foodborne illness outbreaks. Also, these documents can be important when regulators inspect the business, since they demonstrate that sanitation is being properly maintained. For example, understanding the labor conditions, highlighting how labor practices impact overall food safety. Thus, effective record-keeping not only bolsters sanitation efforts but also fosters a culture of continuous improvement in food safety management practices (Figure 4.21).

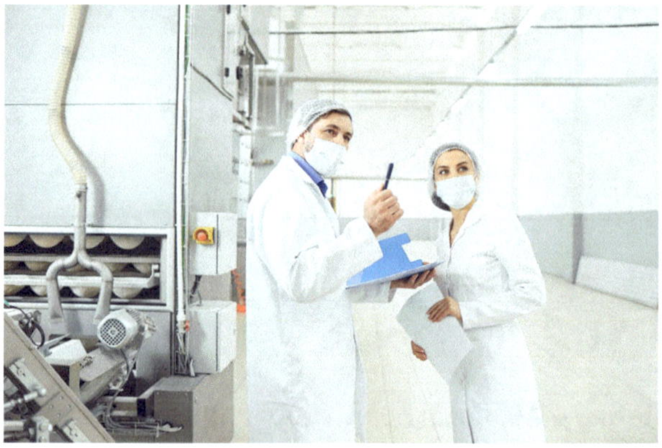

Figure 4.21. Effective documentation and record-keeping requirements play a crucial role in maintaining the sanitation of food equipment and premises.

Source: https://blog.foodsafedrains.com/hs-fs/hubfs/AdobeStock_276342112_web.jpg?width=1000&name=AdobeStock_276342112_web.jpg

4.4.8. Role of Technology in Compliance Monitoring

Technology helps a lot in checking that food equipment and facilities are kept clean according to regulations. Advanced monitoring systems, , such as Internet of Things (IoT) devices and automated sensors, facilitate real-time data collection regarding hygiene levels, temperatures, and equipment functioning. It helps take immediate steps and keeps up with sanitation standards , which results in safer food products. Also, using digital tools to keep records ensures that food service operations are more accountable and transparent. As particularly brought into focus by the COVID-19 pandemic, this technology transition is critical for risk mitigation related to public health with effective compliance frameworks that evolve with emergent issues (OECD, 2020). In the end, using technology has the potential to make compliance monitoring an active process, rather than a passive one, which is critical in a fast-changing environment for coping with the intricate food safety dynamics involved, as emphasized by health policy and resource allocation considerations (Abubakar et al., 2022).

4.4.9. Future Changes in Regulatory Standards

Because the world of food safety is always changing, new regulations will be important for handling new health problems and what consumers expect. Regulatory frameworks need to adapt to incorporate comprehensive public health laws that enhance the protection of food equipment and premises while promoting the right to health, as highlighted in recent findings by experts (Cabrera et al., 2017). Moreover, because people are buying more organic and low-input foods, rules must be updated to guarantee safety, quality and integrity during all stages of processing. Addressing the complexities of these standards will require robust guidance and practical codes of conduct to assist processors in meeting consumer expectations and regulatory requirements (Beck et al., 2006). Accepting these future changes allows regulatory agencies to guard public health and increase trust in the food industry.

A CLOSER LOOK

Listeria monocytogenes

Listeria monocytogenes is the bacterium that leads to the serious disease listeriosis. Pregnant women, newborns, the elderly and people with weak immune systems should be very careful. Most other pathogens do not survive or grow in refrigerated food, but Listeria can , which makes it hard to control in chilled foods.

Common sources of Listeria monocytogenes include:

- Unpasteurized dairy products (e.g., soft cheeses).
- Ready-to-eat deli meats and hot dogs.
- Refrigerated pâtés or meat spreads.
- Smoked seafood.
- Raw sprouts and certain fresh produce.

Symptoms of listeriosis vary from mild flu-like symptoms (, such as fever, muscle aches, and nausea) to more severe complications like meningitis, septicemia, and miscarriage or stillbirth in pregnant women.

Prevention includes:

- Thoroughly cooking food.
- Avoiding high-risk foods during pregnancy.
- Washing fruits and vegetables.
- Practicing good hygiene and food safety (e.g., cleaning surfaces, avoiding cross-contamination).
- Keeping refrigerators below 4°C (40°F).

Food producers and processors use strict HACCP plans to monitor and control Listeria in facilities, as it poses a significant public health risk.

SUMMARY

Keeping food equipment and the premises clean is very important in the food service industry. The recent focus on food safety shows that food premises should be very careful about hygiene. As seen in earlier studies, for instance, the analysis of hygiene habits of Muslim food operators in Malaysia, keeping oneself clean is part of the concept of halal and necessary to avoid foodborne diseases (Lateb et al., 2020). Proper sanitation is reached when operators comprehend hygiene well and are very committed to adhering to these regulations every time. Additionally, increasing monitoring activities by health departments and municipal authorities, as suggested in several environmental health sector assessments, would have a tangible effect on compliance rates and food safety levels in general (Morse et al., 2010). Therefore, prioritizing sanitation will protect customers' health and help in obtaining the public's confidence in food service establishments.

It is very important to keep food equipment and premises clean to protect public health and avoid contamination-related diseases. Following good sanitation guidelines prevents harmful pathogens from growing on surfaces and utensils , which could lead to FBDs. The assessment of current gaps in sanitation efforts is essential, as highlighted in the report emphasizing the importance of identifying research priorities to address these issues (Morse et al., 2010). In addition, the impact of legal rules in public health is very important; they make sure that communities follow sanitation rules and encourage health safety. It is through comprehensive public health legislation that essential practices—ranging from proper waste management to regular equipment maintenance—are enforced, thus creating conditions conducive to overall health and well-being (Cabrera et al., 2017). Food safety is best protected when sound sanitation is combined with strong legal measures.

KEY TERMS FROM THIS CHAPTER

- Medical bills
- Microbial risks
- Operation
- Ownership
- Pollutants
- Proper waste disposal
- Public trust
- Rinse
- Sanitize
- Microbial communities
- Microorganisms
- Organic matter
- Peroxyacetic acid (PAA)
- Pre-clean
- Public health laws
- Quaternary ammonium compounds
- Sanitation protocols

REFERENCES

1. Abd Wahab, S., Anyi, U., Chai, L. C., et al. (2016). *Assessing Staphylococcus aureus in Ready to Eat (Rte) Food and Risk Assessment of Food Premises in Putrajaya*. https://core.ac.uk/download/153824335.pdf (accessed on 29 May 2025).
2. Abdul Lateb, N., & Md Yusof, S. (2020). *The Practice of Halal Concept Among Food Premises in Perlis: The Hygiene Perspective*. https://core.ac.uk/download/322571600.pdf (accessed on 29 May 2025).
3. Abdul Mutalib, N. A., Abdul Rashid, S., Ariffin, H. F., et al. (2020). *Knowledge, Attitude, And Practice on Food Safety Culture Among Kitchen Employees of Malaysian Government Hospitals*. https://core.ac.uk/download/324171185.pdf (accessed on 29 May 2025).
4. Abebe, E., Gugsa, G., & Ahmed, M. (2020). Review on major food-borne zoonotic bacterial pathogens. *Journal of Tropical Medicine, 2020*, Article 4674235. https://doi.org/10.1155/2020/4674235.
5. Abubakar, I., Dalglish, S. L., Angell, B., Sanuade, O. A., Abímbọ́lá, Ṣ., Adamu, A. L., Adetifa, I., et al. (2022). The Lancet Nigeria Commission: Investing in health and the future of the nation. *The Lancet, 399*, 1155–1200. https://doi.org/10.1016/S0140-6736(21)02488-0.
6. Ackah, N. B. (2014). *Developing a Verification Program for Sanitation and Pasteurisation Activities During Pineapple Juice Production* [Master's thesis, Kwame Nkrumah University of Science and Technology]. https://core.ac.uk/download/234683767.pdf (accessed on 29 May 2025).
7. Alberini, A., Mancini, D., Lichtenberg, E., & Galinato, G. I. (2025). *Was it Something I Ate? Implementation of the FDA Seafood HACCP Program*. https://core.ac.uk/download/pdf/6264611.pdf (accessed on 29 May 2025).
8. Asim, S. H. (2017). Initial assessment of environmental microbial hazards in Doha restaurants. https://core.ac.uk/download/84995789.pdf (accessed on 29 May 2025).
9. Beck, A. (2006). *Code of Practice for Organic Food Processing* (U. Kretzschmar, A. Ploeger, & O. Schmid, Contributors). https://core.ac.uk/download/10923324.pdf (accessed on 29 May 2025).
10. Bellini, P., Nesi, P., & Pantaleo, G. (2022). IoT-enabled smart cities: A review of concepts, frameworks and key technologies. *Applied Sciences, 12*, Article 1607. https://doi.org/10.3390/app12031607.
11. Bolton, D., & Meally, A. (2007). *A Risk Assessment and Hazard Analysis and Critical Control Point (HACCP) Study for The Irish Catering Industry*. https://core.ac.uk/download/45656646.pdf (accessed on 29 May 2025).
12. Bottex, B., Gkrintzali, G., García Matas, R., Georgiev, M., Maggiore, A., Merten, C., Rortais, A., et al. (2023). EFSA's activities on emerging risks in 2020. *EFSA Supporting Publications, 20*, e8024. https://doi.org/10.2903/sp.efsa.2023.en-8024.
13. Buchanan, R. L., Gorris, L. G. M., Hayman, M. M., Jackson, T. C., & Whiting, R. C. (2016). A review of *Listeria monocytogenes*: An update on outbreaks, virulence, dose-response, ecology, and risk assessments. *Food Control, 75*, 1–13. https://doi.org/10.1016/j.foodcont.2016.12.016.

14. Cabrera, O. A., Gostin, L. O., Magnusson, R., Nygren-Krug, H., et al. (2017). *Advancing the Right to Health: The Vital Role of Law*. https://core.ac.uk/download/83109641.pdf (accessed on 29 May 2025).

15. Carrascosa, C., Raheem, D., Ramos, F., Saraiva, A., & Raposo, A. (2021). Microbial biofilms in the food industry—A comprehensive review. *International Journal of Environmental Research and Public Health, 18*(4), 2014. https://doi.org/10.3390/ijerph18042014.

16. Chamola, V., Hassija, V., Gupta, V., & Guizani, M. (2020). A comprehensive review of the COVID-19 pandemic and the role of IoT, drones, AI, blockchain, and 5G in managing its impact. *IEEE Access, 8*, 90225–90265. https://doi.org/10.1109/access.2020.2992341.

17. Chopra, V., Toner, E., Waldhorn, R., & Washer, L. (2020). How should U.S. hospitals prepare for Coronavirus Disease 2019 (COVID-19)? *Annals of Internal Medicine, 172*(9), 621–622. https://doi.org/10.7326/m20-0907.

18. Coville, A., Briceño, B., & Martinez, S. (2015). *Promoting Handwashing and Sanitation: Evidence from A Large-Scale Randomized Trial in Rural Tanzania*. https://core.ac.uk/download/75783068.pdf (accessed on 29 May 2025).

19. Crouch, M. L., Jacobs, H. E., & Speight, V. (2021). Defining domestic water consumption based on personal water use activities. *Journal of Water Supply: Research and Technology—AQUA*. https://doi.org/10.2166/aqua.2021.056.

20. De Giovanni, P. (2023). Sustainability of the metaverse: A transition to Industry 5.0. *Sustainability, 15*, Article 6079. https://doi.org/10.3390/su15076079.

21. De Oliveira Mota, J., Kooh, P., Jaffrès, E., Prévost, H., Maignien, T., Arnich, N., Sanaa, M., et al. (2022). First survey about current practices of environmental monitoring programs within French agri-food industries. *Biology, 11*(1), Article 89. https://doi.org/10.3390/biology11010089.

22. Dutta, A., Meijers, H., Ramani, S. V., & Frühauf, T. (2012). *Determinants of the Prevalence of Diarrhoea in Adolescents Attending School: A Case Study of An Indian Village School*. https://core.ac.uk/download/75783133.pdf (accessed on 29 May 2025).

23. Ezzatpanah, H., Gómez-López, V. M., Koutchma, T., Lavafpour, F., Moerman, F., Mohammadi, M., & Raheem, D. (2022). Risks and new challenges in the food chain: Viral contamination and decontamination from a global perspective, guidelines, and cleaning. *Comprehensive Reviews in Food Science and Food Safety, 21*, 868–903. https://doi.org/10.1111/1541-4337.12899.

24. Fair Labor Association. (2004). *Tracking Chart 2004: Nike, Thailand (07037442C)*. https://core.ac.uk/download/33600436.pdf (accessed on 29 May 2025).

25. Fair Labor Association. (2006). *Tracking Chart 2006: Puma, Thailand (07037442CV)*. https://core.ac.uk/download/33603227.pdf (accessed on 29 May 2025).

26. Fair Labor Association. (2008). *Tracking Chart 2008: Asics in Vietnam*. https://core.ac.uk/download/5128900.pdf (accessed on 29 May 2025).

27. Fair Labor Association. (2011). *Tracking Chart 2011: Asics, China (40001537DV)*. https://core.ac.uk/download/33597081.pdf (accessed on 29 May 2025).

28. Faour-Klingbeil, D., Kuri, V., & Todd, E. C. D. (2016). Microbiological quality of ready-to-eat fresh vegetables and their link to food safety environment and handling practices in restaurants. https://core.ac.uk/download/74390081.pdf.

29. Flores Baquero, Ó., Giné Garriga, R., Jiménez Fdez de Palencia, A., & Pérez Foguet, A., et al. (2013). *Post-2015 WASH Targets and Indicators: A Review from a Human Rights Perspective.* https://core.ac.uk/download/41777957.pdf (accessed on 29 May 2025).

30. Himeur, Y., Elnour, M., Fadli, F., Meskin, N., Petri, I., Rezgui, Y., Bensaali, F., et al. (2022). AI-big data analytics for building automation and management systems: A survey, actual challenges and future perspectives. *Artificial Intelligence Review, 56*, 4929–5021. https://doi.org/10.1007/s10462-022-10286-2.

31. Howard, G., Bartram, J., Brocklehurst, C., Colford, J. M., Costa, F., Cunliffe, D., Dreibelbis, R., et al. (2020). COVID-19: Urgent actions, critical reflections and future relevance of 'WaSH': Lessons for the current and future pandemics. *Journal of Water and Health, 18*, 613–630. https://doi.org/10.2166/wh.2020.162.

32. Jeffer, S. B., Kassem, I. I., Kharroubi, S., & Abebe, G. K. (2021). Analysis of food safety management systems in the beef meat processing and distribution chain in Uganda. *Foods, 10*(10), 2244. https://doi.org/10.3390/foods10102244.

33. Jubayer, M. F., Hossain, M. S., Al-Emran, M., & Uddin, M. N. (2022). Implementation of HACCP management system in a cake manufacturing company in Dhaka, Bangladesh: A case study. *Journal of Food Quality, 2022*, Article 5321333. https://doi.org/10.1155/2022/5321333.

34. Kimani-Murage, E., Osogo, D., Nyamasege, C. K., Igonya, E. K., Ngira, D. O., & Harrington, J. (2022). COVID-19 and human right to food: Lived experiences of the urban poor in Kenya with the impacts of government's response measures, a participatory qualitative study. *BMC Public Health, 22*, Article 13638. https://doi.org/10.1186/s12889-022-13638-3.

35. Koutsoumanis, K., Allende, A., Bolton, D., Bover-Cid, S., Chemaly, M., De Cesare, A., Herman, L., et al. (2024). Persistence of microbiological hazards in food and feed production and processing environments. *EFSA Journal, 22*, Article e08521. https://doi.org/10.2903/j.efsa.2024.8521.

36. Lamichhane, B., Mawad, A. M. M., Saleh, M. A., Kelley, W. G., Harrington, P. J., Lovestad, C. W., Amezcua, J., et al. (2024). Salmonellosis: An overview of epidemiology, pathogenesis, and innovative approaches to mitigate the antimicrobial resistant infections. *Antibiotics, 13*(1), 76. https://doi.org/10.3390/antibiotics13010076.

37. Laswai, H., Mukantwali, C., Tiisekwa, B., & Wiehler, C., et al. (2013). *Good Manufacturing and Hygienic Practices at Small and Medium Scale Pineapple Processing Enterprises in Rwanda.* https://core.ac.uk/download/234683640.pdf.

38. Lin, L., Yang, H., & Xu, X. (2022). Effects of water pollution on human health and disease heterogeneity: A review. *Frontiers in Environmental Science, 10*, Article 880246. https://doi.org/10.3389/fenvs.2022.880246.

39. Morse, Tracy and Lungu, Kingsley and Taulo, Steven (2010) Gap Analysis of Environmental Health Research in Malawi : Report to the National Commission of Science and Technology. National Commission for Science and Technology (Malawi), Malawi. (accessed on 29 May 2025).

40. Mazaheri, T., Cervantes-Huamán, B. R. H., Bermúdez-Capdevila, M., Ripolles-Avila, C., & Rodríguez Jerez, J. J. (2021). *Listeria monocytogenes* biofilms in the food industry: Is the current hygiene program sufficient to combat the persistence of the pathogen? *Microorganisms, 9*(1), 181. https://doi.org/10.3390/microorganisms9010181.

41. Nielsen, S. S., Álvarez, J., Bicout, D., Calistri, P., Canali, E., Drewe, J. A., Garin-Bastuji, B., et al. (2021). African swine fever and outdoor farming of pigs. *EFSA Journal, 19*(6), e06639. https://doi.org/10.2903/j.efsa.2021.6639.

42. Olaimat, A. N., Shahbaz, H. M., Fatima, N., Munir, S., & Holley, R. A. (2020). Food safety during and after the era of COVID-19 pandemic. *Frontiers in Microbiology, 11*, 1854. https://doi.org/10.3389/fmicb.2020.01854.

43. Organization for Economic Co-operation and Development (OECD). (2020). *The Territorial Impact of COVID-19: Managing the Crisis Across Levels of Government*. OECD Policy Responses to Coronavirus (COVID-19). https://doi.org/10.1787/d3e314e1-en.

44. Rahman, M. T., Sobur, M. A., Islam, M. S., Ievy, S., Hossain, M. J., El Zowalaty, M. E., Rahman, A. T., et al. (2020). Zoonotic diseases: Etiology, impact, and control. *Microorganisms, 8*, Article 1405. https://doi.org/10.3390/microorganisms8091405.

45. Sant'Ana, A. S., Leitolis, A., Ambiel, C., Habowski, K., da Silva, A. B., Matte, B. F., Perdomo Azeredo, D. R., et al. (2023). Assuring the safety of cultivated meat: HACCP plan development and application to a cultivated meat target-product. *TikiBooks*. https://doi.org/10.22491/application_cultivated_meat.

46. Singh, R., Gehlot, A., Akram, S. V., Thakur, A. K., Gupta, L. R., Priyadarshi, N., & Twala, B. (2024). Integration of advanced digital technologies in the hospitality industry: A technological approach towards sustainability. *Sustainable Engineering and Innovation, 6*(1), 37–56. https://doi.org/10.37868/sei.v6i1.id208.

47. South Carolina Department of Health and Environmental Control. (2005). *Pasteurized Milk and Milk Products Regulation 61-34.1*. https://core.ac.uk/download/588861605.pdf (accessed on 29 May 2025).

48. Stejskal, V., Vendl, T., Aulický, R., & Athanassiou, C. G. (2021). Synthetic and natural insecticides: Gas, liquid, gel and solid formulations for stored-product and food-industry pest control. *Insects, 12*(7), 590. https://doi.org/10.3390/insects12070590.

49. Sudibyo, A., & Yulistia, A. (2011). Studi tentang persepsi, praktek dan sikap terhadap sistem HACCP pada industri pakan dalam mencapai kesesuaian keamanan pakan. https://media.neliti.com/media/publications/140070-EN-studi-tentang-persepsi-praktek-dan-sikap.pdf (accessed on 29 May 2025).

50. Worker Rights Consortium. (2011). *Worker Rights Consortium Assessment Eagle Speed Marketing (Thailand): Findings, Recommendations and Status*. https://core.ac.uk/download/5132576.pdf (accessed on 29 May 2025).

51. Zandona, E., Blažić, M., & Režek Jambrak, A. (2021). Whey utilisation: Sustainable uses and environmental approach. *Food Technology and Biotechnology, 59*(2), 147–161. https://doi.org/10.17113/ftb.59.02.21.6968.

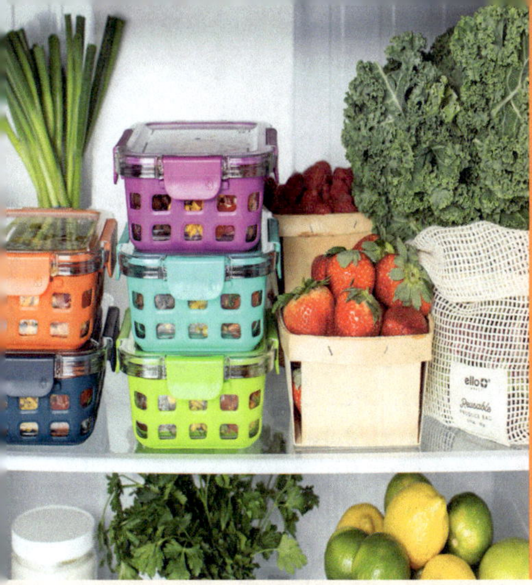

Chapter 5

SAFE FOOD STORAGE AND TEMPERATURE CONTROL

Contents

Introduction 107
5.1. Principles of Safe Food Storage 109
5.2. Temperature Control Guidelines 113
5.3. Food Storage for Different Types of Food 117
5.4. Best Practices for Home and Commercial Storage 121
Summary 126
References 127

Introduction

Food safety is very important because it covers different actions to prevent illnesses from food, which helps to keep the public healthy. Because more people are becoming aware about the hygiene in foodservice establishments, it is especially important to store and keep food at the right temperatures. As emphasized by the Food and Agriculture Organization, effective food safety management involves not only safe food handling but also rigorous training for staff to adhere to these practices (Marule et al., 2024). This training is essential for minimizing contamination risks that arise during food preparation and storage, as evidenced by studies highlighting significant associations between improper temperature control and elevated microbial contamination levels in food products (Bikuba et al., 2025). Food service managers should put in place strong strategies to ensure safe food handling, to avoid health issues and to gain the trust of consumers.

Definition of Food Storage

Food storage is a basic method to maintain the quality and safety of perishable foods , which helps to stop foodborne illnesses and spoilage. This is done by using refrigeration, freezing and storing food in airtight containers , which all help to increase the shelf life of food. Proper food storage is crucial not only for maintaining nutritional value but also for minimizing waste, a concern highlighted in contemporary discussions surrounding sustainability and climate resilience (Intergovernmental Panel on Climate Change, 2023). The importance of effective food storage strategies is further underscored by research indicating that inadequate temperature control can lead to detrimental microbial growth, jeopardizing consumer health (Salminen et al., 2021). Proper methods allow people to ensure their food is safe , which helps improve how food is handled and prepared everywhere. Through such measures, food storage not only safeguards personal health but also contributes to a more sustainable approach to food management (Figure 5.1).

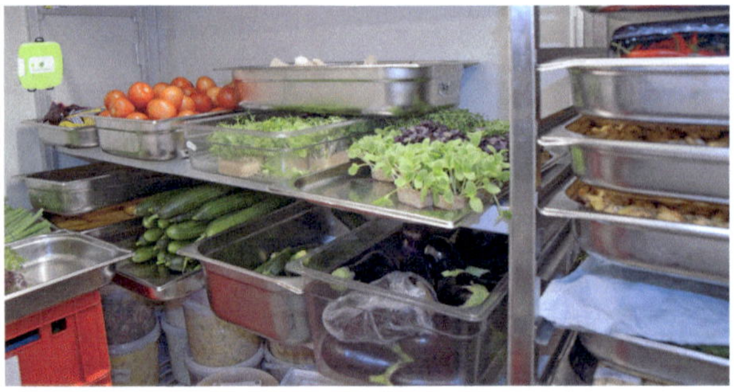

Figure 5.1. Food storage encompasses a fundamental practice aimed at preserving the quality and safety of perishable items, effectively preventing foodborne illnesses and spoilage.

Source: https://compliancemate.com/wp-content/uploads/2025/04/food-storage.png.

Importance of Food Safety

Ensuring food safety is very important, mainly when it comes to storing and maintaining proper temperatures for food. Proper food safety measures stop pathogens from spreading , which helps keep foodborne illnesses away and protects the public. Using various approaches , such as those from the Western Institute for Food Safety and Security, points out the importance of education that covers both food safety and environmental issues. This holistic perspective not only equips students and professionals with the necessary knowledge but also fosters sustainable practices in food production and storage (Angelos et al., 2017). Also, the rules about food safety are not the same in every country, as seen by Australia's strict pasteurization rules that make it hard for artisanal cheese to be produced. These regulations raise pertinent questions about balancing safety with innovation and the benefits of supporting small-scale producers without compromising health (Taylor et al., 2017).

Overview of Temperature Control

Keeping the temperature under control is very important for safe food and the longer shelf life of perishable items. Maintaining the right temperature levels prevents pathogens from growing , which lowers the risk of food poisoning. Recent advancements have shown a growing consumer interest in innovative sustainable processing techniques that enhance the quality and shelf life of various food products, particularly organic items, while aligning with ecological practices (Alminger et al., 2018). Also, adding natural antioxidants from plants can help protect food from spoiling. These substances not only contribute to the health benefits of food products but can also be utilized in active packaging solutions, thereby reinforcing temperature control measures (Alves et al., 2019). As such, a comprehensive understanding of temperature management, combined with these novel approaches, is essential for food safety initiatives in contemporary food storage and handling practices (Figure 5.2).

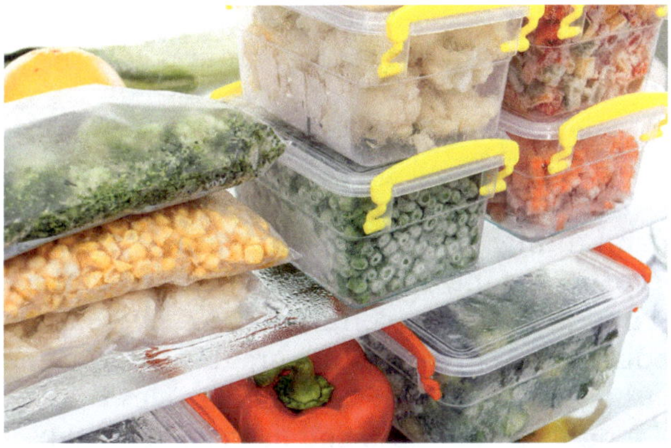

Figure 5.2. Effective temperature control is paramount in ensuring food safety and extending the shelf life of perishable items.

Source: https://www.foodhygienecompany.co.uk/wp-content/uploads/sites/4/2019/06/bigstock-158368310-scaled.jpg.

Role of Proper Storage in Preventing Illness

Keeping food stored properly is very important to avoid illness, since incorrect temperatures can allow harmful pathogens to grow. For instance, *Salmonella enteritidis*, a common foodborne pathogen, exhibits variant growth patterns under different temperature conditions; inadequate storage can enhance its development and subsequently heighten health risks (Baek et al., 2024). Therefore, proper methods are needed to keep food temperatures correct, mainly in items, such as eggs and dairy products. Similarly, in fruit juices, the contamination by mold and the production of toxins like patulin is primarily mitigated through appropriate storage practices that regulate temperature and humidity levels (Singh et al., 2024). Proper storage conditions not only stop microbial growth but also ensure that food retains its nutritional value , which is why careful storage is so important in food safety. Following these storage rules all the time is very important for preventing foodborne illnesses in consumers.

5.1. Principles of Safe Food Storage

Proper food storage helps prevent illnesses from food and keeps products fresh for a long time. The main ideas for safe food storage are to keep food at the right temperature, organize it correctly and use older items first. Following temperature control rules , such as storing perishables below 40°F, helps prevent the growth of dangerous microorganisms. Additionally, the implementation of Hazard Analysis Critical Control Points (HACCP) systems, as required by regulatory authorities, reflects a critical shift toward proactive safety measures in the production and storage of food (Aalberts et al., 2003). Furthermore, understanding the interconnectedness of food safety, security, and environmental impact allows for a comprehensive approach to food management, emphasizing the importance of education within diverse disciplines (Angelos et al., 2017). Adopting these principles leads to a safer system for food and better public health.

5.1.1. Understanding Food Spoilage

It is important to understand food spoilage to use safe food storage and temperature control methods. Bacteria, yeasts and molds grow in food when it is stored at the wrong temperature , which leads to spoilage. They not only make food unsafe but also reduce the nutrients in the food. For instance, a systematic approach employing decision support tools, as seen in the STARTEC project, allows food manufacturers to analyze shelf life along with safety and quality metrics, ensuring that items, such as ready-to-eat (RTE) meals maintain their integrity throughout their intended shelf life (Skjerdal et al., 2017). Moreover, the emerging concept of postbiotics indicates how inactivated microbial components may offer health benefits, thereby fostering an understanding of the balance between beneficial and spoilage microorganisms (Salminen et al.,

2021). Thus, comprehending the mechanisms behind food spoilage is vital for developing robust food safety protocols (Figure 5.3).

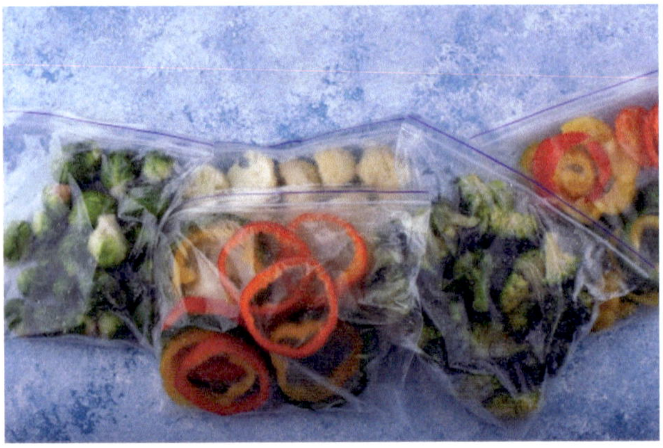

Figure 5.3. Understanding food spoilage is essential for implementing effective, safe food storage and temperature control practices.

Source: https://www.ficsi.in/blog/wp-content/uploads/2022/12/unnamed-6.jpg.

5.1.2. Types of Food Storage Methods

Food safety and quality can be maintained well by using the right storage methods, especially for perishable items. Among all the techniques, keeping food cold or frozen is most important since it slows down bacteria and enzymes that spoil food. Airtight containers are useful because they help keep moisture and air away from the food , which can speed up its spoiling. Recent developments highlight the advantages of edible coatings made from natural extracts, as they serve as barriers against moisture and microorganisms while prolonging shelf life, addressing the high post-harvest losses in fruits and vegetables (Rajial et al., 2024).

Furthermore, as emphasized in research, temperature control is vital in the storage process, allowing for optimal conditions that enhance food longevity and safety (Eze et al., 2024). All these methods together reduce food waste and make sure that consumers get to eat safe and high-quality food products.

5.1.3. Importance of Cleanliness in Storage Areas

Maintaining cleanliness in storage areas is very important, mainly for safe food storage and temperature control. Poor hygiene in food processing can encourage bacteria and pathogens to develop , which increases the risk of foodborne illnesses and makes people doubt the safety of the food supply. Making sure food is safe involves keeping storage areas very clean, since this directly helps maintain the quality of food products. It matters a lot now because the demand for specialized foods , such as halal products, requires strict cleanliness to meet what people expect and what the law requires. By innovating logistics services that prioritize hygiene, companies can effectively address the increasing consumer demand while ensuring that food safety standards are consistently met (Endut et al., 2025). Ultimately, the commitment to cleanliness in storage areas is essential for enhancing food safety and maintaining customer satisfaction in a competitive market (Soong, 2007) (Figure 5.4).

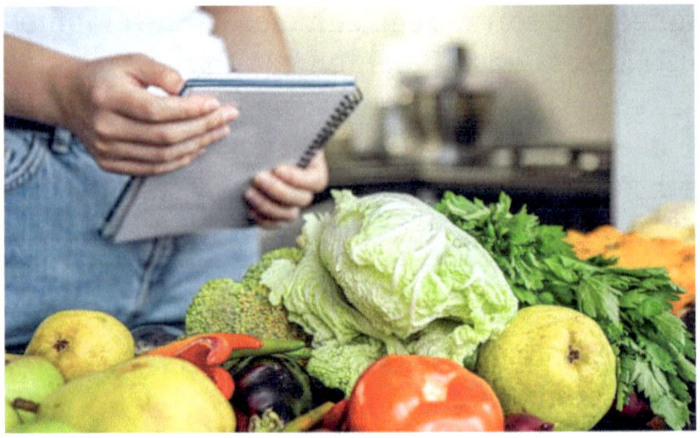

Figure 5.4. The significance of maintaining cleanliness in storage areas cannot be overstated, particularly within the framework of safe food storage and temperature control.

Source: https://cdn.en.ntsquare.com/wp-content/uploads/4-7.jpg.

5.1.4. Role of Packaging in Food Safety

Packaging is very important for food safety, mainly when it comes to proper storage and temperature management. Effective packaging stops food from becoming contaminated, spoiled and helps maintain the quality of food products from the start to the end of the supply chain. As regulatory authorities have shifted towards preventive approaches, such as HACCP, the need for comprehensive packaging solutions that ensure food safety has never been more urgent (Aalberts et al., 2003). New ideas in packaging can save a lot of food from being wasted when it is moved and stored. Because the world's population is rising such advancements are important to ensure food is safe and secure, helping to avoid foodborne illnesses and improve public health.

5.1.5. FIFO (First In, First Out) Method

The FIFO (First In, First Out) method is an essential practice in safe food storage and temperature control, particularly for perishable items. Following this plan helps food establishments use their older food before it becomes spoiled, which reduces waste and makes food safer. Because perishable goods need to be stored properly and quickly, this method is very useful. For example, recent studies highlight that effective temperature management can significantly extend the shelf life of products, , such as the Frafra potato, underscoring the importance of storage techniques in reducing moisture loss and preventing spoilage (Ninfaa et al., 2024). Moreover, optimizing storage temperatures through approaches like those described in optimal control models can ensure the integrity of food products within supply chains, reinforcing the critical nature of FIFO practices in conjunction with temperature regulation (Eze et al., 2024) (Figure 5.5).

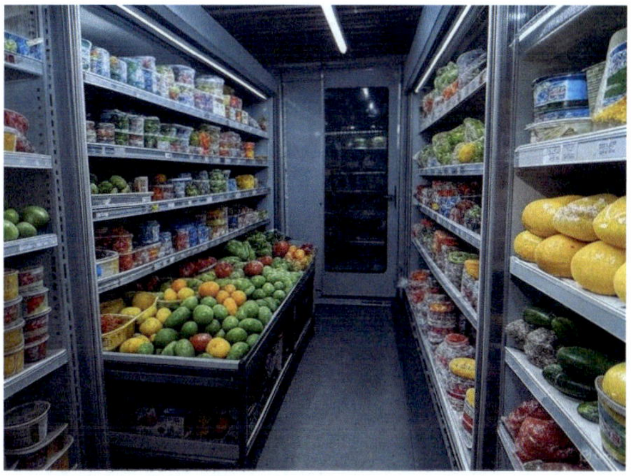

Figure 5.5. The FIFO (First In, First Out) method is an essential practice in safe food storage and temperature control, particularly for perishable items.

Source: https://ordersinseconds.com/wp-content/uploads/2025/03/An-overview-of-perishable-goods-in-storage.-1.jpg.

5.1.6. Temperature Zones for Food Storage

It is very important to control the temperature in food storage, because not doing so can cause serious health issues , such as food poisoning. The best temperature for keeping food fresh in the refrigerator is between 32°F and 40°F, and extremely low temperatures below 0°F are needed to keep food preserved for a long time. Research has shown that the bacterium *Listeria monocytogenes* is particularly sensitive to temperature fluctuations, thriving in temperatures above the recommended thresholds for stored food (EFSA BIOHAZ Panel (EFSA Panel on Biological Hazards), 2020). So, keeping temperatures under control both prevents contamination and helps maintain food quality and safety. Furthermore, innovative preservation methods, such as ionizing radiation, are being explored to enhance the safety of food products in specific regions, such as Alaska, potentially benefiting the local seafood and agricultural industries (Das et al., 1988). So, it is necessary to follow these temperature zones to reduce the risk of food safety problems.

5.1.7. Importance of Labeling and Dating Food

Having clear labels and dates on food helps people store and handle food safely, as it tells them how fresh and safe the food is. Clear labels allow consumers to tell if food is still usable , which leads to less food being wasted and more sustainable eating. Date labels like sell by and use by inform people when to use the food , which helps prevent illness from eating expired products. In the context of climate change and its impact on food systems, as highlighted in the assessment by the IPCC (Intergovernmental Panel on Climate Change, 2023), efficient food management, including precise labeling, can also play a role in mitigating environmental consequences. Furthermore, the exploration of emerging concepts like postbiotics underscores the importance of clear labeling in communicating health benefits and safety standards associated with food products (Salminen et al., 2021) (Figure 5.6).

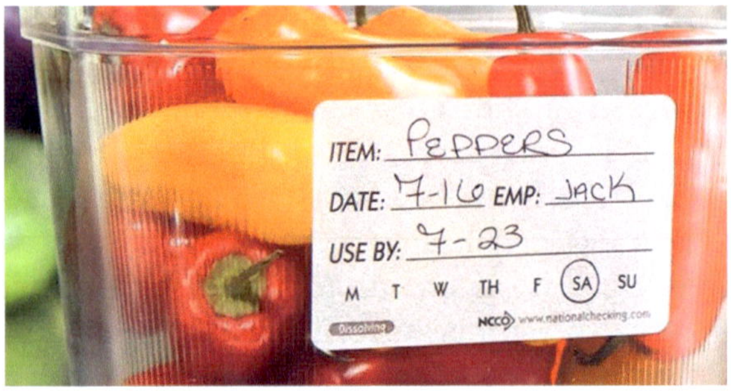

Figure 5.6. Effective food labeling and dating practices are vital components of safe food storage and temperature control, as they provide consumers with critical information regarding the freshness and safety of food products.

Source: https://gfs.com/wp-content/uploads/2022/08/food-safety-labeling-dating.jpg.

5.1.8. Storage of Raw vs. Cooked Foods

It is very important to know how raw and cooked foods should be stored to avoid food illnesses. Storage temperature for poultry and seafood, which are raw, may carry pathogens , such as Salmonella and *Listeria monocytogenes* and these can multiply if the food is not stored at the right temperatures. For instance, the integrity of egg yolk membranes can be compromised at higher temperatures, increasing the probability of contamination, as highlighted in research assessing storage conditions of eggs produced on the island of Ireland (Kelly et al., 2008). By contrast, cooked foods are less likely to be contaminated by bacteria if they are stored and reheated properly. A study revealed that the risk of illness associated with uncooked blanched frozen vegetables was significantly higher than that of their cooked counterparts, indicating the impact of proper temperature management throughout the storage and consumption phases (EFSA BIOHAZ Panel (EFSA Panel on Biological Hazards), 2020). So, using proper storage methods is very important for lowering foodborne illnesses.

5.1.9. Common Mistakes in Food Storage

It looks simple to store food, but many typical mistakes may harm your health and the quality. Many people forget to keep foods cool , which is very important for stopping bacteria growth in perishable foods. Most people do not set the temperature properly in their refrigerators , which can allow food pathogens to grow. If items in the refrigerator or pantry are not kept separate in the right way, raw foods may mix with RTE foods by accident. Another thing often missed is not paying attention to expiration dates or not storing leftovers properly , which can harm your food and your health. Finally, because new ways of storing food make things simpler, users may not follow practices that help maintain the safety of their food. These issues should be handled by remaining more vigilant and sticking to rules, so food storage meets required safety standards for the public's health (Fenster et al., 2019; Stoyanova et al., 2020) (Figure 5.7).

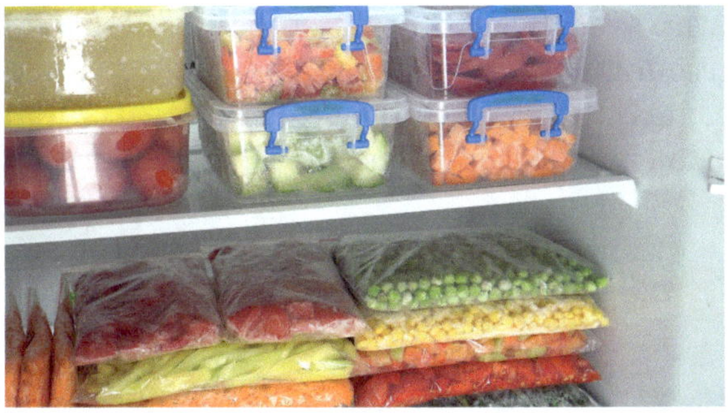

Figure 5.7. Food storage often appears deceptively straightforward, yet numerous common mistakes can compromise both safety and quality.

Source: https://www.aces.edu/wp-content/uploads/2019/08/shutterstock_1228387135.jpg.

5.2. Temperature Control Guidelines

Keeping food at the proper temperature is very important for its safety during both storage and preparation. Keeping food at the proper temperature stops harmful pathogens from growing during the danger zone of 40°F to 140°F. Experts recommend refrigerating perishables at around 40°F or lower so bacteria do not multiply and foods that have been cooked need to remain hotter than 140°F until eaten. Also, specific factors need to be considered for new technologies , such as 3D food printing. Studies suggest that the type of ink used in food packaging can change how well pathogens survive during storage, which underlines the importance of strict temperature control (Hamilton et al., 2024). Because of this, cooling and heating temperatures should be part of food storage to ensure it is safe and to allow for new technology to be used in the food industry (Hamilton et al., 2024).

5.2.1. Recommended Temperature Ranges for Food Storage

Storing food properly is important for its safety and to stop it from spoiling and the right temperature range is very important for this. According to guidelines, perishable foods, , such as meats and dairy products, should be stored at temperatures below 40°F (4°C) to inhibit bacterial growth. Conversely, the freezer should be set at 0°F (–18°C) to preserve the quality of frozen items and prevent the proliferation of pathogens.

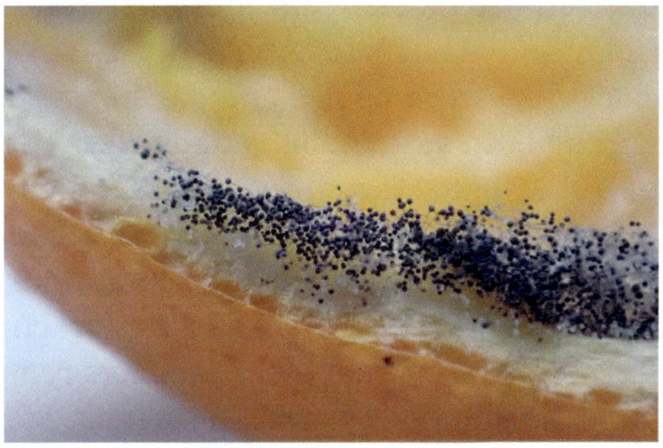

Figure 5.8. Effective food storage is crucial for maintaining food safety and preventing spoilage, with recommended temperature ranges playing a pivotal role in this process.

Source: By Garnhami - Own work, CC BY-SA 4.0, https://commons.wikimedia.org/w/index.php?curid=95145297

For foods like turmeric paste, which require specific storage conditions due to their high moisture content, controlled temperatures can enhance shelf life while mitigating deterioration (Ibadullah et al., 2024). Likewise, citrus fruits , such as mandarins benefit from optimal storage at 10–12 °C, which helps to minimize post-harvest decay and fungal infections (Lemić et al., 2024). Adhering to these temperature recommendations is essential for maximizing food safety and reducing waste within the supply chain (Figure 5.8).

5.2.2. Importance of Refrigeration

Refrigeration plays a major role in keeping food safe, mainly by helping to control food storage and temperature. Refrigeration keeps perishable foods at the right temperature , which delays the growth of bacteria that can cause food poisoning. Cold chains , which play a key role in food distribution today, depend on good refrigeration to maintain a steady temperature throughout the chain.

For instance, studies propose that optimizing cold chain logistics can minimize energy consumption while preserving the quality of products like fresh apples and ice cream, thus enhancing both sustainability and safety (Gallo et al., 2017). Furthermore, advancements , such as high-intensity ultrasound have shown promise in reducing microbial populations in poultry, complementing refrigeration practices by further ensuring that meat products remain safe for consumption (Alarcon-Rojo et al., 2018). All these systems confirm the important part that refrigeration plays in safeguarding public health and food supplies.

5.2.3. Freezing Food Safely

Freezing food safely is very important for food storage because it helps keep it safe and fresh. Proper freezing techniques involve ensuring that food is frozen at temperatures of 0°F (–18°C) or lower, which prevents microbial growth and enzymatic reactions that can lead to spoilage. Wrap or store foods in airtight containers to prevent them from being exposed to air , which can cause freezer burn and change how the food tastes and feels. It is essential to freeze items in portions that facilitate quick thawing, minimizing the time food remains in the "danger zone" between 40°F and 140°F (4°C and 60°C) during the thawing process. In catering environments, where efficiency and food quality are paramount, implementing modern techniques in food freezing can optimize preservation efforts and reduce waste, particularly in regions facing severe food insecurity, as noted in discussions surrounding the challenges of traditional food production practices (Mora et al., 2012) and postharvest losses (Thyrring, 2012) (Figure 5.9).

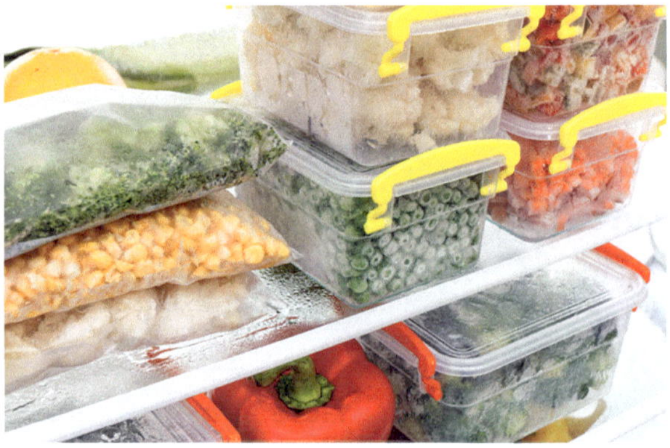

Figure 5.9. The safe freezing of food is a critical aspect of food storage that helps maintain both quality and safety.

Source: https://blogger.googleusercontent.com/img/b/R29vZ2xl/AVvXsEgNaQBfKnunl5c4z-KVrdlU6Deb-L8-2_bDbsdPx1AiyWrVyDZNAiW-nedjQd674OoLuVLAyPq0h4bPajjNCV5bp5dRhsfHjqN5QhZQ2KLQWFoFpibze80QqALJx5PYxfnSCjxCkHLJTSc/s1600/Frozen-food-in-containers.jpg

5.2.4. Temperature Monitoring Tools

Proper temperature monitoring helps keep food safe and prevents it from spoiling , which is key to avoiding foodborne diseases. They start with basic thermometers and go up to digital systems that show the temperature in real time and send alerts. The accuracy of these devices is vital; for instance, improper temperature conditions can lead to the proliferation of harmful pathogens, which pose significant health risks, as emphasized in studies illustrating the adverse effects of food contamination (Kumar et al., 2019).

Furthermore, integrating temperature monitoring systems with food preservation practices can significantly enhance food security by ensuring that products remain within safe temperature thresholds (Intergovernmental Panel on Climate Change, 2023). In this way, having dependable temperature monitoring tools helps keep food safe, supports sustainability in food storage and ensures public health is protected by cutting down on food waste.

5.2.5. Safe Thawing Methods

Knowing how to safely thaw food helps keep it safe and good for eating. The main ways to thaw food are by refrigeration, cold water immersion and microwave thawing. When food is thawed in the refrigerator, it does so slowly and safely , which helps prevent bacteria from forming. Cold water immersion is faster, but it requires frequent temperature checks so the food does not get to the danger zone, where bacteria can grow.

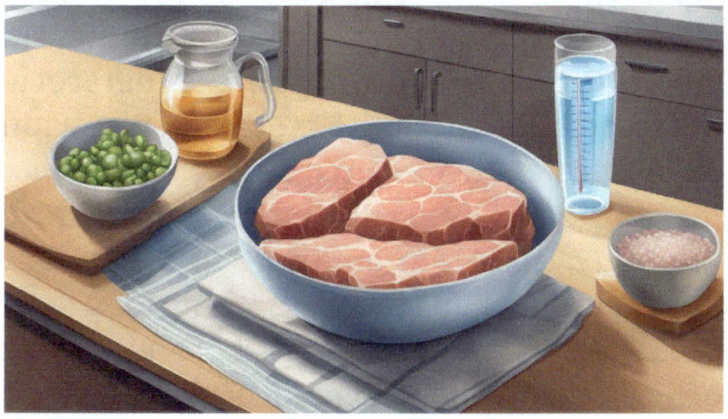

Figure 5.10. Understanding safe thawing methods is essential for preventing foodborne illnesses and maintaining food quality during preparation.

Source: https://images.squarespace-cdn.com/content/v1/62e7a92f066fa3730dcd4604/ebb8e65b-0b30-4c06-bb1b-0bf5f052f0fc/v2-83kvj-c737v.jpg.

Even though microwave thawing is quick, the food must be cooked immediately after to avoid uneven heating and possible bacterial growth. Notably, a significant portion of the population demonstrates unsafe thawing practices, as highlighted in a study where many participants failed to apply appropriate controls during food preparation (Worsfold et al., 1994). Educational initiatives, such as the PEEP Curriculum, aim to enhance understanding of these methods, focusing on informed consumer behaviors related to food safety (Godwin et al., 2019) (Figure 5.10).

5.2.6. Cooking Temperatures for Different Foods

Cooking food at the right temperature is very important for avoiding foodborne illnesses. To eliminate dangerous pathogens, some foods must be cooked to particular temperatures and chicken livers should be heated to at least 70°C. This temperature not only mitigates the risks associated with pathogens like Salmonella and Campylobacter but also allows for the maintenance of desirable textural qualities in the livers, as observed in studies of cooking conditions (Qu et al., 2021). Besides poultry, red meats should be cooked to at least 63°C and ground meats should be cooked to at least 71°C for safety. Also, seafood should be cooked to at least 63°C to prevent the risk of getting sick from bacteria. Following these temperature rules helps keep food safe and lowers the risk of contamination while cooking , which supports healthier meals.

5.2.7. Effects of Temperature Abuse

When food is kept outside the safe temperature range, it can be very dangerous for both food safety and public health. When perishable items are kept in warm temperatures for a long time, it gives pathogenic bacteria a good chance to grow , which can cause food poisoning.

Salmonella and *E. coli*, among others, thrive in temperatures ranging from 40°F to 140°F , which stresses the need for careful cold and hot holding. Poor temperature control can reduce how long food products stay fresh and also affects their quality and nutrients. Moreover, this situation is exacerbated by changes in food packaging technologies, as indicated by recent advancements in smart packaging that aim to extend shelf life and monitor freshness (Salgado et al., 2021). Thus, effective temperature management is essential not only for safeguarding consumer health but also for minimizing food waste, thereby addressing broader environmental concerns related to improper food disposal (Karić et al., 2021) (Figure 5.11).

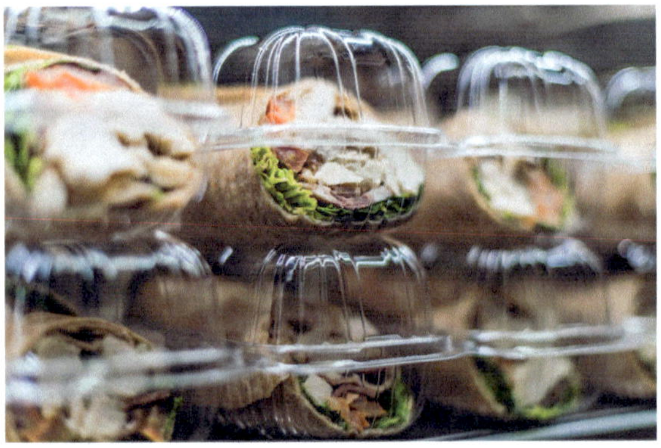

Figure 5.11. Temperature abuse, which occurs when food is stored outside the recommended temperature range, poses significant risks to food safety and public health.

Source: https://www.fooddocs.com/hs-fs/hubfs/Cold-holding%20ready%20to%20eat%20food.jpg.

5.2.8. Guidelines for Transporting Food

The safety and quality of perishable goods depend on proper food transportation , which means following all the set guidelines closely. Temperature control during transportation matters a lot, since poor conditions can result in quick spoilage and more food being thrown away, which can be harmful to people's health. It has been demonstrated that maintaining optimal storage temperatures is essential to prolonging the shelf life of perishable goods, which often possess short windows of usability (Eze et al., 2024). Also, having refrigerated vehicles and insulated packaging ensures that food is kept at the correct temperatures during transport. Failure to regulate these conditions can exacerbate issues related to product integrity, nutritional content, and even the risk of contamination (Osunde et al., 2020). Thus, making sure transportation rules are effective is important for both consumer health and the availability of safe food.

5.2.9. Role of Thermometers in Food Safety

Food thermometers play a very crucial role in maintaining food safety, primarily through assisting in holding food at the correct temperature and in proper storage. Accurate measurement of temperature prevents foodborne diseases by ensuring that food is handled, stored, and cooked at appropriate temperatures. For example, the HACCP scheme places special importance on monitoring temperature as a control point, underscoring the importance of accurate thermometers within food service environments, like schools, where safety protocols are crucial to serving children (Cole et al., 2014). In addition, in areas , such as the Mediterranean, benchmarking food safety practice has established that there is a strong thermal management system required within the fresh produce supply chain, implying that thermometers play a critical role in ensuring quality and safety standards (Martinez et al., 2004). As such, the efficient application of thermometers boosts overall food safety and hence saves public health while enforcing regulatory compliance (Figure 5.12).

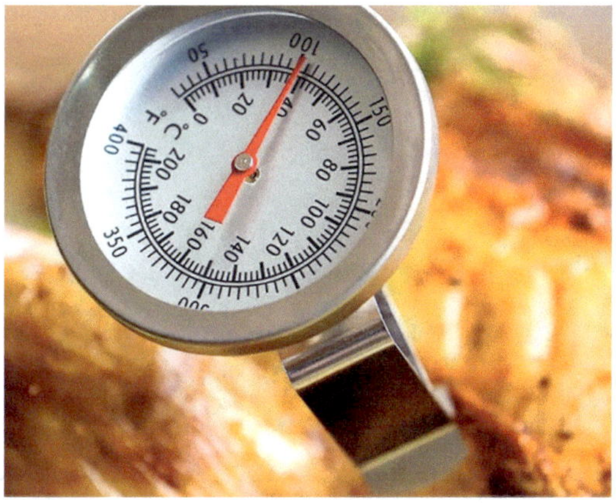

Figure 5.12. Thermometers play a crucial role in ensuring food safety, particularly in maintaining safe storage and temperature control.

Source: https://econtrolsystems.com/wp-content/uploads/2019/11/35-4.27.20-safe-food-temps.jpg

5.3. Food Storage for Different Types of Food

Keeping food safe and fresh is important and this depends on how you store each type of food, as every item has its own needs. For example, meat and dairy should be kept cold at below 40°F to stop bacteria and grains and pasta should be stored in a cool, dark area to prevent moisture and pests. Also, keeping food in airtight containers can help it stay fresh longer by preventing it from coming into contact with air and moisture. Additionally, the expanding application of plastics in packaging food increases concerns of chemicals from additives migrating into food products, requiring thorough consideration of the used packaging materials for protecting consumers' health (Hahladakis et al., 2017). Therefore, it is imperative to comprehend these storage needs not only to protect public health but also to contribute to broader climate-resilient development within food systems (Intergovernmental Panel on Climate Change, 2023).

5.3.1. Meat and Poultry Storage Guidelines

Properly storing meat and poultry is very important for avoiding foodborne illness and sticking to the rules is necessary for food safety. It is important to keep meat and poultry in the fridge at temperatures below 40°F to stop bacteria from growing and raw products should be placed on the bottom shelf to avoid drips from contaminating other foods. Also, packing meat properly is very important; wrapping it tightly in plastic or vacuum-sealing it can help it stay fresh longer. Open dating systems, which educate consumers on product freshness, are worth noting since applying a standardized method could boost the quality of safe purchasing decisions (Labuza and Szybist, 2025). Lastly, applying principles of HACCP to food storage habits can assist in discovering CCPs and compliance with safety measures. Following these recommendations, consumers can avoid a lot of risks linked to unsafely stored meat and poultry (Figure 5.13).

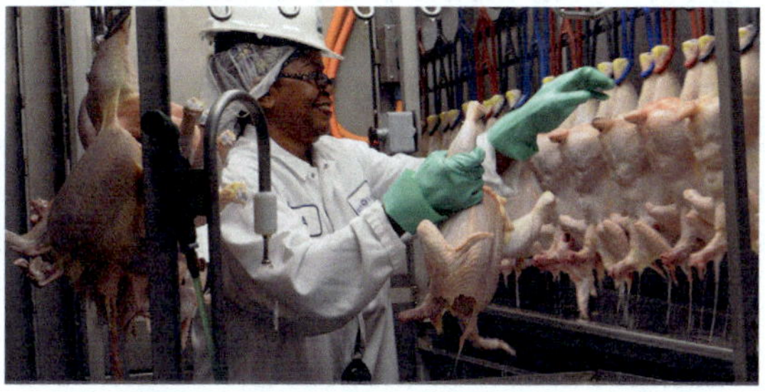

Figure 5.13. The safe storage of meat and poultry is paramount to preventing foodborne illness, and adhering to established guidelines is essential for maintaining food safety.

Source: https://www.fsis.usda.gov/sites/default/files/2024-08/Poultry%20Processing.jpg

5.3.2. Dairy Product Storage

Properly storing dairy products helps keep them safe for people to eat. Milk, cheese and yogurt are perishable and must be kept under special temperature conditions to stop pathogenic microorganisms from growing. Storing dairy products in a cold place below 40°F greatly reduces the chances of them spoiling and causing foodborne illnesses. Implementing a HACCP approach is fundamental for managing potential risks associated with dairy storage, particularly addressing microbiological hazards (Beck et al., 2003).

Also, making sure products are properly packaged and labeled is very important because it helps guarantee their authenticity and traceability, which in turn ensures customers believe in the quality. Making sure dairy products are stored as advised keeps the food chain safe and prevents health problems for the public.

5.3.3. Fruits and Vegetables Storage Tips

Keeping fruits and vegetables in proper storage helps them stay fresh and stops them from spoiling , which makes food safer. It is necessary to understand that some fruits produce ethylene gas , which can cause nearby vegetables to spoil more quickly, so they should be kept apart. Store leafy greens somewhere humid to prevent them from drying out and store root vegetables in a cool, dark place to stop them from sprouting.

Temperature management is important, as most vegetables and fruits are kept in a refrigerator, preferably between 32°F and 40°F, to reduce microbial growth (Koenig et al., 1993). They not only help preserve the life of fruits and vegetables on the shelf but also reduce food loss, a serious problem, as about one in four calories produced on the planet remains uneaten (Lipinski et al., 2013). Through the application of these storage tips, the consumer can greatly improve food safety and sustainability (Figure 5.14).

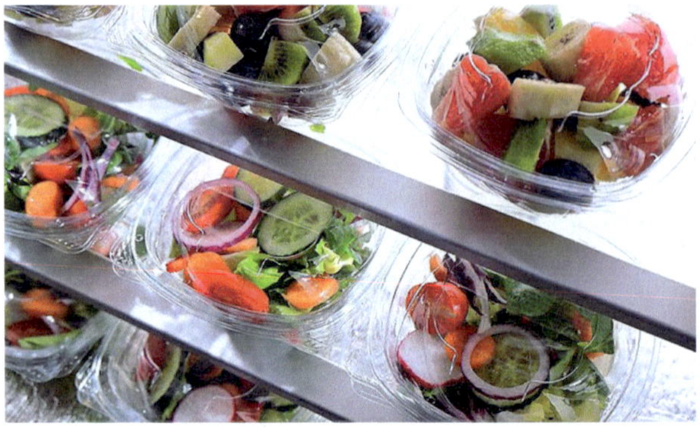

Figure 5.14. Effective storage of fruits and vegetables is crucial for maintaining their freshness and preventing spoilage, ultimately contributing to safe food practices.

Source: https://www.food-safety.com/ext/resources/Images/2024/Jun_Jul/Cat-0624-900-Img1.jpg?height=418&t=1720534531&width=800

5.3.4. Grains and Dry Goods Storage

Proper storage of grains and dry foods is required to protect them and prevent them from spoiling, which can damage food safety. A key part of it is reaching the Safe Moisture Content (SMC), or the maximum safe amount of moisture that permits safe storage without affecting nutritional quality. For grains, this threshold typically falls between 6% and 14%, making it essential for storage facilities to monitor humidity levels closely (Afolabi et al., 2014). Also, keeping food at a cool temperature and well-ventilated helps stop mold and pests from appearing , which could result in food getting contaminated and wasted. Teaching people involved in the food industry about these practices can lead to safer food and better-quality stored grains and dry goods , which is good for public health.

5.3.5. Canned and Preserved Foods

Canned and preserved foods are very important for food safety and storage because global trade brings a wider range of products. Canning includes sterilization , which gets rid of dangerous microorganisms that could make the food unsafe. Still, the safety and quality of these products may be at risk because of inadequate safety rules in different countries. For instance, the U.S. Food and Drug Administration has raised concerns about imported food safety, particularly from regions like China, citing issues , such as inadequate enforcement of food safety regulations and contamination risks associated with additives and labeling (Gale & Buzby, 2009). Additionally, fresh produce, when processed through methods like canning and drying, can enhance shelf life while retaining vital nutrients, though improper handling can lead to contamination, as seen in some fresh fruit products (Olielo et al., 2014). Thus, robust temperature control and stringent quality management are imperative to mitigate food safety risks associated with canned and preserved foods (Figure 5.15).

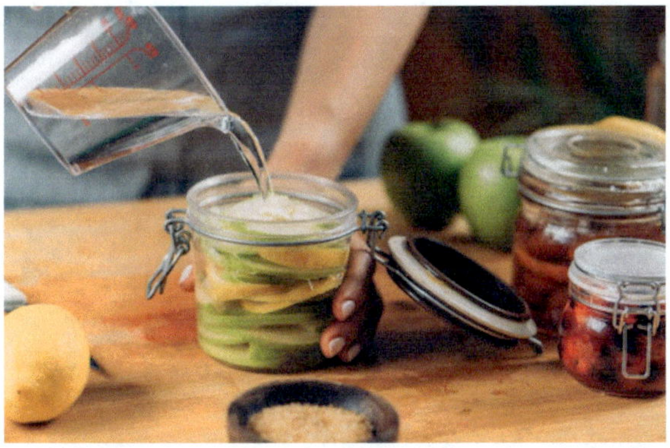

Figure 5.15. Canned and preserved foods represent a crucial component of food safety and storage management, particularly as global trade increases the variety of products available.

Source: https://www.ficsi.in/blog/wp-content/uploads/2022/12/unnamed-4.jpg

5.3.6. Leftovers and Reheating

How you handle leftovers and reheat them is very important for your health and to avoid getting sick from food. Putting your leftovers in the fridge as soon as possible helps to stop bacteria from growing. Research indicates that consumer behaviors surrounding leftovers vary significantly across regions, with findings showing that many individuals leave food at room temperature for extended periods before refrigeration, which can lead to unsafe conditions for consumption (Carbonell-Barrachina et al., 2016). Moreover, when reheating leftovers, it is essential to heat food to a minimum internal temperature of 165°F to effectively eliminate harmful pathogens that may have developed during storage (BC Cook Articulation Committee, 2015). Following these rules allows people to make their meals healthier and tastier. So, it is very important to know about safe food storage and temperature when dealing with leftovers and reheating.

5.3.7. Special Considerations for Allergens

For safe food storage and temperature control, it is very important to pay special attention to allergens to keep consumers safe. Because kitchens handle many different foods, there is a high risk of cross-contamination; that's why strong rules are needed to stop allergens from mixing with other food items. For example, in a multi-use kitchen, it is essential to allocate certain equipment and storage spaces for allergenic foodstuffs, especially in the event of nut-free or gluten-free products, as noted in the guidelines of the industry (Kelliher et al., 2015). In addition, proper temperature management when storing can help avert the risk of spoilage and deterioration of allergenic components, which can otherwise culminate in life-threatening allergic reactions (Janasie et al., 2023). Therefore, practicing these procedures not only meets compliance requirements but also ensures the maintenance of a healthy eating atmosphere for everyone, especially those with increased sensitivity to allergens (Figure 5.16).

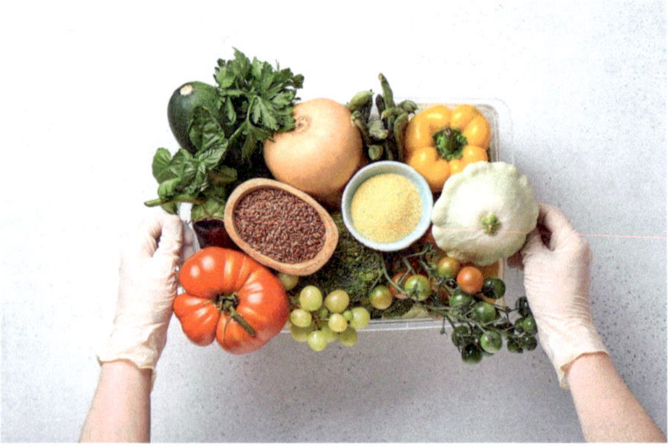

Figure 5.16. In the realm of safe food storage and temperature control, special considerations for allergens are paramount to ensure the health and safety of consumers.

Source: https://cdn.shopify.com/s/files/1/0937/2788/files/female-hands-hold-plastic-box-with-assortment-of-f-2023-11-27-04-58-37-utc.jpg?v=1707489191

5.3.8. Storage of Prepared Meals

It is very important to store prepared meals properly to prevent food poisoning. Food must be kept at the right temperature because Salmonella and similar pathogens can grow if the food is left between 40°F and 140°F , which is known as the danger zone. Research highlights that the integrity of stored food, especially when subjected to varying temperatures, can influence the probability of contamination significantly, as noted in the storage module of the qualitative assessment for Salmonella in eggs (Kelly et al., 2008). Also, cooking methods like sous vide , which rely on precise temperature and vacuum sealing, show that proper chilling and reheating are very important. Refrigerated sous vide meals, for instance, can safely be stored for up to 21 days at temperatures between 0 to 3°C, highlighting how strategic storage practices enhance food safety during extended use (Bourke et al., 2005). So, using safe storage practices is necessary to keep prepared meals fresh.

5.3.9. Seasonal Food Storage Practices

Seasonal food storage practices are very important for safe and proper food storage and temperature control. Because we get different perishable foods from harvests all year, it is necessary to find ways to keep them fresh and avoid wasting them. Using canning, freezing and dehydrating helps keep seasonal produce nutritious and usable for a longer period. Also, understanding the climate in the area can help people and communities change their storage practices to suit the environment. For instance, the need for tailored climate-smart agriculture practices highlights the importance of integrating multiple objectives related to food security and adaptation (Nhiem et al., 2020). In the same way, better food storage helps with disaster management, as can be seen in the practical steps for sanitation and hygiene used in vulnerable areas. These interconnected approaches underscore the significance of adopting effective seasonal food storage practices (Figure 5.17).

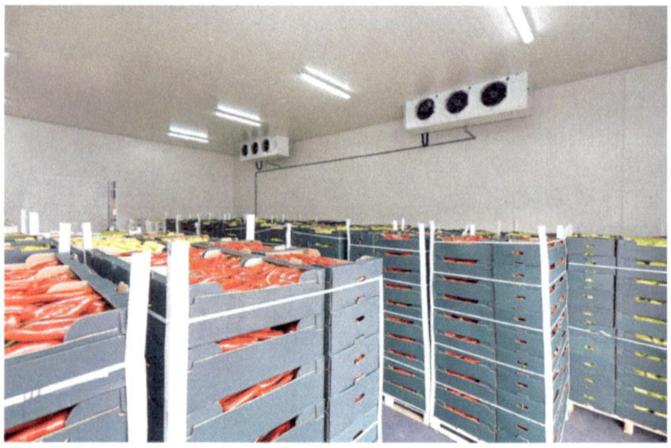

Figure 5.17. The concept of seasonal food storage practices plays a critical role within the framework of safe food storage and temperature control.

Source: https://wareiq-prelogin.s3.ap-south-1.amazonaws.com/wp-content/uploads/2023/11/23123427/cold-storage-warehouse-1124x749.jpeg.

5.4. Best Practices for Home and Commercial Storage

Good storage methods are very important for making sure food is safe both at home and in commercial areas, especially when it comes to proper food storage and temperature control. In residential kitchens, it is essential to store perishable items at temperatures below 40°F to inhibit bacterial growth, particularly for foods susceptible to Salmonella contamination, , such as eggs (Kelly et al., 2008). Commercial businesses can use new packaging ideas to help cut food waste and improve safety. Packaging that is designed correctly shields food during delivery and also helps it stay fresh for longer , which is important as the world's population increases. Using strict temperature rules at home and taking advantage of new packaging methods together helps keep food safe, reduces waste and protects people's health. For this reason, using best practices for storing food in all these areas is a key part of the effort to stop food-related illnesses.

5.4.1. Home Kitchen Organization

Organizing your kitchen at home is important to keep food safe and the temperature correct , which helps prevent illness from food. If you arrange your food properly , such as keeping perishables cold and separating raw from cooked items, you can greatly decrease the chance of cross-contamination at home. Having a tidy refrigerator makes it easy to use the ingredients and helps you check their freshness. This is particularly vital when considering the findings of studies on food safety, which demonstrate that factors like duration and temperature of storage can influence contamination levels (Kelly et al., 2008). Moreover, as indicated in workplace assessments related to food systems, creating designated areas for different food groups can enhance operational efficiency and safety in the kitchen environment (Fair Labor Association, 2006). Ultimately, an organized kitchen facilitates better meal preparation and contributes to overall food safety practices (Figure 5.18).

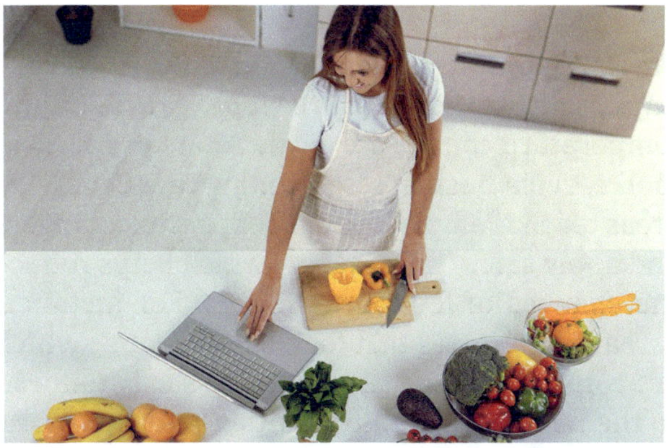

Figure 5.18. Effective home kitchen organization is critical in ensuring safe food storage and maintaining appropriate temperature control, which are essential components in preventing foodborne illnesses.

Source: https://www.ficsi.in/blog/wp-content/uploads/2024/03/Blog-3-6.jpg.

5.4.2. Commercial Kitchen Regulations

Commercial kitchen rules are essential for safe storage and temperature control of food , which is important for public health. Such regulations are in place to reduce the chances of foodborne diseases , which may happen if food is not stored correctly. An example is that keeping food at the right temperature stops microbes from growing during all parts of food handling. The U.S. spends a lot on reducing food waste , which highlights that these rules matter for both health and the economy. Furthermore, specific assessments focus on contamination risks at various stages of food processing, including storage conditions that impact food safety, as noted in (Kelly et al., 2008). When establishments follow strict commercial kitchen rules, they can reduce food waste and make sure that what they sell is safe and high quality , which is good for the community.

5.4.3. Employee Training on Food Safety

Training employees on food safety is very important to make sure food storage and temperature control are always done properly in food service businesses. Training that covers all areas teaches employees to spot possible dangers and apply safety procedures , which helps reduce the chances of foodborne illness. For instance, research indicates that food safety plans , which are commonly used, are not necessarily tailored to the needs of specific facilities, and therefore, other training addressing their specific issues is required. In addition, improper handwashing techniques have been found to be a major issue, with about 60% of food service workers not following recommended hygiene standards (Fair Labor Association, 2006).

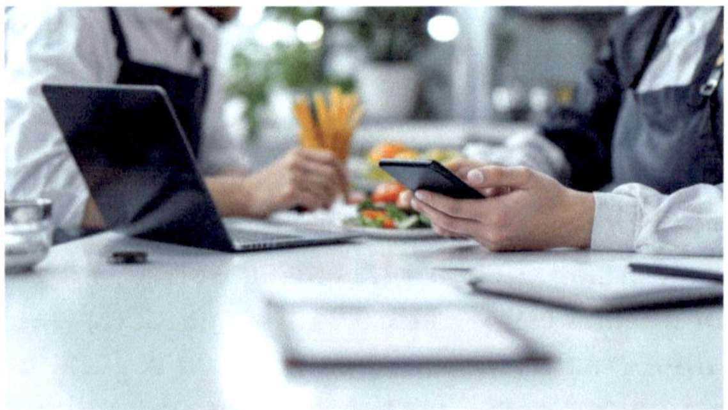

Figure 5.19. Effective employee training on food safety is paramount in ensuring that safe food storage and temperature control practices are consistently followed within food service establishments.

Source: https://framerusercontent.com/images/V3WAGiIHWpZFLmq2C9J4clEBhU.jpg

Thus, strict implementation of training modules on food handling and temperature control needs to be given top priority to ensure employees not only know the theoretical principles but also implement best practices efficiently in actual environments, supporting overall food safety measures (Fair Labor Association, 2006) (Figure 5.19).

5.4.4. Use of Technology in Food Storage

Technological progress in food storage greatly helps to keep food safe and fresh for longer. Using controlled temperature storage and smart sensors greatly lowers the chance of food spoiling. For instance, holding fish at the best temperatures can inhibit histamine formation, which is essential in foodborne illness avoidance, as exemplified from research in the storage of ikan tongkol, where control of the temperature is imperative in minimizing bacterial growth and product quality (Adiputra et al., 2007).

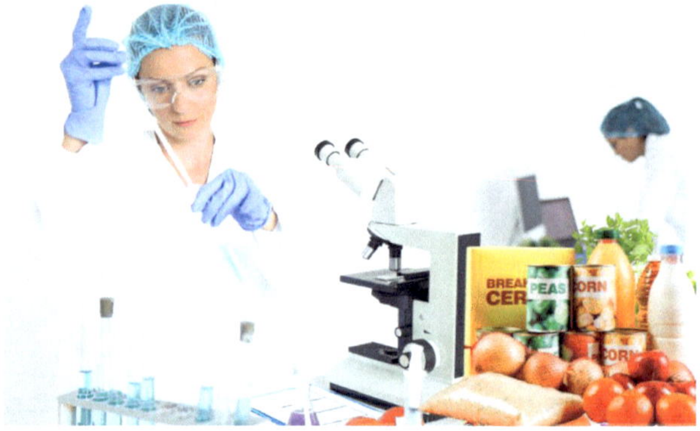

Figure 5.20. The advancement of technology in food storage plays a critical role in enhancing food safety and extending shelf life.

Source: https://envirocarelabs.com/wp-content/uploads/2024/06/Website-Blog-Images-14.jpg

Additionally, organic grain storage highlights the use of energy-efficient drying and cooling systems as emphasized by research, which not only preserves grain quality but also minimizes waste by adopting sustainable production and storage practices (Anon, 2001). Furthermore, the incorporation of advanced technology ensures a holistic means of ensuring safe food storage, ultimately ensuring the protection of public health while meeting the growing need for high-quality food products (Figure 5.20).

5.4.5. Emergency Preparedness for Food Storage

Being prepared to store food in emergencies is highly significant for safety and nutrition. In the event of a natural disaster or other unexpected issue, proper storage of food is highly significant. Proper temperatures for storing foods that are not meant to be kept at room temperature prevent foodborne illnesses , which is significant due to temperature control requirements. Through IoT devices, sophisticated technologies can monitor storage conditions and directly notify of temperature fluctuations that could impact the quality of food. This convergence of technology is highlighted by current research highlighting the value of responsible digitalization to increase food safety measures as well as combat more comprehensive environmental concerns (Dwivedi et al., 2021). In addition, with the dynamic of emergency preparedness changing, food storage systems need to adopt resilient practices that help maintain food integrity against physical and technological hazards (Stoyanova et al., 2020). Through the application of these developments, communities can enhance their capacity in managing emergencies and enhancing public health.

5.4.6. Community Resources for Food Safety

Community resources for food safety are important because they help people follow safe storage and temperature rules , which are needed for public health. Local health departments (LHDs) and cooperative extension services often provide educational programs aimed at increasing awareness of proper food handling and storage techniques. These programs are vital, particularly in areas experiencing high rates of food insecurity, as they can significantly influence community resilience and food security levels (Mittal & Sethi, 2009). Additionally, initiatives aimed at reducing food loss and waste help address the broader implications of food safety, as they reduce the overall demand for food production, which strains local ecosystems (Lipinski et al., 2013). When people in a community get involved with these resources, they learn to be aware and responsible about food safety in their homes and in the community as a whole. Ultimately, strengthening community resources is essential for promoting food safety and enhancing public health outcomes (Figure 5.21).

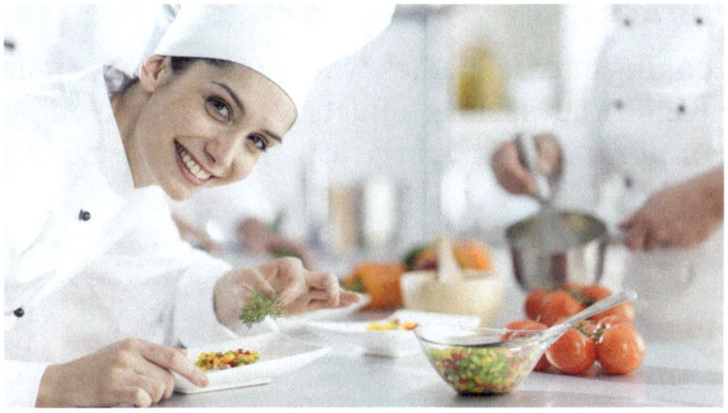

Figure 5.21. Effective community resources for food safety play a crucial role in ensuring safe food storage and temperature control practices, which are imperative for public health.

Source: https://restaurantindia.s3.ap-south-1.amazonaws.com/s3fs-public/content8377.jpg.

5.4.7. Role of Government Regulations

Making sure that food is properly stored and maintained at the correct temperature is largely due to governmental regulations that prevent foodborne diseases. As noted in most studies, poor hygienic practices contribute highly to the risk of microbial contamination of food products, showing the need for strict regulatory mechanisms to implement food safety regulations (Bikuba et al., 2025). Laws require food handlers to be trained properly and outline the rules for CCPs , which include storing and transporting food at the right temperatures. Such measures are vital since inadequate temperature control can lead to the proliferation of harmful pathogens, often exacerbated by inadequate food handling practices (El-Olemy et al., 2008). Government oversight is necessary to ensure that rules are followed and to supply education to food service staff , which improves their food safety knowledge. Thus, strong regulations keep food safe and help people trust the food they buy.

5.4.8. Case Studies of Food Storage Failures

Looking at case studies where food storage fails reveals the serious effects of not controlling temperature properly on food safety. An important example is when frozen meat spoiled due to being kept at the wrong temperature , which caused bacteria to grow and made many people sick. The incident points out that not following temperature rules can be dangerous and that food storage must be regularly checked. Additionally, leveraging technology in storage, say, real-time monitoring of temperature, can notify personnel immediately if temperature changes occur. These technological interventions resonate with the overarching themes identified in the IPCC's (Intergovernmental Panel on Climate Change, 2023) report, which emphasizes the interplay between human practice and ecological consequence. Finally, examination of such failures not only serves to re-emphasize the relevance of food storage in safety but also promotes adjustments that help toward a resilient food supply chain, as implied in emerging responses to global health crises illustrated by Krammer (2020).

A CLOSER LOOK

Storage of Perishable Food Items

Keeping perishable foods in the right way helps keep them safe, stops them from spoiling and lowers the risk of getting sick from food-borne diseases. Meat, dairy products, seafood and fresh produce should be stored in places where the temperature is right to stop harmful microorganisms from growing. Refrigeration at temperatures between 0°C and 4°C (32°F to 40°F) helps preserve freshness, while freezing at –18°C (0°F) or below extends shelf life. Raw meats should be kept in different containers from RTE foods and everything should be stored in clean, airtight containers. Regularly watch the storage conditions, do not forget to check expiration dates and never leave perishable items out at room temperature for a long time. If these methods are used, food will be safe and of good quality.

SUMMARY

The level of safe storage of food and temperature control is very high, as it provides a great support for the safety of food and public health. Employing systems , such as HACCPs prevents food processing and storage risks that enhance food safety. Such a preventive strategy, as remarked by European regulatory agencies, is a significant departure from reactive practices frequently failing to guarantee consumer safety, stressing the importance of stringent control measures (Aalberts et al., 2003). In addition, given the globalization of food distribution, there is a need to have the same high standards of food safety everywhere in order to secure public health and confidence. Therefore, both producers and consumers must prioritize proper food handling practices to minimize foodborne illnesses and promote overall well-being within communities (Fair Labor Association, 2006).

Overall, safe storage of food and temperature control are important because the U.S. food industry generates more than $700 billion annually. Yet, increasing numbers of food safety issues have contributed to lost consumer confidence, and food companies have been forced to tackle these quality problems to stay profitable (Odugbemi et al., 2017). One of the successful approaches is the uptake of stringent certifications , such as the Safe Quality Food (SQF) certification, which is a reliable standard for implementing food safety measures. Research shows that, when properly used, SQF certification can greatly improve food manufacturing practices and reduce failures (Odugbemi et al., 2017). In addition, most operational conditions, like preparing for natural disasters, involve an understanding of how temperature and other environmental factors influence food safety. All of these emphasize the importance of complete strategies to maintain food safety as circumstances evolve.

KEY TERMS FROM THIS CHAPTER

- Airtight containers
- Alaska
- Canning
- Chilling
- Citrus fruits
- Cold chains
- Conjunction
- Contamination risks
- Danger zone
- Date labels
- Dry goods
- FIFO (First In, First Out) method
- Food distribution
- Food safety management
- Frafra potato
- Freezing

REFERENCES

1. Aalberts, C. H. J. (2003). *HACCP Plan Fresh Fish Processing Marituna*. https://core.ac.uk/download/pdf/29294826.pdf (accessed on 29 May 2025).
2. Gallo A, Accorsi R, Baruffaldi G, Manzini R. Designing Sustainable Cold Chains for Long-Range Food Distribution: Energy-Effective Corridors on the Silk Road Belt. *Sustainability*. 2017; 9(11):2044. https://doi.org/10.3390/su9112044 (accessed on 29 May 2025).
3. Adiputra, N., Arka, I. B., Suranaya Pandit, I. G., & Suryadhi, I. G. (2007). *Pengaruh Penyiangan Dan Suhu Penyimpanan Terhadap Mutu Kimiawi, Mikrobiologis Dan Organoleptik Ikan Tongkol (Auxis Tharzard, Lac)*. https://media.neliti.com/media/publications/224812-none-99d878d6.pdf (accessed on 29 May 2025).
4. Afolabi, I. S. (2014). *Moisture Migration and Bulk Nutrients Interaction in A Drying Food Systems: A Review*. https://core.ac.uk/download/95550451.pdf.
5. Alarcon-Rojo, A. D., Luna, L., Mason, T., & Paniwnyk, L. (2018). *Ultrasound for Improving the Preservation of Chicken Meat*. https://core.ac.uk/download/304335332.pdf (accessed on 29 May 2025).
6. Alminger, M. (2018). *Innovative and Eco-Sustainable Processing and Packaging for Safe and High-Quality Organic Products with Enhanced Nutritional Quality: Final Report*. https://core.ac.uk/download/161988934.pdf (accessed on 29 May 2025).
7. Alves, V. D., Lourenço, S. C., & Moldão-Martins, M. (2019). *Antioxidants of Natural Plant Origins: From Sources to Food Industry Applications*. https://core.ac.uk/download/250590170.pdf (accessed on 29 May 2025).
8. Angelos, J. A., Arens, A. L., Johnson, H. A., Cadriel, J. L., & Osburn, B. I. (2017). One Health in food safety and security education: Subject matter outline for a curricular framework. *One health (Amsterdam, Netherlands)*, *3*, 56–65. https://doi.org/10.1016/j.onehlt.2017.04.001(accessed on 29 May 2025).
9. Anon. (2001). *Integrated Grain Storage–Technology Transfer for Organic Farming*. https://core.ac.uk/download/10923913.pdf (accessed on 29 May 2025).
10. Baek, S. H., Lim, C. G., Park, J. I., Seo, Y. B., & Nam, I. (2024). Investigation of *Salmonella enteritidis* growth under varying temperature conditions in liquid whole egg: Proposals for smart management technology for safe refrigerated storage. *Foods, 13*. https://www.semanticscholar.org/paper/c8f1eeb7df519faaea60bbf3f1763f7b64c1ff53 (accessed on 29 May 2025).
11. Beck, A. J., Ferguson, A., & Ropkins, K. (2003). *Development of Hazard Analysis and Critical Control Points (Haccp) Procedures to Control Organic Chemical Hazards in The Agricultural Production of Raw Food Commodities*. https://core.ac.uk/download/60392.pdf (accessed on 29 May 2025).
12. Bikuba, A., Nyamete, F., & Ngungulu, A. W. (2025). Assessment of food safety practices, associated factors and microbial contamination of fried Nile perch in Mwanza City markets: A cross-sectional study. *European Journal of Nutrition & Food Safety*. https://www.semanticscholar.org/paper/4c5d7cf5987a07ccd1cec68de821809155bbe644 (accessed on 29 May 2025).

13. Bourke, P., Carbonell, S., Gormley, R. T., & O'Beirne, D. (2005). *Developing Sous Vide/Freezing Systems for Ready-Meal Components*. https://core.ac.uk/download/45656726.pdf (accessed on 29 May 2025).

14. BC Cook Articulation Committee. (2015). *Food Safety, Sanitation, and Personal Hygiene*. Victoria, B.C.: BCcampus. Retrieved from https://opentextbc.ca/foodsafety/.Garcia Martinez, Marian & Poole, Nigel D. & Briz, Julian & de Felipe, Isabel & Yalcin, Ismet & Koc, A. Ali & Messaho, Driss, 2004. "**Benchmarking International Food Safety Performance in the Fresh Produce Sector**," 84th Seminar, February 8-11, 2004, Zeist, The Netherlands 24998, European Association of Agricultural Economists.(accessed on 29 May 2025).

15. Fred Gale and Jean C. Buzby (2009). *Imports from China and Food Safety Issues*. https://core.ac.uk/download/pdf/6794989.pdf (accessed on 29 May 2025).

16. Carbonell-Barrachina, A. A., Cardinal, P., Chambers, E., IV, et al. (2016). *Food Leftover Practices Among Consumers in Selected Countries in Europe, South and North America*. https://core.ac.uk/download/141472164.pdf (accessed on 29 May 2025).

17. Coastal Response Research Center. (2020). *NOS Hurricane Preparedness Summit Series 2020*. https://core.ac.uk/download/389382413.pdf (accessed on 29 May 2025).

18. Cole, K., Kwon, J., Olds, D., & Roberts, K. (2014). *Analysis of School Food Safety Programs Based on HACCP Principles*. https://core.ac.uk/download/77977698.pdf (accessed on 29 May 2025).

19. Das, D. K., Hok, C. I., Lewis, C. E., & Logan, T. (1988). *Circular 64*. https://core.ac.uk/download/162574814.pdf (accessed on 29 May 2025).

20. Dwivedi, Y. K., Hughes, L., Kar, A. K., Baabdullah, A. M., Grover, P., Abbas, R., Andreini, D., et al. (2021). Climate change and COP26: Are digital technologies and information management part of the problem or the solution? An editorial reflection and call to action. *International Journal of Information Management, 63*, Article 102456. https://doi.org/10.1016/j.ijinfomgt.2021.102456.

21. El-Olemy, A., & Fouda, L. (2008). Health education intervention program of food services staff for provision of safety food in Tanta hospitals, *38*, 439–458. https://www.semanticscholar.org/paper/8557a707861699054312b84d843274804039111d (accessed on 29 May 2025).

22. Endut, I. R., Faisol, N., Jaafar, H. S., & Omar, M. (2025). *Innovation in Logistics Services–Halal Logistics*. https://core.ac.uk/download/pdf/6643402.pdf (accessed on 29 May 2025).

23. Eze, J., Duan, Y., Eze, E., Ramanathan, R., & Ajmal, T. (2024). Machine learning-based optimal temperature management model for safety and quality control of perishable food supply chain. *Scientific Reports, 14*. https://www.semanticscholar.org/paper/04d5d30b2a76df10b319cfbf31870044ecd6b27b (accessed on 29 May 2025).

24. Fair Labor Association. (2006). *Tracking Chart 2006 Adidas Group, Guatemala 010028420E*. https://core.ac.uk/download/33596236.pdf (accessed on 29 May 2025).

25. Fenster, K., Freeburg, B., Hollard, C., Wong, C., Rønhave Laursen, R., & Ouwehand, A. C. (2019). The production and delivery of probiotics: A review of a practical approach. *Microorganisms, 7*(3), 83. https://doi.org/10.3390/microorganisms7030083.

26. Godwin, S. L., & Ricketts, J. (2019). *Poultry and Egg Education Project (PEEP) Curriculum Resource*. https://core.ac.uk/download/479060111.pdf (accessed on 29 May 2025).

27. Hahladakis, J. N., Velis, C. A., Weber, R., Iacovidou, E., & Purnell, P. (2017). An overview of chemical additives presents in plastics: Migration, release, fate and environmental impact

during their use, disposal and recycling. *Journal of Hazardous Materials, 344*, 179–199. https://doi.org/10.1016/j.jhazmat.2017.10.014.

28. Hamilton, A. N. (2024a). *Determination of Factors Influencing Microbial Food Safety Risks of Additive Manufacturing and 3d Printing of Food*. https://core.ac.uk/download/613694278.pdf (accessed on 29 May 2025).

29. Hamilton, A. N. (2024b). *Determination of Factors Influencing Microbial Food Safety Risks of Additive Manufacturing And 3d Printing of Food*. https://core.ac.uk/download/619597376.pdf (accessed on 29 May 2025).

30. Ibadullah, W., Brishti, F. H., Ab Rashid, N. K. M., Rashedi, I., Abedin, N. H. Z., Shukri, R., & Mohd Dzomir, A. Z. (2024). Effect of gamma irradiation and salt on the physical properties and microbiological quality of turmeric paste (*Curcuma longa*). *Journal of Biochemistry, Microbiology and Biotechnology*. https://www.semanticscholar.org/paper/24c9a6bba4f2a5a1466397cba71709a85b7550d4 (accessed on 29 May 2025).

31. Intergovernmental Panel on Climate Change. (2023). *Climate Change 2022–Impacts, Adaptation and Vulnerability*. https://doi.org/10.1017/9781009325844.

32. Janasie, C. M. (2023). *Federal Food Safety Framework: Where Does Seaweed Fit in?* https://core.ac.uk/download/556225924.pdf (accessed on 29 May 2025).

33. Karić, N., Maia, A. S., Teodorović, A., Atanasova, N., Langergraber, G., Crini, G., Ribeiro, A. R., et al. (2021). Bio-waste valorization: Agricultural wastes as biosorbents for removal of (in)organic pollutants in wastewater treatment. *Chemical Engineering Journal Advances, 9*, 100239. https://doi.org/10.1016/j.ceja.2021.100239.

34. Kelliher, K., Matsunami, K., & Sheffield, T. (2015). *A Reference Guide for Identifying the Technical Details of a Commercial, Shared-Use Kitchen in Bates Mill No. 5*. https://core.ac.uk/download/230690070.pdf (accessed on 29 May 2025).

35. Kelly, L., Madden, R. H., Murchie, L., et al. (2008). *Qualitative Exposure Assessment for Salmonella spp. In Shell Eggs Produced on The Island of Ireland*. https://core.ac.uk/download/9023098.pdf (accessed on 29 May 2025).

36. Koenig, B., Rohrs, B. A., Rupp, M. J., et al. (1993). *Parent Resource Packet–A Guide for New Parents*. https://core.ac.uk/download/286359687.pdf (accessed on 29 May 2025).

37. Krammer, F. (2020). SARS-CoV-2 vaccines in development. *Nature, 586*, 516–527. https://doi.org/10.1038/s41586-020-2798-3.

38. Kumar, P., Lee, S. S., Zhang, M., Tsang, Y. F., & Kim, K. H. (2019). Heavy metals in food crops: Health risks, fate, mechanisms, and management. *Environment International, 125*, 365–385. https://doi.org/10.1016/j.envint.2019.01.067.

39. Labuza, T. P., & Szybist, L. M. (2025). *Current Practices and Regulations Regarding Open Dating of Food Products*. https://core.ac.uk/download/pdf/7025298.pdf (accessed on 29 May 2025).

40. Lemić, D., Galešić, M. A., Bjeliš, M., & Virić Gašparić, H. (2024). Ozone treatment as a sustainable alternative for suppressing blue mold in mandarins and extending shelf life. *Agriculture*. https://www.semanticscholar.org/paper/a7c2b9342d0184ed702c7a126e3a5841c59d2e2f (accessed on 29 May 2025).

41. Lipinski, B., Hanson, C., Lomax, J., Kitinoja, L., Waite, R., & Searchinger, T. (2013). *Creating a*

Sustainable Food Future: Reducing Food Loss and Waste (Installment 2). https://core.ac.uk/download/71362194.pdf (accessed on 29 May 2025).

42. Marule, N. L., du, G., & Marx-Pienaar, N. (2024). Gauteng's managers' implementation of food safety protocols and practices in their QSR environments. *Journal of Consumer Sciences.* https://www.semanticscholar.org/paper/506df82b5101cd300059e28908a5d233ff44c5d6 (accessed on 29 May 2025).
43. Mora, J. (2012). *An Examination of Modernist Culinary Techniques and Equipment and Their Application in Catering Operations.* http://digitalscholarship.unlv.edu/cgi/viewcontent.cgi?article=2350&context=thesesdissertations (accessed on 29 May 2025).
44. Nguyen, D. N., Nguyen-Duy, N., Rubiano, F., & Talsma, T. (2020). *CSA Practices for Sustainable Cocoa Farming Systems.* https://core.ac.uk/download/294831730.pdf (accessed on 29 May 2025).
45. Ninfaa, D. A. W., Anyindana, A., & Lenia. (2024). Evaluating the impact of various storage techniques on longevity of Frafra potato (*Solenostemon rotundifolius*) in the Upper East Region of Ghana. *Journal of Applied Sciences and Environmental Management.* https://www.semanticscholar.org/paper/9a2c5ec8935cf39ef18f33f3d6965758912cc03e (accessed on 29 May 2025).
46. Odugbemi, A. A. (2017). *Safe Quality Food Certification and Producing Safe and Quality Food Products.* https://core.ac.uk/download/147841284.pdf (accessed on 29 May 2025).
47. Olielo, T. K. (2014). *Microbial and Preservative Safety of Fresh and Processed Fruit Salads, Fruit Soft Drinks and Jam in Kenya.* https://core.ac.uk/download/478343015.pdf (accessed on 29 May 2025).
48. Osunde, Z., & Adepoju, L. (2020). Changes in quality of pawpaw (*Carica papaya*) fruit dried under different pretreatments and drying. *Journal of Engineering in Agriculture and the Environment.* https://www.semanticscholar.org/paper/8dc99165ee68497d2b99fb79b53f08cdbe9c56ce (accessed on 29 May 2025).
49. Qu, Z., Tang, J., Sablani, S. S., Ross, C. F., Sankaran, S., & Shah, D. H. (2021). Quality changes in chicken livers during cooking. *Poultry Science, 100*, Article 101316. https://doi.org/10.1016/j.psj.2021.101316.
50. Rajial, H., & Varma, S. (2024). Edible coatings: A novel approach to extending the shelf life of fruits and vegetables. *Journal of Advances in Biology & Biotechnology.* https://www.semanticscholar.org/paper/85c1a6c4ee75a40eae52af9062d2f467abbc80b1 (accessed on 29 May 2025).
51. Salgado, P. R., Di Giorgio, L., Musso, Y. S., & Mauri, A. N. (2021). Recent developments in smart food packaging focused on biobased and biodegradable polymers. *Frontiers in Sustainable Food Systems, 5*, 630393. https://doi.org/10.3389/fsufs.2021.630393.
52. Salminen, S., Collado, M. C., Endo, A., Hill, C., Lebeer, S., Quigley, E. M. M., Sanders, M. E., et al. (2021). The International Scientific Association of Probiotics and Prebiotics (ISAPP) consensus statement on the definition and scope of postbiotics. *Nature Reviews Gastroenterology & Hepatology, 18*, 649–667. https://doi.org/10.1038/s41575-021-00440-6.
53. Mittal, S. Sethi, D. (2009). *Food Security in South Asia: Issues and Opportunities.* Working Paper No. 240. https://core.ac.uk/download/pdf/6257149.pdf (accessed on 29 May 2025).

54. Shanbari, B. (2024). Describing the Kingdom of Saudi Arabia's efforts in controlling foodborne illnesses during Hajj seasons. *International Journal of Medicine in Developing Countries*. https://www.semanticscholar.org/paper/5df4e4fdd09f34f750838aa772f3cfb85c533239 (accessed on 29 May 2025).

55. Singh, S. P., Sharma, R., Suthar, P., & Thakur, M. (2024). Emerging innovative pre- and post-harvest management practices to mitigate patulin-linked food safety risks in apple and its products. *Journal of Food Safety*. https://www.semanticscholar.org/paper/4f5eb5d2f23b76588fa5f84ec9a725edf7f22fb4 (accessed on 29 May 2025).

56. Skjerdal, T., Gefferth, A., Spajic, M., Gaston, E., De Cesare, A., Vitali, S., Pasquali, F., et al. (2017). The STARTEC decision support tool for better tradeoffs between food safety, quality, nutrition, and costs in production of advanced ready-to-eat foods. *BioMed Research International, 2017*, Article 6353510. https://doi.org/10.1155/2017/6353510.

57. Soong, S. F. V. (2007). *Managing Halal Quality in Food Service Industry* [Master's thesis, University of Nevada, Las Vegas]. https://digitalscholarship.unlv.edu/cgi/viewcontent.cgi?article=1702&context=thesesdissertations (accessed on 29 May 2025).

58. Staffell, I., Scamman, D., Velazquez Abad, A., Balcombe, P., Dodds, P. E., Ekins, P., Shah, N., et al. (2018). The role of hydrogen and fuel cells in the global energy system. *Energy & Environmental Science, 12*, 463–491. https://doi.org/10.1039/c8ee01157e.

59. Stoyanova, M., Nikoloudakis, Y., Panagiotakis, S., Pallis, E., & Markakis, E. (2020). A survey on the Internet of Things (IoT) forensics: Challenges, approaches, and open issues. *IEEE Communications Surveys & Tutorials, 22*(2), 1191–1221. https://doi.org/10.1109/comst.2019.2962586.

60. Taylor, M., & Van Caenegem, W. (2017). *Real Deal or No Deal? A Comparative Analysis of Raw Milk Cheese Regulation in Australia and France*. https://core.ac.uk/download/196605026.pdf (accessed on 29 May 2025).

61. Thyrring, J. (2012). *Ensuring Water and Food Security in a Developing Sub-Saharan Africa*. https://core.ac.uk/download/10932506.pdf (accessed on 29 May 2025).

62. Worsfold, D. (1994). *An Evaluation of Domestic Food Hygiene and Food Preparation Practices*. https://core.ac.uk/download/161771547.pdf.

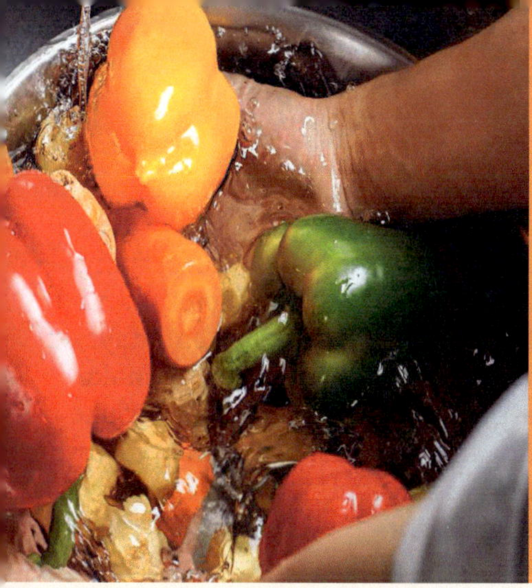

Chapter 6

COMMON FOODS AND ADULTERATION

Contents

Introduction 133
6.1. Common Foods Prone to Adulteration 136
6.2. Methods of Adulteration 140
6.3. Health Implications of Food Adulteration 144
6.4. Regulatory Measures and Consumer Protection 148
Summary 153
References 154

Introduction

The importance of knowing about adulteration in food comes from its wide effects on people's health and the honesty of markets, mainly for popular foods. Food can be adulterated by adding cheaper things or by using complex chemical methods. For instance, olive oil is often adulterated with hazelnut oil, where analytical methods have revealed that even minor adulterations, as low as 2%, can be detected through careful composition analysis of phytosterols (Azadmard-Damirchi, 2007). In addition, advances in electrical property measurement offer other approaches for differentiating types of fats, including being able to tell lard from tallow and palm oil by conductance and impedance (Djatna et al., 2013). This demonstrates that having knowledge of what to search for and employing reliable testing is crucial for maintaining food safety and quality, since adulteration is still a significant issue.

Definition of Food Adulteration

Food adulteration is basically when food is changed, either accidentally or on purpose , which leads to a drop in the food's quality or safety. Food can be manipulated by adding poor-quality materials or taking out important ingredients , which weakens the food supply. Food adulteration is not only a problem for consumers but it can also cause food poisoning and nutritional problems for the public. Because food systems are complex and food is now traded worldwide, it is harder to find and stop adulteration.

As noted in food system safety discussions, a broader understanding of food safety includes both the short-term hazards of consumption as well as the long-term health and environmental effects of food production procedures (Leib et al., 2019). Efficient detection and monitoring are necessary in evading economically driven adulteration and ensuring food products' safety (Manning & Soon, 2025) (Figure 6.1).

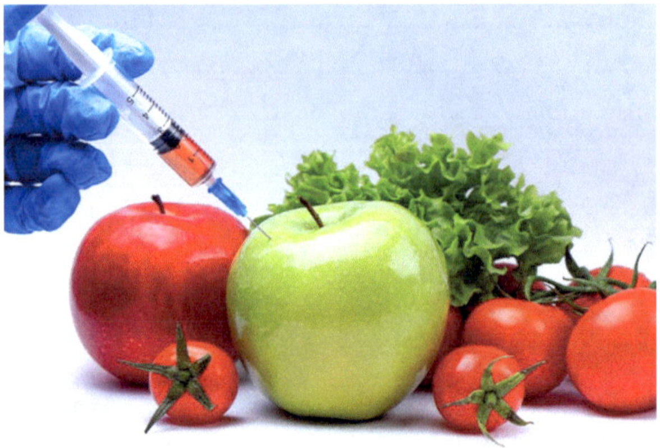

Figure 6.1. Food adulteration refers to the intentional or unintentional alteration of food products, resulting in a lowered quality or safety standard.

Source: https://thenorthlines.com/wp-content/uploads/2024/08/1_l_xcnLM0Eb0DjYj672jJ_A.jpg

Historical Context of Food Adulteration

Food adulteration in history shows a worrying trend that follows changes in society and the needs of the market. Since ancient days, people began adulterating food mainly to make more money, even if it put consumers at risk. Industrialization made it easier for people to add lower-quality ingredients to staple foods , which increased the amount produced. In the late 1800s and early 1900s, new regulations appeared because of health problems and concerns from consumers. Strong laws were put in place to stop these problems, but they still occur in today's food systems. The objective of this study is to explore the current strategies available to monitor and detect the economically and criminally motivated adulteration of food, identifying their strengths and weaknesses and recommending new approaches and policies to strengthen future capabilities to counter adulteration in a globalized food environment (Manning & Soon, 2025). Understanding this historical backdrop is crucial for framing current challenges and responses to food integrity (French & Phillips, 2002).

Importance of Studying Common Foods

There is more to studying common foods than just wanting to cook them; it also concerns health, the economy and society. It is necessary to know what coffee is made of and how it is produced to protect consumers from adulteration , which is happening more in the food industry. For instance, methodologies using high-performance liquid chromatography have demonstrated their effectiveness in assessing the authenticity of coffee by identifying common adulterants like chicory and barley, particularly highlighting how such techniques can provide essential insights into food quality (Burcio et al., 2021). Also, what foods people buy and eat , which is affected by their availability and price, has a major impact on both eating habits and health outcomes. For example, research on sucrose solutions reveals how taste modification through adulterants can affect consumption rates, reinforcing the necessity of studying food integrity to ensure public well-being and informed choices in food consumption (Valyear, 2014) (Figure 6.2).

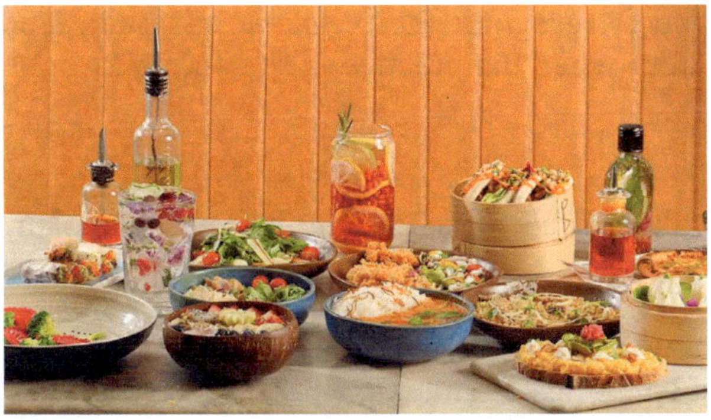

Figure 6.2. The significance of studying common foods extends beyond mere culinary interest; it encompasses critical health, economic, and social dimensions.

Source: https://restaurantindia.s3.ap-south-1.amazonaws.com/s3fs-public/2025-04/Daisy%20maa.jpg.

Overview of Common Food Items Affected

A lot of common foods are at risk from food adulteration , which affects both their quality and safety. Fats and oils are often affected and lard is a common example. It may be cut with cheaper alternatives , such as tallow or palm oil. Recent studies have demonstrated that specific electrical properties can help differentiate these fats, thereby enhancing detection methods for adulteration (Djatna et al., 2013). Seafood also raises concerns because 84% of seafood eaten in the United States is imported. The Food and Drug Administration (FDA) oversees the safety of these products, yet the prevalence of adulteration in seafood, particularly from lower-middle-income exporting countries, has led to increased detentions and import refusals as a response to regulatory challenges (Anders and Westra, 2025). They illustrate why it is important to closely watch food production to protect people.

Impact of Adulteration on Health

Besides affecting the economy, food adulteration can have major effects on public health and the safety of those who eat these products. Because of adulterants, the nutritional quality of food products can be reduced , which may cause nutritional deficiencies in children and the elderly. For instance, the adulteration of olive oil with lower-quality oils, as indicated by analyses that provide detailed insights into phytosterol profiles, can introduce harmful substances, jeopardizing cardiovascular health (Azadmard-Damirchi, 2007).

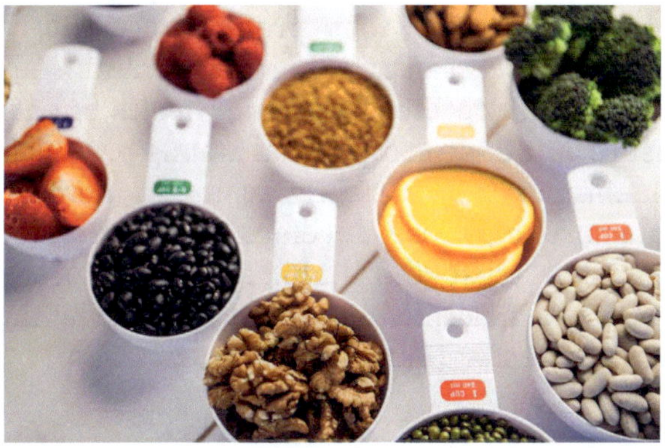

Figure 6.3. The ramifications of food adulteration extend far beyond economic implications, significantly impacting public health and consumer safety.

Source: https://www.godigit.com/content/dam/godigit/directportal/en/portion-cups-of-healthy-ingredients.jpg.

Additionally, as the adoption of legislation like the 1906 Pure Food and Drugs Act reflects, both public interest and regulatory mechanisms address these risks by aiming to ensure the authenticity and quality of food (Libecap et al.,

2025). However, these regulatory efforts may fall short if specific interests manipulate the systems for their gain, ultimately endangering consumer health and exposing the population to substandard products that may harbor unforeseen health risks (Figure 6.3).

Economic Implications of Food Adulteration

Food adulteration not only tricks consumers, but it can also cause problems in the market and change the prices in the agri-food sector. Since adulterated food causes people to distrust the market, fewer people buy genuine products , which results in financial losses for producers and retailers. Manufacturers may have to pay more for regulatory compliance and technology to detect problems , which can place a financial burden on them. DNA barcoding is one method that addresses this problem by helping to identify food products accurately , which supports safety and prevents fraud. These steps not only protect consumer health but also ensure equitable competition among producers (Manning & Soon, 2025). By facilitating increased transparency, these developments can revive consumer trust and stabilize market prices, creating a healthier economic climate within the food sector (Barcaccia et al., 2015).

6.1. Common Foods Prone to Adulteration

The problem of food adulteration seriously affects consumer safety and trust, mainly because many common ingredients are often changed. Honey, olive oil and many types of spices are often targets of economic adulteration, when cheaper substitutes are used or mixed with them. A survey conducted within the food and beverage industry reveals that 88.9% of participants acknowledge certain ingredients as being at higher risk for adulteration, with 55.6% identifying it as a top concern for food safety and quality assurance (Murphy et al., 2016). This vulnerability is exacerbated by factors like the origin of ingredients and supplier reliability, leading to a heightened risk of adulteration from regions associated with lower regulatory standards (Capps et al., 2025). For this reason, it is very important for everyone involved in food to recognize these risks to maintain food safety when malpractice is so common.

6.1.1. Milk and Dairy Products

Milk and dairy products are important in many diets because they are nutritious and also work well in a variety of recipes. Still, these foods are more likely to be adulterated , which can harm people's health and make people less confident in the food they buy.

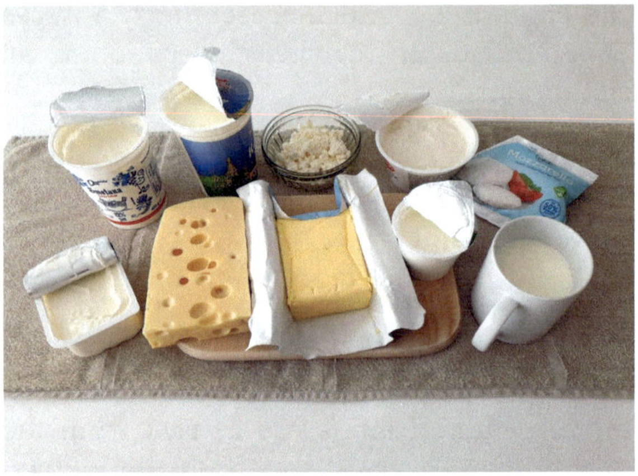

Figure 6.4. Milk and dairy products serve as staple components of many diets globally, not only for their nutritional value but also for their versatility in culinary applications.

Source: https://upload.wikimedia.org/wikipedia/commons/3/35/DairyProductsGermany.jpg

Milk may be adulterated by adding water, starch or chemicals , which reduces its quality and nutrients. Due to DNA barcoding and other emerging technologies, it is now feasible to authenticate the source of dairy products. The process capitalizes on the distinct genetic markers in plant and animal species, thus facilitating food piracy detection as well as adherence to health regulations (Archives Glasgow City et al., 2002). Moreover, the harmonization of DNA barcoding methodologies enables it to be successfully used in the protection of food quality and safety in the continually changing food sector (Barcaccia et al., 2015) (Figure 6.4).

6.1.2. Grains and Cereals

Despite being important foods in many diets, grains and cereals have been questioned because of concerns about their safety and quality due to more cases of food adulteration. In regions , such as China, public anxiety regarding the safety of food grains, including rice and wheat, is heightened by fears surrounding GMOs and environmental contamination (Jackson et al., 2016). More and more people are worried about food safety because social media often spreads news of food scandals and safety issues. In Ghana, a notable disparity exists between food production and consumption, with staple crops like maize and rice dominating diets while underutilized foods remain neglected (Aryeetey et al., 2022). Because of this, it is necessary to have reliable food safety systems and to educate the public to decrease the risk of adulteration and make consumers more confident about the quality of grain. Because of this, dealing with these issues is very important for keeping food secure and encouraging healthy eating.

6.1.3. Spices and Herbs

Because spices and herbs are of importance and incorporated in processed products, their authenticity is currently an important factor in food fraud. As highlighted by current studies, the vulnerability of spices like paprika provides an opportunity for fraud, and hence, there have been developed innovative analytical tools for their detection (Oliveira, 2020). These methods, in particular, near-infrared (NIR) spectroscopy and chemometrics, have shown potential to identify adulterants rapidly and in a non-destructive manner, playing a significant role in maintaining product quality. Moreover, evidence is that a high percentage of retail samples have been found to contain various forms of adulteration, which signifies the significance of rigorous testing procedures (Black et al., 2016). Together, these developments not only improve the safety of consumers but also support assurance in the integrity of the spice and herb supply chain, highlighting the continuous fight against food fraud on global markets (Figure 6.5).

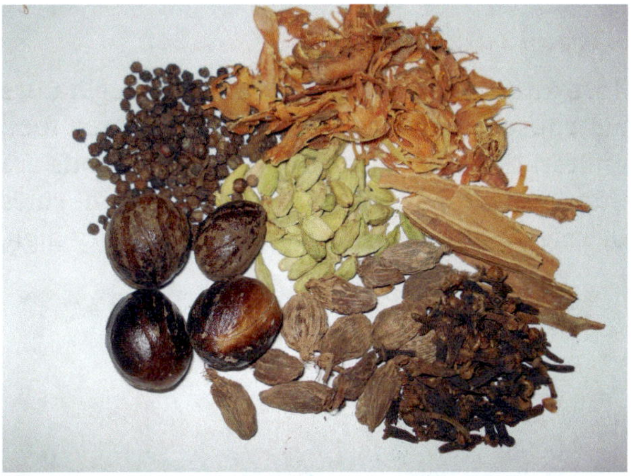

Figure 6.5. The integrity of spices and herbs has become a pressing concern in the context of food adulteration, particularly due to their significant economic value and widespread use in processed foods.

Source: https://upload.wikimedia.org/wikipedia/commons/a/a7/Garam_Masala.JPG

6.1.4. Oils and Fats

Oils and fats are important for nutrition as well as being easy targets for adulteration in the food industry. Because of the rise in unethical activities in the food industry, both consumers and producers are worried about the real quality and authenticity of the products. Many high-value oils are mixed with cheaper oils , which affects their quality and safety. To counteract these illegitimate practices, novel analytical tools like vibrational spectroscopy (VS) combined with chemometrics have come up as critical instruments for oil and fat authentication. VS methods, notably Fourier transform infrared (FTIR) spectroscopy, have proved to be highly effective in the analysis of quality factors and rapid detection of adulteration and safety of oils. The integration of VS with chemometric analysis not only facilitates the identification of genuine products but also promises a future where the integrity of oils and fats can be more reliably maintained (Li et al., 2018; Rohman, 2023).

6.1.5. Fruits and Vegetables

More international trade in fruits and vegetables has caused people to worry more about food adulteration and safety. Because these foods are often brought in from places with different rules for safety, the risk of contamination is very high.

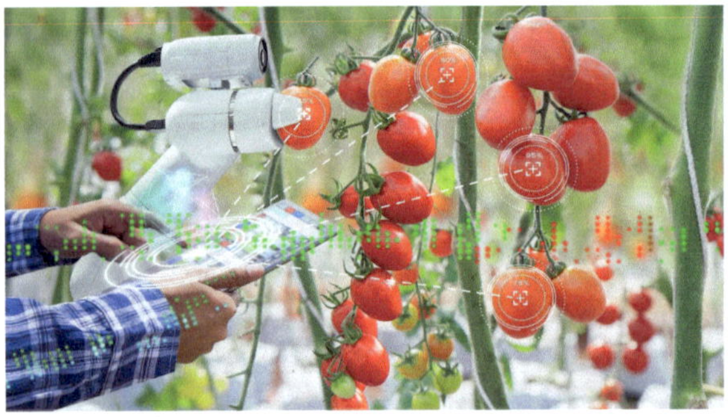

Figure 6.6. The growing global trade in fruits and vegetables has significantly increased concerns about food adulteration and safety.

Source: https://static.toiimg.com/thumb/resizemode-4,width-1280,height-720,msid-105187889/105187889.jpg.

Specifically, the U.S. FDA has raised alarms regarding food imports from countries like China, where lax enforcement of food safety measures can lead to the introduction of unsafe additives and residues (Gale & Buzby, 2009). The problems with these imports stress the importance of thinking about food safety in a wider way than only what we eat. This encompasses nutritional integrity and environmental considerations, collectively termed "Food System Safety" (Leib et al., 2019). Addressing these challenges is crucial, as ensuring the safety of fruits and vegetables will contribute to healthier diets and overall public health (Figure 6.6).

6.1.6. Meat and Poultry

The safety of meat and poultry is extremely significant for the public, but meat and poultry are usually adulterated which can be harmful to health. The numerous challenges in meat production, like the use of additives and errors in labeling, indicate why we should enact stricter food safety regulations. The expanded definition of food safety, encompassing evaluation of risk across the food supply chain, is vital to meeting these issues, as discussed in Leib et al. (2019). In addition, DNA barcoding and other technologies assist in verifying that meat and poultry foods are authentic , which combats food fraud and guarantees labels are proper. This approach has been found effective in the detection of species employed in food processing, enabling agencies to effectively track and control possible adulteration of the meat industry, validating its imperative in maintaining food safety and quality in the market, according to Barcaccia et al. (2015).

6.1.7. Fish and Seafood

The industry has to deal with serious problems of adulteration and mislabeling , which reduce people's trust and the integrity of the market. As a high-value sector, certain fish species, such as the red mullet (*Mullus barbatus*) and striped red mullet (*Mullus surmuletus*), are particularly susceptible to fraudulent practices due to their economic demand and morphological similarities with less valuable species like the Goldband goatfish (*Upeneus moluccensis*) and the imported

West African goatfish (*Pseudupeneus prayensis*) (Giantsis et al., 2023). It causes financial harm to consumers and also makes people worry about the safety of their food. As a result, new methods , such as multiplex PCR assays have been created to help tell different fish species apart. Moreover, advancements in analytical methodologies, such as MALDI-TOF MS, have shown promise in detecting adulteration across various food products, including seafood, thereby supporting the efforts to maintain quality standards in the industry (Zambonin, 2021) (Figure 6.7).

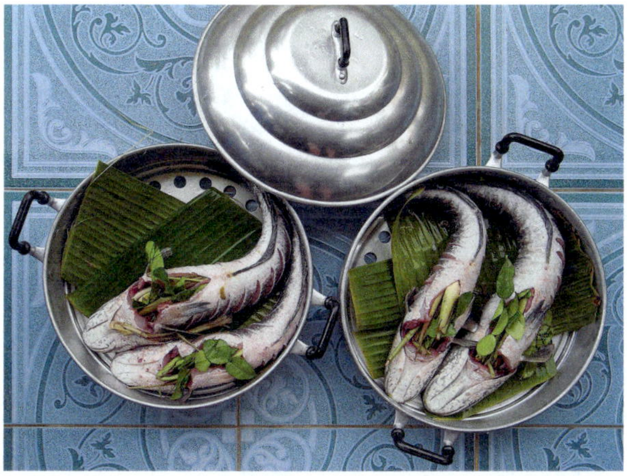

Figure 6.7. The fish and seafood industry faces significant challenges related to adulteration and mislabeling, which undermine consumer trust and market integrity.

Source: https://upload.wikimedia.org/wikipedia/commons/thumb/1/19/Fish_stuffed_with_Thai_herbs.jpg/1200px-Fish_stuffed_with_Thai_herbs.jpg

6.1.8. Sugar and Sweeteners

Because sugar and sweeteners are common ingredients in many foods, they are a major concern in the area of food adulteration. Many industries add high fructose corn syrup or invert sugar to fruit juices to reduce the cost , which can make the juice less authentic and of lower quality. This issue is elucidated through studies that developed methods for detecting these unauthorized sweeteners in juices, revealing how robust chromatographic techniques can identify their presence even at low concentrations, from 0.5% to 3% (Willems, 2017). Moreover, honey, an equally well-known sweetener, can also be adulterated similarly. Even with a definition that is set by strict regulations within the European Union, cases of adulteration with rice syrup and fructose are nevertheless perennial issues, and this calls for sophisticated detection techniques like visible and NIR spectroscopy to guarantee product quality (Aliaño González et al., 2019).

6.1.9. Beverages

A large portion of the food industry is made up of beverages and these can easily be adulterated , which can harm their quality and consumers' trust. The rise in health consciousness has led to an increased demand for beverages that are low in sugar, prompting manufacturers to incorporate high-intensity sweeteners (HIS) to cater to this market trend.

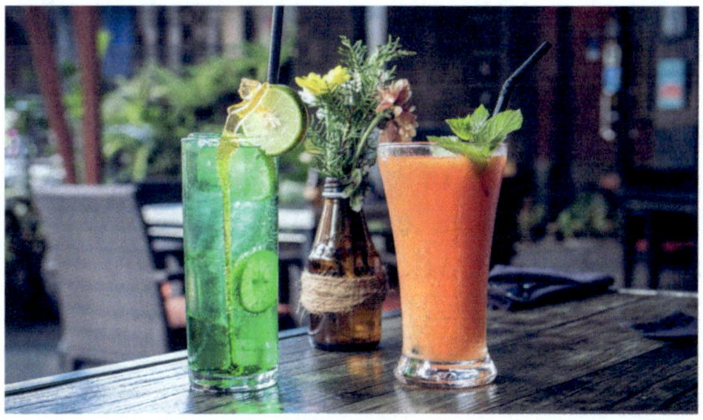

Figure 6.8. Beverages represent a significant category within the food industry, often subject to adulteration that can compromise both quality and consumer trust.

Source: https://indian-retailer.s3.ap-south-1.amazonaws.com/s3fs-public/2022-05/pexels-artem-beliaikin-452737.jpg.

Consequently, ensuring the accurate measurement of HIS levels in commercial products has become paramount, as evidenced by a study that established an analytical method using LC-MS/MS for the simultaneous determination of nine such compounds in various beverages, revealing that all samples complied with legal limits (Nicoluci et al., 2025). It is also common for the purity of liquid dairy products , such as milk, to be questioned, so new ways of detecting adulteration are needed. For example, a potentiometric electronic tongue has proven effective in rapidly identifying milk types and detecting common adulterants, showcasing the need for reliable methods to safeguard beverage integrity (Perez-Gonzalez et al., 2024) (Figure 6.8).

6.2. Methods of Adulteration

The ways food is adulterated matter a lot for the safety and honesty of food , which can affect consumer health and trust. Dilution is a common way food is adulterated by adding cheaper ingredients to boost the volume or weight , which reduces its quality. For example, for extra virgin olive oil, strict standards determine its chemical composition, such as low acidity and the absence of perceptible defects, which renders it vulnerable to fraudulent operations , such as blending with lower-quality oils (Cénez-López et al., 2020). Additionally, technology like the Internet of Things (IoT) that comes with this technology can be a double-edged sword in that it's intended to make farming more efficient, but at the same time reveals the possibility of high-tech adulteration methods that bypass conventional methods of detection (Elijah et al., 2018). Therefore, understanding the various methods through , which food may be adulterated is crucial in establishing effective regulations as well as ensuring food safety.

6.2.1. Chemical Adulteration

Chemically altering food can be very harmful, often ruining the quality of products people usually consume. It usually means adding chemicals or fake ingredients to make food look better or last longer , which often makes the food less nutritious and unsafe. An example is when olive oil is mixed with hazelnut oil , which is often difficult to discover unless it is properly examined. Specific markers , such as 4,4′-dimethylsterols can be traced back to identify this adulteration, revealing how refined hazelnut oil can mimic the characteristics of virgin olive oil at minimal concentrations, thus complicating quality assurance efforts (Azadmard-Damirchi, 2007). Moreover, regulatory frameworks, such as the 1906 Pure Food and Drugs Act, aim to address these issues by introducing standards intended to protect consumers from misleading practices, driven by both public interest and industry manipulation (Libecap et al., 2025) (Figure 6.9).

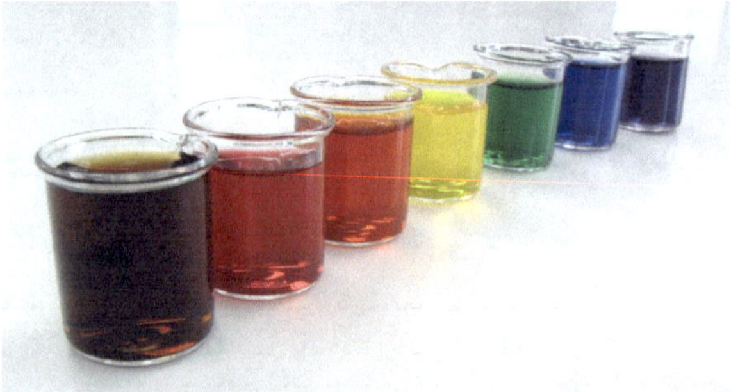

Figure 6.9. The practice of chemical adulteration poses significant challenges to food safety, often undermining the integrity of commonly consumed products.

Source: https://upload.wikimedia.org/wikipedia/commons/f/f0/Rainbow_of_food_natural_food_colors.jpg

6.2.2. Biological Adulteration

Biological adulteration happens when harmful substances are added to food, either by accident or intentionally , which reduces the quality and safety of the food. A good example is when olive oil is mixed with hazelnut oil, because the special phytosterol content in both oils can help identify the mixture. Studies demonstrate that using advanced methods like solid-phase extraction (SPE) can effectively identify this adulteration at levels as low as 2%, thereby ensuring food authenticity and consumer protection (Azadmard-Damirchi, 2007).

Also, using DNA barcoding and other molecular methods helps address the problem of biological adulteration. This technology enables the precise identification of species in food products, thereby aiding in the prevention of food fraud and enhancing food security (Barcaccia et al., 2015). This means that analyses of phytochemicals and genetic profiles are very important for developing strategies to handle the risks of biological adulteration in common foods.

6.2.3. Physical Adulteration

Physical adulteration makes food safety difficult, often affecting both the quality and honesty of foods that many people eat. Adulteration in this way includes the addition of things like stones, dirt or other substances that are not part of the food , which can change the taste and nutrients of the food. Besides affecting consumer health, such practices also play a role in keeping the food industry stable economically. Various techniques have been developed to detect these contaminants, relying heavily on the known identities of possible adulterants and the availability of analytical methods (Manning & Soon, 2025).

Furthermore, advancements in omics technologies have emerged as promising tools for enhancing food authenticity, which is crucial in mitigating the risks associated with physical adulteration (Allen et al., 2016). By implementing these innovative approaches, stakeholders can strengthen food safety measures and promote greater transparency in food supply chains (Figure 6.10).

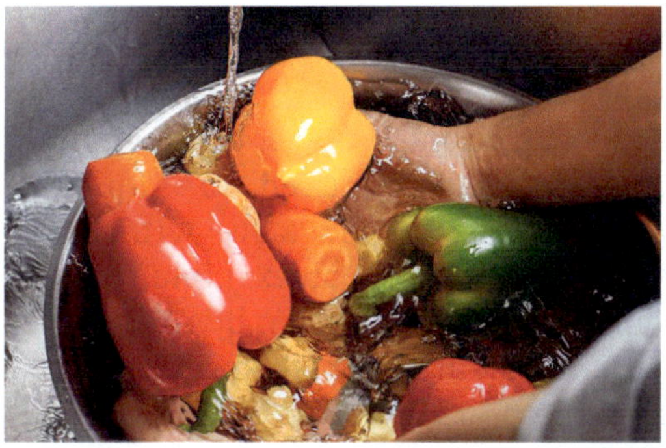

Figure 6.10. Physical adulteration presents a significant challenge within the broader issue of food safety, often compromising both the quality and integrity of commonly consumed products.

Source: https://www.godigit.com/content/dam/godigit/directportal/en/hands-wash-vegetables-in-basin.jpg.

6.2.4. Intentional vs. Unintentional Adulteration

The difference between on-purpose and accidental changes in food greatly impacts both food safety and how regulations are made. People may add harmful materials to products on purpose to make more profit , which can harm the public. Sometimes, food is adulterated by accident because people do not know or follow the correct ways to handle and produce food. Because of this gap, people question the effectiveness of present monitoring methods , which usually only find well-known adulterants. Research highlights the inadequacies of existing detection methods, noting that they rely on the adulterant being known, limiting their effectiveness (Manning & Soon, 2025). Also, the many steps in global food supply chains can result in accidental contamination because different production methods can cause problems without anyone trying to cheat. Addressing these challenges requires a comprehensive understanding of both forms of adulteration to formulate robust preventative measures (Aued-Pimentel et al., 2018).

6.2.5. Common Additives used in Adulteration

Food adulteration is more common because many additives are used to improve the appearance, texture or taste without really providing nutrition. As an example, low-quality ingredients are often hidden by using synthetic colors and flavors , which makes consumers believe the food is better than it really is. Bringing in products from countries where regulations are not as strict , such as China, is a major food safety issue. The U.S. FDA has pointed out consistent problems with unsafe additives and misbranding in such imports, which can be of serious health concern for consumers (Buzby et al., 2025). Additionally, the complexities of international food safety regulations reflect the challenge of maintaining compliance across different supply chains, which the FDA continues to tackle through collaboration with foreign regulatory bodies (Horton et al., 1997). Consequently, knowledge of such additives is key to both public health and food safety campaigns (Figure 6.11).

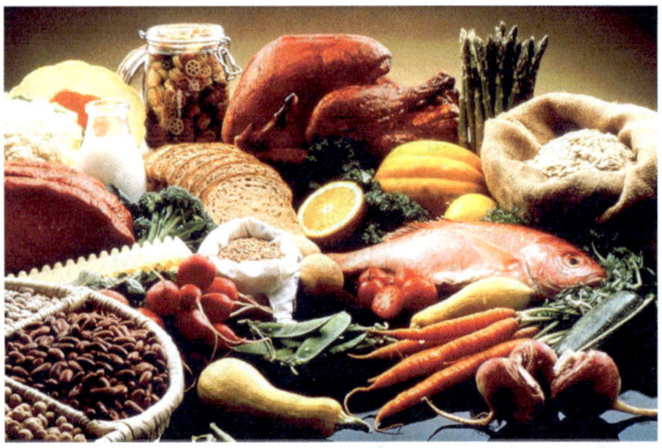

Figure 6.11. The prevalence of food adulteration is often exacerbated by the use of common additives that serve to enhance the appearance, texture, or flavor of products without adding genuine nutritional value.

Source: https://upload.wikimedia.org/wikipedia/commons/6/6d/Good_Food_Display_-_NCI_Visuals_Online.jpg.

6.2.6. Techniques for Detecting Adulteration

Different approaches to analysis need to be employed to discover whether the usual foods contain adulterants and are still safe. Luminescent assays are a popular method and they have helped determine whether virgin olive oil has been contaminated. For example, a model of regression utilizing different luminescent frequencies that have been associated with minor oils can accurately determine the purity of oils, thus exposing any adulteration blending with lower-cost alternatives, e.g., hazelnut oil (Recamales et al., 2019). An even broader strategy for combating food adulteration includes applying chemical analysis and verifying the source of products, searching for evidence of adulteration and guaranteeing the integrity of the food chain. This integrated approach not only improves detection capacity but also reinforces policies to address economically driven food fraud (EMA) globally (Manning & Soon, 2025).

6.2.7. Role of Technology in Adulteration

Technology has numerous impacts on food adulteration, with both new challenges and solutions in the contemporary food safety environment. Progress in molecular technologies like DNA barcoding enables regulators and industry players to trace and identify sources of food products with great accuracy, thus minimizing cases of food piracy and guaranteeing authenticity (Barcaccia et al., 2015). It aids in identifying adulterants that have the potential to reduce food quality, which aids in consumer safety and confidence. Additionally, various detection methods have been developed to combat economically motivated fraud, enabling the authentication of claims regarding food provenance, breed, and geographic origin (Manning & Soon, 2025). Whereas these technologies offer essential tools in the fight against food adulteration, they also highlight the need for ongoing monitoring and updating of regulatory systems to keep abreast of changing techniques utilized by fraudsters (Figure 6.12).

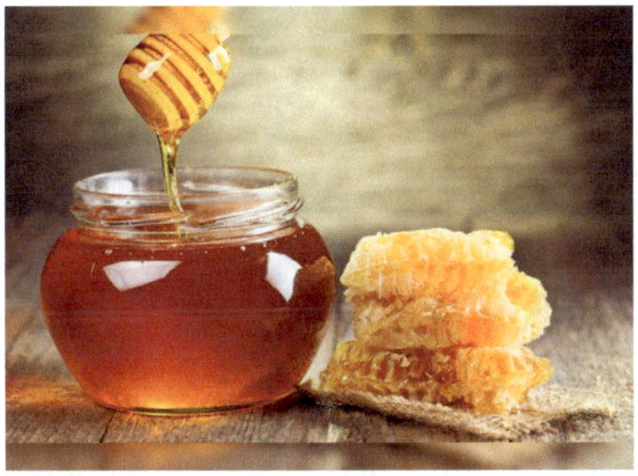

Figure 6.12. Role of technology in adulteration.

Source: https://img.etimg.com/thumb/width-1200,height-900,imgsize-1325353,resizemode-75,msid-79551460/industry/cons-products/food/fssai-seeks-details-of-cse-tests-on-honey-questions-body-for-not-conducting-smr-test.jpg

6.2.8. Case Studies of Notorious Adulteration Incidents

Many historical cases show that food adulteration has consistently threatened the health and safety of people. In the early 20th century, milk was often diluted with water to make more , which often resulted in people becoming very sick. Such cases highlight the systemic vulnerabilities within food supply chains, exacerbated by external crises like the COVID-19 pandemic, which has illuminated the fragility of these systems (Do et al., 2021). Another critical instance involves the adulteration of spices with heavy metals, such as lead and arsenic, which not only diminishes quality but poses serious health risks, including genetic instability and carcinogenicity (M-Mood et al., 2021). They prove that tough regulations and thorough monitoring are needed to prevent food adulteration and make sure food is safe and of good quality.

6.2.9. Consumer Awareness and Education

As more people worry about the safety and authenticity of food, consumer education is very important in preventing food adulteration. A study assessing Nigerian consumers revealed that a significant portion of respondents lacked familiarity with the term food fraud, despite their awareness of specific high-profile incidents , such as plastic rice and counterfeit dairy products (Onyeaka et al., 2024). This divergence highlights that there is a need for further efforts to make people aware of the ways to identify forged or adulterated foods. In addition, with increasing awareness among consumers regarding nutritional facts, they are willing to pay extra for healthier products, which indicates the need for awareness about food quality (Gale & Buzby, 2009. By creating an enlightened consumer market, stakeholders are able to promote improved purchasing habits, eventually contributing towards a safer and healthier food system focusing on wellbeing and safety (Figure 6.13).

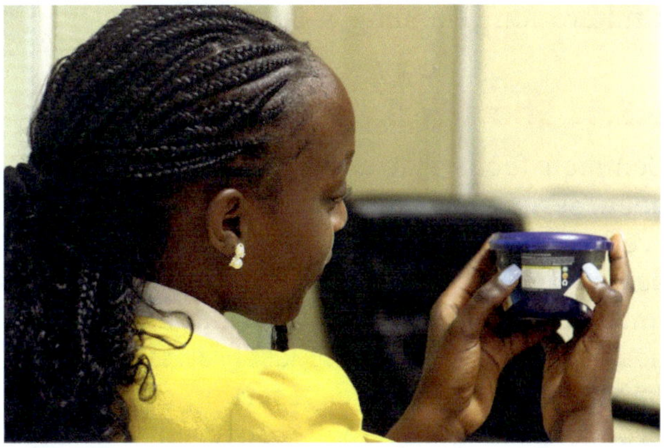

Figure 6.13. In an era marked by increasing concern over food safety and authenticity, consumer awareness and education play pivotal roles in combating food adulteration.

Source: https://kenaff.org/wp/wp-content/uploads/2023/10/IMG_1852-scaled.jpg

6.3. Health Implications of Food Adulteration

More and more cases of contaminated food are being discovered worldwide , which has made the health risks of adulteration more serious. Adulteration can result in food that contains harmful substances, whether they are toxic chemicals or allergens , which can endanger people's health. By doing this, companies trick consumers about the quality of their food , which can result in both short-term and long-term health problems. To combat this dilemma, advanced techniques like DNA barcoding are being employed in the food industry to ensure safety and authenticity; this method identifies species based on genetic material, thus supporting food labeling efforts and uncovering food piracy (Barcaccia et al., 2015). In addition, overall strategies to monitor food adulteration should be established with an emphasis on identifying intentional adulterants as well as authenticating declared claims of provenance, which can reduce health hazards from economically motivated adulteration (Manning & Soon, 2025).

6.3.1. Short-Term Health Effects

Common foods that are adulterated can bring about serious and quick health problems. If there are harmful substances in food, it can result in acute stomach problems, allergies and nutritional imbalances, mainly in groups like infants who need a high-quality diet for fast growth. As noted, unbalanced diets and exposure to unsafe food products are particularly concerning for this demographic due to their reliance on limited food choices in the early stages of life (Agostoni et al., 2012). Moreover, the influence of regulatory and industry practices on food quality can exacerbate these risks; stakeholders may prioritize market advantages over public health, leading to the introduction of potentially hazardous substances into the food supply (Libecap et al., 2025). Thus, the intersection of food adulteration and short-term health effects underscores the urgent need for stringent food safety regulations to protect consumers (Figure 6.14).

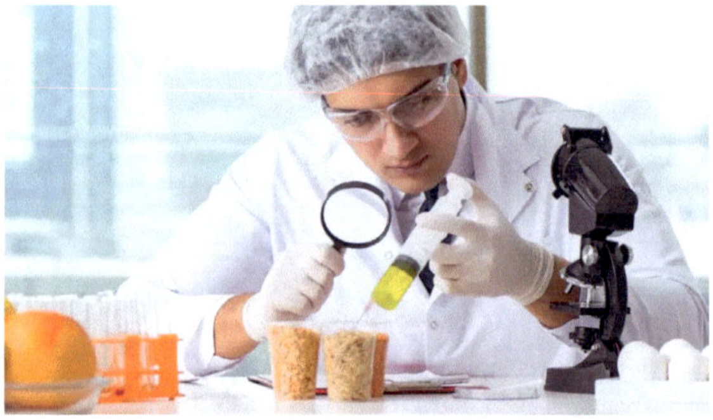

Figure 6.14. The adulteration of common foods poses significant short-term health effects that can manifest rapidly and severely.

Source: https://static.toiimg.com/thumb/msid-112419148,width-1280,height-720,imgsize-43342,resizemode-6,overlay-toi_sw,pt-32,y_pad-40/photo.jpg.

6.3.2. Long-Term Health Consequences

The lasting health risks of food adulteration are very worrying, since they affect both people's health and the overall functioning of the food supply chain. Consuming adulterated foods may result in chronic health problems , such as obesity, heart disease and cancer, and these diseases can take years to appear. Furthermore, because there are not many regulations, dangerous substances can remain in food , which increases these health problems over time. A detailed knowledge of food safety, as contended in Leib et al. (2019), is imperative to managing acute and cumulative dangers of food intake. It emphasizes how regulation, as explained in Libecap et al. (2025), can be used by the interests of industry to make it ineffective at maintaining public health. Maintaining food safety and combating adulteration is extremely important for our health as well as for avoiding future health issues.

6.3.3. Vulnerable Populations at Risk

Food adulteration is dangerous for people who do not have enough access to safe and healthy foods. Often, low-income families, children and the elderly are more likely to be harmed by adulterated foods because they tend to buy the cheapest and sometimes contaminated products. For example, in a survey of wheat flour adulteration in Gorakhpur, India, it was found to be shockingly contaminated, with more than 31% of samples coming positive for toxic adulterants like chalk powder and starch, which are responsible for causing grave health conditions, ranging from gastrointestinal diseases to irreversible organ damage (Singh et al., 2024). In addition, food fraud, a financially driven technique, accentuates health hazards for such groups, since they might not know about the risk implicated in such adulteration (Jayasena et al., 2023). Therefore, food safety must be addressed and public awareness improved in order to guard vulnerable communities (Figure 6.15).

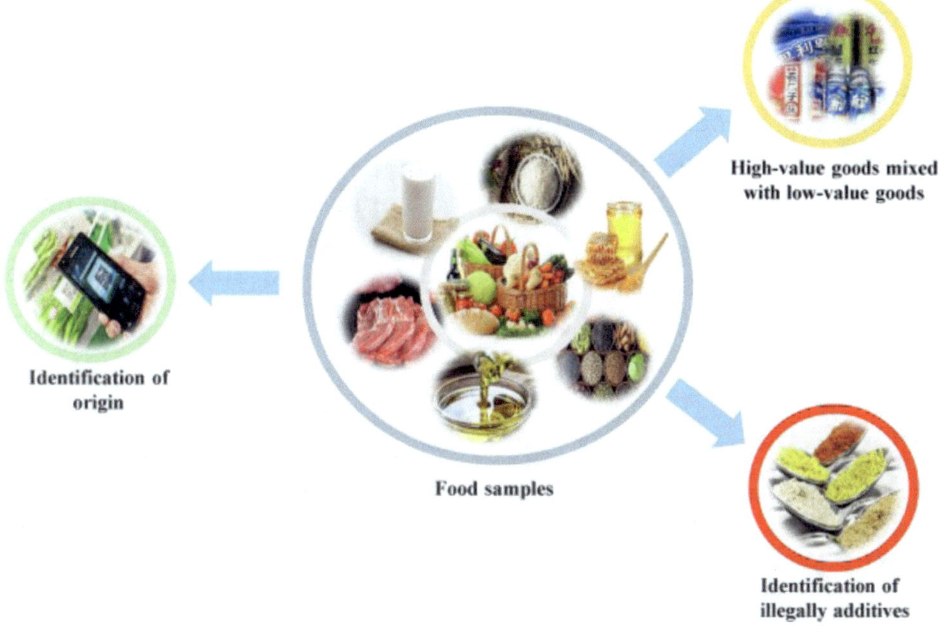

Figure 6.15. The phenomenon of food adulteration poses significant risks to vulnerable populations, particularly those with limited access to safe and nutritious food sources.

Source: https://ars.els-cdn.com/content/image/1-s2.0-S0308814624017205-gr1.jpg

6.3.4. Allergic Reactions and Sensitivities

More people experiencing allergic reactions and sensitivities is causing major concerns in food production and adulteration. People usually believe that the foods they buy are safe and properly labeled, but this belief can be very risky. Reports of food contamination, which may include allergens, are frequent, as various factors , such as microbial or chemical adulteration can exacerbate allergic reactions among sensitive individuals (Boys, 2025). Also, the rules for labeling food allergens are not the same in every country , which makes it difficult to handle these allergens well. For instance, Ireland has established relatively robust labeling regulations under the supervision of the FSAI, while India struggles with inconsistent standards and enforcement through the FSSAI (Machha et al., 2020). Such differences make it more dangerous for people with food allergies, so food safety and labeling must be stricter to protect them everywhere.

6.3.5. Impact on Nutritional Value

When common foods are adulterated, it reduces the nutritional value and many of the benefits people hope to get from them. Mixing hazelnut oil with virgin olive oil changes both the taste and the nutrition of the oil. Studies reveal that processing methods, such as refining and bleaching, can drastically reduce the levels of critical phytosterols, compounds essential for cardiovascular health, in these oils (Azadmard-Damirchi, 2007).

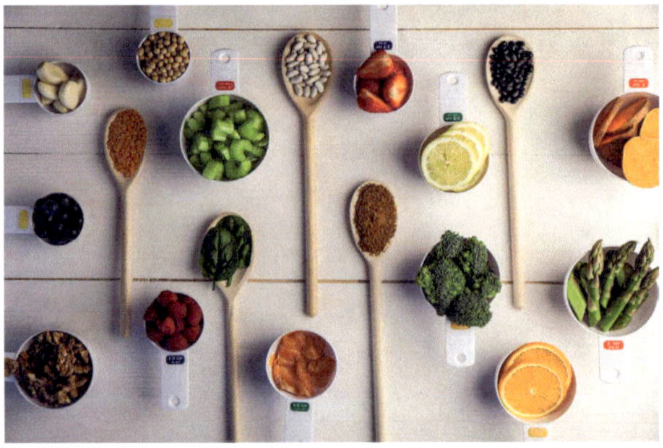

Figure 6.16. The adulteration of common foods significantly impacts their nutritional value, often diminishing the beneficial properties that consumers expect.

Source: https://www.godigit.com/content/dam/godigit/directportal/en/portion-cups-and-spoons-of-healthy-ingredients.jpg.

Furthermore, the use of advanced methodologies like DNA barcoding in the food industry enhances food safety and quality, allowing for the detection of adulterants that can compromise nutritional integrity (Barcaccia et al., 2015). Ultimately, the prevalence of food adulteration invokes significant concern regarding the true quality of commonly consumed products, emphasizing the need for vigilance in food labeling and regulatory measures to protect consumer health and nutritional interests (Figure 6.16).

6.3.6. Psychological Effects of Food Safety Concerns

Because of food safety concerns, people today tend to feel more anxious, afraid and suspicious about their food. When people learn more about food adulteration and contamination, they might become more worried about the safety of what they eat , which can cause them to avoid certain foods or take extra safety measures. This anxiety can be exacerbated by statistics revealing the prevalence of food-borne illnesses—approximately 76 million cases occur annually in the United States alone, emphasizing the staggering impact of microbial contamination on public health (Bondi et al., 2014). It is also possible for psychological distress to arise when people learn that even safe-looking foods can carry dangerous germs , which can have wider effects on mental health. This interrelation between food safety perceptions and psychological health underscores the necessity for effective communication and education on food safety protocols and risk management (Abraham et al., 2008).

6.3.7. Role of Public Health Organizations

Organizations in public health are important for ensuring the safety of common foods that might be contaminated. Their job includes checking food safety and setting up rules to keep consumers safe from heavy metals that might end up in food products. Research indicates that exposure to contaminants like mercury and lead can lead to serious health issues, emphasizing the need for vigilant oversight by public health entities (Barcaccia et al., 2015). Also, using new technologies like blockchain, these organizations can make food traceability and transparency better. By leveraging such innovations, public health organizations can create more efficient supply chains that mitigate risks associated with food adulteration, thereby promoting better health outcomes and fostering consumer trust in the safety of their food (Barcaccia et al., 2015) (Figure 6.17).

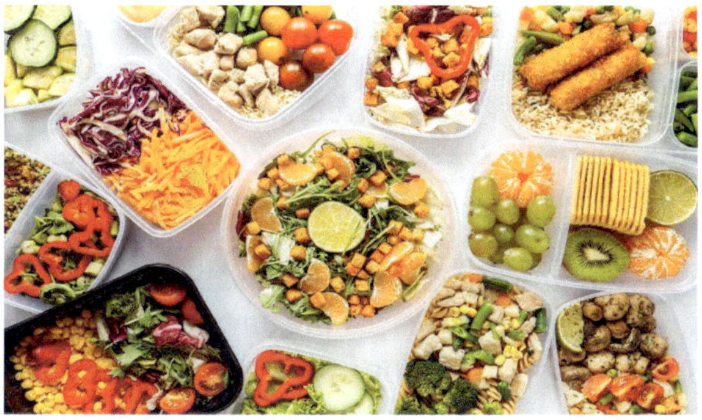

Figure 6.17. Public health organizations play a crucial role in safeguarding the integrity of food supply chains, particularly in the context of common foods that may be subject to adulteration.

Source: https://indian-retailer.s3.ap-south-1.amazonaws.com/s3fs-public/2021-09/flat-lay-batch-cooking-composition.jpg.

6.3.8. Case Studies of Health Crises Due to Adulteration

The consequences of food adulteration can be seen in several ways and show how it harms public health and safety. A major issue is the decline in food quality in Bangladesh , which happens because of many social, economic and environmental factors working together. For instance, the unchecked practices in shrimp farming near coastal areas have not only compromised the local environment but have also severely affected the health of consumers who unknowingly ingest contaminated products (Sanyal et al., 2006). When food safety systems fail, it makes these problems worse, as people start to doubt the quality of food , which may cause health risks. Additionally, asymmetric information about production processes creates low incentives for maintaining food quality, leaving consumers vulnerable to ingestion of adulterated foods (Hennessy et al., 2025). They show that strong rules and public awareness are needed to stop the widespread problem of food adulteration.

6.3.9. Preventive Measures for Consumers

As people try to stay safe with their food, using preventive strategies is very important to fight against adulteration. Being aware of where food comes from and being able to check its authenticity helps people decide what to buy. Techniques for detecting adulterants, while essential, often rely on existing knowledge of what to look for in food items, highlighting the importance of consumer education in this arena (Manning & Soon, 2025).

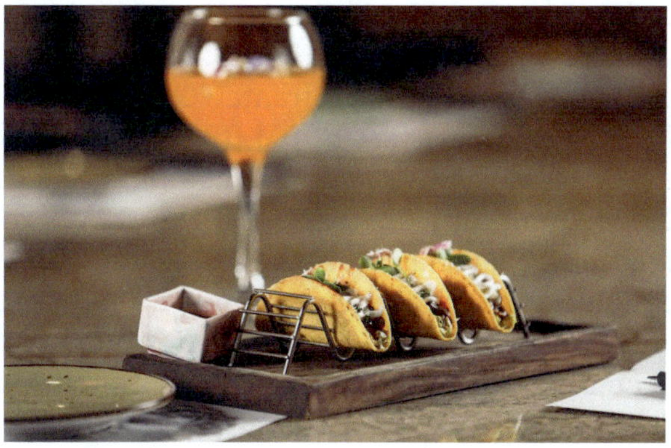

Figure 6.18. Awareness of food origins, coupled with the ability to verify authenticity, empowers consumers to make informed choices about the products they purchase.

Source: https://www.winsavvy.com/wp-content/uploads/2023/10/food-and-drink-8076626_1280-1.webp.

Also, knowing about food safety in terms of illness, the environment and nutrition helps consumers be more careful. This comprehensive perspective enables individuals to recognize the interconnectedness of different risks within the food system, thereby fostering safer eating habits and advocating for better regulatory policies (Leib et al., 2019). By embracing these preventive strategies, consumers can play a pivotal role in minimizing the prevalence of food adulteration and ensuring a healthier food environment (Figure 6.18).

6.4. Regulatory Measures and Consumer Protection

Laws and regulations help to ensure that food is safe and not altered , which is important for consumer health. Law No. 8 of 1999 on Consumer Protection and Law No. 18 of 2012 on Food give a basis for protecting consumers from consuming food that is not properly labeled or has been altered. These laws not only emphasize the ethical responsibilities of businesses but also highlight the regulatory framework mandated by authorities , such as BPOM (Indonesian Food and Drug Authority) to ensure compliance with safety standards (Marheni, 2025). Moreover, the right to safe and nutritious food, as articulated in various international human rights frameworks, underscores the need for stringent regulations to combat food insecurity and malnutrition, which often arise from inadequate food safety practices (Muwanga & Korsten , 2024). Stronger regulations are needed to ensure that the market puts consumer welfare above making money.

6.4.1. Overview of Food Safety Regulations

In food safety, regulations help protect the public by controlling the risks that come from food adulteration. These regulations are designed to establish standards that ensure the integrity and safety of food products, which is paramount given the various forms of adulteration, such as the addition of inferior substances or misleading labeling practices that jeopardize consumer well-being (Anagaw et al., 2024). Different places have different laws for food safety and this gets more complicated when food supplements are involved, since they are often not regulated as strictly as pharmaceuticals. This lapse can lead to the illegal inclusion of unregulated substances in products, posing significant health risks, such as hepatotoxicity or other adverse effects stemming from adulteration (Zhivikj et al., 2024). Therefore, strengthening enforcement mechanisms and increasing consumer awareness are essential in developing an effective food safety regulatory paradigm that addresses the ongoing challenges posed by adulteration (Figure 6.19).

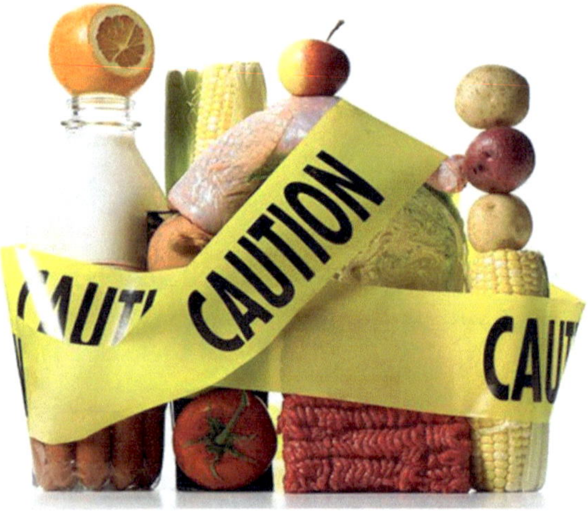

Figure 6.19. In the realm of food safety, regulations serve as a critical framework aimed at safeguarding public health from the hazards associated with food adulteration.

Source: https://static.wixstatic.com/media/f774cd_eaa19385e3dc42e2a7d8414e7800fa65~mv2.jpg/v1/fill/w_722,h_406,al_c,q_80,enc_avif,quality_auto/f774cd_eaa19385e3dc42e2a7d8414e7800fa65~mv2.jpg

6.4.2. Role of Government Agencies

Government agencies are very important in overseeing food safety and stopping adulteration, especially in light of existing laws. The FDA was formed because society needed more oversight as industrialization grew , which was made clear by the 1906 Pure Food and Drugs Act. This legislation emerged from a confluence of interests, where public demand for safe food intersected with industry motivations to stabilize quality standards, illustrating the multifaceted drivers of regulatory action (Libecap et al., 2025). Furthermore, the FDA's authority extends beyond domestic concerns, involving cooperation with international entities to address global food safety challenges, such as the risks associated with bovine spongiform encephalopathy (BSE) (Horton et al., 1997). In the end, government agencies are responsible for protecting public health by making sure food is safe and by responding to new issues in the food supply chain.

6.4.3. International Standards for Food Safety

An awareness of the international food safety standards is extremely crucial in dealing with the increasing problem of food adulteration. They are established to ensure consumer health protection and ensure fair trade, bringing about the importance of rigorous food safety practices in all aspects of the global supply chain. Institutions like the World Health Organization (WHO) and the Food and Agriculture Organization (FAO) have key roles in formulating these standards, which act as guidelines for countries to set their food safety regulations. Adhering to these standards minimizes opportunities for contamination of food and maximizes the confidence of consumers in the products. As noted by contemporary studies, the common and in some cases uncontrolled consumption of dietary supplements may result in unforeseen effects , such as exposure to contaminated substances (Maughan et al., 2018). In addition, the sudden growth of academic literature on sports nutrition emphasizes the need to comprehend and assess food safety protocols to provide evidence that athletes and consumers are protected from the dangers of food adulteration (Kerksick et al., 2018) (Figure 6.20).

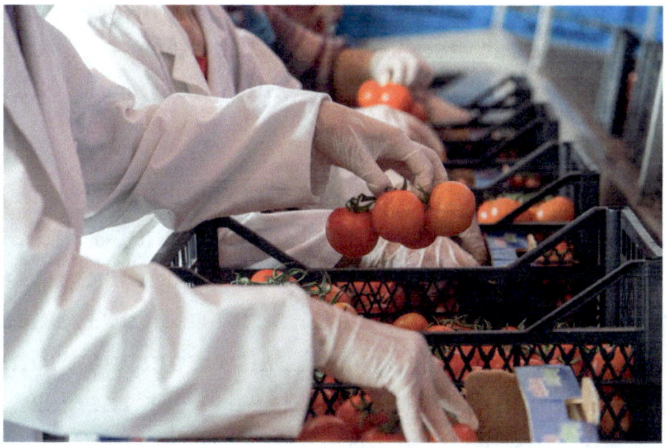

Figure 6.20. Understanding international standards for food safety is crucial in addressing the growing concerns related to food adulteration.

Source: https://cdn.wikifarmer.com/images/detailed/2024/03/iStock-813073702.jpg

6.4.4. Importance of Food Labeling

It is very important to label food, mainly because common foods are often adulterated. Making sure labels are accurate helps protect people and helps them make better choices. It helps consumers check the ingredients and nutritional facts of products , which lets them avoid allergens or harmful substances that might be added through adulteration. Also, labeling makes the food industry more transparent and this can be improved further by using blockchain. This technology not only ensures the integrity of the supply chain but also provides real-time access to information about product origins, thereby increasing consumer trust and accountability (Antonucci et al., 2019). So, food labeling helps prevent food fraud and protects public health , which is why consumers should look for well-labeled products to avoid the risks of adulterated foods.

6.4.5. Consumer Rights and Advocacy

Because food adulteration is common, it seriously affects consumer rights , which means more people need to be aware of this issue. Consumers are often unwitting victims of EMA, which involves the substitution or addition of harmful substances to food products for financial gain, jeopardizing health and safety (Onyeaka et al., 2024).

Although there are strict laws against adulterating food, enforcement is not regular , which results in many people ignoring the rules. In Bangladesh, alarming statistics revealed that 1000s suffer from health complications attributed to adulterated foods, yet the issue garners insufficient attention (Ali et al., 2013). Because of this gap, it is clear that people should be educated about food safety and there should be tough laws to punish those who break them. Empowering consumers through knowledge not only fortifies their rights but also cultivates a healthier food environment, fostering greater accountability in the food industry (Figure 6.21).

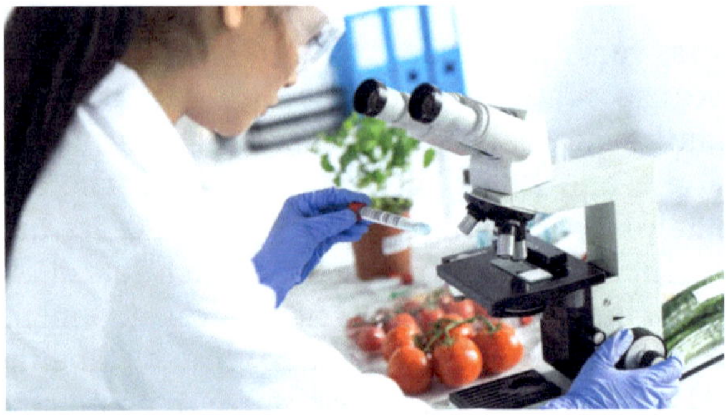

Figure 6.21. The prevalence of food adulteration poses a significant threat to consumer rights, highlighting the urgent need for advocacy and awareness among the public.

Source: https://static.toiimg.com/thumb/imgsize-23456,msid-105187905,width-600,resizemode-4/105187905.jpg.

6.4.6. Challenges in Enforcement of Regulations

It is difficult for food safety regulations to be enforced , which can make it harder to fight food adulteration. A significant problem is caused by the complexity of global supply chains , which means food products may be handled in several different countries before they reach people. Being so connected can make it harder to identify who is responsible , which makes it harder to control food safety. For example, the increasing volume of imported seafood into the United States, which rose from 66% in 1999 to over 84% in 2009, exemplifies the difficulty of maintaining stringent quality standards (Anders et al.). Also, if regulatory agencies lack the needed resources, it becomes difficult for them to do thorough inspections and enforcement. The FDA uses Import Alerts to select certain countries for more careful inspections and these countries , which are often from the lower-middle-income group, may be subjected to more scrutiny and retaliation because of import refusals and detentions. Thus, the enforcement landscape remains precarious and challenging.

6.4.7. Role of NGOs in Food Safety

In the context of food safety, non-governmental organizations (NGOs) play a pivotal role by advocating for enhanced standards and promoting transparency throughout the food supply chain. They act as links between those who eat food, those who make it and the authorities, promoting rules that stop adulteration and keep foods safe. By fostering information sharing among stakeholders, NGOs facilitate the development of systems like the Food Integrity Information Sharing System (FI-ISS), which enhances early detection and prevention of food integrity issues, as evidenced by the strong support from food industry stakeholders for participating in such initiatives (Luijckx et al., 2019). Moreover, NGOs often provide educational resources to empower consumers about food safety practices, effectively bridging the gap between scientific research and public awareness (Solaiman, 2024). Through these efforts, NGOs not only contribute to improved food quality but also advocate for accountability and transparency in food production, thereby enhancing overall public health outcomes (Figure 6.22).

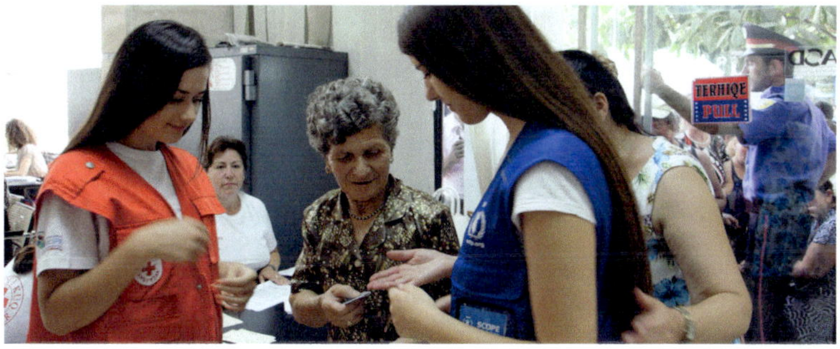

Figure 6.22. In the context of food safety, non-governmental organizations (NGOs) play a pivotal role by advocating for enhanced standards and promoting transparency throughout the food supply chain.

Source: https://www.wfp.org/sites/default/files/images/ngo_hero_wfp-carlos_munoz_cropped.jpg

6.4.8. Innovations in Food Safety Practices

Because food adulteration continues to be a problem, there is now greater attention on new food safety measures, mainly in the meat and spice industries. New technologies, such as duplex polymerase chain reaction (PCR), have emerged as vital tools in detecting adulteration, as demonstrated in studies where over 95% of minced meat samples labeled as beef contained no mutton, revealing considerable discrepancies between product labeling and actual contents (Doroudian et al., 2024). Similarly, the adulteration of spices with harmful substances poses significant health risks, necessitating advanced monitoring techniques to ensure purity and safety (Sahoo & Sama, 2024). Such innovations help testing methods work better and encourage consumers to have more trust in food products. With new food safety regulations being introduced, it is necessary to use such technologies to secure public health and maintain the integrity of food systems worldwide , which helps to control the risks from food adulteration.

6.4.9. Future Directions for Food Safety Legislation

Since concerns regarding food safety and contamination continue to rise, food safety law must enhance its rules to counter new issues. Since food production, globalization and consumer demand continually change, it is essential to rethink our existing policies. For example, FDA modernization could give the agency more ability to track and control risk, especially in the case of dietary supplements and foods imported from other countries, where current law is frequently inadequate (Horton et al., 1997). Also, forethought collaboration with global regulatory agencies can support food safety measures, as can be seen through continued partnerships with the European Union to address food safety matters that extend beyond countries (Noah et al., 2006). Ultimately, the merging of rigorous risk assessment and cooperation with other nations will be critical to safeguarding public health and gaining the confidence of consumers in food supplies.

A CLOSER LOOK

Food Quality

The qualities of food , such as taste, appearance and freshness, determine how much consumers will value and accept it. Such attributes are taste, texture, color, aroma, nutritional value, freshness and safety. Good food quality means it is healthy, clean and clearly labeled. Ensuring food quality is important for both making customers happy and for the health and trust of the public. Things that influence food quality are the selection of raw materials, the methods used to process food, the way it is packaged, how it is stored and how it is transported. Maintaining food quality means using strict quality control at every step of the food supply chain.

SUMMARY

A look at everyday food items and the widespread problem of adulteration, one can see that the purity of food items is crucial for consumer safety and public health. The complexities imposed by globalization have already had a massive impact on the quality and handling of food supplies, even mirroring trends seen in other industries like drug manufacturing. This requires strong policy guidelines to strengthen oversight mechanisms and shield consumers from deceptive actions that erode confidence in food systems. Case studies also show that developing nations could be subject to increased challenges in implementing food safety due to limited resources and regulatory frameworks. Finally, tackling food adulteration takes a concerted effort from stakeholders, governments, industries, and consumers, to promote accountability so that quality is never compromised and the basic right to safe and nutritious food is protected.

Food adulteration is a complex and widespread issue that raises high-profile food safety and public health concerns. The key facts surrounding this problem are the steps required to modify standard foodstuffs so that profitability is achieved at the expense of quality, thus defrauding the consumers. Research determines new ways of detecting illegal adulterants through immunoassays that attack broad-specific antibody recognition mechanisms critical for accurate identification (Yu et al., 2025). Furthermore, studying systemic conditions provides critical information on the design of structures that prioritize safety measures, as seen in infrastructure development initiatives where systematic study is critical in responding to recurrent issues (Hui, 2024). Through synthesis of these perspectives, it is evident that addressing food adulteration involves a multi-faceted strategy that harmonizes scientific advancements and robust regulatory frameworks to protect consumers and purity of food stocks.

KEY TERMS FROM THIS CHAPTER

- Near-infrared (NIR) spectroscopy
- Nutritional deficiencies
- Olive oil
- Phytosterol profiles
- Polymerase chain reaction (PCR)
- Red mullet
- Solid-phase extraction (SPE)
- Staple foods
- Sucrose
- Sweeteners
- Non-governmental organizations (NGOs)
- Oils
- Physical adulteration
- Phytosterols
- Pseudupeneus prayensis
- Seafood
- Spices
- Starch
- Sugar
- Vegetables

REFERENCES

1. Abraham, S., Grace, D., Parambi, T., & Pahuja, S. A. (2008). Milestones in development of Good Clinical Practice. *The Internet Journal of Health, 9*. https://www.semanticscholar.org/paper/467f393702a2af5a6b97809c14f029a3654c1001 (accessed on 29 May 2025).
2. Agostoni, C., Aris, B., Koletzko, B., Bier, D. M., Birlouez-Aragon, I., et al. (2012). *Quality and Safety Aspects of Infant Nutrition*. https://core.ac.uk/download/16432924.pdf (accessed on 29 May 2025).
3. Akinsemolu, A. A., Chukwugozie, D. C., David, K., Ghosh, P., et al. (2024). *Combatting Food Fraud in Sub-Saharan Africa: Strategies for Strengthened Safety and Security*. https://core.ac.uk/download/614712545.pdf (accessed on 29 May 2025).
4. Onyeaka, H., Anyogu, A., Odeyemi, O. A., Ukwuru, M. U., Eze, U., Isaac-Bamgboye, F. J., Anumudu, C. K., Akinwunmi, O. O., Sotayo, O. P., & Jeff-Agboola, Y. A. (2024). Navigating Food Fraud: A Survey of Nigerian Consumer Knowledge and Attitudes. *Foods (Basel, Switzerland), 13*(20), 3270. https://doi.org/10.3390/foods13203270Ali, A. N. M. A., & Solaiman, S. M. (2013). *Rampant Food Adulteration in Bangladesh: Gross Violations of Fundamental Human Rights with Impunity*. https://core.ac.uk/download/37016885.pdf (accessed on 29 May 2025).
5. Aliaño González, M. J., Espada Bellido, E., Fernández Barbero, G., Ferreiro González, M., et al. (2019). A screening method based on Visible-NIR spectroscopy for the identification and quantification of different adulterants in high-quality honey. https://core.ac.uk/download/599470329.pdf (accessed on 29 May 2025).
6. Al-Jaroodi, J., & Mohamed, N. (2019). Blockchain in industries: A survey. *IEEE Access, 7*, 36500–36515. https://doi.org/10.1109/access.2019.2903554.
7. Allen, D. P., Elliott, C. T., Ellis, D. I., Goodacre, R., et al. (2016). A flavor of omics approaches for the detection of food fraud. https://core.ac.uk/download/144581233.pdf (accessed on 29 May 2025).
8. Anagaw, Y. K., Ayenew, W., Limenh, L. W., Geremew, D. T., Worku, M., Tessema, T. A., Simegn, W., et al. (2024). Food adulteration: Causes, risks, and detection techniques—Review. *SAGE Open Medicine, 12*. https://www.semanticscholar.org/paper/6bde09b50e1e42312135b45aec0108307728ce87 (accessed on 29 May 2025).
9. Anders, S., & Westra, S. (2025). *A Review of FDA Imports Refusals–US Seafood Trade 2000–2010*. https://core.ac.uk/download/pdf/6502886.pdf (accessed on 29 May 2025).
10. Antonucci, F., Figorilli, S., Costa, C., Pallottino, F., Raso, L., & Menesatti, P. (2019). A review on blockchain applications in the agri-food sector. *Journal of the Science of Food and Agriculture, 99*(14), 6129–6138. https://doi.org/10.1002/jsfa.9912.
11. French, M. and Phillips, J. ORCID logo (2002) Food safety regimes in Scotland, 1899-1914. Journal of Scottish Historical Studies, 22(2), pp. 134-157. (doi: 10.3366/jshs.2002.22.2.134) Aryeetey, R., Boadi, P., & Gyimah, F. T. (2022). *Descriptive Analysis of Changes in Ghana's Food Availability and Food Safety Information Between 2010 and 2020*. https://core.ac.uk/download/544237259.pdf (accessed on 29 May 2025).
12. Aued-Pimentel, S., Badia-Melis, R., Bera, D., Brito, M. L., et al. (2018). Economically motivated food fraud and adulteration in Brazil: Incidents and alternatives to minimize occurrence. https://core.ac.uk/download/212594601.pdf (accessed on 29 May 2025).

13. Azadmard-Damirchi, S. 2007. Olive Oil: Phytosterols, Tracing of Adulteration with Hazelnut Oil and Chemical Interesterification. Doctor's dissertation. ISSN 1652-6880, ISBN 91-576-7335-0 Balali-Mood, M., Naseri, K., Tahergorabi, Z., Khazdair, M. R., & Sadeghi, M. (2021). Toxic mechanisms of five heavy metals: Mercury, lead, chromium, cadmium, and arsenic. *Frontiers in Pharmacology, 12*, Article 643972. https://doi.org/10.3389/fphar.2021.643972.

14. Barcaccia G, Lucchin M, Cassandro M. DNA Barcoding as a Molecular Tool to Track Down Mislabeling and Food Piracy. *Diversity*. 2016; 8(1):2. https://doi.org/10.3390/d8010002Bhattacharjee, D., & Dey, M. (2016). Evaluation of determinant awareness factors for the purchase decision of food items in Bangladesh: An empirical study. https://core.ac.uk/download/234694192.pdf (accessed on 29 May 2025).

15. Black, C., Chevallier, O. P., Elliott, C. T., & Galvin-King, P. (2016). A comprehensive strategy to detect the fraudulent adulteration of herbs: The oregano approach. https://core.ac.uk/download/33595879.pdf (accessed on 29 May 2025).

16. Bondi, M., Messi, P., Halami, P., Papadopoulou, C., & de Niederhausern, S. (2014). Emerging microbial concerns in food safety and new control measures. *BioMed Research International, 2014*, Article 251512. https://www.semanticscholar.org/paper/4b64843548520cfe5300268041b1cdf1d686f72f (accessed on 29 May 2025).

17. Boys, K. A. (2025). *From Contamination to Climate Change: Emerging Risks at The Nexus of Food Safety and Nutrition, And Their Implications for Public Health*. https://core.ac.uk/download/647992949.pdf (accessed on 29 May 2025).

18. Broad Leib, E. M., & Pollans, M. J. (2019). *The New Food Safety*. https://core.ac.uk/download/231832064.pdf (accessed on 29 May 2025).

19. Fred Gale and Jean C. Buzby (2009). *Imports from China and Food Safety Issues*. https://www.ers.usda.gov/publications/pub-details?pubid=44392(accessed on 29 May 2025).

20. Capps, O., Jr., Fairchild, G. F., & Nichols, J. P. (2025). *Observations on Economic Adulteration of High-Value Food Products: The Honey Case*. https://core.ac.uk/download/pdf/6995148.pdf (accessed on 29 May 2025).

21. Singh, K., Dwivedi, A. K., Samuel, C., & Dixit, S. (2024). Exploring the Prevalence and Risks of Wheat Adulteration in Gorakhpur City, Uttar Pradesh, India. *South Eastern European Journal of Public Health*, 1920–1927. https://doi.org/10.70135/seejph.vi.2750Djatna, T., Fauzi, A. M., I, T. T., et al. (2013). Application of electrical properties to differentiate lard from tallow and palm oil. https://media.neliti.com/media/publications/156673-EN-application-of-electrical-properties-to.pdf (accessed on 29 May 2025).

22. Do, Q., Mishra, N., Wulandhari, N. B. I., Ramudhin, A., Sivarajah, U., & Milligan, G. (2021). Supply chain agility responding to unprecedented changes: Empirical evidence from the UK food supply chain during COVID-19 crisis. *Supply Chain Management: An International Journal, 26*, 737–752. https://doi.org/10.1108/scm-09-2020-0470.

23. Doroudian, M., Soezi, M., Rasouli, M., Arshadi Far, M., Yousefi Dehbidi, M., Maafi, P., Yousefi, F., et al. (2024). Identification of meat adulteration in minced meat samples labeled as beef and mutton in Tehran stores using duplex PCR. *Food Science & Nutrition, 12*(14), 7504–7511. https://www.semanticscholar.org/paper/460c19842b14db7491fa2592c43b2e1197189f46 (accessed on 29 May 2025).

24. Fernández Recamales, Á., González Domínguez, R., Morales Millán, M. T., Sayago Gómez, J., et al. (2019). Assessment of virgin olive oil adulteration by a rapid luminescent method. https://core.ac.uk/download/227043576.pdf (accessed on 29 May 2025).

25. Giantsis, I., Tokamani, M., Triantaphyllidis, G., Tzatzani, S., Chatzinikolaou, E., Toros, A., Bouchorikou, A., et al. (2023). Development of multiplex PCR and melt–curve analysis for the molecular identification of four species of the Mullidae family, available in the market. *Genes, 14*(5), Article 1015. https://www.semanticscholar.org/paper/1e36a0dfdd4ac7792a5b293ababa422c385a867f (accessed on 29 May 2025).

26. Hennessy, D. A., Jensen, H. H., & Roosen, J. (2025). Systemic failure in the provision of safe food. https://core.ac.uk/download/pdf/6643009.pdf (accessed on 29 May 2025).

27. Horton, L. (1997). The United States Food and Drug Administration: Its role, authority, history, harmonization activities, and cooperation with the European Union. https://core.ac.uk/download/5079826.pdf (accessed on 29 May 2025).

28. Jackson, P. A., Wang, W., & Zhu, H. (2016). Consumer anxieties about food grain safety in China. https://core.ac.uk/download/46665136.pdf (accessed on 29 May 2025).

29. Jayasena, V., Karnpanit, W., & Kemsawasd, V. (2023). Incidents and potential adverse health effects of serious food fraud cases originated in Asia. https://core.ac.uk/download/587863071.pdf (accessed on 29 May 2025).

30. Jiménez-López, C., Carpena, M., Lourenço-Lopes, C., Gallardo-Gómez, M., Lorenzo, J. M., Barba, F. J., Prieto, M. A., et al. (2020). Bioactive compounds and quality of extra virgin olive oil. *Foods, 9*, Article 1014. https://doi.org/10.3390/foods9081014.

31. Jugreet, S., Mahomoodally, M. F., Zengin, G., & Maggi, F. (2021). Essential oils as natural sources of fragrance compounds for cosmetics and cosmeceuticals. *Molecules, 26*(3), 666. https://doi.org/10.3390/molecules26030666.

32. Kerksick, C. M., Wilborn, C., Roberts, M. D., Smith-Ryan, A. E., Kleiner, S. M., Jäger, R., Collins, R., et al. (2018). ISSN exercise & sports nutrition review update: Research & recommendations. *Journal of the International Society of Sports Nutrition, 15*, Article 38. https://doi.org/10.1186/s12970-018-0242-y.

33. Li, Q., Chen, J., Huyan, Z., Kou, Y., Xu, L., Yu, X., & Gao, J. (2018). Application of Fourier transform infrared spectroscopy for the quality and safety analysis of fats and oils: A review. *Critical Reviews in Food Science and Nutrition, 59*, 3597–3611. https://www.semanticscholar.org/paper/4a34c317ebd79619184267a1bee49d67fc91fafd (accessed on 29 May 2025).

34. Libecap, G. D., & Law, M. T. (2025). The determinants of Progressive Era reform: The Pure Food and Drugs Act of 1906. https://core.ac.uk/download/pdf/6690770.pdf (accessed on 29 May 2025).

35. Luijckx, N. L., Minnens, F., & Verbeke, W. (2019). Food supply chain stakeholders' perspectives on sharing information to detect and prevent food integrity issues. https://core.ac.uk/download/227040542.pdf (accessed on 29 May 2025).

36. Machha, N. (2020). Comparison of allergen legislation between India and Ireland. https://core.ac.uk/download/385853952.pdf (accessed on 29 May 2025).

37. Manning, Louise & Soon, Jan Mei, 2014. "**Developing systems to control food adulteration**," Food Policy, Elsevier, vol. 49(P1), pages 23-32. (accessed on 29 May 2025).

38. Marheni, L. (2025). Analysis of the study of consumer protection law against expired food products and medicines from a business law perspective. *Kajian Pendidikan, Seni, Budaya, Sosial dan Lingkungan*. https://www.semanticscholar.org/paper/3f48038f83a7f5678d58f5103bf017c4b57b3a0a (accessed on 29 May 2025).

39. Maughan, R. J., Burke, L. M., Dvořák, J., Larson-Meyer, D. E., Peeling, P., Phillips, S. M., Rawson, E. S., et al. (2018). IOC consensus statement: Dietary supplements and the high-performance athlete. *British Journal of Sports Medicine, 52*, 439–455. https://doi.org/10.1136/bjsports-2018-099027.

40. Murphy, L. C. (2016). The food industry's perception of economically motivated adulteration and related risk factors. https://core.ac.uk/download/268805566.pdf (accessed on 29 May 2025).

41. T.S.N. Muwanga & L. Korsten 'The right to food in South Africa: A consumer protection perspective' (2024) 24 African Human Rights Law Journal 632-658. http://dx.doi.org/10.17159/1996-2096/2024/v24n2a10.(accessed on 29 May 2025).

42. Nicoluci, Í. G., da Silva, B. S., Braga, P. A. C., & Arisseto-Bragotto, A. P. (2025). Nine high-intensity sweeteners in beverages in a single LC-MS/MS analysis. *Food Additives & Contaminants: Part B, Surveillance*. https://www.semanticscholar.org/paper/ce3e20a0592398e39e010511e55058229989b3ef (accessed on 29 May 2025).

43. Noah, B. A., & Noah, L. (2006). *A Drug by Any Other Name ...? Paradoxes in Dietary Supplement Risk Regulation*. https://core.ac.uk/download/267160615.pdf (accessed on 29 May 2025).

44. Núñez Burcio, O., Núñez, N., & Saurina, J. (2021). Authenticity assessment and fraud quantitation of coffee adulterated with chicory, barley and flours by untargeted HPLC-UV-FLD fingerprinting and chemometrics. https://core.ac.uk/download/419530775.pdf (accessed on 29 May 2025).

45. Olakunle, E., Abdul Rahman, T., Orikumhi, I., Leow, C. Y., & Hindia, M. H. D. N. (2018). An overview of Internet of Things (IoT) and data analytics in agriculture: Benefits and challenges. *IEEE Internet of Things Journal, 5*, 3758–3773. https://doi.org/10.1109/jiot.2018.2844296.

46. Oliveira, M. M. de. (2020). *Detection and Quantification of Paprika Powder Adulteration by Near Infrared (NIR) Spectroscopy*. https://core.ac.uk/download/326804290.pdf (accessed on 29 May 2025).

47. Perez-Gonzalez, C., García-Hernández, C., García-Cabezón, C., Rodríguez-Méndez, M., Dias, L., & Martín-Pedrosa, F. (2024). Analysis of milk adulteration by means of a potentiometric electronic tongue. *Journal of Dairy Science*. https://www.semanticscholar.org/paper/cbc48a6c587922de34b0f96727dab77ee8ae6d7c (accessed on 29 May 2025).

48. Rohman, A. (2023). The progress of authentication analysis of fats and oils using vibrational spectroscopy and chemometrics analysis: Narrative review. *Journal of Oil Palm Research*. https://www.semanticscholar.org/paper/8efbbe3b8d6b6dbd41d84fa869411f75ad8a8b60 (accessed on 29 May 2025).

49. Sahoo, J. P., & Sama, K. C. (2024). Adulteration in Indian spices: An alarming concern and a silent health hazard. *International Journal of Adulteration*. https://www.semanticscholar.org/paper/e31d123d447f4275ee9eb852dc970d373ac4b581 (accessed on 29 May 2025).

50. Sanyal, N. (2006). *Political Ecology of Environmental Crises in Bangladesh*. https://core.ac.uk/download/6116391.pdf (accessed on 29 May 2025).

51. Solaiman, S. M. (2024). *Fight for the Right to Safe Food in Bangladesh—Viewed through the Prisms of International and Indian Laws: Mice Will Play While the Cat Stays Away*. https://core.ac.uk/download/641674077.pdf (accessed on 29 May 2025).

52. Valyear, M. D. (2014). *A Bittersweet Investigation of Availability and Nutritive Value as Determinants of Volitional Sucrose Consumption*. https://core.ac.uk/download/143687545.pdf (accessed on 29 May 2025).

53. Wang, H. (2024). Research on the same direction separation and common board problem of freeways based on tolerance system design. *Frontiers in Traffic and Transportation Engineering*. https://www.semanticscholar.org/paper/14bf76d4bfaeb205cc9b203848fb02d81cf0f32b (accessed on 29 May 2025).

54. Willems, J. L. (2017). *Development of Authenticity Methods for Apple and Pear Juices*. https://core.ac.uk/download/226153757.pdf (accessed on 29 May 2025).

55. Yu, X., Zhou, T., Pan, K., Fan, M. H., Yan, X., Huang, X. A., Zhang, H., et al. (2025). Structure profiling of broad-specificity immunoassays: Multitarget recognition for sulfonylurea adulteration in food. *Journal of Agricultural and Food Chemistry*. https://www.semanticscholar.org/paper/5d73fb7ab81eb49cf51c0c1f04a92879225bf0c4 (accessed on 29 May 2025).

56. Zambonin, C. (2021). MALDI-TOF mass spectrometry applications for food fraud detection. *Applied Sciences, 11*, 3374. https://www.semanticscholar.org/paper/f138fdfa626d665f4381c68a1efb9c6db10814d5 (accessed on 29 May 2025).

57. Zhivikj, Z., Petreska-Ivanovska, T., Karapandzova, M., Kulevanova, S., Kadifkova-Panovska, T., & Petrushevska-Tozi, L. (2024). Safety issues of herbal weight loss dietary supplements: Hepatotoxicity and adulteration. *Arhiv za Farmaciju*. https://www.semanticscholar.org/paper/43614af5bd6e217da5d78c221ada085c970fa2da (accessed on 29 May 2025).

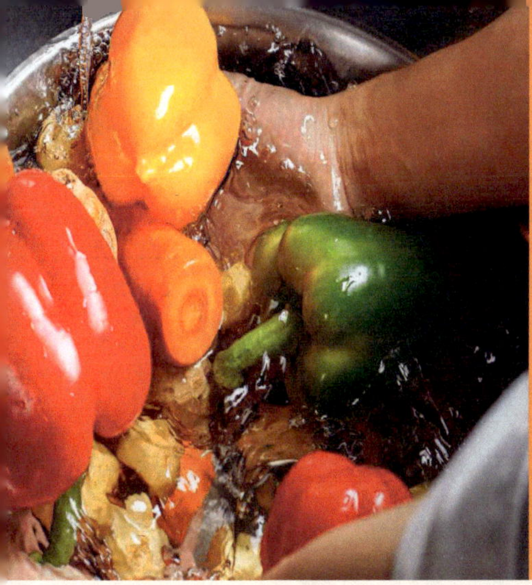

Chapter 7

DETECTION OF ADULTERANTS

Contents

Introduction....159
7.1. Methods of Detection....160
7.2. Current Laws and Regulations....164
7.3. Impact of Adulteration Laws on Society....168
Summary....174
References....175

Introduction

In the past few years, food safety has become very important because of more cases of food adulteration , which endangers people's health and damages the market's integrity. Finding adulterants in food helps maintain public health, increases people's trust in the food and ensures the food meets regulations. Combat against food adulteration , which is usually motivated by money, needs a variety of approaches. A strong food safety system is built by using knowledge from different areas of education. Based on recent research, Western Institute for Food Safety and Security underscores the requirement for curricula that address the interconnections of disciplines so as to guide experts confronted with the dilemma of ensuring food safety while not undermining environmental resources (Angelos et al., 2017). Additionally, effective monitoring of food adulteration demands robust methods to assess both known and unknown adulterants, ensuring the integrity of food products in a globalized market (Manning & Soon, 2025).

7.1. Methods of Detection

Because of the need for safer and better quality food, finding adulterants in food has improved a lot. Many techniques have been created, starting with chemical methods and going up to advanced sensor systems. For example, sensors have helped a lot in finding out if milk has been adulterated with urea or melamine. These techniques not only provide rapid results but also enhance accuracy compared to conventional methods, which can be time-consuming and less reliable (Sharma, 2024). Also, in the struggle against food fraud, one needs to understand the various types of adulteration and the vulnerabilities of the food supply system. The assessment methods are crucial here in order to identify the risks that are possible and to apply preventive steps (Battell, 2023). Because science keeps advancing, it is important to keep finding new ways to detect adulteration to protect the public and maintain trust with consumers.

7.1.1. Sensory Evaluation Techniques

The use of sensory evaluation is very important for finding food adulterants, especially in coffee, since adulterants can look very similar to the original product. In a study exploring the adulteration of roasted coffee, trained sensory analysts utilized their refined palates to distinguish between pure and adulterated samples, achieving significant correlation with spectroscopic methods (Barrios-Rodriguez et al., 2022). Using sensory analysis helped to understand the coffee's qualities and it worked together with advanced technology, giving a complete evaluation of the coffee's authenticity. Additionally, with widespread use of digital technologies, further improving techniques that escalate sensory analysis capacity is vital to close the gap between subjective perception and objective measurement (Alves et al., 2024). This two-pronged strategy enhances the trustworthiness of adulterant detection, giving consumers quality products in addition to ensuring food supply chains remain uncompromised (Figure 7.1).

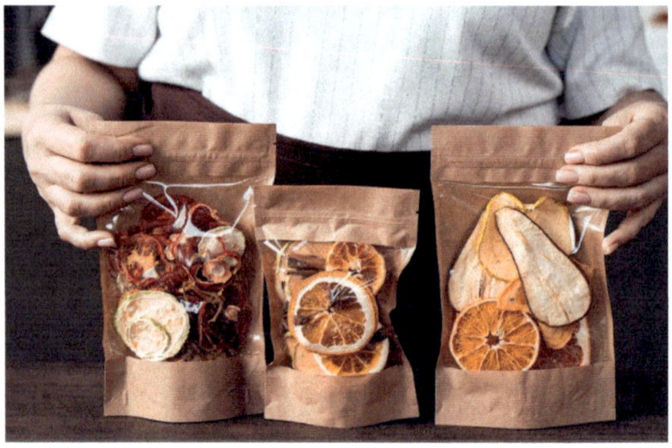

Figure 7.1. The integration of sensory evaluation techniques serves as a crucial component in the detection of food adulterants, particularly in products like coffee, where visual inspection alone is insufficient due to the deceptive similarity in color and texture among adulterants.

Source: https://www.ficsi.in/blog/wp-content/uploads/2023/09/blog-1.jpg.

7.1.2. Chemical Tests for Adulterants

Checking food for adulterants with chemical tests is very important for keeping food safe and genuine. Spectroscopic methods, chromatography and tests using specific reagents are used to find unwanted substances. They are used to identify certain compounds and also to check if food products are genuine, dealing with the issue of economic or criminal adulteration. As established in the monitoring strategies study, the validity of these chemical tests relies on having analytical methods that are able to distinguish pure products from adulterated ones using set standards (Manning & Soon, 2025). In addition, incorporating these test approaches into educational models, as described by the Western Institute for Food Safety and Security, can promote public awareness of food safety issues and stimulate inter-disciplinary collaborations to maintain food integrity while not sacrificing environmental assets (Angelos et al., 2017).

7.1.3. Spectroscopic Methods

Using spectroscopic methods is now very important for finding adulterants in food, especially in herbal and dietary supplements, where fraud is more likely. With these techniques, researchers can quickly and accurately identify the chemicals in food, helping them determine the purity and what is in the food.

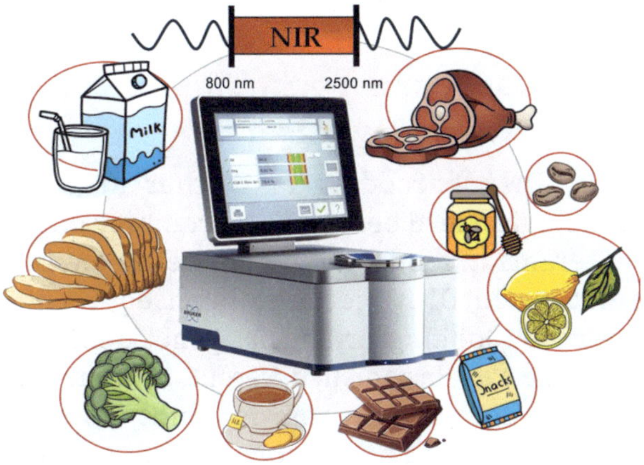

Figure 7.2. The application of spectroscopic methods has become increasingly vital in the detection of adulterants in food.

Source: Fodor M, Matkovits A, Benes EL, Jókai Z. The Role of Near-Infrared Spectroscopy in Food Quality Assurance: A Review of the Past Two Decades. *Foods*. 2024; 13(21):3501. https://doi.org/10.3390/foods13213501

For instance, Fourier-transform infrared spectroscopy (FT-IR) coupled with chemometric analysis has demonstrated robustness in screening for adulterants, revealing that over 24% of tested samples contained some form of contamination, as reported in recent studies (Black et al., 2016). Moreover, the integration of liquid chromatography-high-resolution mass spectrometry (LC-HRMS) enhances this methodology by allowing for biomarker identification, further supporting the need for effective analytical approaches in combating food fraud. As highlighted in discussions on food safety, the implementation of such advanced spectroscopic techniques is essential for protecting consumers and maintaining the integrity of the food supply (Amaral et al., 2016) (Figure 7.2).

7.1.4. Chromatographic Techniques

Because food adulteration is happening more often, it is now very important to have reliable ways to detect it and chromatography is a key tool for this. They make it possible to separate and identify complex mixtures , which is why they are effective for finding adulterants in food. Techniques , such as Thin Layer Chromatography (TLC), Gas Chromatography (GC), and High-Performance Liquid Chromatography (HPLC) have been widely employed due to their ability to accurately differentiate between pure and contaminated samples.

Lately, scientists have combined chromatography with chemometric analysis , which makes it possible to find multiple adulterants at the same time and strengthens the reliability of testing methods. For instance, a two-tier testing approach by LC-HRMS has revealed that more than 24% of herbal samples were adulterated, highlighting the role chromatographic methods play in maintaining food quality and safety (Black et al., 2016).

7.1.5. Microbiological Methods

Using microbiological methods to find food adulterants is now very important for maintaining food safety and quality. Using culture-based assays, molecular approaches and rapid detection systems helps identify the specific microbes that show the food has been adulterated. For example, in milk, the use of traditional microbiology can show if urea or formalin is present by observing how microorganisms and enzymes behave. These are supported by evidence reporting widespread milk adulteration in countries , such as Pakistan, where poor handling and processing heavily impair product safety (Khan et al., 2016).

Additionally, innovations in sensor technologies highlight the promise of evolving intelligent detection systems that integrate optical and biochemical analysis, enabling more accurate quality evaluations (Baloch et al., 2021). Therefore, the inclusion of microbiological techniques into food safety measures is crucial for safeguarding consumer health and improving food quality control (Figure 7.3).

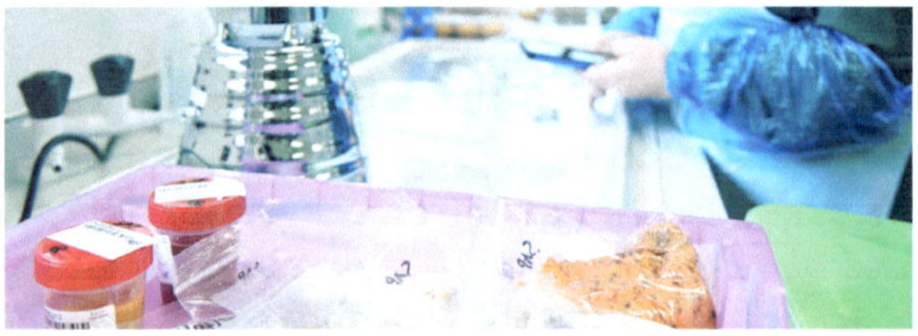

Figure 7.3. Utilizing techniques , such as culture-based assays, molecular methods, and rapid detection systems facilitates the identification of specific microbial contaminants that indicate adulteration.

Source: https://sciex.com/adobe/dynamicmedia/deliver/dm-aid--8ddb61e4-8774-48d4-95d6-0c6ef87e1182/food-fraud-main-2880x1024.jpg?quality=75&width=1920.

7.1.6. Rapid Testing Kits

Thanks to rapid testing kits, it is now much easier to detect food safety issues and adulterants in a short period. In the past, checking the authenticity of food often meant running many laboratory tests , which took a lot of time and money. Rapid testing kits use new technologies to provide results quickly , which helps with faster decisions in the food industry. For instance, the development of a single HyBeacon(®) probe assay for identifying Atlantic cod exemplifies how these kits can pinpoint specific species, ensuring authenticity and reducing fraud in seafood markets (Court et al., 2025).

In addition, the necessity for effective detection mechanisms is highlighted by the identification of some pathogenic *Escherichia coli* serogroups as ground meat adulterants, which requires effective detection measures to ensure public health protection (Baker et al., 2015). Therefore, these quick tests are significant in food safety today since they provide both speed and accuracy in detecting adulterants.

7.1.7. Advanced Technologies (e.g., DNA Barcoding)

Lately, DNA barcoding and other advanced technologies have become important for finding adulterants in food. The method relies on using standardized DNA pieces to precisely identify species by looking at special genetic markers that make each organism different. Its usefulness in food safety comes from its ability to check raw materials and detect contaminants in many food types , which is why it is important for herbal medicine and food production.

For instance, studies have demonstrated the successful application of DNA barcoding methods to screen commercial products for specific species, revealing instances of adulteration even at low DNA concentrations (Hill et al., 2019). In addition, the strength of DNA barcoding is promoted by choosing suitable genetic markers, which promote high species discrimination (Aseema et al., 2024). Going forward, we are likely to face challenges of food adulteration, and it will be crucial to utilize such technologies in ensuring food safety and quality (Figure 7.4).

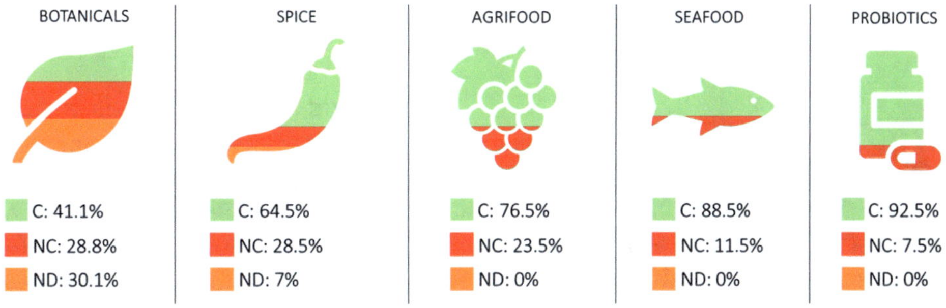

Figure 7.4. The effectiveness of DNA barcoding in food safety lies in its ability to authenticate raw materials and detect contaminants across various matrices.

Source: Gorini T, Mezzasalma V, Deligia M, De Mattia F, Campone L, Labra M, Frigerio J. Check Your Shopping Cart: DNA Barcoding and Mini-Barcoding for Food Authentication. *Foods*. 2023; 12(12):2392. https://doi.org/10.3390/foods12122392

7.1.8. Role of Food Laboratories

Food laboratories are very important in the effort to stop food adulteration , which can threaten both safety and quality. They depend on advanced methods to verify food products, making sure they follow safety rules and that consumers are not tricked by fake products. As highlighted in the studies, the detection of common adulterants in staple foods is crucial, as items like wheat flour are particularly susceptible to unethical modifications that can adversely affect health (Singh et al., 2024).

Furthermore, food laboratories not only conduct detailed analyses but also support regulatory authorities in monitoring food authenticity and purity (Hendri et al., 2016). Because of this teamwork, people can trust what they buy and the food system remains reliable. Effective detection is made possible by food laboratories , which helps reduce the risks of adulterated foods and reassures the public about food safety.

7.1.9. Limitations of Current Detection Methods

It is still very difficult to detect food adulterants because current methods have their own limitations. Although many popular techniques are useful for detecting some contaminants, they tend to be quite limited in their ability to detect adulterants in complex foods. It is sometimes hard for conventional methods to find very low levels of adulterants that are like real products. This is particularly evident in olive oil testing, where existing authentication models have demonstrated only moderate success rates, identifying 86.8% of adulterated samples but still leaving room for error with 81.1% of genuine products misclassified (Bendini et al., 2021). In addition, although DNA barcoding has been promising for the identification of plant material, its use in food products is controversial due to the heterogeneity in DNA quality and fragment size , which makes detection unreliable (Hill et al., 2019). Such drawbacks indicate the urgent need for the development of stronger methods , which can be used with confidence to guarantee food authenticity (Figure 7.5).

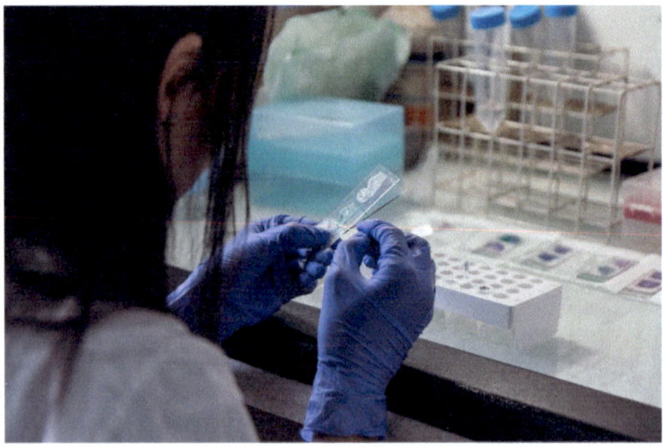

Figure 7.5. Conventional methods may struggle to detect low levels of adulterants that share similar properties with genuine products.

Source: https://smsla.global/wp-content/uploads/2025/01/lab-2813958_1280.jpg.

7.2. Current Laws and Regulations

Current legislation and statutes on food adulteration guarantee that consumers are safeguarded and that products of quality are maintained. Different areas have implemented laws that define what can be done in food, and transparency and compliance with rules at the point of manufacture are key. Within the European Union, the treatment and definition of novel foods like coffee and microalgae are constantly under scrutiny. As emphasized in recent summaries, some coffee wastes, despite being conventionally ingested in non-EU nations, need to undergo stringent safety assessments prior to authorizing them as novel foods (Klingel et al., 2020). Even the legal regulations encompassing microalgae, particularly their carotenoid synthesis, reflect how much regulation there is for food additives and nutritional supplements. These advancements highlight the need to maintain compliance with laws that reduce risks of adulteration and improve the safety profile of foodstuffs (Novoveská et al., 2019).

7.2.1. Overview of National Laws on Adulteration

Since food adulteration is a serious problem globally, stringent national legislation and regulations are necessary to safeguard the public. In America, the Food and Drug Administration (FDA) is at the forefront of enforcing adulteration laws, holding manufacturers responsible for maintaining the purity of their products. They address the use of toxic materials as well as the production of products and labeling. In Europe and elsewhere, the same has been established, usually on the basis of international trade regulations, to manage food safety and quality in the same manner. Importantly, while industries move to incorporate new substances like microalgae for nutritional value, the regulatory environment shifts to address legalities surrounding these advancements and their possible effects on consumer safety (Novoveská et al., 2019). In addition, the speedy growth in the market of dietary supplements fuels concern about the regulation of such products and their impact on consumer protection (Kerksick et al., 2018) (Figure 7.6).

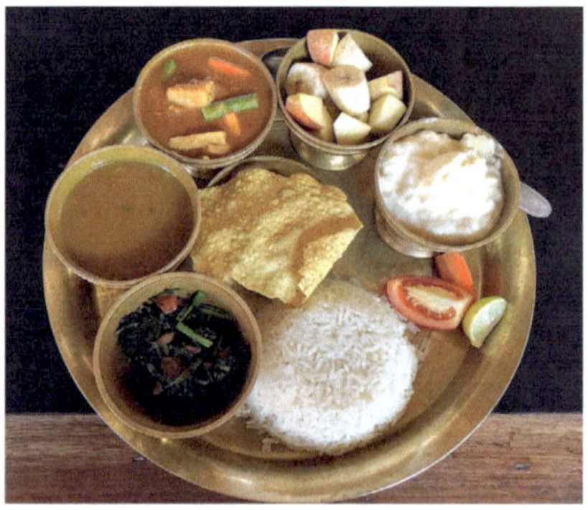

Figure 7.6. Adulteration of food products remains a significant concern globally, necessitating stringent national laws and regulatory frameworks to safeguard public health.

Source: By Subhashish Panigrahi - Own work, CC BY-SA 4.0, https://commons.wikimedia.org/w/index.php?curid=75816881

7.2.2. Role of the Food and Drug Administration (FDA)

The FDA helps to keep food safe and makes sure that adulteration is properly managed in the market. Since it is a federal agency, the FDA sets tough rules and checks food safety closely to make sure regulations are being followed for the benefit of the public. These regulations extend to innovative food products derived from microalgae and other novel sources, which can be potentially beneficial yet come with their own regulatory challenges, particularly in terms of commercial production and safety assessments (Novoveská et al., 2019). Moreover, the agency's oversight includes evaluating the bioactive compounds in food items, such as curcumin derived from turmeric, ensuring that they meet safety and efficacy standards before reaching consumers (Kotha & Luthria, 2019). Because of this complete set of rules, the food industry can avoid adulteration and ensure its products are safe , which helps build trust among consumers and improves health.

7.2.3. State-Level Regulations and Enforcement

Laws and actions at the state level are very important for adulteration, since they have a direct effect on food safety and public health. Every state makes its own rules about food safety and quality , which are tailored to the needs and interests of that region. Because of the diversity in farming and what people want to eat, these regulations are made to deal with problems of adulteration in great detail. Routine checks and fines for not following the rules are necessary to make sure companies follow the set standards. Furthermore, the interaction of state regulations with federal guidelines creates a layered approach to food safety, as illustrated by the challenges of regulating the production of microalgae-derived carotenoids (Novoveská et al., 2019). Moreover, effective enforcement is necessary to eliminate food safety hazards, as evidenced by the various stakeholders involved in the food supply chain, from producers to consumers (Jaffee et al., 2018) (Figure 7.7).

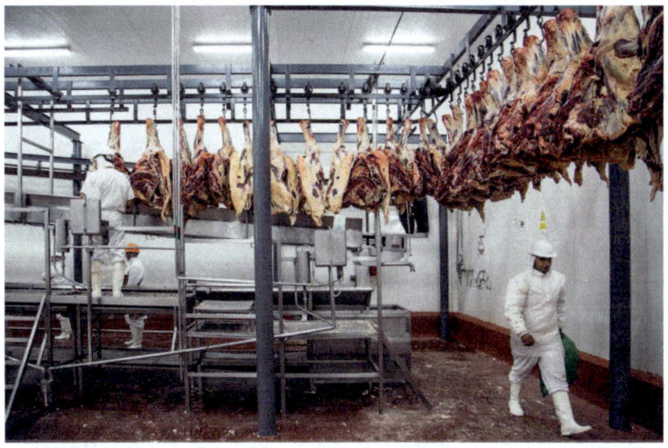

Figure 7.7. The role of state-level regulations and enforcement in the context of adulteration is crucial, as these local frameworks directly influence food safety and public health outcomes.

Source: https://foodforwardndcs.panda.org/content/uploads/2024/02/ww241043.jpg.

7.2.4. International Standards and Agreements

Addressing adulteration in the world's food supply chain depends greatly on having international standards and agreements. By bringing regulations together, these standards guarantee food is safe and high quality , which helps both consumers and traders. For example, the Codex Alimentarius, which was established by the World Health Organization and the Food and Agriculture Organization, is a key reference for countries to use, which assists in reducing risks of adulterated products (Novoveská et al., 2019).

In addition, with digital technologies revolutionizing the food and agriculture industries, new opportunities are available for promoting better compliance and easier alignment with standards, which reduces trade-related transaction costs (Jouanjean, 2019). The blend of regulations and emerging technologies indicates that nations must collaborate in combating food adulteration to guarantee the safety and stability of the international market.

7.2.5. Penalties for Adulteration Violations

Such violations are a major risk to the health and safety of the public, so strong laws are needed to stop them. These actions are often punished very severely, with criminal and civil consequences that vary depending on the area. As an example, those convicted of adulterating food products may be required to pay large fines, make restitution and could be sentenced to prison for the people involved. The purpose of these legal frameworks is to punish offenders and also to stop future incidents by making sure companies follow strict procedures. However, challenges remain in enforcing these laws effectively; for instance, the absence of clear implementing regulations can create a legal vacuum, hindering authorities from imposing penalties effectively (Asyyere et al., 2025). Also, making sure these penalties are enforced properly depends on agencies working together, but this can be difficult because of inefficiencies and conflicts within the system. Thus, for laws against adulteration to be truly effective, they must be both comprehensive and enforceable (Figure 7.8).

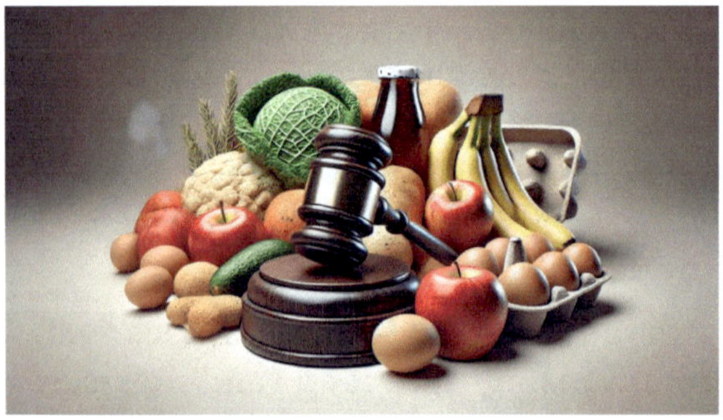

Figure 7.8. Penalties for adulteration violations.

Source: https://www.digicomply.com/hubfs/Food%20Fraud%20Penalties.png.

7.2.6. Recent Amendments to Existing Laws

Laws covering food safety and adulteration have been updated lately , which has greatly changed the rules to better protect consumers in a global market. Because of the challenges in international supply chains, these new regulations are needed, as recent studies on pharmaceutical manufacturing point out that better oversight is important for ensuring both the quality and safety of products. Besides, the new ways of defining and handling food safety laws encourage people to see all risks linked to food systems. This is crucial because traditional interpretations often overlook cumulative and environmental safety concerns, which are integral to public health (Leib et al., 2019). The amendments cover both detailed and broad meanings of safety , which leads to better use of resources and a unified policy that can reduce risks and improve health across the food and drug supply chains.

7.2.7. Comparison of Laws Across Different Countries

It is clear from comparing laws on food adulteration in different countries that there are many differences in how laws are made and enforced. For example, the European Union and the United States put strong rules in place for food safety and adulteration, but China and Japan have developed their own laws that fit their cultures and economies. In Europe and the USA, existing laws are rigorously enforced, focusing on protecting consumer health and ensuring transparency in food production systems, highlighting the role of stakeholders in maintaining food safety standards, as noted in Jaffee et al. (2018). Conversely, despite its high potential for carotenoid production from microalgae, China faces challenges in regulatory compliance that may hinder the commercialization of such innovations, as discussed in Novoveská et al. (2019).

This disparity illustrates how differing legal approaches shape the dynamics of food safety and adulteration across nations, ultimately affecting public health outcomes and market integration (Figure 7.9).

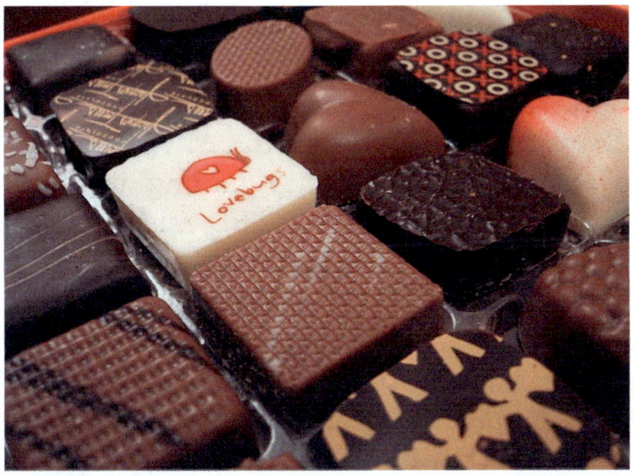

Figure 7.9. Legal approaches shape the dynamics of food safety and adulteration across nations.

Source: By John Hritz from Ann Arbor, MI, USA - Flickr, CC BY 2.0, https://commons.wikimedia.org/w/index.php?curid=348696

7.2.8. Role of Consumer Protection Agencies

Consumer protection agencies are important for public health since they enforce rules against food adulteration and make sure food products are safe. These agencies are tasked with monitoring food safety standards and addressing violations that compromise consumer health, particularly in light of rising instances of foodborne diseases, which affect an estimated 600 million people globally each year (D-Klingbeil et al., 2019). Using strict food laws and regulations, they try to lower the chances of adulterated food substances. Consumer protection agencies also provide education and training to ensure people understand why food safety is important , which helps the community resist food fraud. As the regulatory landscape evolves, particularly in response to globalization and emerging risks, the effectiveness of these agencies will significantly depend on their ability to adapt and integrate scientific advancements into their enforcement practices (Novoveská et al., 2019). So, they are important for both quick consumer protection and for encouraging people to trust the food system over time.

7.2.9. Challenges in Enforcing Adulteration Laws

It is very difficult to enforce adulteration laws , which can seriously harm both public health and the safety of consumers. Detecting adulterants in large-scale products is a major problem because the process can be very complicated.

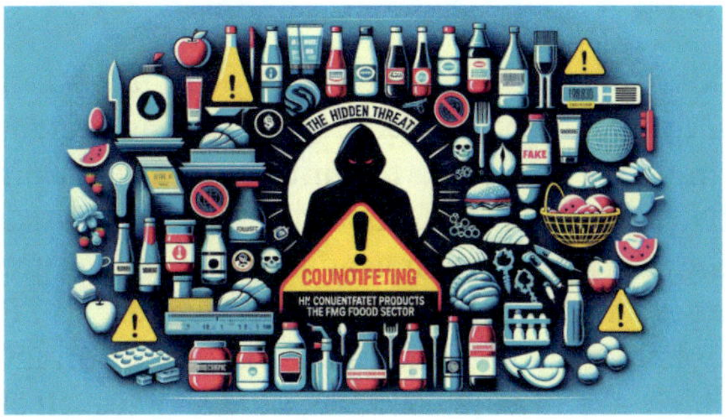

Figure 7.10. The enforcement of adulteration laws faces numerous challenges that significantly affect public health and consumer safety.

Source: https://media.licdn.com/dms/image/v2/D5612AQGonp8k4dazGg/article-cover_image-shrink_720_1280/article-cover_image-shrink_720_1280/0/1705809843493?e=2147483647&v=beta&t=NKq0nUDU9Bt4iOfB-VArTtiuYX1rFSZbUJ1XEuht2sE.

Even though regulations are tough, the way they are enforced usually does not keep up with the latest changes in food and product production. In addition, not having enough resources for regulatory agencies makes it difficult for them to enforce rules and monitor manufacturers , which opens the door for unethical companies. The incentivization of exploiting these regulations is illustrated in sectors , such as the carotenoid market, where complexities in the legal framework impede proper oversight (Novoveská et al., 2019). Furthermore, issues related to institutional racism can exacerbate disparities in the enforcement of health regulations, disproportionately impacting marginalized communities who often lack adequate access to safe products (Williams, 2018). Consequently, addressing these multifaceted challenges is crucial for ensuring robust enforcement of adulteration laws (Figure 7.10).

7.3. Impact of Adulteration Laws on Society

Adulteration laws have greatly improved the health and safety of people by creating a strong framework to stop harmful and misleading activities. In the past, food and pharmaceuticals being adulterated so often adulterated, posing great dangers and causing many health crises, making people lose trust in them. New adulteration laws , which are always being updated, place strong emphasis on quality control and regulation to tackle these problems. These laws make the supply chain more open , which helps both consumers and the market as a whole. Recent studies have pointed out that the growing globalization of markets makes it much harder to enforce these standards, mainly in the pharmaceutical sector. Effectively implementing robust adulteration laws thus plays a vital role in promoting public health and maintaining the ethical standards of commerce, reflecting society's growing demand for accountability in food and drug manufacturing (French & Phillips, 2002).

7.3.1. Public Health Implications

Because food and product adulteration can be very harmful to public health, it is important for policymakers and regulators to address it right away. Having hazardous substances in foods risks people's health and makes people question the safety of the food they eat. As noted, numerous incidents of food adulteration and associated disease outbreaks have led to a significant decline in consumer confidence, emphasizing the urgent need for efficient traceability systems in the food supply chain (Haleem et al., 2019). With these systems, it would be easier to keep track of things and hold people responsible , which would reduce the risks of contaminated products. Furthermore, the variability in quality among non–FDA-approved products, such as CBD, raises concerns about unregulated substances entering the market, often carrying unknown health risks (White, 2019). Addressing these issues through stringent laws and enforcement can ultimately protect public health and enhance the integrity of food safety frameworks (Figure 7.11).

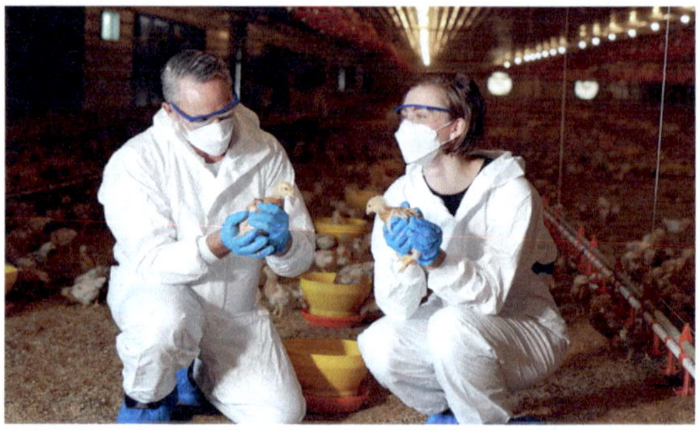

Figure 7.11. The implications of food and product adulteration on public health are profound, warranting immediate attention from policymakers and regulatory bodies.

Source: https://www.food-safety.com/ext/resources/Images/2024/Jun_Jul/Spot-0624-900-Img1.jpg?height=740&t=1721141055&width=auto.

7.3.2. Economic Consequences for Consumers

Consumers may experience many economic problems because of adulteration , which can affect their finances and make them lose trust in the food industry. When food is adulterated, both its quality and the price for consumers increase , which can go unnoticed by those buying the products. Such deceptive practices can distort market dynamics, where consumers are left vulnerable to fraudulent activities, including species substitution and other manipulations in food supply chains, particularly evident in commodities like seafood (Fox et al., 2018). Also, as noted in food safety discussions, the consequences go further than just losing money; they also affect people's health and the ethical standards surrounding food. Acknowledging that consumers rely on the integrity of food products to secure nutritional needs emphasizes the necessity for effective regulations and awareness campaigns aimed at mitigating these risks (Jaffee et al., 2018). Therefore, dealing with adulteration matters for both public safety and fairness in food markets.

7.3.3. Impact on Food and Drug Industries

The connection between food safety laws and the food and drug sectors points out the major effect of adulteration rules on both health and the economy. They help to guarantee that food is not contaminated or contains any harmful additives , which encourages people to trust the products. According to Jaffee et al. (2018), food safety is intricately linked to achieving Sustainable Development Goals, particularly in enhancing nutritional security and health outcomes. Simultaneously, the use of antibiotics in food production has raised significant concerns regarding drug residues and antimicrobial resistance, as pointed out in Kirchhelle (2018). There are many ways countries regulate antibiotics , which shows the difficulties in making food safety standards the same. Consequently, the enforcement of stringent adulteration laws not only protects consumer health but also encourages agricultural practices that align with global safety standards, promoting overall growth within the food and drug industries (Figure 7.12).

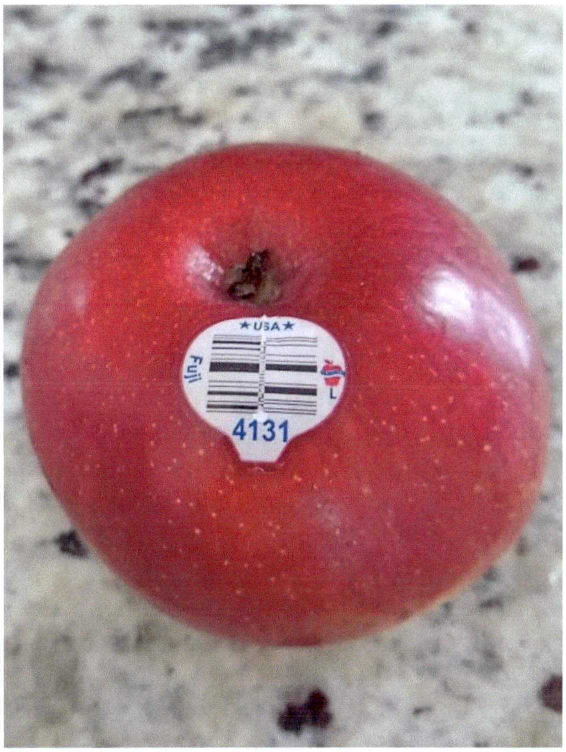

Figure 7.12. The intricate relationship between food safety regulations and the food and drug industries highlights the profound impact of adulteration laws on public health and economic stability.

Source: By Whoisjohngalt - Own work, CC BY-SA 4.0, https://commons.wikimedia.org/w/index.php?curid=95335760

7.3.4. Consumer Trust and Confidence

For laws and procedures on adulterated food to work, people must trust and believe in them. If people think the food they get is safe and genuine, they are much more likely to participate in the market. With blockchain, the food supply chain becomes more transparent and traceable , which helps build trust. By verifying the integrity of claims regarding product authenticity, such as organic or sustainably sourced designations, blockchain can alleviate consumer concerns related to adulteration, ultimately enhancing their confidence in food products (Rejeb et al., 2020). However, putting this technology into practice may meet several problems , such as rules from regulators and technological issues. According to researchers, the way people view food and technology is very important for future food safety and trust in the market.

7.3.5. Role of Advocacy Groups

Shaping food safety rules and dealing with adulteration are important roles played by advocacy groups. They help consumers talk to regulatory bodies about any public health issues related to food safety. Advocacy groups can help ensure that policy changes are made and producers and suppliers are more responsible by educating people about the risks of contaminated and adulterated food. For instance, in the context of rapidly changing regulatory frameworks, such as those observed in China, advocacy groups contribute to the development of a governance model , which promotes cooperation among government entities, businesses, and civil stakeholders to enhance food safety standards (Liu et al., 2019).

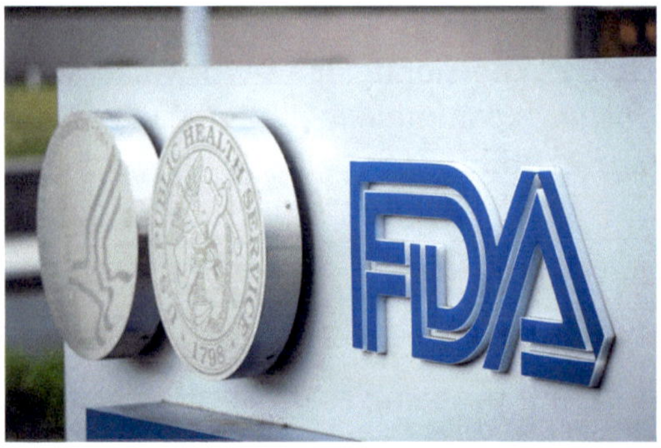

Figure 7.13. Advocacy groups play a pivotal role in shaping food safety regulations and combating the challenges posed by adulteration.

Source: https://www.digicomply.com/hubfs/FDA%202023%20SGS.png.

Furthermore, as these groups facilitate transparency and provide crucial information to consumers, they empower individuals to make informed choices, thereby driving demand for safer, higher-quality food products and prompting more stringent adherence to quality control measures (Salem et al., 2020) (Figure 7.13).

7.3.6. Social Justice Issues Related to Adulteration

Because adulteration affects so many consumers and mostly impacts the most vulnerable, it is a social justice concern as well as a safety issue. Marginalized groups are more likely to receive items that are dangerous for their health , such as food that is not clean or health-related products that are unsafe , which leads to more health problems for them. In places where regulation is weak, laws against adulteration may not be followed , which allows dishonest vendors to make money at the expense of these communities. Strong legal rules are needed, but they must be backed by effective actions to help these groups. As seen in the context of smokeless tobacco in India, where 21.4% of adults are affected and significant health impacts are observed, addressing such issues requires a multistakeholder approach aiming for systemic change in policy enforcement and public health initiatives (Yadav et al., 2020). Furthermore, the ongoing crisis of synthetic opioid-related deaths accentuates the urgency for reform in controlling adulterated substances to mitigate harm to marginalized populations (Pardo et al., 2019).

7.3.7. Global Implications of Local Laws

The way local laws affect global matters , such as food adulteration rules, is becoming more important. In regions like Bangladesh, the trustworthiness of halal food products, governed by local laws, directly influences consumer behavior and purchasing decisions, showcasing how domestic regulations can resonate on a global scale (Ashraf, 2019). Additionally, as the market for products like cannabidiol (CBD) expands, the legal status and variation in quality of non–FDA-approved CBD products underscore the complexities of local laws affecting international commerce and consumer safety (White, 2019). So, local laws, made to address regional issues, end up shaping global rules and earning consumer trust. The divergence in regulations not only impacts local markets but also poses challenges and opportunities for international trade, where conformity to varying standards becomes crucial for maintaining product integrity and consumer confidence across borders (Figure 7.14).

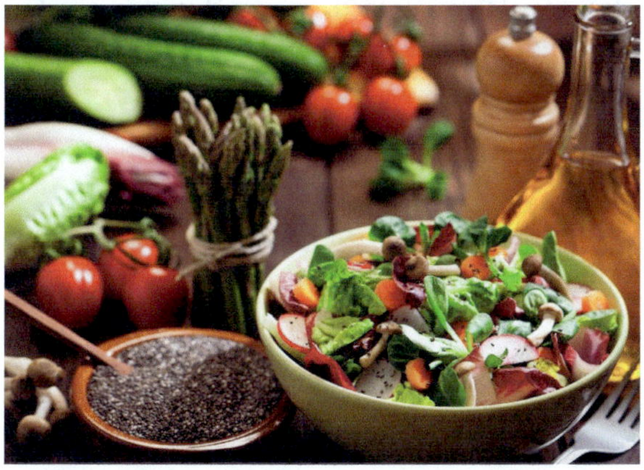

Figure 7.14. The interplay between local laws and global implications becomes increasingly significant, particularly regarding food adulteration regulations.

Source: https://consumer-voice.org/wp-content/uploads/2022/06/Eat-Right-India-Steadily-Reforming-Indias-Food-Ecosystem.jpg.

7.3.8. Trends in Consumer Behavior

People have started expecting more transparency and quality from the food they buy , which is linked to worries about adulteration. Many people now want to know where their food comes from and how it is processed, mainly because of the growth of digital technology. The integration of information and communication technologies (ICTs), such as blockchain and artificial intelligence, has provided consumers with unprecedented access to data about product safety and authenticity, thus mitigating fears of fraud (Guruswamy et al., 2022). In addition, as people become more informed about food safety, many are urging authorities to put in place tougher rules and laws about food quality and adulteration. This evolving consumer landscape necessitates a response from regulatory bodies to ensure that laws and procedures are not only current but also capable of adapting to the rapidly changing market dynamics fueled by informed and conscientious consumers (Hui et al., 2020).

7.3.9. Future Outlook on Adulteration Laws

Since food safety is always changing, laws against adulteration must be ready to handle new issues that arise in the agri-food sector. More and more, those making food policy understand that advanced technology and data integration are important for fighting food fraud. The adoption of the Farm to Fork Strategy exemplifies this shift, emphasizing the need for enhanced traceability and better coordination among stakeholders to effectively address fraudulent practices in the food chain (Andrea et al., 2024). Digital traceability systems play a major role in making regulations more effective , which protects consumers and guarantees the quality of products.

Also, using data analytics to spot possible adulteration risks will strengthen the laws in place and encourage cooperation between authorities and companies. Ultimately, a robust and adaptable legal framework, informed by technological innovations, will be crucial in evolving the landscape of food safety and protecting public health in the future (Figure 7.15).

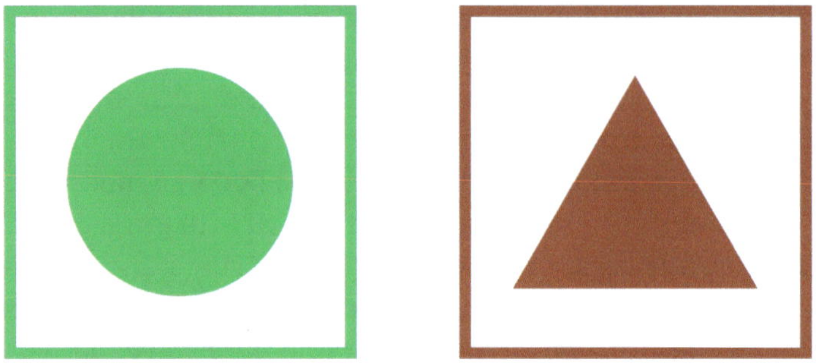

Figure 7.15. Policymakers are increasingly recognizing the importance of advanced technologies and data integration in combating food fraud.

Source: By Food Safety and Standards Authority of India - https://www.fssai.gov.in/upload/uploadfiles/files/Compendium_Labelling_Display_23_09_2021.pdfOwn work based on: Current FSSAI Veg and Non-veg Labels.png:, Public Domain, https://commons.wikimedia.org/w/index.php?curid=141453300

A CLOSER LOOK

Food Safety

Food safety means taking steps and maintaining conditions to prevent food from being contaminated by bacteria, viruses, parasites and chemicals. It requires handling, preparing, storing and moving food properly to stop food-borne illnesses and keep the public healthy. Some key things in food safety are cleanliness, cooking food at the right temperature, avoiding cross-contamination and obeying food safety rules and standards. Food safety depends on both consumers and food industry workers following the best practices and safety rules. Food safety protects people's health, earns their trust and makes sure the food supply is dependable (Abebaw, 2019).

SUMMARY

It is very important to use advanced techniques to find adulterants in food to maintain food safety and public trust. DNA barcoding and other new methods are important for spotting contaminants , which supports both accurate labeling and helps stop food piracy. As noted in the exploration of DNA barcoding, its application extends to uncovering the authenticity of various agricultural products, making it an invaluable tool in the industry (Barcaccia et al., 2015). Additionally, the adaptation of specific PCR tests for commercial products demonstrates the efficacy of molecular techniques in detecting adulteration at multiple levels (Hill et al., 2019). As these methods are improved and standardized, both regulations and consumer awareness grow. Working on these detection methods will make food safer and more reliable for consumers.

It is now a serious public health concern that adulterants are found in food, as recent studies have shown many staples are contaminated. For instance, in a study conducted in Gorakhpur, India, it was revealed that nearly 31.25% of wheat flour samples contained harmful adulterants, including starch and chalk powder, which pose significant health risks , such as gastrointestinal distress and long-term kidney damage (Singh et al., 2024). Milk , which is a key part of many diets, is easily adulterated, so it requires both destructive and non-destructive methods to be checked for safety. Techniques like Lactoscan and hyperspectral imaging have shown promising results, with advanced deep learning models achieving up to 97% accuracy in identifying adulteration (Aqeel et al., 2024). All of these studies point out that we need more awareness, stronger regulations and advanced testing to stop food adulteration and safeguard consumer health.

KEY TERMS FROM THIS CHAPTER

Adulterated samples
Carotenoid production
Chemometric analysis
Commercialization
DNA barcoding
Enforcement
Food adulterants
Fragment size
Authenticity
Chemical methods
Chromatography
Culture-based assays
DNA quality
Fake products
Food laboratories
Gas Chromatography (GC)

REFERENCES

1. Abebaw, Bamlaku. "Analytical Authentication and Determination of Adulteration in Branded Honey Samples Collected from Selected Areas in Ethiopia." Food Science and Quality Management, International Institute for Science, Technology and Education, 2019.Aiswarya, S., Meenu, L., Menon, K. U., Donelli, M., & Menon, S. (2024). A novel microstrip sensor based on closed loop antenna for adulteration detection of liquid samples. *IEEE Sensors Journal, 24*(2), 1405–1414. https://www.semanticscholar.org/paper/b124b8c1b12d788b5d18eef75b39b4edb8a0c636 (accessed on 29 May 2025).
2. Al-Jaroodi, J., & Mohamed, N. (2019). Blockchain in industries: A survey. *IEEE Access, 7*, 36500–36515. https://doi.org/10.1109/access.2019.2903554.
3. Alves, E. A., Baqueta, M. R., Diniz, P. H. G. D., et al. (2024). Authentication of indigenous Brazilian specialty Canephore coffees using smartphone image analysis. https://core.ac.uk/download/643634260.pdf (accessed on 29 May 2025).
4. Amaral, J. S., Oliveira, B., & Rocha, T. (2016). Adulteration of dietary supplements by the illegal addition of synthetic drugs: A review. https://core.ac.uk/download/153416605.pdf (accessed on 29 May 2025).
5. Angelos, J. A., Arens, A. L., Johnson, H. A., Cadriel, J. L., & Osburn, B. I. (2017). One Health in food safety and security education: Subject matter outline for a curricular framework. *One health (Amsterdam, Netherlands), 3*, 56–65. https://doi.org/10.1016/j.onehlt.2017.04.001Aouadi, B., Zaukuu, J.-L. Z., Vitális, F., Bodor, Z., Fehér, O., Gillay, Z., Bázár, G., et al. (2020). Historical evolution and food control achievements of near infrared spectroscopy, electronic nose, and electronic tongue—Critical overview. *Sensors, 20*(19), 5479. https://doi.org/10.3390/s20195479.
6. Aqeel, M., Iqbal, M., Ullah, S., Syed, S., et al. (2024). Hyperspectral identification of milk adulteration using advance deep learning. https://core.ac.uk/download/639873499.pdf (accessed on 29 May 2025).
7. French, M. and Phillips, J. (2002) Food safety regimes in Scotland, 1899-1914. *Journal of Scottish Historical Studies*, 22(2), pp. 134-157. (doi: 10.3366/jshs.2002.22.2.134)Ashraf, M. (2019). Islamic marketing and consumer behavior toward halal food purchase in Bangladesh. *Journal of Islamic Marketing, 10*(3), 893–910. https://doi.org/10.1108/JIMA-03-2018-0051.
8. Asyyere, K., Siagian, H., Pahlevi, S., Simanulllang, Y., & Riady. (2025). Implementation of corporate criminal sanctions enforcement in arrears of BPJS employment contributions. *Contemporary Journal of Applied Sciences.* https://www.semanticscholar.org/paper/ccaa00e2c0ba58124929871fed2356d07c17f90e (accessed on 29 May 2025).
9. Baker, C. A. (2015). Shiga toxin-producing *Escherichia coli* (STEC) detection strategies with formalin-fixed STEC cells. https://core.ac.uk/download/84120148.pdf (accessed on 29 May 2025).
10. Baloch, A., Latif, A., Bhanger, M., & Baloch, S. (2021). Detection of milk impureness. https://core.ac.uk/download/614034298.pdf (accessed on 29 May 2025).
11. Barcaccia G, Lucchin M, Cassandro M. DNA Barcoding as a Molecular Tool to Track Down Mislabeling and Food Piracy. *Diversity*. 2016; 8(1):2. https://doi.org/10.3390/d8010002Barrios-Rodriguez, Y. F., Devia-Rodriguez, Y., & Guzmán, N. G. (2022). Detection of adulterated coffee by Fourier-transform infrared (FTIR) spectroscopy associated with sensory analysis. https://

core.ac.uk/download/653735685.pdf (accessed on 29 May 2025).

12. Bateman, B., Heide-Jørgensen, U., Einarsdóttir, K., Engeland, A., Furu, K., Gissler, M., Hernández-Díaz, S., et al. (2018). β-Blocker use in pregnancy and the risk for congenital malformations. *Annals of Internal Medicine, 169*(10), 665–673. https://www.semanticscholar.org/paper/54b8ce2f0c930b754324752c2d3ef7a571c62ea3 (accessed on 29 May 2025).
13. Battell, S. E. (2023). *On the Threshold*. https://doi.org/10.3366/batt5686.
14. Bendini, A., Alonso, J. B., Toschi, T. G., et al. (2021). Large-scale evaluation of shotgun triacylglycerol profiling for the fast detection of olive oil adulteration. https://core.ac.uk/download/387863385.pdf (accessed on 29 May 2025).
15. Bhat, S. A., Huang, N. F., Sofi, I. B., & Sultan, M. (2021). Agriculture-food supply chain management based on blockchain and IoT: A narrative on enterprise blockchain interoperability. *Agriculture, 12*(1), 40. https://doi.org/10.3390/agriculture12010040.
16. Black, C., Chevallier, O. P., Elliott, C. T., et al. (2016). A comprehensive strategy to detect the fraudulent adulteration of herbs: The oregano approach. https://core.ac.uk/download/33595879.pdf (accessed on 29 May 2025).
17. Black, C., Chevallier, O., & Elliott, C. (2016). The current and potential applications of ambient mass spectrometry in detecting food fraud. https://core.ac.uk/download/74404921.pdf (accessed on 29 May 2025).
18. Bocchino, A., Siligato, R., & Ulberth, F. (2024). An information-based risk analysis IT tool protecting the European food system(s). https://core.ac.uk/download/642862754.pdf (accessed on 29 May 2025).
19. Broad Leib, E. M., & Pollans, M. J. (2019). The new food safety. https://core.ac.uk/download/231832064.pdf (accessed on 29 May 2025).
20. Cadot, O., & Gourdon, J. (2014). Assessing the price-raising effect of non-tariff measures in Africa. *Journal of African Economies, 23*(4), 425–463. https://doi.org/10.1093/jae/eju007.
21. Cama-Moncunill, R., Casado-Gavalda, M. P., Cullen, P. J., Markiewicz-Keszycka, M., et al. (2019). Laser-induced breakdown spectroscopy for food authentication. https://core.ac.uk/download/482671896.pdf (accessed on 29 May 2025).
22. Capps, O., Jr., Fairchild, G. F., & Nichols, J. P. (2025). Observations on economic adulteration of high-value food products: The honey case. https://core.ac.uk/download/pdf/6995148.pdf (accessed on 29 May 2025).
23. Casadei, E., Valli, E., Panni, F., Donarski, J., Farrús Gubern, J., Lucci, P., Conte, L. S., et al. (2021). Emerging trends in olive oil fraud and possible countermeasures. *Food Control, 124*, Article 107902. https://doi.org/10.1016/j.foodcont.2021.107902.
24. Costa, J. G., Vidović, B., Saraiva, N., Costa, M. do C., Del Favero, G., Marko, D., Oliveira, N., et al. (2019). Contaminants: A dark side of food supplements? *Free Radical Research, 53*(10), 1113–1135. https://doi.org/10.1080/10715762.2019.1636045.
25. Court, D. S., Dawnay, N., Duxbury, N., Hughes, T., et al. (2025). Species detection using HyBeacon® probe technology: Working towards rapid onsite testing in non-human forensic and food authentication applications. https://core.ac.uk/download/42478088.pdf (accessed on 29 May 2025).

26. Crişan, I., Ona, A., Vârban, D., Muntean, L. S., Vârban, R., Stoie, A., Mihăiescu, T., et al. (2023). Current trends for lavender (*Lavandula angustifolia* Mill.) crops and products with emphasis on essential oil quality. *Plants, 12*(3), Article 357. https://doi.org/10.3390/plants12020357.

27. Da Rocha, T. S., Amaral, J. S., & Oliveira, M. B. P. P. (2015). Adulteration of dietary supplements by the illegal addition of synthetic drugs: A review. *Comprehensive Reviews in Food Science and Food Safety, 15*(1), 43–62. https://doi.org/10.1111/1541-4337.12173.

28. Singh, K., Dwivedi, A. K., Samuel, C., & Dixit, S. (2024). Exploring the Prevalence and Risks of Wheat Adulteration in Gorakhpur City, Uttar Pradesh, India. *South Eastern European Journal of Public Health*, 1920–1927. https://doi.org/10.70135/seejph.vi.2750Faour-Klingbeil, D., & Todd, E. C. D. (2019). Prevention and control of foodborne diseases in Middle-East North African countries: Review of national control systems. *International Journal of Environmental Research and Public Health, 17*(1), Article 70. https://doi.org/10.3390/ijerph17010070.

29. Fitzgerald, M., Heinrich, M., & Booker, A. (2020). Medicinal plant analysis: A historical and regional discussion of emergent complex techniques. *Frontiers in Pharmacology, 10*, 1480. https://doi.org/10.3389/fphar.2019.01480.

30. Fox, M., Mitchell, M., Dean, M., Elliott, C. T., & Campbell, K. (2018). The seafood supply chain from a fraudulent perspective. *Food Security, 10*(4), 939–963. https://doi.org/10.1007/s12571-018-0826-z.

31. Guruswamy, S., Pojić, M., Subramanian, J. V., Mastilović, J., Sarang, S., Subbanagounder, A., Stojanović, G., et al. (2022). Toward better food security using concepts from Industry 5.0. *Sensors, 22*(21), 8377. https://doi.org/10.3390/s22218377.

32. Haleem, A., Khan, S., & Khan, M. I. (2019). Traceability implementation in food supply chain: A grey-DEMATEL approach. *Information Processing in Agriculture, 6*(3), 335–348. https://doi.org/10.1016/j.inpa.2019.01.003.

33. Hassoun, A., Måge, I., Schmidt, W., Temiz, H. T., Li, L., Kim, H. Y., Nilsen, H., et al. (2020). Fraud in animal origin food products: Advances in emerging spectroscopic detection methods over the past five years. *Foods, 9*(8), 1069. https://doi.org/10.3390/foods9081069.

34. Hendri, R., Jaswir, I., Mirghani, M. E. S., Salleh, M., et al. (2016). An overview of the current analytical methods for halal testing. https://core.ac.uk/download/300435937.pdf (accessed on 29 May 2025).

35. Hill, E., Howard, C., Kreuzer, M., Mali, S., et al. (2019). DNA authentication of St John's Wort (*Hypericum perforatum* L.) commercial products targeting the ITS region. https://core.ac.uk/download/287585220.pdf (accessed on 29 May 2025).

36. Hong, E., Lee, S. Y., Jeong, J. Y., Park, J. M., Kim, B. H., Kwon, K., & Chun, H. S. (2017). Modern analytical methods for the detection of food fraud and adulteration by food category. *Journal of the Science of Food and Agriculture, 97*(12), 3877–3896. https://doi.org/10.1002/jsfa.8364.

37. Horton, L. (1997). The United States Food and Drug Administration: Its role, authority, history, harmonization activities, and cooperation with the European Union. https://core.ac.uk/download/5079826.pdf (accessed on 29 May 2025).

38. Hossain, A., Skalický, M., Brestič, M., Mahari, S., Kerry, R. G., Maitra, S., Sarkar, S., et al. (2021). Application of nanomaterials to ensure quality and nutritional safety of food. *Journal of Nanomaterials, 2021*, 1–19. https://doi.org/10.1155/2021/9336082.

39. Hui, T., Mohammed, B. I., Donyai, P., McCrindle, R., & Sherratt, R. S. (2020). Enhancing pharmaceutical packaging through a technology ecosystem to facilitate the reuse of medicines and reduce medicinal waste. *Pharmacy, 8*(2), 58. https://doi.org/10.3390/pharmacy8020058.
40. Jaffee, S., Henson, S., Unnevehr, L. J., Grace, D., & Cassou, E. (2018). *The Safe Food Imperative: Accelerating Progress in Low- And Middle-Income Countries.* World Bank. https://doi.org/10.1596/978-1-4648-1345-0.
41. Johnston, L. D., Miech, R. A., & O'Malley, P. M. (2020). *Monitoring the Future National Survey Results on Drug Use, 1975–2019: Overview, Key Findings on Adolescent Drug Use.* https://doi.org/10.3998/2027.42/162579.
42. Jouanjean, M. A. (2019). *Digital Opportunities for Trade in The Agriculture and Food Sectors.* OECD Food, Agriculture and Fisheries Working Papers. https://doi.org/10.1787/91c40e07-en.
43. Kamalapreetha, B., Gopi, K. G., Gayathiri, R., et al. (2023). An overview on the impact of food fraud incidences in various countries and its detection methods, assessment techniques and preventive measures. https://core.ac.uk/download/588484397.pdf (accessed on 29 May 2025).
44. Karajovic, M., Kim, H., & Laskowski, M. (2019). Thinking outside the block: Projected phases of blockchain integration in the accounting industry. *Australian Accounting Review, 29*(2), 319–330. https://doi.org/10.1111/auar.12280.
45. Kendall, H., Kuznesof, S., Dean, M., Chan, M.-Y., Clark, B., Home, R., Stolz, H., et al. (2018). Chinese consumers' attitudes, perceptions and behavioral responses towards food fraud. *Food Control, 95*, 339–351. https://doi.org/10.1016/j.foodcont.2018.08.006.
46. Kerksick, C. M., Wilborn, C., Roberts, M. D., Smith-Ryan, A. E., Kleiner, S. M., Jäger, R., Collins, R., et al. (2018). ISSN exercise & sports nutrition review update: Research & recommendations. *Journal of the International Society of Sports Nutrition, 15*, Article 38. https://doi.org/10.1186/s12970-018-0242-y.
47. Khan, M. I., Shehzadi, R., & Tang, Y. Q. (2016). Composition and adulteration analysis of milk samples from ten different towns of Lahore. https://core.ac.uk/download/234684175.pdf (accessed on 29 May 2025).
48. Kirchhelle, C. (2018). Pharming animals: A global history of antibiotics in food production (1935–2017). *Palgrave Communications, 4*, Article 96. https://doi.org/10.1057/s41599-018-0152-2.
49. Klingel, T., Kremer, J. I., Gottstein, V., Rajcic de Rezende, T., Schwarz, S., & Lachenmeier, D. W. (2020). A review of coffee by-products including leaf, flower, cherry, husk, silver skin, and spent grounds as novel foods within the European Union. *Foods, 9*(5), 665. https://doi.org/10.3390/foods9050665.
50. Kotha, R. R., & Luthria, D. L. (2019). Curcumin: Biological, pharmaceutical, nutraceutical, and analytical aspects. *Molecules, 24*(16), 2930. https://doi.org/10.3390/molecules24162930.
51. Kushlick, D., Murkin, G., Powell, M., Rolles, S., et al. (2016). *Alternative World Drug Report.* https://core.ac.uk/download/34724856.pdf (accessed on 29 May 2025).
52. Leon, C. (2017). *The Botany and Macroscopy of Chinese Materia Medica: Sources, Substitutes and Sustainability.* https://core.ac.uk/download/161105681.pdf (accessed on 29 May 2025).
53. Liu, Z., Mutukumira, A. N., & Chen, H. (2019). Food safety governance in China: From supervision to coregulation. *Food Science & Nutrition, 7*(12), 4127–4139. https://doi.org/10.1002/fsn3.1281.

54. Manning, L., & Soon, J. M. (2016). Food safety, food fraud, and food defense: A fast-evolving literature. *Journal of Food Science, 81*(4), R823–R834. https://doi.org/10.1111/1750-3841.13256.

55. Manning, Louise & Soon, Jan Mei, 2014. "**Developing systems to control food adulteration**," Food Policy, Elsevier, vol. 49(P1), pages 23-32.(accessed on 29 May 2025).

56. Motherway, M. O., O'Connor, L., Smith, S., Bolton, D., Cormican, M., De Waal, T., Gutierrez, M., et al. (2024). Assessment of the safety of "probiotics" in food supplements. *Food Risk Assess Europe.* https://www.semanticscholar.org/paper/2eeef58d0c41e4631747a3d5f2574fb259a210b9 (accessed on 29 May 2025).

57. Murphy, L. C. (2016). *The Food Industry's Perception of Economically Motivated Adulteration and Related Risk Factors.* https://core.ac.uk/download/268805566.pdf (accessed on 29 May 2025).

58. Novoveská, L., Ross, M., Stanley, M. S., Pradelles, R., Wasiolek, V., & Sassi, J. F. (2019). Microalgal carotenoids: A review of production, current markets, regulations, and future direction. *Marine Drugs, 17*(11), 640. https://doi.org/10.3390/md17110640.

59. Pardo, B., Taylor, J., Caulkins, J. P., Kilmer, B., Reuter, P., & Stein, B. D. (2019). *The Future of Fentanyl and Other Synthetic Opioids.* RAND Corporation. https://doi.org/10.7249/rr3117.

60. Pareeda, A., Nair, V. D., & Saini, K. C. (2024). DNA barcoding: An effective molecular tool for species identification, molecular authentication and phylogeny studies in plant science research. https://core.ac.uk/download/622344256.pdf (accessed on 29 May 2025).

61. Peiper, N. C., Clarke, S., Vincent, L., Ciccarone, D., Kral, A. H., & Zibbell, J. E. (2018). Fentanyl test strips as an opioid overdose prevention strategy: Findings from a syringe services program in the Southeastern United States. *International Journal of Drug Policy, 63*, 122–128. https://doi.org/10.1016/j.drugpo.2018.08.007.

62. Putri, S. A. (2022). *Regulation of Food Safety by the National Agency for Drug and Food Control (NADFC) in Indonesia: A Quest for Effectiveness.* https://core.ac.uk/download/611832272.pdf (accessed on 29 May 2025).

63. Rahimi, F., Chatzimichail, S., Saifuddin, A., Surman, A. J., Taylor-Robinson, S. D., & Salehi-Reyhani, A. (2020). A review of portable high-performance liquid chromatography: The future of the field? *Chromatographic, 83*(10), 1165–1195. https://doi.org/10.1007/s10337-020-03944-6.

64. Rejeb, A., Keogh, J. G., Zailani, S., Treiblmaier, H., & Rejeb, K. (2020). Blockchain technology in the food industry: A review of potentials, challenges and future research directions. *Logistics, 4*(4), 27. https://doi.org/10.3390/logistics4040027.

65. Rejeb, A., Rejeb, K., Zailani, S., & Kayıkçı, Y. (2022). Knowledge diffusion of halal food research: A main path analysis. *Journal of Islamic Marketing, 14*(9), 1715–1743. https://doi.org/10.1108/jima-07-2021-0229.

66. Sacco, S., Merki-Feld, G., Ægidius, K., Bitzer, J., Canonico, M., Kurth, T., Lampl, C., et al. (2017). Hormonal contraceptives and risk of ischemic stroke in women with migraine: A consensus statement from the European Headache Federation (EHF) and the European Society of Contraception and Reproductive Health (ESC). *The Journal of Headache and Pain, 18*, Article 108. https://www.semanticscholar.org/paper/f73dac713e67aed38ed2239e2ff588062de2508d (accessed on 29 May 2025).

67. Sahoo, S., & Chatterjee, A. (2009). Consumer protection–Problems and prospects. *Political Economy: Structure & Scope of Government eJournal.* https://www.semanticscholar.org/paper/ba1b1436bdc4276179bb70ebcee6dae2ddc290b7 (accessed on 29 May 2025).

68. Salem, M. A., Perez de Souza, L., Serag, A., Fernie, A. R., Farag, M. A., Ezzat, S. M., & Alseekh, S. (2020). Metabolomics in the context of plant natural products research: From sample preparation to metabolite analysis. *Metabolites, 10*(1), 37. https://doi.org/10.3390/metabo10010037.

69. Shafiq, M., Anjum, S., Hano, C., Anjum, I., & Abbasi, B. H. (2020). An overview of the applications of nanomaterials and nanodevices in the food industry. *Foods, 9*(2), 148. https://doi.org/10.3390/foods9020148.

70. Sharma, N. V. (2024). *A Review on Various Sensors Employed for Detecting Adulterants (Urea and Melamine) In Milk and Milk Products.* https://core.ac.uk/download/613698492.pdf (accessed on 29 May 2025).

71. Valand, R., Tanna, S., Lawson, G., & Bengtström, L. (2019). A review of Fourier Transform Infrared (FTIR) spectroscopy used in food adulteration and authenticity investigations. *Food Additives & Contaminants: Part A, 37*(1), 19–38. https://doi.org/10.1080/19440049.2019.1675909.

72. Wang, H., Chen, Y., Wang, L., Liu, Q., Yang, S., & Wang, C. Q. (2023). Advancing herbal medicine: Enhancing product quality and safety through robust quality control practices. *Frontiers in Pharmacology, 14*, Article 1265178. https://doi.org/10.3389/fphar.2023.1265178.

73. White, C. M. (2019). A review of human studies assessing cannabidiol's (CBD) therapeutic actions and potential. *The Journal of Clinical Pharmacology, 59*(7), 923–934. https://doi.org/10.1002/jcph.1387.

74. Widad, E., El Bakkali, M., Amenzou, N., Touhami, M., Fouad, T., & Amar, H. (2025). Detection of adulteration in Moroccan and Egyptian sesame oil using isotopic analysis and infrared spectroscopy. *Journal of Applied and Natural Science.* https://www.semanticscholar.org/paper/d549a462fa2b08f7e5a0fc7790caad0bb043cba3 (accessed on 29 May 2025).

75. Williams, D. R. (2018). Stress and the mental health of populations of color: Advancing our understanding of race-related stressors. *Journal of Health and Social Behavior, 59*(4), 466–485. https://doi.org/10.1177/0022146518814251.

76. Yadav, A., Singh, P. K., Yadav, N., Kaushik, R., Kumar, C., Chandra, A., Singh, S., et al. (2020). Smokeless tobacco control in India: Policy review and lessons for high-burden countries. *BMJ Global Health, 5*(2), e002367. https://doi.org/10.1136/bmjgh-2020-002367.

77. Zhao, J., Yang, W., Cai, H., Cao, G., & Li, Z. (2025). Current progress and future trends of genomics-based techniques for food adulteration identification. *Foods, 14.* https://www.semanticscholar.org/paper/0cab54e85c3c4c15530520b4949aefc770000539 (accessed on 29 May 2025).

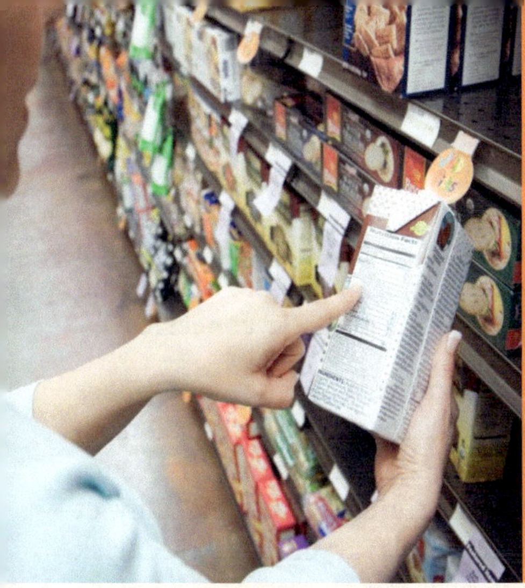

Chapter 8

CONSUMER AWARENESS AND FOOD LABELING

Contents

Introduction 181
8.1. The Importance of Food Labeling 185
8.2. Regulations Governing Food Labeling 189
8.3. Consumer Behavior and Food Labeling 193
8.4. Challenges in Food Labeling 197
Summary 203
References 204

Introduction

With the economy nowadays globalized, food labeling has become more significant, shaping consumer choice and promoting quality awareness of food. With more discerning consumers calling for more transparency in the makeup of what they eat, quality marking remains an effective tool for education-driven consumer choice. Current debates highlight that labeling is an important driver of consumer behavior, necessitating the need for transparency and honesty in labeling in marketing (Armbruster and Henneberry, 2025). Furthermore, geographical origin labels have also gained significance as indicators of quality, with consumers showing greater willingness to pay for products carrying a specific origin, for instance, geographical indications (GI) and protected designation of origin (PDO) labeling (Colson et al., 2025). The trend in consumer preference necessitates the need for food labeling in bringing consumers together with the quality and authenticity of the chosen product, leading to greater awareness of food consumption.

Definition of Consumer Awareness

Consumer awareness is an integral part of an informed society, particularly in food labeling. It refers to the awareness and knowledge of consumers about the implications of their shopping behavior, e.g., nutritional content, sustainability, and ethical considerations of food products. The more informed consumers are about their shopping behavior, the more accountable producers become, and the lower the food wastage in society. For instance, the United States of America alone wastes approximately $218 billion worth of food annually, an appeal for greater consumer awareness and conscious consumption habits. Programs in vogue to inform consumers through open and educational food labeling can enable consumers to make decisions that not only benefit their health but also facilitate environmental sustainability, thus developing a multilateral market for food recovery and reduction schemes (Figure 8.1).

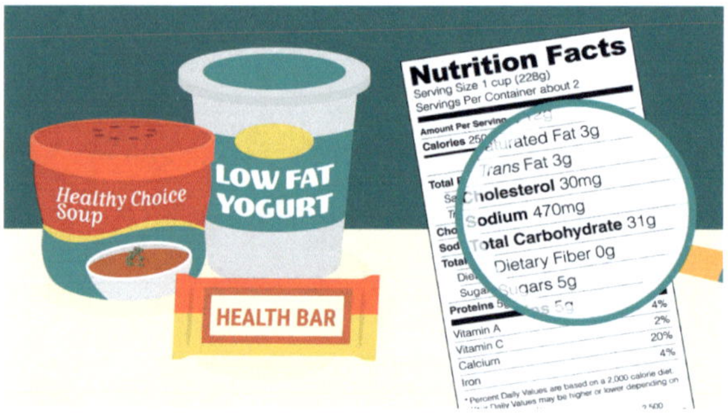

Figure 8.1. Consumer awareness is a critical component of an informed society, particularly in the context of food labeling.

Source: https://foodsafetyworks.com/wp-content/uploads/2023/02/CleanLabel.png.

Importance of Food Labeling

Food labeling is a significant method of promoting consumer education to allow for the making of educated choices about their diet. Descriptive and clear labeling not only gives significant information about nutrients but also allows consumers to identify potential allergens and additives that may affect health outcomes. Most significantly, the distinction between genetically modified (GM) food and organic food has been a point of concern.

Research has indicated that consumers prefer locally sourced foods that are free from artificial additives, reflecting a general preference for natural foods in the diet (Govindasamy et al., 2025). In addition, fear of perceived risk originating from agro-biotechnology, such as long-term health effects and environmental hazards, affects consumers' purchasing behavior, opting for organic foods over GM foods (Rimal et al., 2006). Effective food labeling not only enhances transparency but also allows consumers to make health- and value-driven purchases.

Overview of Food Labeling Regulations

The regulatory landscape of food labeling in the United States has evolved tremendously since the enactment of the Nutrition Labeling and Education Act (NLEA) in 1990, which established uniform nutritional standards to advance consumer awareness. The law mandates proper disclosures on the label to inform the consumer of proper information regarding the nutritional content of food products. The labels' effectiveness has also been found to be a function of consumer information processing and hence includes message form and context variables in interpreting NFP (Andrews et al., 2017). In addition, the complex nature of food waste and its economic consequences require effective labeling practices that increase transparency and reduce food discarding. Through the interaction of logical labeling practices and human cognition, policymakers can ensure consumer empowerment, navigation proficiency, and ultimately influence healthier lifestyle choices in a more complex food environment (Figure 8.2).

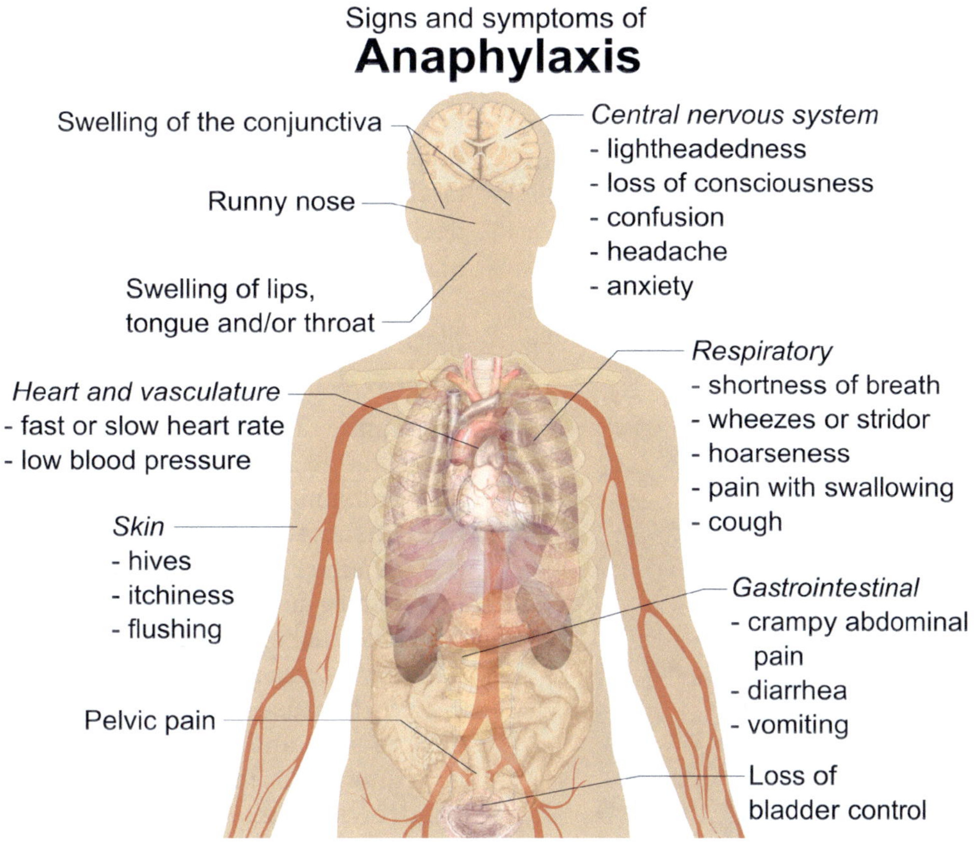

Figure 8.2. Nutritional Labeling Education Act (NLEA).

Source: By Trounce - self-made based on Image:Nutritionfacts.png and typographic specfifications outlined here, Public Domain, https://commons.wikimedia.org/w/index.php?curid=3871981

Role of Consumers in the Food Market

Consumers are more empowered in today's food market via their shopping behavior, which is most visibly driven by food label awareness and knowledge. Past research has shown that consumer attitudes and opinions toward food labels are key drivers of shopping behavior, with a complex interplay between market forces and consumer awareness (Jadi et al., 2022). Furthermore, this awareness is non-preference-based; it is an influential driver of conformity toward healthier diets, such as the Mediterranean diet. One study provided evidence that consumers with food access issues for foods characteristic of this diet have lower levels of conformity, which suggests that economic factors and food security are closely tied to consumer behavior. Promoting greater awareness of food labels by consumers, therefore, not only empowers consumers to make better choices but can redirect market trends toward the consumption of healthier, sustainable foods.

Significance of Informed Choices

Informed decision-making plays an important role in affecting consumer behavior and preference regarding food labeling, with an emphasis on the pivotal role of awareness in affecting sustainable consumption patterns. Given that consumers are confronted with a very complex marketplace, the ability to read food labels is important in affecting informed decision-making associated with health issues and self-values.

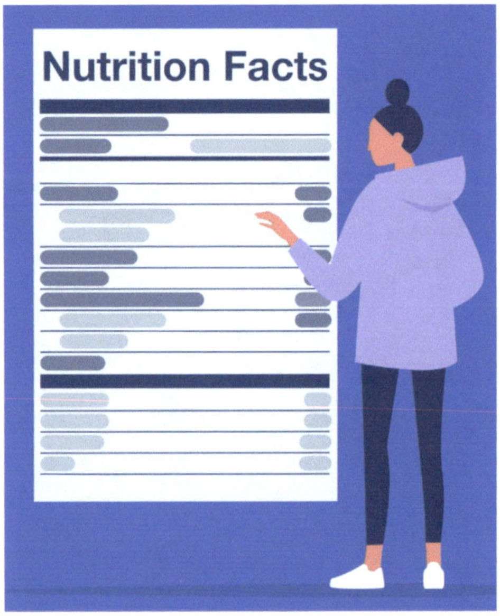

Figure 8.3. Informed choices significantly impact consumer behavior and preferences in the context of food labeling, highlighting the essential role of awareness in promoting sustainable consumption practices.

Source: https://cdn.prod.website-files.com/63050ce148a3f9607b3c5464/65f46f072a16a177382e5ad6_iStock-1213797475.webp.

Empirical evidence shows that demographic factors contribute to decision-making; women and higher-income households, for instance, are found to have a greater probability of using eco-labels due to the health and environmental impacts of food production systems (Armah, 2025). An example of another study on the risk attitude of GM foods illustrates polarized views of consumers, citing that while most perceive minimal risk, a significant minority strongly protest GM ingredients (Veeman et al., 2025). Enhancing consumer awareness of food labeling is therefore significant in shaping informed decision-making and, by implication, shaping market trends (Figure 8.3).

Impact of Consumer Awareness on Health

Consumer awareness is a major factor in determining health, particularly how it affects food consumption and food choice. The greater the consumer's awareness of nutrient content and its effect on food choice, the healthier the food choice and the improved public health. The Nutrition Labeling Education Act (NLEA) has had a great impact on consumers' food labeling reading because it made nutritional information easy to read and understand, thereby enabling consumers to make informed food choices (Andrews et al., 2017). More knowledge is needed because the staggering $218 billion yearly wastage of food is a testament to the need for more responsible consumption patterns in the United States. Encouraging consumer knowledge thus not only results in individual health but also solves more social problems , such as food wastage, attesting to the interdependence of informed consumerism and public health matters.

Connection Between Labeling and Consumer Rights

As consumer awareness matures under the canopy of food labeling, the interdependence between proper labeling and consumer rights assumes greater significance. Food labels are not only nutritional value signifiers but also tools for encouraging transparency in food production and food safety processes. Informed choice is protected by law through mandates for transparent labeling, thus enabling consumers to make choices that satisfy their health and ethical requirements. This empowerment is essential in the context of a digital era where advertising campaigns have a propensity to suffocate the truth, backed by evidence that suggests consumer behavior is heavily determined by labeling practices and online product debates (Dwivedi et al., 2020). Further, the potential for misinformation makes ongoing and honest labeling a necessity, which goes towards eliminating trust issues that may emerge in the market (Dwivedi et al., 2022). The protection of consumer rights through proper food labeling is hence essential in the development of a responsible and respectful market (Figure 8.4).

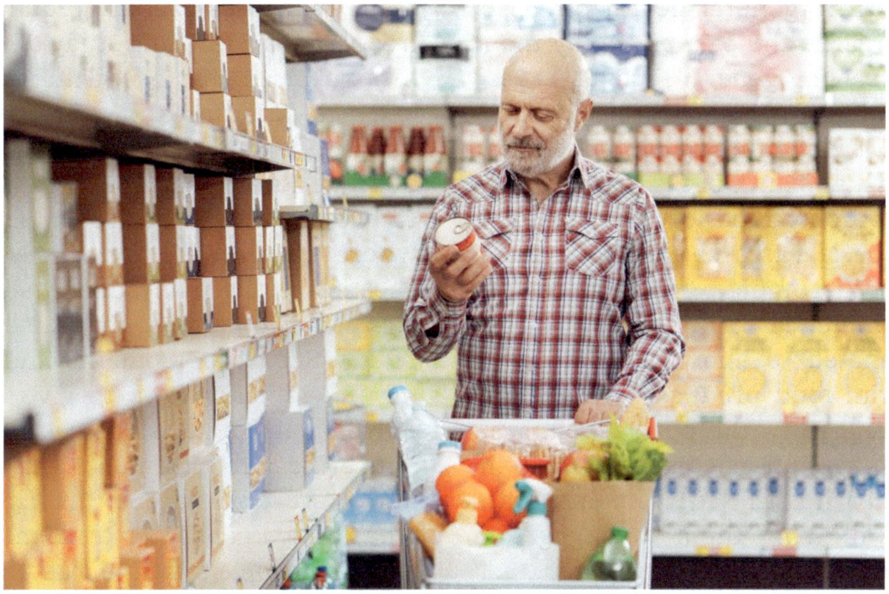

Figure 8.4. Food labels serve not only as guides for nutritional value but also as instruments for promoting transparency in food production and safety standards.

Source: https://cdn.cpdonline.co.uk/wp-content/uploads/2024/10/21135913/The-Role-of-Food-Labels-in-Promoting-Health-and-Safety.jpg.

8.1. The Importance of Food Labeling

Food labeling is critical to facilitate consumer education through the provision of important information regarding the nutritional content, ingredients, and allergens of food products. As consumers attempt to make informed food choices, proper labeling allows them to understand the health implications of their food intake, which can lead to healthful options. The connection between food consumption and personal health is particularly relevant, as evidenced by growing per capita meat consumption and health implications; proper labeling can inspire consumers towards healthier options and moderation of consumption patterns (Godfray et al., 2018). Proper labeling also allows for not only personal health but also environmental factors, as informed consumers can make decisions that support sustainable practices (Mach et al., 2019). Food labeling is thus part and parcel of making an educated population, which consequently results in personal well-being and community health levels.

8.1.1. Nutritional Information and Its Relevance

Nutritional awareness is necessary for the consumer to make an informed food choice, particularly in a time when food labeling regulations are so varied. Appropriate nutritional information not only allows individuals to take charge of their general health but also allows them to realize the part played by their food choices in solving general societal issues, including animal welfare and environmental sustainability. As highlighted by recent studies, increasing consumer sentiment is that welfare-friendly food is not only superior and better but also healthier (de la Varga et al., 2020). Such awareness is also promoted by the potential revolutionary influence of digital interfaces, which are estimated to allow consumers to engage more with food products (Dwivedi et al., 2022). Consequently, the open labeling of nutritional information becomes critical in uniting consumer health requirements with ethical issues, allowing them to engage in the food system responsibly and informed. Therefore, consumer awareness of nutritional information is necessary to allow a more ethical food environment (Figure 8.5).

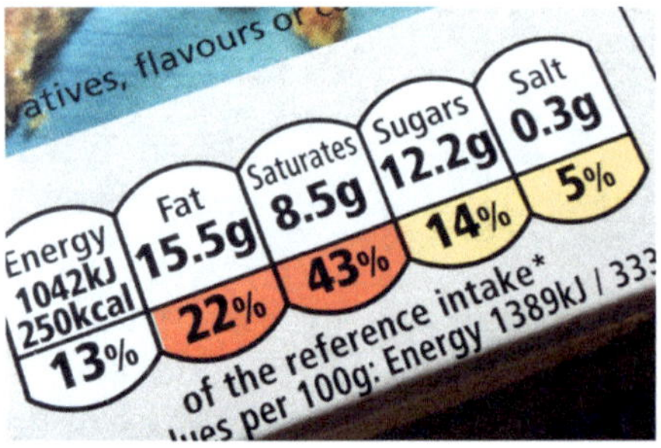

Figure 8.5. Understanding nutritional information is crucial for consumers aiming to make informed dietary choices, particularly in an age where food labeling regulations vary significantly.

Source: https://cdn.shopify.com/s/files/1/0655/6414/7950/files/untitled-design-14-2.jpg?v=1718191243.

8.1.2. Ingredient Lists and Transparency

The demand for ingredient lists transparency is a reaction to a rising consumer need for informed decision-making regarding food products. As health concerns increase, one must know what the ingredients are composed of, particularly for those with specific dietary requirements. Gluten-free pasta is a learning study on how ingredient lists can be applied to food literacy since it shows extreme differences in terms of nutrients and quality between brands and types (Boukid et al., 2025). These can be observed in other product categories, as well, such as menstrual products, where ingredient disclosures only recently became required in some states, reflecting a lack of consumer knowledge and safety (Spitzer, 2024). Such developments illustrate the need for full labeling laws to give consumers the power to make decisions based on their health and ethical requirements. At the end of the day, more transparency in ingredient lists is what builds consumer trust in manufacturers, allowing people to be the masters of their health and nutrition.

8.1.3. Allergen Information and Safety

The increased prevalence of food allergies necessitates strict allergen labeling for consumer protection and education. Precautionary allergen labeling has been critical in minimizing risks for food-allergic consumers, facilitating informed food selection in the diet. Although the advent of precautionary allergen labeling, intended to minimize the level of trace allergens, has been intended to minimize exposure to these allergens, it has created confusion for consumers due to the myriad of labels with varying implications (Allen et al., 2014). The inconsistency reflects the need for standardized regulations globally, given the intricacy of global food production and supply. Moreover, as new diet trends, such as gluten-free diets, become trendy, consumers require detailed information beyond simple allergen disclaimers in order to appreciate health impacts and safety in depth (McCabe et al., 2010). An effective labeling system must therefore strike a delicate balance between consumer protection and effective communication to attain ultimate overall food safety (Figure 8.6).

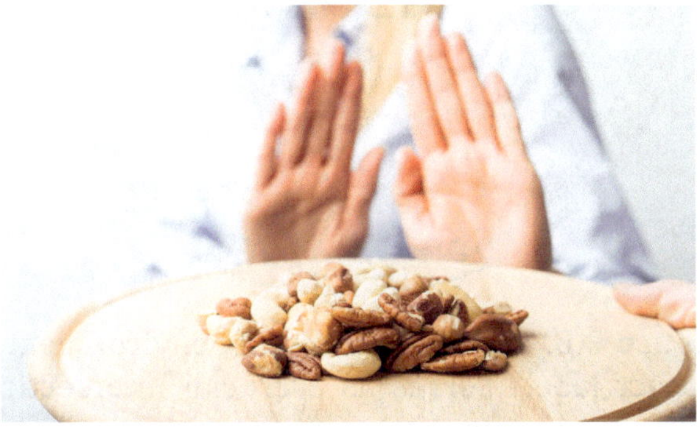

Figure 8.6. The increasing prevalence of food allergies necessitates robust allergen labeling to ensure consumer safety and awareness.

Source: https://5845715.fs1.hubspotusercontent-na1.net/hub/5845715/hubfs/allergen%20control.jpg.

8.1.4. Claims and Certifications (e.g., Organic, Non-GMO)

The prevalence of claims and certifications , such as organic and non-GMO, on food products is a significant driver of consumer knowledge and purchasing behavior. Such claims are a sign of farm practices that resonate with the increasing number of health- and environmentally conscious consumers. Studies show that more than half of consumers consider producers' certification while determining the quality of the product, and health benefits play a significant role in the choice of organic products (Melovi et al., 2020). Prior to organic production benefits in cost of production and market price, but there are obstacles in consumer attitude and product availability (Durham et al., 2021). Moreover, the success of such labels relies on customers' capacity to obtain credible information on the certification process, which can aid their confidence in the health benefits offered by such products. Therefore, with consumers calling for healthy food, the role of proper labeling is all the more necessary.

8.1.5. Serving Sizes and Portion Control

The issue of portion control and serving size is of utmost importance in making consumers aware and improving diet choices. Optimal nutrition labeling facilitates this awareness since it allows consumers to estimate appropriate portions in the context of their overall diet needs.

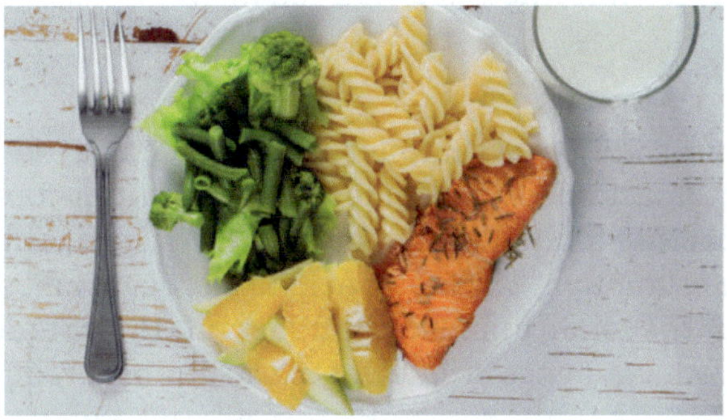

Figure 8.7. The issue of serving sizes and portion control is critical in fostering consumer awareness and improving dietary choices.

Source: https://thegoodbug.com/cdn/shop/articles/Picture1_e181ff1e-9954-4dac-80b4-2668231c2210.png?v=1723704654.

8.1.6. Date Labeling (e.g., Sell By, Use By)

Date labeling, including the utilization of terms like sell by and use by, is of utmost significance in food safety and consumer education, but causes confusion among consumers. Most consumers misinterpret the labels, believing they denote absolute food safety as opposed to optimal freshness. This misunderstanding makes a major contribution to wastage as products past their labeled dates are substantially discarded even when still fit for human consumption. Literature shows that varying labeling practices across the food sector are a reason for this trend, causing confusion among consumers about the quality and safety of food choices (Dwivedi et al., 2022).

Applying new technologies, for instance, employing artificial intelligence, would improve customer experience in comprehending such labels by providing more accurate representations of food freshness and safety, hence reducing wastage and satisfaction in general (Puntoni et al., 2020). In this context, we are reminded that labeling transparency and consumer education are required to help enable informed decision-making.

8.1.7. Environmental Impact Labels

Environmental impact labeling is a key intersection of consumer education and food labeling policy, thus facilitating sustainable consumption. The labels help to alert consumers to the environmental impact of their food products, hence facilitating market transparency. Even though consumers are still worried about the sustainability of their diet, there is increasing demand for such labels, primarily carbon footprints and other environmental metrics.

Nevertheless, when demand for the labels is increasing, the real effect of such labels on consumer behavior is uncertain, where strong drivers , such as price and habit, override sustainability concerns (Mehta et al., 2020). Second, while manufacturers seek to offer better guidance in labeling, there are concerns about establishing trust and transparency in the system (Mehta et al., 2020). Generally, the success of environmental impact labeling relies on how well they are able to offer useful information in the midst of consumer behavior and competition in the market (Figure 8.8).

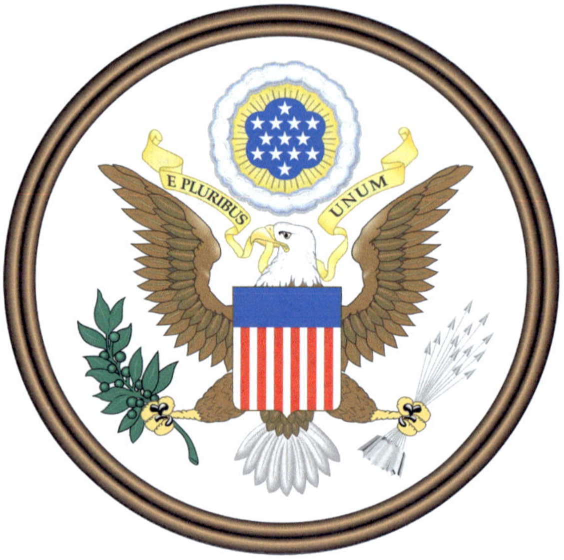

Figure 8.8. The phenomenon of environmental impact labels serves as a crucial intersection between consumer awareness and food labeling practices, thereby promoting sustainable consumption.

Source: By U.S. Government - Extracted from PDF version of Our Flag, available here (direct PDF URL here.), Public Domain, https://commons.wikimedia.org/w/index.php?curid=41373752

8.1.8. Ethical Considerations in Food Labeling

Ethical food labeling is a core point of concern in food culture today, affecting consumer awareness and brand reputation. Ethical labeling not only ensures transparency but also strengthens consumer-producer trust. Labels emphasizing sustainable production, animal welfare, and fair trade push consumers towards value-driven choices. With increasingly growing demand for ethically produced food, particularly from sophisticated consumer segments, food manufacturers are increasingly compelled to adopt thorough labeling standards consistent with such ethical labels. For instance, approaches like biofortification, as discussed in (Consultation Working Groups et al., 2017), focus on the convergence of nutrition and ethics, where food security is quantified in terms of open-label measurement. Once again, research in various markets, including South Africa, demonstrates how consumer assessments of food quality encompass both conventional and sophisticated ethical traits, which attests to the central significance of ethical labeling in food consumption (Biénabe et al., 2010).

8.1.9. Consumer Trust and Brand Loyalty

Today's marketplace, consumer trust, and brand loyalty have emerged as key drivers fueling purchasing behavior, especially for food items. As consumers increasingly understand the complexity of food labeling and its implications on health and sustainability, the trust that consumers place in a brand is often determined by the clarity of such labels.

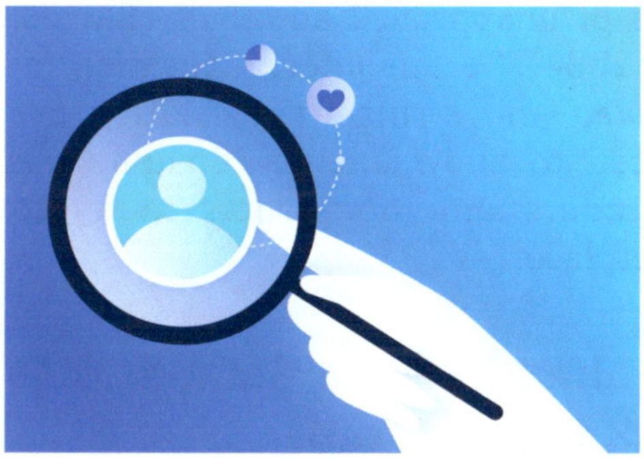

Figure 8.9. In the contemporary marketplace, consumer trust and brand loyalty have emerged as critical components influencing purchasing behaviors, particularly concerning food products.

Source: https://www.similarweb.com/blog/wp-content/uploads/2024/08/Consumer-Behaviour_-Types-Examples-Analysis.png.

Brands that can articulate what they represent and drive home the quality aspect tend to be better emotionally connected with consumers, thus leading to loyalty and repeat purchase behavior. This is also supported by studies that reveal that what consumers evaluate as value, e.g., emotional bonding with a brand, plays an important role in determining what they plan to purchase and overall brand trust. Transparency and ethical labeling in food thus not only create consumer trust but also play a core role in building long-term brand loyalty in today's marketplace, where what consumers are most concerned with is sustainability and health (Nekmahmud et al., 2020) (Figure 8.9).

8.2. Regulations Governing Food Labeling

The regulatory environment of food labeling has significantly altered since the enactment of the Nutrition Labeling and Education Act (NLEA) in 1990, which was a milestone in the display of nutritional facts to consumers. Recent research shows that transparent communication through the use of nutrition facts panels (NFPs) and front-of-pack (FOP) labels will have a direct influence on consumer behavior and health impacts for food choice and obesity prevention. Recent evidence shows that further consideration is needed to consider the effects of various labeling formats, including non-FDA-regulated formats, on consumer information and choice (Andrews et al., 2017).

Industry incentives, particularly to employ FOP labels, are also most frequently stimulated by competitive pressures and anticipated regulatory activity, which suggests that the dynamic relationship between consumer demands and industry responses is complex (Caldeira et al., 2025). These are the findings that are most relevant to policymakers attempting to increase consumer awareness and encourage healthier food choices, ultimately guiding public health action.

8.2.1. Overview of the FDA and Its Role

The Food and Drug Administration (FDA) takes the lead in food safety regulation, offering consumers products up to standards of high health and safety. Through regulation, the FDA keeps food labeling accurate and informative, enhancing consumer education and good judgment. This is particularly crucial in an era when innovations, , such as those developed through advancements in nanotechnology, are transforming food products and agricultural practices. As noted, nanotechnology offers limitless means of improving food quality and security, but needs tight regulation to correct possible hazards from novel nanomaterials (He et al., 2018). Additionally, while the FDA dictates guidelines on labeling and public health programs, it is equally essential that health experts exercise prudence and consider patient-specific requirements when offering advice on food choices, strengthening the argument in favor of consumer information needing to be supplemented with regulation (Mach et al., 2019) (Figure 8.10).

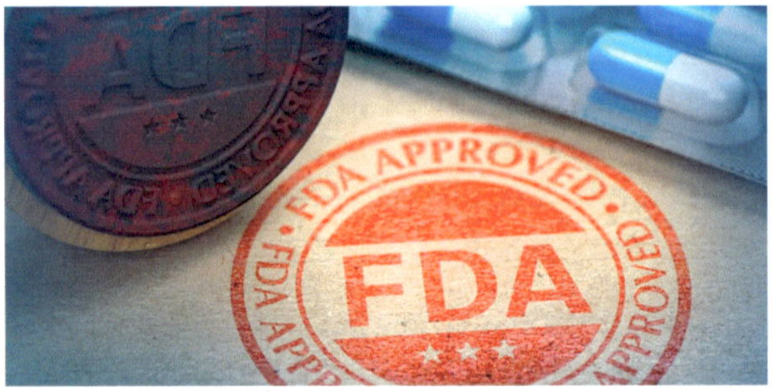

Figure 8.10. The Food and Drug Administration (FDA) plays a pivotal role in regulating food safety, ensuring that consumers have access to products that meet strict health and safety standards.

Source: https://www.digicomply.com/hubfs/what%20makes%20enforcing%20safety%20standards%20a%20challenge%20for%20the%20food%20and%20drug%20administration.webp.

8.2.2. Key Regulations (e.g., Nutrition Labeling and Education Act)

The efficacy of food labeling acts, for instance, the Nutrition Labeling and Education Act (NLEA), is crucial in encouraging consumer knowledge and awareness of nutritional information. Food has to be labeled clearly due to this act, allowing one to make healthy food choices regarding what to consume. But research shows that even though the majority of participants are knowledgeable about food labels, technical jargon and false labeling mislead people, as evident with recent research highlighting that consumers cannot utilize nutritional information (Uzoma et al., 2025). Similarly, the situation of artificial food colorants (AFCs) is also the same; even when regulated, the majority of consumers still lack knowledge of the International Numbering System for Food Additives and the health effects of unapproved additives (Rameshbabu et al., 2024). To this effect, education must be improved and stringent legislation must be enforced to allow one to consume healthily and understand food labels in a crowded marketplace.

8.2.3. International Standards (e.g., Codex Alimentarius)

Development of international standards, , such as the Codex Alimentarius, is essential in promoting consumer awareness and shaping global food labeling policies. Such standards, under the common auspices of the Food and Agriculture Organization (FAO) and the World Health Organization (WHO), offer guidelines that guarantee food safety, promote fair trade, and safeguard public health. To this end, the Codex prioritizes open labeling, e.g., declaring ingredients, nutritional content, and allergens, which help empower consumers to make informed choices about their foods (Huang, 2024). However, processes toward such standards reflect inherent tensions, particularly between trade facilitation and the promotion of public health. Notably, involvement in the development of such guidelines leans toward industry interests rather than consumer health interests, and hence, public health interests need more representation to ensure that labeling measures truly enhance consumer empowerment and protection (Boatwright et al., 2024) (Figure 8.11).

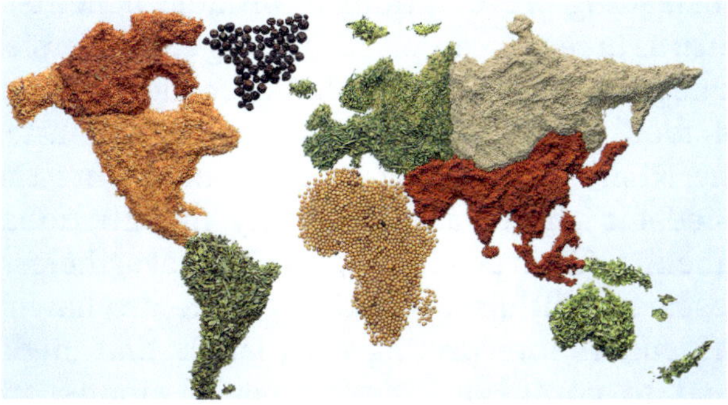

Figure 8.11. The establishment of international standards, , such as those set by the Codex Alimentarius, plays a pivotal role in enhancing consumer awareness and guiding food labeling practices globally.

Source: https://images.squarespace-cdn.com/content/v1/5e0e1d15dcd662506441ff4b/089e96f9-e309-480d-8ebd-8f1112dd2da7/0423_SPI_Codex+Blog+Image_1200x667.jpeg.

8.2.4. State vs. Federal Regulations

The federal-state divide between consumer education and food labeling is essential to providing transparency and protecting public health. Federal statute, as enacted by the FDA, provides a uniform code attempting to facilitate interstate commerce while protecting consumers from deceptive assertions. State statute, however, generally emerges from local consumer pressures and environmental concerns, thus creating a mosaic of statutes complementing or contradicting federal codes. The evolution of deceptive environmental advertising, as uncovered through current public debate surrounding eco-labeling schemes, demonstrates the necessity for more stringent federal regulation to promote consumer confidence and counteract confusion generated by contradictory state statutes (Fliegelman et al., 2011). Furthermore, the intersection between agricultural policy and consumer rights only further complicates the matrix, necessitating coordinated measures weighing federal uniformity against state sensitivity (Phillips, 2025).

8.2.5. Enforcement and Compliance Issues

Effective enforcement and compliance measures are crucial in ensuring that food labeling achieves its role of protecting consumer rights and public health. Regulators like the FDA have moved towards punitive measures against non-compliance, but the shift has been accompanied by limited success.

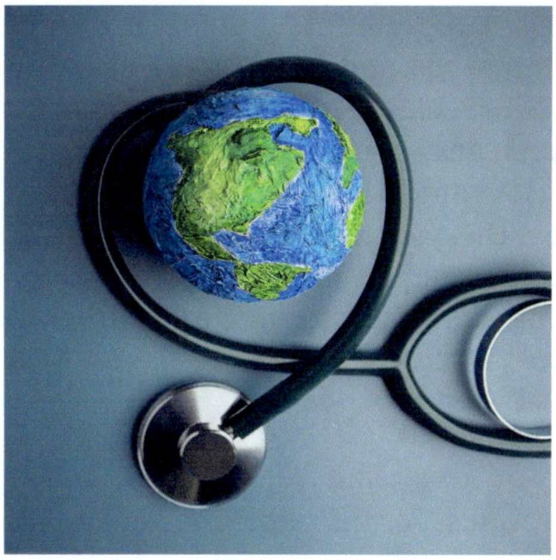

Figure 8.12. Regulatory agencies like the Food and Drug Administration (FDA) have increasingly adopted punitive measures against non-compliance, but this shift has had mixed results.

Source: https://www.ppd.com/wp-content/uploads/2023/12/regulatory-compliance-in-healthcare_ss1936522507-min.jpg.

For instance, while fines and pursuing individual liability for managers under the Park doctrine aim to deter illegal behavior, such actions have been accompanied by limited success in meeting compliance (Girard, 2012). Similarly, the prevalence of misleading environmental statements in product advertising shows the necessity of stricter regulations in protecting consumers from deception while ensuring true transparency (Fliegelman et al., 2011). Therefore, the challenge is in finding the correct balance between punitive and correctional measures that ensure compliance while sensitizing consumers, hence building an informed public that can effectively monitor and shape corporate behavior (Figure 8.12).

8.2.6. Labeling for Dietary Supplements

In consumer information, dietary supplement labeling has become a chief pillar in informing consumers about the products in question. Dietary supplements, including vitamins, minerals, herbs, and amino acids, may often lack stringent regulatory control for pharmaceutical products and hence become a necessity for proper labeling to inform consumers and provide choice. FOP systems of nutritional labeling seek to simplify complex nutrition information, hence enabling consumers to make healthier choices on time (Andrews et al., 2014).

Transparency is also a need in the diverse dietary needs arising from religious and cultural backgrounds. For instance, consumers adopting some dietary restrictions should be facilitated in the identification of inappropriate ingredients simply; thus, labeling becomes a chief aspect in ensuring adherence to medical needs as well as flavor (Hashmi, 2012). Improved labeling practices are hence needed to ensure an informed consumer base with improved public health.

8.2.7. Misleading Labels and Consumer Protection

Misleading labeling poses a significant threat to consumer protection, mainly because advertising increasingly includes environmental and nutritional content. Recurring instances of misleading environmental labeling, for instance, brought about calls for stronger regulatory mechanisms to safeguard consumers against misleading presentations of product benefits, , such as in recent carbon advertising controversies (Fliegelman et al., 2011). Moreover, the evolution of food labeling standards, particularly after the NLEA became law in 1990, highlights the need for clarity and simplicity in nutritional labeling (Andrews et al., 2017). Nevertheless, research still discovers that people are having difficulties interpreting such labels that might lead to confusion as to what the foods are composed of and how they might affect health. Thus, regulatory agencies must adapt to the complexity of labeling practices to better serve informed consumers and, in turn, better public health outcomes (Figure 8.13).

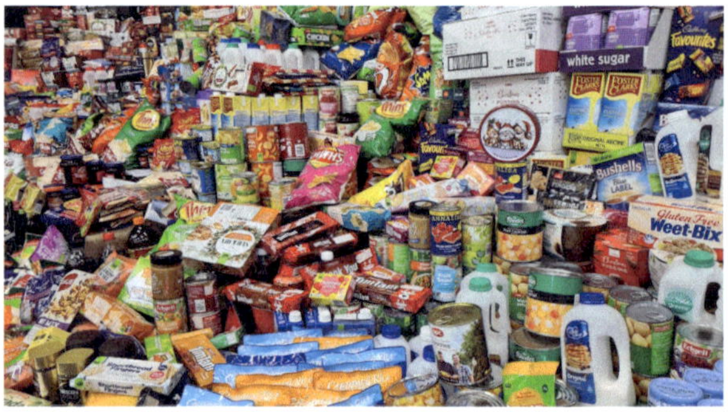

Figure 8.13. Misleading labels pose a significant challenge to consumer protection, particularly in an era where environmental claims and nutritional information are increasingly prominent in marketing strategies.

Source: https://www.deskera.com/blog/content/images/2023/03/nico-smit-MrQs5dCGyno-unsplash.jpg.

8.2.8. Recent Changes in Labeling Laws

Paradigm changes in food labeling legislation over the last ten years have led the way in meeting increased consumer demands for transparency and accountability in the food industry. The changes have been driven by increased public health consciousness, environmental awareness, and ethical consumption. For instance, new laws now require more open disclosure of genetically modified organisms (GMOs) and agrochemical applications, thereby enabling consumers to make informed food choices. As observed, agrochemicals have doubled food production within a century, but their impact on food quantity and safety has led to the shift towards better labeling practices (Carvalho, 2017). Additionally, with increased trends towards the consumption of meat worldwide, the health and environmental effects of livestock production are being questioned and policymakers are left struggling with more informative labeling legislation to address such issues (Godfray et al., 2018). The changes are a landmark towards increased consumer awareness and better food labeling laws.

8.2.9. Future Trends in Food Labeling Regulations

With increasing consumer demand for health-driven eating choices, future directions in food labeling regulation will change significantly. The increased scrutiny of nutritional information, fueled by earlier legislations , such as the NLEA, indicates a movement toward greater focus on legibility and readability in labeling. Retailers are already responding to this increased consumer demand by embracing FOP labeling formats that are easy to read, thereby making consumer choice easier and forestalling future regulation (Caldeira et al., 2025). Nevertheless, there are still issues regarding the market impact and performance of the labels, an indicator of an evolving dynamic between consumer demand and business interests. Furthermore, with the recent advances in research on NFPs and their impact on consumer selection, regulatory bodies , such as the FDA have the mandate to respond to key policy questions, including the performance of various labeling formats and their impact on public welfare (Andrews et al., 2017) (Figure 8.14).

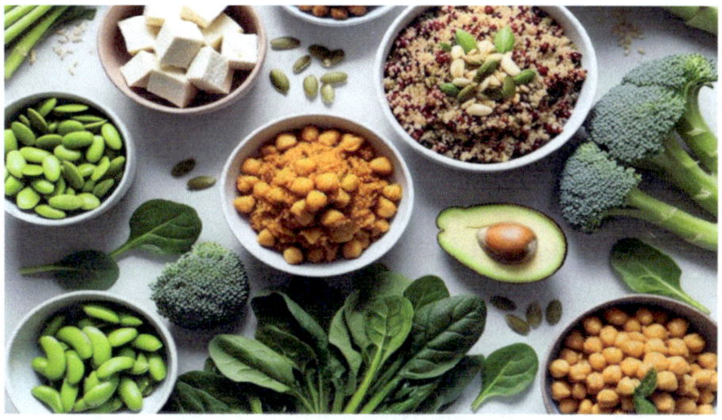

Figure 8.14. As consumer awareness regarding health-related dietary choices continues to rise, future trends in food labeling regulations are likely to evolve significantly.

Source: https://globalwellnessinstitute.org/wp-content/uploads/2025/04/Screenshot-2025-04-02-at-3.09.22%E2%80%AFPM.png.

8.3. Consumer Behavior and Food Labeling

How consumers look at and use food labels is a key topic in researching how people choose what to eat. Since the introduction of the NLEA in 1990, research has sought to understand how various labeling formats—, such as NFPs, FOP symbols, and health claims, affect consumer decisions. It is evident that aspects , such as ingredient labeling on packages and nutritional labeling have a considerable influence on attitudes towards meat foods and frequency of eating, necessitating effective labeling in promoting healthy consumption patterns (Rimal et al., 2006). Further, the moderation of these labeling factors and the key moderating variables , such as motivation of the consumer and information processing ability, links labeling and consumer behavior complex (Andrews et al., 2017). As policies continue to change, it is interesting to note these dynamics to refine the way people are aware of their health and play a role in public health.

8.3.1. Factors Influencing Consumer Choices

Many things affect what people choose to buy , such as health concerns, being environmentally aware and social trends. Eco-labels are a good example of how branding can change people's shopping habits, since they both describe the product and encourage consumers to buy things that are socially responsible.

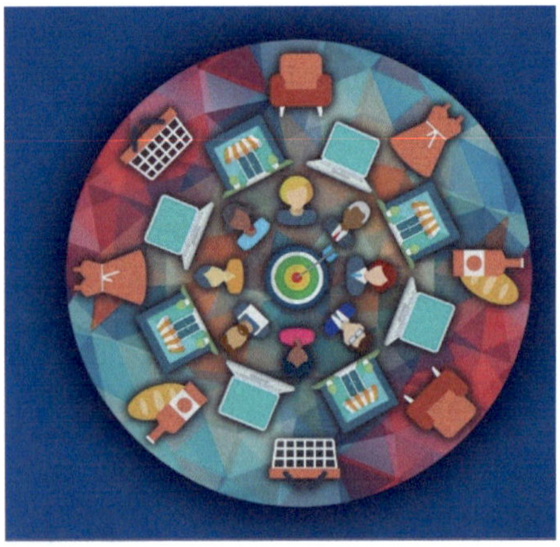

Figure 8.15. Consumer choices are significantly shaped by a multitude of factors, including health consciousness, environmental awareness, and social influences.

Source: https://www2.deloitte.com/content/dam/insights/us/articles/4822_The-consumer-is-changing/images/4822_banner.png/_jcr_content/renditions/cq5dam.web.1440.660.jpeg

Research suggests that successful eco-labels leverage behavioral insights, thereby influencing not only eco-minded consumers but also a broader audience by framing sustainable choices as social norms (Czarnezki et al., 2018). Moreover, the perceived quality of organic products often plays a pivotal role in consumer decision-making, as expectations regarding taste and health benefits can motivate purchases (Asioli et al., 2009). As consumers navigate increasing information complexities in food labeling, the effectiveness of labels in conveying these attributes directly influences their purchasing habits, ultimately underscoring the intricate interplay between consumer awareness, perceived value, and labeling in the food market (Figure 8.15)..

8.3.2. The Role of Education in Consumer Awareness

Education is at the center of consumer awareness, particularly in food labeling. By creating critical thinking and nutrition literacy, education creates informed consumers who are able to adapt to the contemporary-day complex market system. As observed from the rise in digital marketing campaigns, companies have never had a bigger potential and challenge in communicating messages to consumers through social media platforms, and for this reason, education programs are effective in enabling people to differentiate between fact and misinformation (Dwivedi et al., 2020). Research also illustrates the impact of awareness in food waste, demonstrating that consumers should be exposed to the connection between their actions and the overall environmental impact (Schanes et al., 2018). An education system rooted in consumer awareness is, therefore, a solution to healthier behavior and more sustainable food consumption decision-making.

8.3.3. Impact of Marketing on Food Labeling

The convergence of marketing and food labeling has a profound effect on consumer information and purchasing behavior. Retailers employ FOP labels as a way of establishing customer knowledge and facilitating food choice, ultimately as a response to competitive market pressures and regulatory requirements (Caldeira et al., 2025). This marketing, in possessing a functional purpose, also aims to generate perceived value that can distinguish products in a competitive market. Moreover, research reveals that point-of-purchase (POP) signage works well to promote consumer awareness of organic foods, changing purchasing behavior in various store environments (Fishman et al., 2025). These types of marketing stimulate consumer participation and can lead to higher sales, although their success can vary by store type and population. Ultimately, the way in , which products are labeled and marketed has a profound effect on consumer attitudes, stimulating informed choice-making and shaping industry practice in food labeling (Figure 8.16).

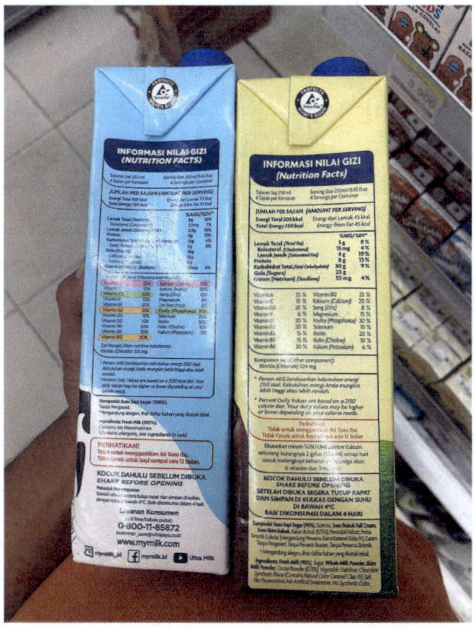

Figure 8.16. Retailers often adopt front-of-package (FOP) labels to enhance customer understanding and assist in food choice, responding both to market competition and regulatory pressures.

Source: By Rantemario - Own work, CC BY-SA 4.0, https://commons.wikimedia.org/w/index.php?curid=151891372

8.3.4. Demographic Differences in Label Interpretation

The way people interpret and use food labels is affected by their demographics , which highlights differences in how aware and how they decide what to buy. Research indicates that while the majority of consumers report utilizing nutrition labels, there has been a notable decline in the use of specific components, particularly among younger adults under 30 years old, who exhibit diminishing engagement with the Nutrition Facts panel and nutritional information on key ingredients (Todd and Variyam, 2025). Conversely, older consumers, especially those aged 50 to 59, and individuals with health concerns, emerge as more vigilant label users, motivating dietary decisions and shopping choices alike (Andrews et al., 2017). This variety points out that special educational plans are needed to meet the needs and preferences of different groups. When strategies are adjusted to suit various age, education and health situations, stakeholders help people understand labels and pick healthier foods.

8.3.5. The Influence of Social Media on Consumer Perceptions

Because social media is everywhere today, what people think about food labeling is greatly affected by the information they see online. Many users look to social media to learn about what is in a product and to check the truth of health statements , which affects their buying decisions. For example, the way social media is used by communities means that people can discuss food products and their labels , which may influence their knowledge of nutrition. Research highlights that consumers process NFPs differently based on social influences, which can either clarify or confuse product information (Andrews et al., 2017). Additionally, varying consumer perceptions around food attributes, , such as the preference for naturalness and resistance to GM foods, as noted in studies involving South

Korean consumers, further reveal how social media can amplify concerns about food safety and quality (Govindasamy et al., 2025). This dynamic underscores the necessity for clear and effective labeling practices to navigate consumer expectations (Figure 8.17).

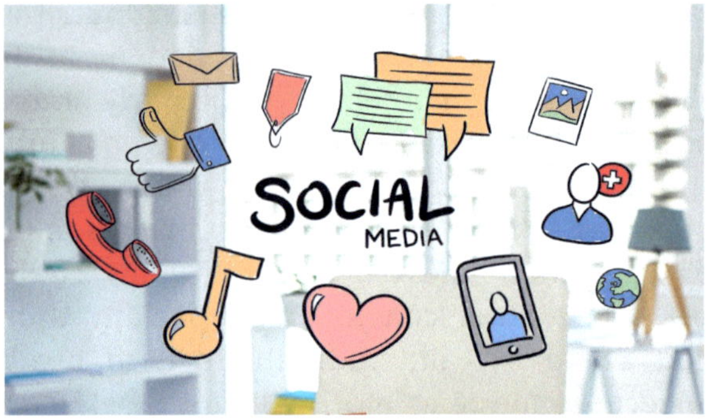

Figure 8.17. Users often rely on social media to gather insights into product attributes, , such as nutritional content and the authenticity of health claims, thus shaping their purchasing decisions.

Source: https://indian-retailer.s3.ap-south-1.amazonaws.com/s3fs-public/2022-05/hand-drawn-illustrations-social-media.jpg.

8.3.6. Case Studies of Consumer Reactions to Labeling

The consumer responses to the labeling of food reflect important trends that point towards the need for better awareness and education of food products. For example, a case study of the acceptance of genome-edited foods in Nigeria concluded that while the respondents declared familiarity with such foods at a mere 30.1%, a considerable 36.8% showed acceptance of them, given that the benefits were well explained and communicated (Adeboye et al., 2024). This shows that consumers' acceptance depends on transparent labeling and educational campaigns. In India, too, awareness of AFCs reflects consumers' lack of knowledge of labeling, as most of them are not aware of the INS (Rameshbabu et al., 2024). These results reflect the importance of inclusive labeling practices in influencing consumers' attitudes and suggest the need for prompt regulatory steps and education programs for informed choice and awareness of food safety.

8.3.7. The Role of Taste vs. Health in Purchasing Decisions

More and more, people consider both taste and health when making food purchases, especially because of food labeling. Some consumers have to decide between enjoying tasty meals and being aware of the health problems linked to those foods. As products are promoted as healthier by manufacturers, people often check if these claims are true, especially since many want clear information on food labels. This complexity is further inflamed by the influence of social media, where marketing strategies frequently emphasize taste and appeal, potentially overshadowing essential health-related information (Hudders et al., 2020). Although people are generally eating healthier, many still choose what tastes best , which means flavor can be more important than health in many situations. Thus, understanding this balance is crucial for both marketers and consumers navigating the landscape of food products (Dwivedi et al., 2022) (Figure 8.18).

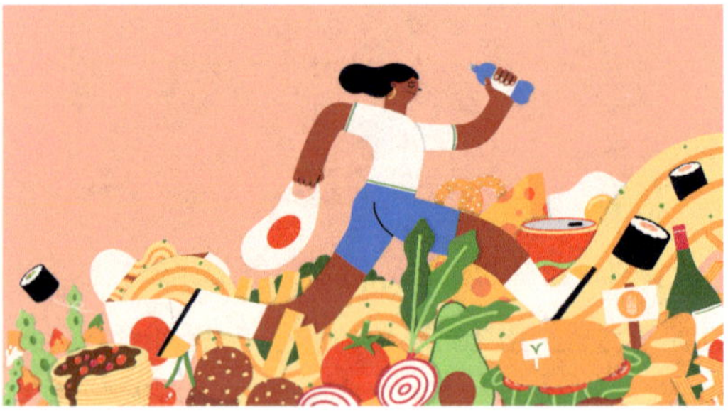

Figure 8.18. In consumer purchasing decisions, the interplay between taste and health considerations is increasingly pertinent, particularly in the context of food labeling.

Source: https://researchleap.com/wp-content/uploads/2023/08/FoodAndBeverage.png.

8.3.8. Consumer Advocacy Groups and Their Impact

Consumer advocacy groups are very important in influencing public consciousness and the demand for change in the food labeling sector. Through corporate accountability campaigns, advocacy groups encourage openness and keep consumers on their toes as they make informed decisions about their food. The influence of advocacy is immense, as witnessed in campaigns against food waste, a challenge costing the U.S. economy over $218 billion per year, a figure , which underscores the demand for effective labeling practices to minimize waste and optimize resource utilization. Globalization also created room for the establishment of advocacy groups, enabling consumers to call for more social and environmental accountability from producers. Campaigns like the Forest Stewardship Council and Fair Trade certification are evidence of how concerted consumer action can lead to fair market conditions while increasing consciousness of sustainable practices (Conroy, 2025). Consumer advocacy groups are therefore key in leading the demand for accountability and better food labeling standards.

8.3.9. Trends in Consumer Demand for Transparency

People today want more information about what is in their food , which shows a major change in what consumers expect. As people learn more about what they eat, they look for information about the sources, ways of producing and types of ingredients in their food. This trend is evident in the rising popularity of organic produce, despite comprising a small segment of total agricultural output in the European Union, is noted for its larger farm sizes and a comparatively younger demographic of farmers engaged in sustainable practices (Kasperowicz-Stępień et al., 2016). Further, the engagement of stakeholders in the policy process has been shown to foster innovation in organic food markets and address consumer demands for transparency well through evidence from the efforts of various European nations to strengthen the food policy frameworks (Dabbert et al., 2025). Such evidence indicates the strong drive towards more accountable and informed food systems (Figure 8.19).

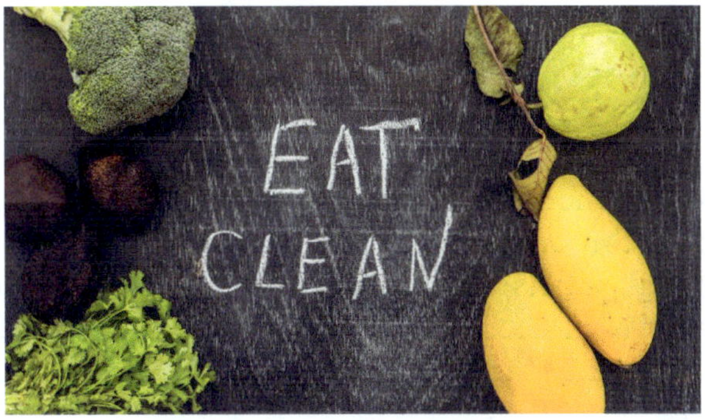

Figure 8.19. As consumers become more educated about the implications of their food choices, they actively seek clarity regarding sourcing, production methods, and ingredient origins.

Source: https://indian-retailer.s3.ap-south-1.amazonaws.com/s3fs-public/2024-05/eat-clean-la-gi-10-cong-dng-ca-ch-d-an-eat-clean-ma-bn-cn-bit_51133e3a%20%281%29.jpg.

8.4. Challenges in Food Labeling

The problems with food labeling extend beyond mere consumer confusion; they have a profound impact on food waste and sustainability efforts as well. In the United States, food labels generally contain misleading expiration dates, like sell by or best before, that lead consumers to discard perfectly good products. This confusion is partly to blame for the stratospheric figure that the U.S. waste system squanders $218 billion on never-eaten food, representing roughly 1.3% of the GDP. Unharvested crops, over-servings, and label confusion are all contributing factors.

ReFED, and other stakeholders, advocate for clear labeling practices as one piece of a comprehensive strategy to combat food waste, create local jobs, and protect the environment. Clarity and transparency in food labeling is, therefore, not merely a consumer education problem, but a step in the right direction to address serious environmental issues.

8.4.1. Complexity of Food Labeling Information

Because food labeling is so detailed, it can be hard for consumers to understand it. Even though labels are important for telling people what is in their food, many find it difficult to understand the different ways and terms labels use.

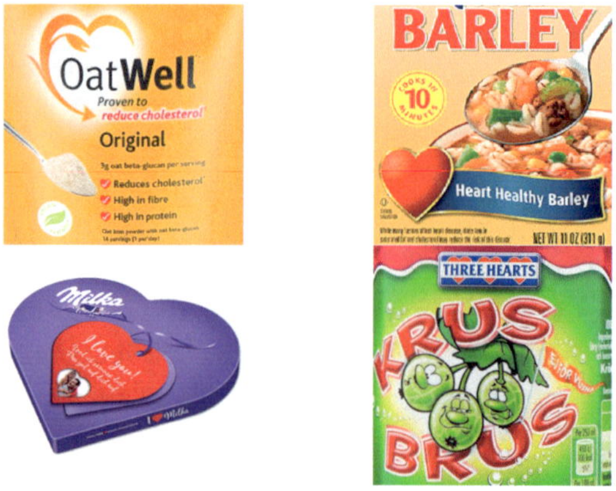

Figure 8.20. Despite the essential role that labels play in informing consumers about nutritional content and ingredients, many individuals struggle to decipher the complex language and varying formats employed.

Source: Miklavec K, Hribar M, Kušar A, Pravst I. Heart Images on Food Labels: A Health Claim or Not? *Foods*. 2021; 10(3):643. https://doi.org/10.3390/foods10030643

Because of this complexity, people might misunderstand what the labels mean , which goes against their purpose. Initiatives , such as updating the Nutrition Facts Panel and developing uniform FOP labeling systems aim to enhance clarity and reduce cognitive overload for consumers (Khandpur et al., 2014). In addition, as research is initiated, consumer sentiment towards labeling procedures also has an immense impact on consumer demand for transparency, with numerous individuals calling for labeling to be made compulsory due to health concerns related to the application of biotechnology in food production (Han and Harrison, 2025). Simplifying the information outlined on food labels, therefore, becomes an intense area of enhancing consumer decisions and informing a better food culture (Figure 8.20).

8.4.2. Misinterpretation of Labels by Consumers

Misinterpretation of food labels by consumers is a significant barrier to informed dietary choice. As discussed in studies, while nutritional labeling aims to promote healthier food choices, consumers are unable to interpret the information presented, leading to an uninformed choice of foods (Andrews et al., 2017). Complexity of NFP and variation in preference for simplified versions of the label, like the Guideline Daily Amount (GDA) and Traffic Light, also lead to confusion. For instance, a study revealed that consumer acceptability was determined by sociodemographic characteristics and individuals' beliefs in the efficiency of the labels in driving choice in Germany and Belgium (Hoefkens et al., 2025). This variation suggests that usability of nutritional labeling can be significantly different across regions and populations, and therefore, the necessity for region- and population-specific label designs maximizing clarity and use. Enhancing consumer familiarity with food labels is at the heart of healthy dietary behavior promotion in a diverse population.

8.4.3. The Issue of Food Fraud and Mislabeling

Because of food fraud and mislabeling, consumers are less sure about the safety and quality of the food they buy. As demonstrated in the seafood sector, mislabeling, particularly through species substitution, can severely undermine effective stock management and consumer choice, with studies revealing that up to 58% of products from certain retailers were fraudulent (Tartre, 2016). Such an adulteration is not only ethically incorrect but is also economically driven, characteristic of a broader trend of economically driven food fraud (EMA), in which foodstuffs are intentionally contaminated, potentially at the expense of consumer health (Onyeaka et al., 2024). Furthermore, a lack of awareness surrounding food fraud persists among consumers; for instance, in a study involving over 2,000 respondents in Nigeria, many were unfamiliar with the term food fraud despite being aware of local scandals (Onyeaka et al., 2024). Thus, enhancing consumer education about food labeling practices is essential to mitigate the risks associated with fraudulent food products (Figure 8.21).

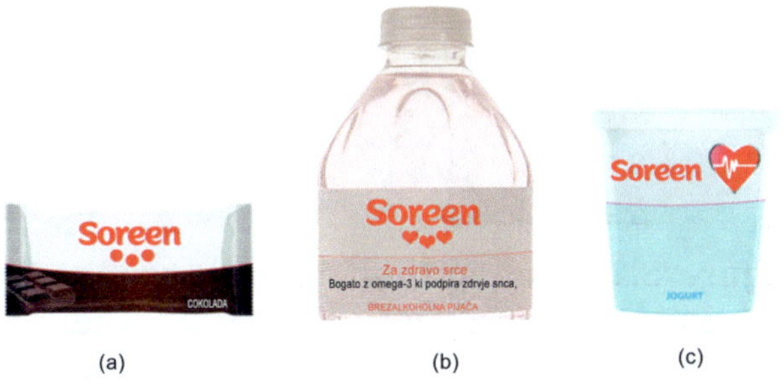

Figure 8.21. The prevalence of food fraud and mislabeling poses significant challenges to consumer safety and trust in the food supply.

Source: Miklavec K, Hribar M, Kušar A, Pravst I. Heart Images on Food Labels: A Health Claim or Not? *Foods*. 2021; 10(3):643. https://doi.org/10.3390/foods10030643

8.4.4. Balancing Information Overload and Simplicity

In the modern-day information age, a balance between the intricacy of food labeling and consumer simplicity is required to support informed decision-making. Consumers are typically presented with an excess of information that can undermine the necessary messages that are communicated on food labels. To this extent, it is necessary to distill key information while preserving the integrity of informative content. For instance, education programs that incorporate environmental standards and open labeling processes not only support food literacy but also meet legislative requirements, thus supporting consumer understanding (Stangland, 2002). Furthermore, the application of simple labeling processes can avert ambiguity, emphasizing key characteristics—, such as nutritional value and the source of ingredients, while refraining from excessive information. In developing conditions that support clarity, , such as in research on effective technologies (Fisher et al., 2011), stakeholders can enhance the development of a model that empowers consumers to make healthier, more sustainable choices without the burden of excessive information.

8.4.5. The Role of Technology in Labeling

Technology has greatly changed food labeling , which has helped people become more aware and make better choices. Now, QR codes, augmented reality and mobile applications allow people to get quick details on food products, like what they are made of, where they come from and what allergens they might contain. By being more open, companies help consumers and also meet the increased need for accountability among food producers. ReFED points out that the U.S. spends $218 billion each year on food that is not eaten , which stresses the importance of having better labeling to cut down on waste and improve how food is distributed. Smart labeling systems can also help ensure food safety and lower the chance of contamination , which is good for public health. Ultimately, technology in labeling serves as a pivotal mechanism in bridging the gap between consumer knowledge and responsible food consumption (Figure 8.22).

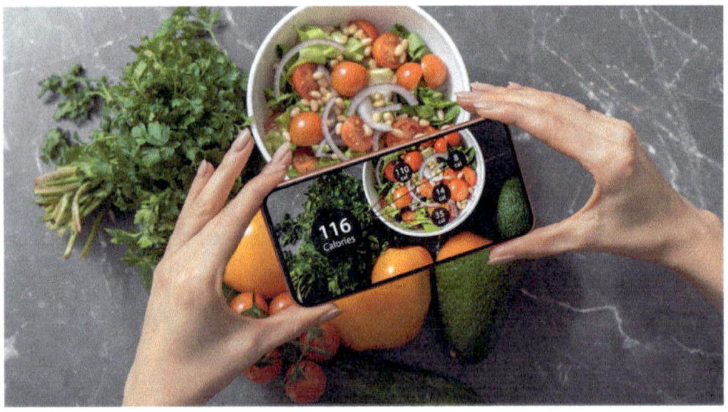

Figure 8.22. Innovations , such as QR codes, augmented reality, and mobile applications now provide consumers with immediate access to detailed information about food products, including nutritional content, sourcing practices, and potential allergens.

Source: https://program-ace.com/wp-content/uploads/augmented-reality-in-the-food-industry-preview.jpg.

8.4.6. Globalization and Labeling Challenges

The intricacy of globalization is a major challenge to food labeling, and its direct impact is on purchasing behavior and awareness of consumers. Because the process of food production transcends borders, label simplicity and consistency are paramount to allow consumers to make quality choices. Moreover, the intersection of factors , such as agricultural practice, health impact, sociocultural, environmental, and socioeconomic factors converges to determine the sustainability of diets and hence complicates labeling (Cogill et al., 2015). Processors make millions of foods in the United States, and this calls for mass-scale labeling that responds to diverse consumer needs and requirements. Research illustrates labeling impacts on consumer behavior, illustrating the role played by the private and public sectors in delivering credible information (Armbruster and Henneberry, 2025). These interplays, thus, necessitate investments in effective labeling standards, which facilitate transparency, hence consumer awareness in the age of globalization.

8.4.7. Cultural Differences in Food Labeling

People's perceptions of food labels are shaped by their culture , which makes it necessary to adjust approaches to help people understand them better. In Europe, consumers in countries like France and Germany exhibit a higher trust and value for government-mandated labels compared to their counterparts in the United Kingdom, where private brands are more prevalent and preferred (Fox et al., 2025).

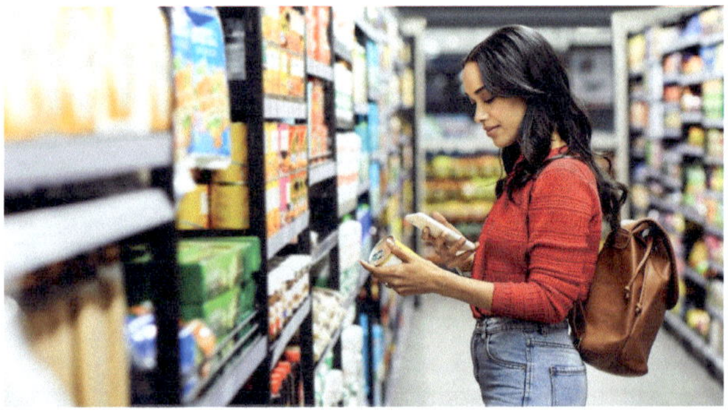

Figure 8.23. Cultural differences significantly influence the perceptions and effectiveness of food labeling, highlighting the need for tailored approaches in enhancing consumer awareness.

Source: https://www.pwc.com/gx/en/issues/c-suite-insights/shrinking-the-consumer-trust-deficit/voice-of-consumer-survey-hero.jpeg.

The perception gap explains why there are people who are more concerned about food safety and quality than others. Additionally, the success of fair trade and organic products explains why social values are not the same in different cultures. For instance, while consumers in Europe may be drawn to labels that indicate ethical consumption, which is a commitment to sustainability, their counterparts in other regions may not be concerned much about such a feature, showing that there is a complicated food labeling dynamics environment (Codron et al., 2025). These are factors to take into account to enhance food labeling communication globally (Figure 8.23).

8.4.8. Economic Factors Affecting Labeling Practices

Labeling strategies within the food sector are significantly influenced by a chain of economic drivers that determine consumer attitudes and market direction. As consumers become increasingly conscious, particularly of food safety and health concerns, food manufacturers are required to adapt labeling schemes to demonstrate transparency and credibility. The economic drive of marketing within a rapidly growing, saturated market compels manufacturers to prioritize perceived benefits, for instance, organic certification or non-GMO, as selling points. Perceived risk factors of agro-biotechnology, for instance, environmental and health concerns, are supported by studies to influence consumer decision-making, often taking precedence over possible benefits (Rimal et al., 2006). Expansion of the organic foods market also relies on consumers' willingness to adopt quality, which can be promoted by effective labeling strategies that prioritize health attributes and sensory attributes (Asioli et al., 2009). Economic drive, therefore, underlies the demand for new labeling schemes that respond to evolving consumer attitudes.

8.4.9. Future Challenges in Food Labeling

The more people learn about food labeling, the more issues become obvious in this field. An important difficulty is that labeling systems are becoming more complicated , which may confuse people and prevent them from making good decisions. Furthermore, the environmental impact of food production is often obscured by traditional labels, as highlighted by the limited effectiveness of carbon labeling in influencing consumer behavior (Fearne et al., 2013). It means that giving information alone is not enough; the information must be clear and easy to understand for consumers to truly understand. Food waste is still closely tied to the way food is labeled. In America, $218 billion worth of food is wasted each year , which proves that clear labels indicating freshness and expiration are needed. So, to deal with these issues, we need a plan that brings together educating consumers, standardizing labels and openly communicating about food sustainability.

A CLOSER LOOK

Genetically Modified (GM) Foods

GM foods are food items produced from organisms whose genetic composition has been altered using biotechnology to introduce desirable features. The alterations are carried out to enhance qualities , such as resistance to diseases and pests, tolerance to stress, enhanced nutrition, and extended shelf life. GM crops , such as corn, soybean, and cotton are produced commercially worldwide, and this contributes to increased agricultural productivity and food security. GM foods have, however, been controversial regarding potential health effects, environmental concerns, and ethics. The regulatory agencies in most nations test the safety of GM foods by exposing them to rigorous testing prior to approval for human use.

SUMMARY

The interface between consumer knowledge and food labeling is more crucial than ever in influencing purchasing behavior and encouraging healthier food choices. As demonstrated, consumers demonstrate a stronger preference for the choice of green- or health-stamped products, reflecting a strong aspiration to align purchases with perceived health and environmental value. For instance, evidence suggests that a large proportion of households are prepared to pay more for green-stamped milk, demonstrating a latent awareness of the effect of their food choices (Wei et al., 2006). Moreover, the success of health-based claims, , such as low in salt or light, demonstrates the complex interface between labeling and consumer interpretation, leading them to assess products differently based on information alone (Bourdeaudhuij et al., 2015). Such evidence demonstrates that effective labeling not only informs but also improves consumers' ability to make healthier choices, ultimately leading to a healthier and better-informed population.

A holistic conceptualization of consumer awareness and food labeling uncovers some general issues informing modern debates and policies within the agri-food sector. First, consumer behavior in combating food waste is evident, particularly in developed nations , such as Greece, where recent studies emphasize how socioeconomic factors and growing awareness of waste conditions consumer behavior from 2012 to 2024 (Zacharatos & Theodoridis, 2025). Second, the application of labeling technology, e.g., blockchain and QR codes, identifies a new consumer requirement for greater transparency in response to food quality, safety, and sustainability issues, particularly in traditional marketplaces like Italy (Petrontino et al., 2024). These outcomes identify a significant change in consumers' willingness to pay a premium for value-based foods. Overall, additional consumer education and awareness through labeling can address genuine issues about food loss and food safety as well as encourage more sustainable consumption behaviors.

KEY TERMS FROM THIS CHAPTER

- Additives
- Allergens
- Communication
- Consumer awareness
- Consumer knowledge
- Date labeling
- Digital interfaces
- Economy
- Food consumption
- Agro-biotechnology
- Animal welfare
- Consumer attitudes
- Consumer empowerment
- Consumer rights
- Decision-making
- Eco-labels
- Environmental sustainability
- Food label awareness

REFERENCES

1. Veeman, Michele M. & Adamowicz, Wiktor L. & Hu, Wuyang, 2005. "Risk Perceptions, Social Interactions and the Influence of Information on Social Attitudes to Agricultural Biotechnology," Project Report Series 24052, University of Alberta, Department of Resource Economics and Environmental Sociology. (accessed on 29 May 2025).
2. Adeboye, S., Asala, S. W., Adeshina, D., Yusuf, H. O., & Ogbimi, E. R. (2024). Consumer awareness and perception of genome-edited food: A case study in the Federal Capital Territory, Abuja, Nigeria. Journal of Agriculture and Food Sciences. https://www.semanticscholar.org/paper/2bcdf766215cc75cad281bd9a3b9f7c645792668 (accessed on 29 May 2025).
3. Onyeaka H, Anyogu A, Odeyemi OA, Ukwuru MU, Eze U, Isaac-Bamgboye FJ, Anumudu CK, Akinwunmi OO, Sotayo OP, Jeff-Agboola YA. Navigating Food Fraud: A Survey of Nigerian Consumer Knowledge and Attitudes. Foods. 2024; 13(20):3270. https://doi.org/10.3390/foods13203270(accessed on 29 May 2025).
4. Allen, K. J., Beyer, K., Ebisawa, M., et al. (2014). Precautionary Labelling of Foods for Allergen Content: Are We Ready for A Global Framework? https://core.ac.uk/download/76995503.pdf (accessed on 29 May 2025).
5. Alonso de la Varga, M., González Montaña, J. R., & Lomillos Pérez, J. M. (2020). Consumers' concerns and perceptions of farm animal welfare. Animals, 10(3), 385. https://doi.org/10.3390/ani10030385.
6. Andrews, J. C., Burton, S., & Cook, L. A. (2017). Nutrition Labeling in The United States and The Role of Consumer Processing, Message Structure, And Moderating Conditions. https://core.ac.uk/download/213088885.pdf (accessed on 29 May 2025).
7. Andrews, J. C., Chen, J. T., Levy, A. S., et al. (2017). How do Consumers Use Nutrition Labels on Food Products in the United States? https://core.ac.uk/download/213087624.pdf (accessed on 29 May 2025).
8. Andrews, J. C., Levy, A. S., Lin, C. T. J., et al. (2014). Consumer Research Needs from The Food and Drug Administration on Front-of-Package Nutritional Labeling. https://core.ac.uk/download/67757133.pdf (accessed on 29 May 2025).
9. Armah, P. W. (2025). The Determinants of Eco-Label Usage in The Organic Produce Market of Northeast Arkansas. https://core.ac.uk/download/pdf/7089132.pdf (accessed on 29 May 2025).
10. Armbruster, W. J., & Henneberry, S. R. (2025). Emerging Roles for Food Labels: Inform, Protect, Persuade. https://core.ac.uk/download/pdf/6988113.pdf (accessed on 29 May 2025).
11. Asioli, D., Bendini, A., Buchecker, K., et al. (2009). Summary Report on Sensory-Related Socio-Economic and Sensory Science Literature About Organic Food Products. https://core.ac.uk/download/10929728.pdf (accessed on 29 May 2025).
12. Biénabe, E., & Vermeulen, H. (2010). The Quality Turn In South Africa: Insights from A Comprehensive Investigation into The Food Quality Behaviors, Perceptions and Knowledge of South African Consumers with A Focus on Middle and Upper Socioeconomic Groups. http://agritrop.cirad.fr/558660/1/document_558660.pdf (accessed on 29 May 2025).
13. Boatwright, M., Lawrence, M., Carriedo, A., Slater, S., McCoy, D., Northcott, T., & Baker, P. (2024). Understanding the politics of food regulation and public health: An analysis of Codex standard-

setting processes on food labelling. International Journal of Health Policy and Management, 13. https://www.semanticscholar.org/paper/b885e653a5d921d8237248d838f7ac075e03ca2a (accessed on 29 May 2025).

14. Boukid, F., Gasparre, N., & Rosell, C. M. (2025). Guiding Trust: The Role of Labeling Information in The Market for Gluten-Free Pasta (2019–2023). https://core.ac.uk/download/650673714.pdf (accessed on 29 May 2025).

15. Brown, K., Harris, F., Potter, C., & Knai, C. (2020). The future of environmental sustainability labelling on food products. The Lancet Planetary Health, 4(3), e137–e138. https://doi.org/10.1016/S2542-5196(20)30074-7.

16. Caldeira, M., Sottomayor, M., & Souza Monteiro, D. M. (2025). Portuguese Retailers' Motivations to Adopt Front of Pack Nutrition Labels: A Qualitative Analysis. https://core.ac.uk/download/pdf/6615150.pdf (accessed on 29 May 2025).

17. Carvalho, F. P. (2017). Pesticides, environment, and food safety. Food and Energy Security, 6(2), 48–60. https://doi.org/10.1002/fes3.108.

18. Codron, J. M., Sirieix, L., & Reardon, T. (2025). Social and Environmental Attributes of Food Products in An Emerging Mass Market: Challenges of Signaling and Consumer Perception, With European Illustrations. https://core.ac.uk/download/pdf/9314571.pdf (accessed on 29 May 2025).

19. Cogill, B., Fanzo, J. C., & Johnston, J. L. (2015). Understanding Sustainable Diets: A Descriptive Analysis of The Determinants and Processes That Influence Diets and Their Impact on Health, Food Security, And Environmental Sustainability. https://core.ac.uk/download/132676312.pdf (accessed on 29 May 2025).

20. Colson, G. J., Facendola, M., Grebitus, C., et al. (2025). Consumer Preferences for Country-of-Origin, Geographical Indication, and Protected Designation of Origin Labels. https://core.ac.uk/download/pdf/6642980.pdf (accessed on 29 May 2025).

21. Conroy, M. E. (2025). Can Advocacy-Led Certification Systems Transform Global Corporate Practices? Evidence, And Some Theory. https://core.ac.uk/download/pdf/6548888.pdf (accessed on 29 May 2025).

22. Consultation Working Groups, De Steur, H., Garcia-Casal, M. N., Giyose, B., et al. (2017). Staple Crops Biofortified with Increased Vitamins and Minerals: Considerations for A Public Health Strategy. https://core.ac.uk/download/84044266.pdf (accessed on 29 May 2025).

23. Jason J. Czarnezki, K. Ingemar Jonsson & Katrina Kuh, Crafting Next Generation Eco-Label Policy, 48 Envtl. L. 409 (2018), https://digitalcommons.pace.edu/lawfaculty/1100/.Dabbert, S., Haring, A. M., Vairo, D., Zanoli, R., et al. (2025). Policies Supporting Organic Food and Farming in The Eu: Assessment and Development by Stakeholders In 11 European Countries. https://core.ac.uk/download/pdf/7055588.pdf (accessed on 29 May 2025).

24. De Bourdeaudhuij, I., De Pelsmaeker, S., De Steur, H., Gellynck, X., et al. (2015). Impact of Health Labels on Flavor Perception and Emotional Profiling: A Consumer Study on Cheese. https://core.ac.uk/download/55743341.pdf (accessed on 29 May 2025).

25. Durham, T. C., & Mizik, T. (2021). Comparative economics of conventional, organic, and alternative agricultural production systems. Economies, 9(2), 64. https://doi.org/10.3390/economies9020064.

26. Dwivedi, Y. K., Hughes, L., Baabdullah, A. M., Ribeiro-Navarrete, S., Giannakis, M., Al-Debei, M. M., Dennehy, D., et al. (2022). Metaverse beyond the hype: Multidisciplinary perspectives on emerging challenges, opportunities, and agenda for research, practice and policy. International Journal of Information Management, 66, 102542. https://doi.org/10.1016/j.ijinfomgt.2022.102542.

27. Dwivedi, Y. K., Ismagilova, E., Hughes, D. L., Carlson, J., Filieri, R., Jacobson, J., Jain, V., et al. (2020). Setting the future of digital and social media marketing research: Perspectives and research propositions. International Journal of Information Management, 59, 102168. https://doi.org/10.1016/j.ijinfomgt.2020.102168.

28. Fearne, A., Hornibrook, S. A., & May, C. A. (2013). Sustainable Development and The Consumer: Exploring the Role of Carbon Labelling in Retail Supply Chains. https://core.ac.uk/download/16702275.pdf (accessed on 29 May 2025).

29. Fisher, D., Hand, J., Liesen, R., Wilson, E., et al. (2011). Screening of Energy Efficient Technologies for Industrial Buildings' Retrofit. https://core.ac.uk/download/9033399.pdf (accessed on 29 May 2025).

30. Fishman, A., Reicks, M., & Splett, P. (2025). Shelf Labeling of Organic Foods: Effects on Customer Perceptions and Sales. https://core.ac.uk/download/pdf/7025310.pdf (accessed on 29 May 2025).

31. Fletcher, S. M., & Rimal, A. (2025). Understanding Consumers' Attitude Toward Meat Labels and Meat Consumption Pattern. https://core.ac.uk/download/pdf/6553422.pdf (accessed on 29 May 2025).

32. Fliegelman, J. E. (2011). The Next Generation of Greenwash: Diminishing Consumer Confusion Through a National Eco-Labeling Program. https://core.ac.uk/download/144227842.pdf (accessed on 29 May 2025).

33. Fox, J. A., Lusk, J. L., & Roosen, J. (2025). Consumer Demand for and Attitudes Toward Alternative Beef Labeling Strategies in France, Germany, and the UK. https://core.ac.uk/download/pdf/7083315.pdf (accessed on 29 May 2025).

34. Girard, V. W. (2012). Reducing Unlawful Prescription Drug Promotion: Is the Public Health Being Served by An Enforcement Approach That Focuses on Punishment? https://core.ac.uk/download/70374920.pdf (accessed on 29 May 2025).

35. Godfray, H. C. J., Aveyard, P., Garnett, T., Hall, J. W., Key, T. J., Lorimer, J., Pierrehumbert, R. T., et al. (2018). Meat consumption, health, and the environment. Science, 361(6399). https://doi.org/10.1126/science.aam5324.

36. Govindasamy, R., Hallman, W. K., Jang, H. M., Onyango, B., et al. (2025). Consumer Acceptance of Genetically Modified Foods in South Korea: Factor and Cluster Analysis. https://core.ac.uk/download/pdf/6813941.pdf (accessed on 29 May 2025).

37. Han, J. H., & Harrison, R. W. (2025). A Multinomial Logit Model of Consumer Perceptions for Biotech Food Labeling. https://core.ac.uk/download/pdf/7075644.pdf (accessed on 29 May 2025).

38. Hashmi, M. (2012). To Take or Not to Take: Bioethical Conflicts with Non-Adherence to Medications Due to Religious Beliefs. https://core.ac.uk/download/28938491.pdf (accessed on 29 May 2025).

39. He, X., Deng, H., & Hwang, H. M. (2018). The current application of nanotechnology in food and agriculture. Journal of Food and Drug Analysis, 27(1), 1–21. https://doi.org/10.1016/j.jfda.2018.12.002.

40. Hoefkens, C., Moeser, A., Van Camp, J., Verbeke, W., et al. (2025). Nutrient Profile Labelling: Consumers' Perceptions in Germany and Belgium. https://core.ac.uk/download/pdf/6689729.pdf (accessed on 29 May 2025).

41. Huang, H. (2024). Comparative analysis of pre-packaged food labeling regulations between China, the European Union and the United States. Lecture Notes in Education Psychology and Public Media. https://www.semanticscholar.org/paper/14063d704762437e6e6a5908e3bdd119a2f651bc (accessed on 29 May 2025).

42. Hudders, L., De Jans, S., & De Veirman, M. (2020). The commercialization of social media stars: A literature review and conceptual framework on the strategic use of social media influencers. International Journal of Advertising, 40(3), 327–375. https://doi.org/10.1080/02650487.2020.1836925.

43. Jadi, R., Bepari, Z., & Birje, R. (2022). Assessment of consumer awareness on food labels and the effect of the level of awareness on purchasing behavior of consumers in Belgaum District. GBS Impact: Journal of Multi-Disciplinary Research. https://www.semanticscholar.org/paper/1208b4efb111df3137aeafe04e557bfd6e9c4cf6 (accessed on 29 May 2025).

44. Kasperowicz-Stępień, A., & Stabryła-Chudzio, K. (2016). Development of Organic Farming in Poland After 2013 In Terms of Common Agricultural Policy. https://core.ac.uk/download/322516243.pdf (accessed on 29 May 2025).

45. Khandpur, N., & Roberto, C. A. (2014). Improving the Design of Nutrition Labels to Promote Healthier Food Choices and Reasonable Portion Sizes. https://core.ac.uk/download/28950220.pdf (accessed on 29 May 2025).

46. Mach, F., Baigent, C., Catapano, A. L., Koskinas, K. C., Casula, M., Badimón, L., Chapman, M. J., et al. (2019). 2019 ESC/EAS guidelines for the management of dyslipidemias: Lipid modification to reduce cardiovascular risk. European Heart Journal, 41(1), 111–188. https://doi.org/10.1093/eurheartj/ehz455.

47. McCabe, M. S. (2010). Balancing Consumer Protection and Scientific Integrity in The Face of Uncertainty: The Example of Gluten-Free Foods. https://core.ac.uk/download/72051983.pdf (accessed on 29 May 2025).

48. Mehta, N., Cunningham, E., Roy, D., Cathcart, A., Dempster, M., Berry, E., & Smyth, B. (2020). Exploring perceptions of environmental professionals, plastic processors, students and consumers of bio-based plastics: Informing the development of the sector. Sustainable Production and Consumption, 26, 574–587. https://doi.org/10.1016/j.spc.2020.12.015.

49. Melović, B., Ćirović, D., Backović, T., Dudić, B., & Gubíniová, K. (2020). Attracting green consumers as a basis for creating sustainable marketing strategy on the organic market—Relevance for sustainable agriculture business development. Foods, 9(11), 1552. https://doi.org/10.3390/foods9111552.

50. Rimal, Arbindra & Moon, Wanki & Balasubramanian, Siva K., 2006. "Perceived Risks of Agro-Biotechnology and Organic Food Purchases in the United States," Journal of Food Distribution Research, Food Distribution Research Society, vol. 37(2), pages 1-10, July.Nekmahmud, M., & Fekete-Farkas, M. (2020). Why not green marketing? Determinants of consumers' intention

to green purchase decision in a new developing nation. Sustainability, 12(19), 7880. https://doi.org/10.3390/su12197880.

51. Petrontino, A., Frem, M., Fucilli, V., Tria, E., Campobasso, A. A., & Bozzo, F. (2024). Consumers' purchase propensity for pasta tracked with blockchain technology and labelled with sustainable credence attributes. Frontiers in Sustainable Food Systems. https://www.semanticscholar.org/paper/4d6a05e9d5b88294490b61f6ade481a67090fc4b (accessed on 29 May 2025).
52. Phillips, M. J. (2025). Perspectives on Consumers, Industry, And Regulations in The Food Sector. https://core.ac.uk/download/pdf/6988100.pdf (accessed on 29 May 2025).
53. Puntoni, S., Reczek, R. W., Giesler, M., & Botti, S. (2020). Consumers and artificial intelligence: An experiential perspective. Journal of Marketing, 85(1), 131–151. https://doi.org/10.1177/0022242920953847.
54. Rameshbabu, J., & Swaminathan, U. (2024). Consumer awareness and contemporary policy regulations on artificial food colorant safety in India. Current Research in Nutrition and Food Science Journal. https://www.semanticscholar.org/paper/4b482b30afedbea1e8afd9d104e4b97c19727279 (accessed on 29 May 2025).
55. Schanes, K., Dobernig, K., & Gözet, B. (2018). Food waste matters–A systematic review of household food waste practices and their policy implications. Journal of Cleaner Production, 182, 978–991. https://doi.org/10.1016/j.jclepro.2018.02.030.
56. Spitzer, E. (2024). What is in Your Tampon? Increasing Transparency in Menstrual Products. https://core.ac.uk/download/622347132.pdf (accessed on 29 May 2025).
57. Stangland, T. L. (2002). Integrating Environmental Education with Family and Consumer Science Education. https://core.ac.uk/download/541934002.pdf (accessed on 29 May 2025).
58. Tartre, R. J. (2016). Testing Potential Fish Fraud in Community-Supported Fisheries. https://core.ac.uk/download/84397725.pdf (accessed on 29 May 2025).
59. Todd, J. E., & Variyam, J. N. (2025). The Decline in Consumer Use of Food Nutrition Labels, 1995–2006. https://core.ac.uk/download/pdf/6435264.pdf (accessed on 29 May 2025).
60. Uzoma, C. M., Uwugiaren, N. J., Ugwunze, C. A., Abdullah, Y. D., & Umaru, H. M. (2025). Assessing the impact of food labeling policies on consumer behavior, non-communicable disease risks, and machine learning-driven insights: Analyzing purchasing patterns and health outcomes in central Lagos, Nigeria. World Journal of Advanced Research and Reviews. https://www.semanticscholar.org/paper/f6024a691882d497cbd6a1425ced6020bb7310a0 (accessed on 29 May 2025).
61. Wei, X., & Zeng, Y. (2006). Consumer's Attitudes and Willingness-To-Pay for Green Food in Beijing. https://core.ac.uk/download/10930440.pdf (accessed on 29 May 2025).
62. Zacharatos, T. V., & Theodoridis, P. K. (2025). Consumer behavior and food waste in Greece: Insights from 2012 to 2024. Encyclopedia. https://www.semanticscholar.org/paper/e75b1c22757f2b202191c6ecfc1a4c46ecba06c3 (accessed on 29 May 2025).

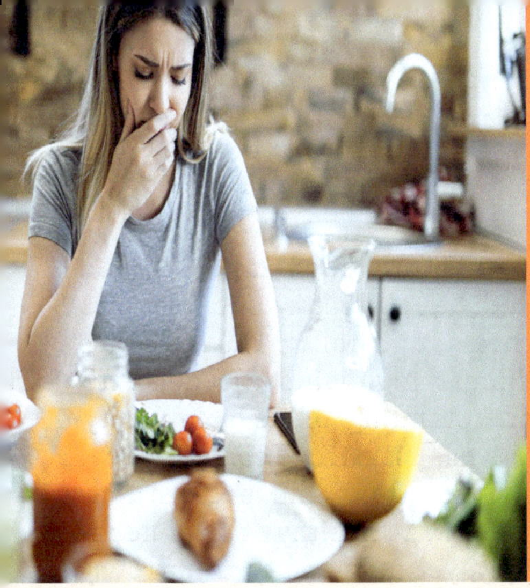

Chapter 9

UNDERSTANDING FOOD POISONING

Contents

Introduction 209
9.1. Causes of Food Poisoning 212
9.2. Symptoms and Diagnosis 216
9.3. Treatment and Management 220
Summary 226
References 227

Introduction

Millions of people around the world are affected by food poisoning, which is a problem that affects food production, preparation and consumption. Pathogenic microorganisms appearing due to poor hygiene in farming and cooking make it more likely for people to get sick from food. As highlighted by literature, some of the factors behind such toxicity that underlies such health issues include heavy metals in crop environments, a pointer to the complexity of food safety (Blundell et al., 2016). Moreover, pesticide application controversy highlights other hazards in food production; while organic production has been shown to reduce some risk of pathogens, it will unintentionally raise others, posing a delicate balance in food safety management (Brandt, 2007). Because many factors are involved, understanding food poisoning well is necessary to reduce its risks and protect the public.

Definition of Food Poisoning

Food poisoning is primarily described as a disease caused by the intake of contaminated food or drinks, which leads to a variety of symptoms, such as nausea, vomiting, diarrhea, and abdominal discomfort. The dangerous impact is primarily caused by pathogens, such as bacteria, viruses, and parasites, or the presence of toxic chemicals, such as chemical residues and natural food toxins in some foods. The incidence of foodborne disease is an indicator of major loopholes in food safety practices, which means the necessity for tight control in food production and handling. Effective management practices, such as enhanced sanitation processes and rigorous monitoring, are required to reduce the incidence of food poisoning. The food safety culture is also advanced, with organic farming signifying a decrease in risks and some special concerns regarding contamination, signifying the necessity for a high level of understanding of agricultural processes (Brandt, 2007; Bergsten et al., 2018) (Figure 9.1).

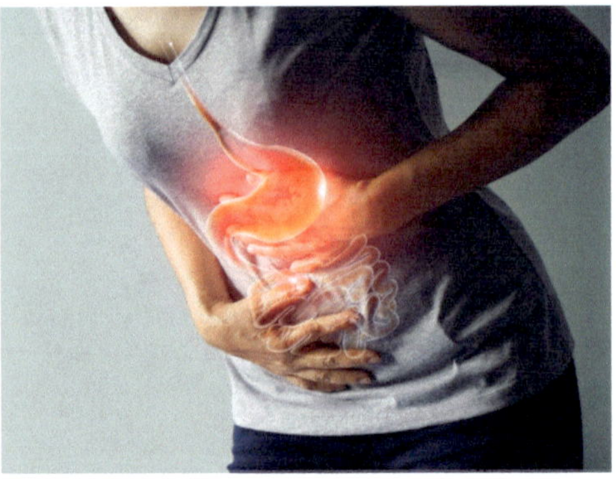

Figure 9.1. Food poisoning is broadly defined as an illness resulting from the consumption of contaminated food or beverages, which can cause a range of symptoms including nausea, vomiting, diarrhea, and abdominal pain.

Source: https://www.cdc.gov/food-safety/media/images/2024/06/GettyImages-1052976746-16x9-1.jpg.

Importance of Understanding Food Poisoning

It is paramount to be cognizant of food poisoning for individual health, but it is also vital for public health and policy. The incidence of foodborne illness highlights the need for a complete understanding of its complexity. Foodborne illness has disastrous consequences on susceptible populations and overburdens the healthcare system. A healthy society needs a safe food supply, yet food safety is narrowly conceived as simply foodborne illness (Leib et al., 2019). The narrow conception may lead to inefficient resource allocation and exclusion of broader public systemic risks of food production and consumption. Regardless of this, this realization of the interdependence of food safety and neurological disease also calls for increased public awareness and knowledge of food issues (Ngudi et al., 2014). Being more aware of the cause of food poisoning allows policymakers and the public to make better choices, ultimately improving public health and enhancing social welfare.

Prevalence of Food Poisoning Cases

There are still many cases of food poisoning, which shows how difficult it is to ensure food safety. Each year, numerous individuals suffer from foodborne illnesses, driven by various pathogens, including *B. cereus* and *S. aureus*, which remain prevalent in ready-to-eat (RTE) foods. A comprehensive study evaluating 21,822 microbiological test results from RTE food samples in Western Australia from 2009 to 2022 indicated a troubling trend, revealing an increase in the prevalence of *B. cereus*, while *S. aureus* and non-STEC -*E. coli* showed a decline (Foxcroft et al., 2024). This volatility heightens the need for ongoing observation and research in a bid to gain a comprehensive understanding of the determinants of such fluctuations, as well as the potential impact of ecological factors, such as climate change and recent global pandemics on food safety policy (The Writing Committee of the Report on Cardiovascular in China and Hu, 2023). The dynamic nature of these pathogens highlights the importance of robust food safety protocols to minimize risks to public health (Figure 9.2).

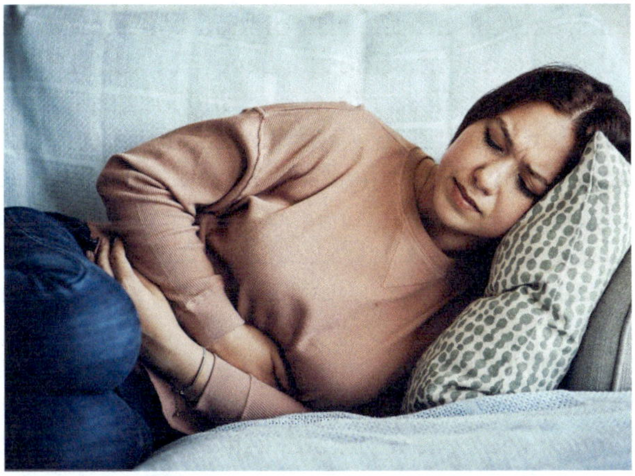

Figure 9.2. The prevalence of food poisoning cases continues to be a significant public health concern, reflecting the complexities involved in food safety management.

Source: https://media.self.com/photos/62968716cafa033ae66f8aa1/4:3/w_2560%2Cc_limit/food-poisoning-contagious.jpg.

Common Misconceptions About Food Poisoning

The prevalence of myths regarding food poisoning can greatly undermine public health interventions at preventing outbreaks. For example, one such myth is the belief that food poisoning results from spoilt or rotten food alone, when many of these disease-causing pathogens are found on fresh produce, such as fruits and vegetables. Misconceptions also arise in believing that home cooking removes all risks, when improper handling and cooking temperatures join conditions that favor bacterial growth. For example, most individuals wrongly believe geckos to be poisonous carriers of diseases based on local myths, which leads to unnecessary fear and avoidance that interferes with food safety measures (Ceríaco et al., 2011). In addition, most individuals undervalue the role of cross-contamination in food handling, which easily transfers pathogenic microbes from one food to another, making efforts in food safety futile (Ackerman et al., 2007). Education and awareness are, therefore, crucial in eliminating the myths.

Impact on Public Health

Besides making people sick, food poisoning points out the wider problems of poverty and poor food safety policies. A lot of foodborne illnesses can burden healthcare services, cause people to miss work and increase economic differences. Vulnerable populations, particularly those living in impoverished conditions, are disproportionately affected due to limited access to safe food and healthcare resources, as outlined in Bergsten et al. (2018).

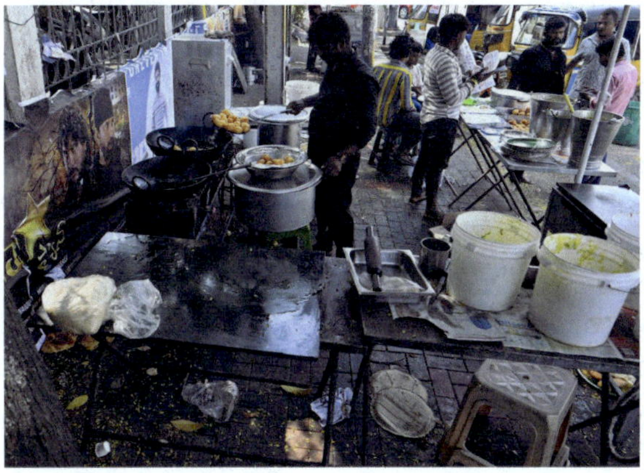

Figure 9.3. The impact of food poisoning on public health extends beyond immediate illness, highlighting systemic issues, such as poverty and inadequate food safety protocols.

Source: https://th-i.thgim.com/public/incoming/odxc6l/article68924613.ece/alternates/FREE_1200/28112024_%20food%20poisoning%20cases%20%2003.jpg.

It is very important to manage food safety properly to prevent these health issues; international food safety standards set by the

Codex Alimentarius help fill in gaps in food hygiene and protect people worldwide. Yet, earlier controversies around the formulation of such standards mirror the difficulty of achieving a balance between qualitative and quantitative food safety measures, as discussed by Ramsingh (2014). Preventing food poisoning is a multidisciplinary process that integrates health, economic, and social interventions (Figure 9.3).

Economic Costs Associated with Food Poisoning

The cost of food poisoning to the economy is enormous, with direct medical expenses, lost business, and social effects. The food poisoning victims typically get huge medical expenses for treatment and hospitalization, which mount rapidly, particularly for serious complications requiring hospitalization. Secondly, trickle-down effects also occur in the economy, as sick workers lose days at work, resulting in loss of business revenues and lower economic production. This is then followed by the social effect of food poisoning, which hit targeted public health clinics and overwhelmed prevention and education efforts. Efficient management practices, like IPM programs, can cut these costs by restricting the application of toxic pesticides and thus decreasing the rate of foodborne diseases caused by contaminated agricultural produce (Resosudarmo, 2025). Additionally, localized economic disparities highlight how food poisoning disproportionately impacts marginalized communities, resulting in health and economic disparities (Bergsten et al., 2018).

9.1. Causes of Food Poisoning

Bacteria, viruses and parasites are the main causes of food poisoning, which disrupts the health of the digestive system. Some of the most well-known bacteria that cause food poisoning are Salmonella and *Escherichia coli* and they are found in foods that are not cooked or stored properly. Additionally, less recognized conditions, such as pica, an eating disorder characterized by the consumption of non-food items, can elevate the risk of food contamination and subsequent illness (Lacey et al., 1989). Furthermore, *Clostridium perfringens* has gained attention for its role in foodborne outbreaks, particularly in settings where food is prepared in large quantities, such as cafeterias (Modi & Wilcox, 2001). It is necessary to learn about all these factors to develop good prevention plans, which should highlight safe food handling, the right cooking temperatures and informing people about eating disorders that could result in dangerous eating habits. All of these reasons add to the difficulty of food poisoning.

9.1.1. Bacterial Pathogens

Bacterial pathogens are the main causes of food poisoning and greatly affects the health of many people. *Clostridium perfringens* is a well-known example because it plays a part in both foodborne and antibiotic-related diarrheal diseases. While traditionally associated with contaminated meats, recent evidence suggests that enterotoxigenic strains of *C. perfringens* may also play a substantial part in cases not linked to food sources, such as hospital-acquired infections (Modi & Wilcox, 2001). They have a greater effect than only causing infections; they also challenge health systems and how resources are assigned, mainly in the field of laboratory diagnostics. Bacterial pathogens also respond to and reflect changes in the environment and in ecology. For instance, determinants of wildlife mortality, as identified by various pathogens and toxicants, reiterate the association between wildlife health and food safety practice among humans (Garbriel et al., 2015). It is important to value these associations as a basis for the formulation of efficient prevention strategies in food poisoning (Figure 9.4).

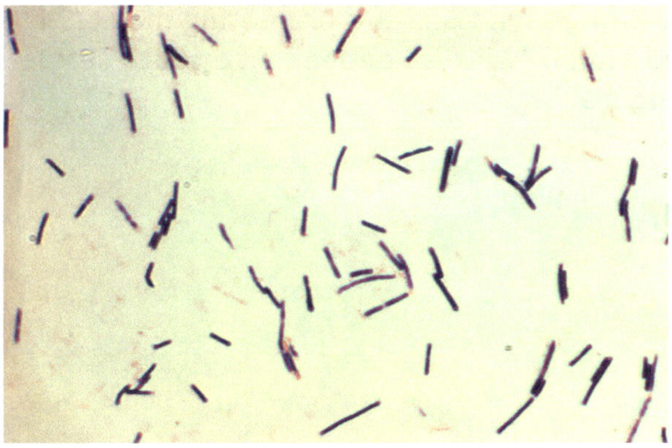

Figure 9.4. *Clostridium perfringens*, recognized for its role in both foodborne and antibiotic-associated diarrheal diseases.

Source: https://upload.wikimedia.org/wikipedia/commons/5/5e/Clostridium_perfringens.jpg.

9.1.2. Viral Pathogens

The role of viral pathogens in food poisoning is typically overshadowed by that of bacterial contaminants but is of significant public health importance. Norovirus and hepatitis A are among the viruses that are often associated with foodborne outbreaks in raw or undercooked shellfish and fresh contaminated fruits and vegetables. Infection from these viruses may lead to gastrointestinal illness, expressed in the form of vomiting, diarrhea, and abdominal cramps, lasting for a few days to weeks. Recent studies highlight that compared to bacterial pathogens, viral pathogens require limited infectious material to cause disease, making prevention a challenge. The viral strain research, in line with case studies on *Salmonella enterica*, indicates a high level of understanding of foodborne disease, considering the genetic diversity and virulence determinants involved (Hou et al., 2024). Additionally, new approaches, such as the application of computational tools in the identification of natural antiviral compounds, are presented as alternative ways of reducing the impact of these pathogens on food safety (Garbriel et al., 2015).

9.1.3. Parasitic Infections

Many foodborne illnesses are caused by parasites, which are not always given enough attention in discussions about food poisoning. Most of these infections are caused by eating contaminated foods, especially undercooked meats, unwashed vegetables and water that is not clean. These infections are capable of causing severe problems, leading to belly pain and body-wide complications. Environmental factors, including the use of pesticides, also lead to these infections through disruption of local ecosystems and the initiation of parasitic pathogen amplification (Sánchez-Bayo, 2021). The interaction between health and climate change has also prompted additional research into how changes in ecological systems could be influencing the transmission dynamics of these parasites (Dén et al., 2021). Ultimately, a comprehensive understanding of parasitic infections within the context of food poisoning requires an integration of ecological, microbial, and public health perspectives to mitigate risks effectively (Figure 9.5).

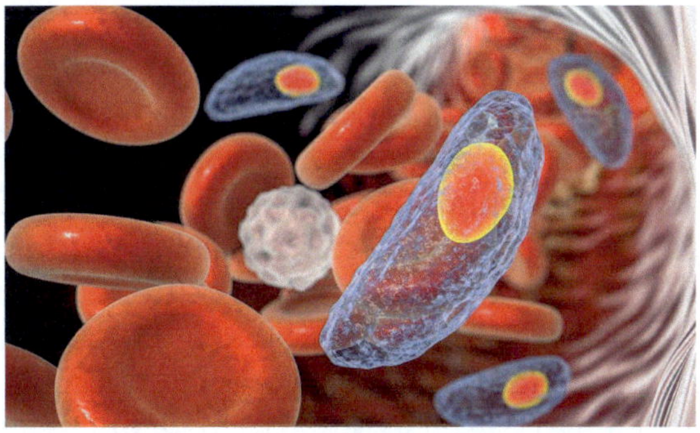

Figure 9.5. Parasitic infections represent a significant, yet often underappreciated, portion of foodborne illnesses, contributing to the broader understanding of food poisoning.

Source: https://www.food-safety.com/ext/resources/Images/2024/Apr_May/B2B-0424-900-Img1.jpg?1716907254.

9.1.4. Chemical Contaminants

The widespread problem of chemical contaminants in our food supply is a key factor in understanding food poisoning. A case in point is lasalocid, an ionophore antibiotic employed in poultry that, despite its growth-promoting efficacy, is highly dangerous when residues persist in eggs, which are commonly undetected because of poor regulatory knowledge and testing measures (Roxburgh et al., 2010). The risk of human exposure to such contaminants is of grave public health concern because the precise toxic levels of lasalocid in humans remain unknown. Furthermore, the ubiquity of pesticides in conventional agriculture adds another dimension to risk; although organic farming minimizes this type of contamination, it never eliminates the risk of exposure to natural toxins (Brandt, 2007). Therefore, the multifaceted nature of chemical contaminants highlights the necessity for stringent testing and better food safety regulations to ensure consumer protection from the covert risks of foodborne disease.

9.1.5. Improper Food Handling

Not handling food properly can seriously harm public health, mainly in places where food is made for children or people with special needs, such as day care centers and restaurants. Research indicates that children attending day care are three times more likely to contract foodborne illnesses than their peers not in such environments, primarily due to inadequate food safety measures and the susceptibility of their developing immune systems (Seabela, 2020). Other than that, a restaurant food handlers' study revealed appalling gaps in personal hygiene and sanitation, where 87.5% of them had never received adequate training in food hygiene (Neme et al., 2017). Inadequate knowledge regarding food safety and dirty habits raises the chances of food contamination. Adhering to stringent training and following safety guidelines is of the highest priority in avoiding such risks and promoting the health of individuals who are dependent on such services (Figure 9.6).

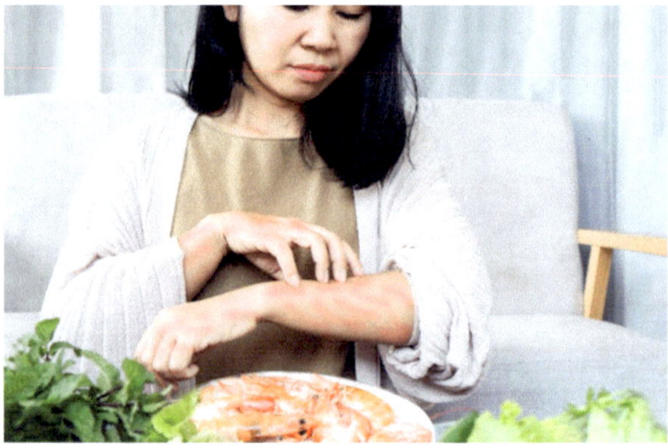

Figure 9.6. Improper food handling practices pose a significant threat to public health, particularly in settings where food is prepared for vulnerable populations, such as day care centers and restaurants.

Source: https://allieddigestivehealth.com/wp-content/uploads/2024/01/Woman-has-allergic-reaction-to-shrimp.jpg.

9.1.6. Cross-Contamination

In the context of food safety, cross-contamination is a critical concern that significantly contributes to food poisoning incidents. This phenomenon occurs when harmful pathogens, such as bacteria and viruses, transfer from one food item to another, often facilitated by improper handling or inadequate sanitation practices. For instance, using the same cutting board for raw meat and vegetables without proper cleaning can lead to the spread of zoonotic pathogens that pose severe health risks to consumers (Brandt et al., 2007). Furthermore, emerging research highlights the implications of climate change on the prevalence of waterborne pathogens, which can exacerbate foodborne illnesses through contaminated water supplies (Heaviside et al., 2018). As such, understanding the dynamics of cross-contamination is essential for mitigating food poisoning risks. Implementing rigorous hygiene standards and educating food handlers about safe practices can drastically reduce the chances of cross-contamination, thereby improving public health outcomes.

9.1.7. Inadequate Cooking Temperatures

Not cooking food at the right temperature is a major reason for food poisoning, which means handling food properly is very important. It has been found that improper ways of cooking food are a main reason for foodborne diseases, so proper temperature control is necessary during preparation. For instance, many individuals lack awareness of the necessary cooking temperatures for various foods, leaving them susceptible to contamination by pathogens (Perkins et al., 2021). Moreover, a study analyzing domestic food preparation practices reveals alarming statistics, with over 40% of participants exhibiting temperature abuse during food transport and storage, and 19% of individuals holding cooked food at ambient temperatures for excessive periods (Worsfold, 1994).

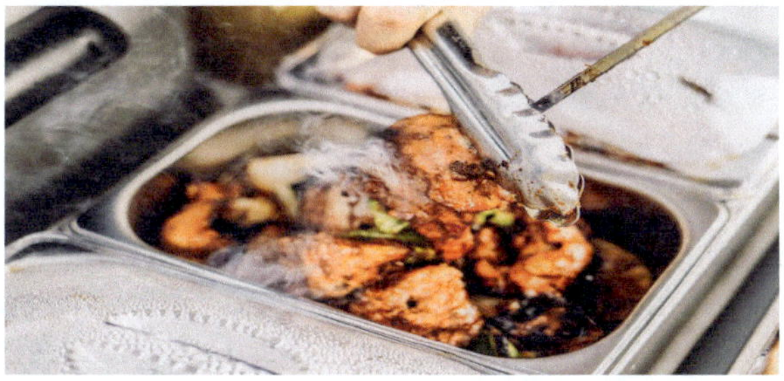

Figure 9.7. Inadequate cooking temperatures emerge as a critical factor in the prevalence of food poisoning, underscoring the importance of proper food handling practices.

Source: https://images.squarespace-cdn.com/content/v1/5b35d983c3c16a60c7dc8168/1667300269472-LT69ZUF2M51ZCS902FP8/Why-food-hygiene-and-safety-is-important-to-reduce-food-poisoning.

The study shows that cooking food at too low a temperature greatly increases the risk of foodborne illnesses. Hence, ensuring food is cooked to the appropriate temperatures is vital in mitigating the risk of food poisoning and protecting public health (Figure 9.7).

9.1.8. Food Storage Practices

Correct food storage is necessary to avoid food poisoning, because bacteria can grow in improperly stored food. For instance, the International Codex Alimentarius, established by the FAO and WHO, highlights the importance of adherence to both qualitative and quantitative standards in food hygiene, which directly impacts how food is stored and handled (Ramsingh, 2014). Also, organic farming brings a special aspect; while some steps reduce risks of contamination, managing storage conditions like temperature and humidity is still key to safety. Notably, some research suggests that higher levels of plant defense mechanisms in organic products can lead to reduced quality loss during storage and transport, promoting safer consumption (Brandt, 2007). So, learning how to store food properly helps prevent both wasting food and the spread of foodborne diseases.

9.1.9. Risk Factors in Food Production

Food production is beset by various risk factors that play a significant role in food safety and are the causes of food poisoning incidence. One of the problems is the use of synthetic pesticides, efficient as they are in managing pests, but they can lead to toxic food residues. As shown, organic food pesticide residues are always lower than in conventional food, which means that organic production may lower some of the risks of these chemicals (Brandt, 2007). Issues, such as improper handling in post-harvest activities or poor storage can exacerbate the risk of contamination and spoilage as well. Additionally, environmental impacts of conventional methods of farming, e.g., water source contamination, can lead to long-term impacts on health in addition to short-term food safety (Ngudi et al., 2014). More understanding of these risk factors is necessary in order to formulate effective measures in containing the occurrence of foodborne disease as well as making food systems safer (Figure 9.8).

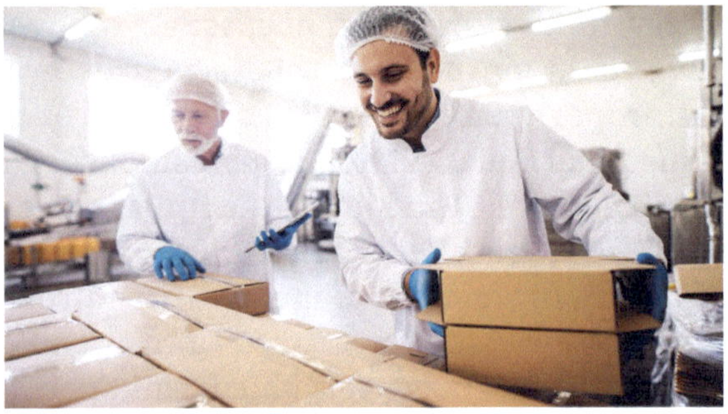

Figure 9.8. Food production is fraught with various risk factors that significantly influence food safety and contribute to the prevalence of food poisoning.

Source: https://goaudits.com/wp-content/uploads/2023/12/HACCP-audits.jpg.

9.2. Symptoms and Diagnosis

A range of symptoms can appear with food poisoning, which can influence how the condition is diagnosed. Typical symptoms are nausea, vomiting, diarrhea and stomach cramps, and they usually start within hours of eating or drinking contaminated food or water. What causes these symptoms often decides how long and how severe they are, which makes it more complicated to diagnose. For instance, while Clostridium difficile can lead to antibiotic-associated diarrhea, it comprises only a fraction of food poisoning cases, necessitating careful differentiation through laboratory testing (Modi & Wilcox, 2001). Also, even though heavy metal poisoning is not common, it adds another challenge. Exposure to toxic elements like cadmium and mercury can present overlapping gastrointestinal symptoms with foodborne illnesses, underscoring the importance of comprehensive diagnostic evaluations (Blundell et al., 2016). It is very important to know the symptoms well for accurate diagnosis and to direct proper treatment in cases of food poisoning.

9.2.1. Common Symptoms of Food Poisoning

Recognizing the common signs of food poisoning allows for fast treatment, which can lessen how much someone is affected. It usually takes hours to days for symptoms to appear after eating or drinking contaminated food or drinks and these symptoms may be nausea, vomiting, diarrhea and abdominal cramps.

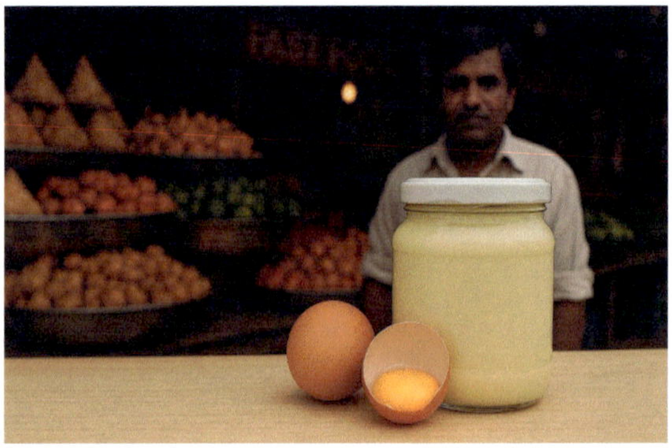

Figure 9.9. The recognition of common symptoms associated with food poisoning is essential for prompt diagnosis and treatment, which can significantly mitigate illness severity.

Source: https://medicircle.in/uploads/2025/april2025/whatsapp_image_2025-04-25_at_17.10.59.jpeg.

When the body is attacked by harmful bacteria, viruses or parasites, these are the symptoms it shows. Notably, infections caused by organisms like *Clostridium perfringens* can mimic food poisoning but may originate from toxic elements related to antibiotic use, emphasizing the complexity of diagnosing these symptoms accurately (Modi & Wilcox, 2001). Moreover, the impacts of food poisoning extend beyond immediate health concerns, as they can disrupt agricultural practices, given the potential links between pest management strategies and food safety (Labarta and Swinton, 2025). Understanding these symptoms enables affected individuals to seek timely medical assistance, ultimately contributing to better public health outcomes (Figure 9.9).

9.2.2. Duration of Symptoms

Variability in the timeline of food poisoning symptoms is contingent on the causative microorganism, underlying health issues, and patient reaction. For instance, whereas symptoms caused by prevalent pathogens like Salmonella resolve after days, others are longer, and it is challenging to diagnose and treat them. Notably, *Clostridium perfringens*, which is a prevalent cause of foodborne illnesses, may induce episodes of diarrhea for over a week and mask the identification of the cause, ultimately affecting recovery interventions (Modi & Wilcox, 2001). Awareness of the timeline of symptoms is beneficial, particularly in heavy metal poisoning, which, as rare as it is, can significantly extend morbidity from continuous exposure (Blundell et al., 2016). Furthermore, awareness of variability in symptomatology timelines allows health professionals to provide early interventions and tailor treatment to the specific foodborne illness, thereby maximizing patient outcomes and public health interventions.

9.2.3. Variability of Symptoms by Pathogen

The symptoms of food poisoning can vary a lot because each pathogen can cause its own set of clinical signs. For instance, *Clostridium perfringens*, known for its rapid proliferation and toxin secretion, may lead to symptoms ranging from mild gastrointestinal distress to severe abdominal cramps and diarrhea, depending on the individual and the strain of the pathogen involved (Cavalieri et al., 2018). Similarly, other pathogens, such as *Vibrio cholerae* and certain strains of *Escherichia coli*, can result in varying degrees of severity in symptoms, occasionally culminating in life-threatening dehydration or systemic infections (Heaviside et al., 2018). Since the symptoms can be different, it is harder to diagnose and treat, so a detailed knowledge of what the pathogen does is essential. Recognizing these differences is critical for timely intervention and can directly influence public health strategies aimed at prevention and education regarding foodborne illnesses (Figure 9.10).

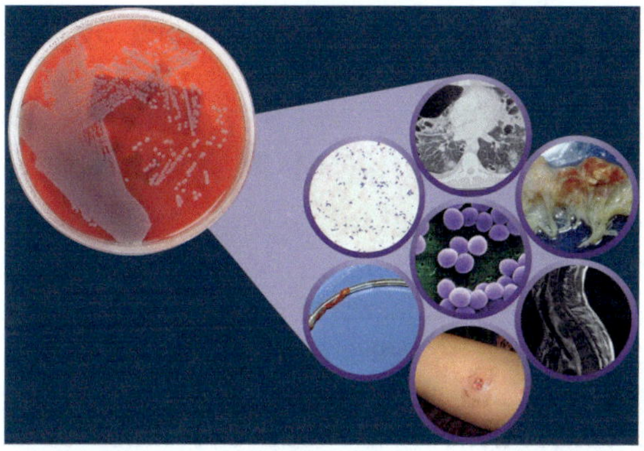

Figure 9.10. The variability of symptoms associated with food poisoning is significantly influenced by the specific pathogens involved, each of, which can elicit distinct clinical manifestations.

Source: https://journals.asm.org/cms/asset/897bde9f-c463-485c-9c07-751e64608e3b/cmr.2015.28.issue-3.largecover.jpg.

9.2.4. Diagnostic Methods Used

Various techniques are used to find food poisoning pathogens, which are key for managing outbreaks. With the help of new molecular methods like PCR-based pulsed-field gel electrophoresis and nucleotide sequencing, it has become easier to spot and describe pathogens involved in foodborne illnesses. For instance, these methods have successfully identified outbreaks caused by Staphylococcus aureus and Enteropathogenic *Escherichia coli* among cooking employees in Chungcheongnam-do, Republic of Korea, revealing the important link between food handlers and illness transmission (Park et al., 2024).

Furthermore, when examining chronic exposure to toxins, traditional approaches underscore the relevance of thorough patient histories and symptomology to diagnose conditions like Dushi Visha, which often elude immediate detection (Pandhare et al., 2024). They help put together a clear picture of food poisoning, which supports actions by public health and prevention.

9.2.5. Importance of Medical History

A person's medical background is important for understanding food poisoning, because it shows what infections they might be more likely to get. If a patient has a pre-existing health condition like a heart or immune problem, the consequences of foodborne illnesses may be more severe, so a detailed medical check-up is important during the diagnosis. Because of this personalized assessment, treatment is adapted to each person, which is very useful as lifestyle-related health problems are becoming more common. Furthermore, understanding an individual's dietary habits and previous instances of food poisoning can reveal patterns that help healthcare providers identify specific sources or types of food that may pose risks, as shown by the advancements in machine learning applications in healthcare for predicting and diagnosing such conditions (Qayyum et al., 2020). In essence, a detailed medical history not only aids in immediate treatment but also informs preventive measures against future occurrences (Figure 9.11).

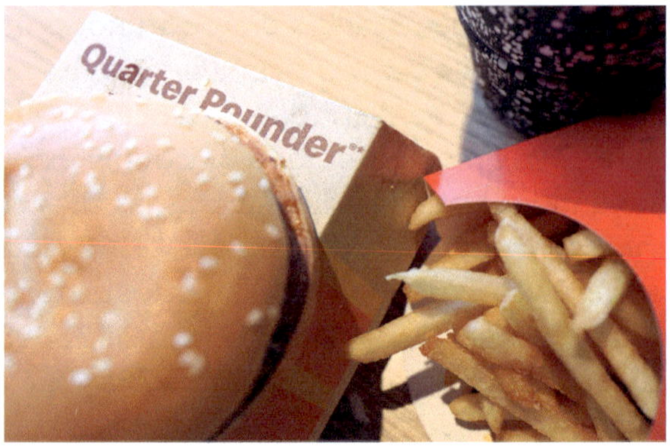

Figure 9.11. An individual's medical history plays a crucial role in understanding food poisoning, as it provides significant insights into predispositions and potential vulnerabilities to various pathogens.

Source: https://platform.vox.com/wp-content/uploads/sites/2/2024/10/gettyimages-2180538535.jpg?quality=90&strip=all&crop=0%2C0%2C100%2C100&w=2400.

9.2.6. Laboratory Tests for Pathogens

The use of laboratory tests for pathogens is also significant in the case of food poisoning, as they are utilized to determine the implicated microorganisms responsible for gastrointestinal illness. In the clinical setting, accurate diagnosis can distinguish among a number of pathogens, i.e., bacteria and viruses, that express a range of symptoms and potential complications. The detection of enterotoxins of *Clostridium perfringens*, for instance, is of specific significance in the diagnosis of antibiotic-associated diarrhea, although tests of this type are not used routinely despite their use in some instances (Modi & Wilcox, 2001).

The IID survey stresses the significance of advanced laboratory data in addressing the high rates of morbidity and mortality of foodborne pathogens and the necessity for improved surveillance systems and research in assessing the overall disease burden (Gauci et al., 2006).

The strengthening of laboratory test protocols, therefore, is essential for public health action against food poisoning.

9.2.7. Differentiating Food Poisoning from Other Illnesses

It is very important to tell food poisoning apart from other illnesses in gastrointestinal cases for the correct diagnosis and care. Common symptoms, such as nausea, vomiting, diarrhea and abdominal pain are found in viral gastroenteritis, pancreatitis and appendicitis, which makes it difficult to assess patients. Doctors need to pay attention to when the symptoms started and how long they last, as food poisoning usually appears shortly after eating, but other conditions may develop more slowly.

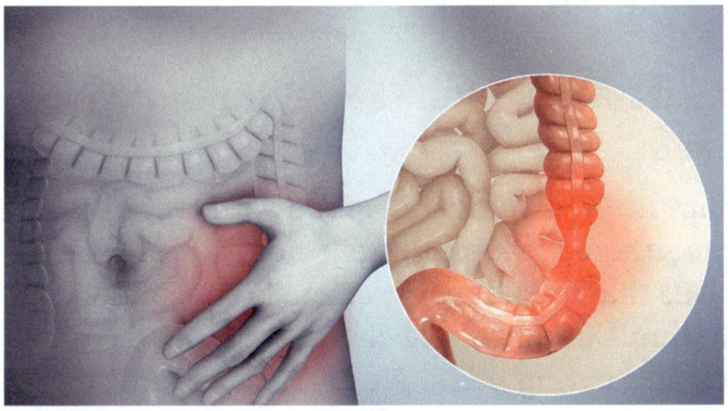

Figure 9.12. Symptoms, such as nausea, vomiting, diarrhea, and abdominal pain overlap significantly with conditions like viral gastroenteritis, pancreatitis, and even appendicitis, complicating clinical assessments.

Source: https://upload.wikimedia.org/wikipedia/commons/thumb/1/1a/Irritable_bowel_syndrome.jpg/1200px-Irritable_bowel_syndrome.jpg

Also, a patients health background and recent meals can be very helpful; for instance, eating undercooked or contaminated food may indicate food poisoning. In addition, understanding these conditions now depends a lot on gut microbiota. Recent studies highlight how alterations in gut flora can influence gastrointestinal health, thereby complicating diagnoses (Cryan et al., 2019). Thus, healthcare providers must evaluate these nuances to effectively differentiate between food poisoning and other gastrointestinal disorders (Yatham et al., 2018) (Figure 9.12).

9.2.8. When to Seek Medical Attention

Knowing when to appear for medical evaluation following the manifestations of food poisoning symptoms is the key to successful treatment and healing. Signs of severe cramping of the abdomen, persistent vomiting, fever, or dehydration are indications for immediate medical evaluation. Complicated cases can lead to impaired functioning of vital organs if not immediately treated, requiring hospitalization for intravenous treatment or other interventions. Moreover, high-risk groups, children six years or younger, older adults, and immunocompromised patients, have a higher risk and need to be closely monitored for exacerbated symptoms. Not only the severity of symptoms, but also their duration, needs to be assessed; symptoms lasting longer than 48 hours need to be evaluated to determine if more serious conditions exist. As healthcare professionals go about developing their treatment plans, they need to carefully monitor patient symptoms and experiences so that intervention can be made on time and the risk of ill effects with long-term implications is avoided (Annandale et al., 2005; Ghosh et al., 2010).

9.2.9. Complications Arising from Food Poisoning

There are other effects from food poisoning besides the usual gastrointestinal problems. A lot of individuals may suffer from lasting health issues, such as the risk of neurodegenerative symptoms, because of the pathogens and toxins present in contaminated food. For instance, the ingestion of high levels of certain chemicals, such as hydrogen sulfide, has been linked to significant brain damage and cognitive deficits, reflecting the need for awareness regarding chemical food safety in both everyday and specialized contexts, such as space missions (Anantharam et al., 2016). Moreover, chemical agents that compromise food safety pose serious public health challenges, necessitating stringent safety protocols to protect consumers from illness (Pier et al., 2025). Understanding these complications is crucial for developing effective interventions and educational strategies to minimize the risks associated with food poisoning and ensure long-term health outcomes for affected individuals (Figure 9.13).

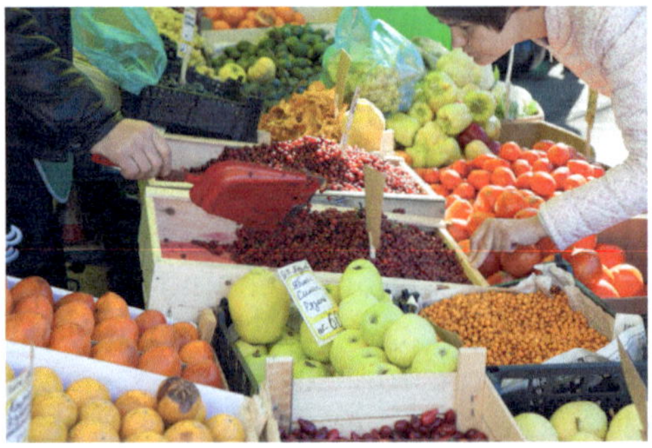

Figure 9.13. Many individuals experience severe long-term health effects, including the risk of neurodegenerative symptoms, which can arise from various pathogens and toxins found in contaminated food.

Source: https://cdn.who.int/media/images/default-source/impact-sheets/food-at-a-market.png?sfvrsn=360f608b_14.

9.3. Treatment and Management

Proper treatment and control of food poisoning are important in reducing the negative health impacts of this condition. First, rehydration is paramount, especially in diarrhea and vomiting conditions, since fluid loss can result in severe dehydration. Oral rehydration solutions or electrolyte beverages are thus usually recommended. In some instances, especially with bacterial causation, antibiotics can be used, although the practice in most cases is dependent on some pathogens involved, as some bacteria worsen conditions if not well-treated. Second, public education on food safety measures is paramount. The adoption of organic farming methods is believed to minimize the occurrence of foodborne diseases through minimal exposure to illicit pesticides and pathogens in conventional farming, leading to improved food safety and better overall public health (Brandt, 2007). Additionally, ongoing neurological research could shed more light on the long-term impact of food poisoning, further guiding treatment procedures (Ngudi et al., 2014).

9.3.1. Home Remedies for Mild Cases

The high number of food poisoning cases encourages people to try home remedies for cases that are not very serious. Some of the usual methods are drinking clear fluids, having ginger tea and eating bland foods, such as toast or rice to help the stomach. Even so, using some folk remedies can slow down recovery; for example, Hispanic people may use traditional remedies that include substances that are harmful. A study highlighted that 8.5% of respondents used Azarcón, a folk remedy associated with lead exposure, linking such practices to increased health risks in children suffering from digestive ailments (Castillo-Couch et al., 2011). Even though home remedies can give quick relief, you should check if they are safe for you. Public awareness of the risks associated with certain traditional treatments is crucial in preventing adverse effects and ensuring that individuals make informed choices in their quest for relief from food-related illnesses (Schultz et al., 2016) (Figure 9.14).

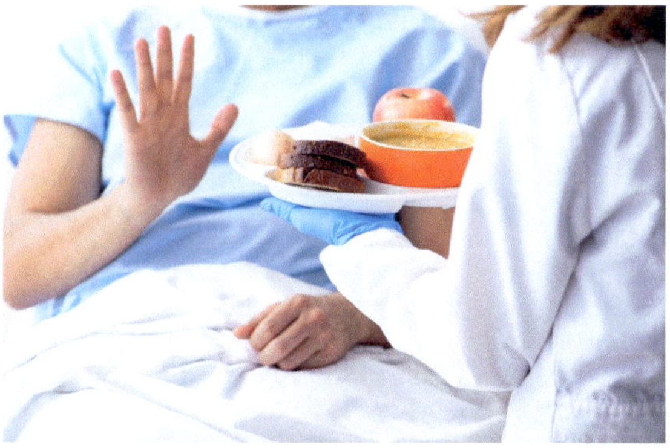

Figure 9.14. Common approaches include hydration with clear fluids, ginger tea, and incorporating bland diets, such as toast or rice to reduce gastrointestinal discomfort.

Source: https://arizonapremiersurgery.com/wp-content/uploads/2023/10/What-To-Eat-After-Hernia-Surgery.jpg.

9.3.2. Importance of Hydration

Hydration is a key element of overall health and is specifically crucial when managing symptoms of food poisoning. Proper fluid intake is essential to avoid dehydration that can worsen gastrointestinal symptoms of foodborne diseases.

When pathogens invade the body, it reacts with dehydration through diarrhea and vomiting, resulting in possible electrolyte and essential nutrient imbalances. Proper hydration comes into play here; it assists in the restoration of fluid balance as well as the natural detoxification processes. Secondarily, awareness of the hydration factor function can reverse oxidative stress, usually elevated during illnesses due to the production of excess harmful free radicals. The synergistic effects of hydration play to maintaining a good defense against food poisoning complications, highlighting the importance of fluid balance during such health emergencies (Raghu et al., 2020; Qaderi et al., 2023).

9.3.3. Over-the-Counter Medications

The role of over-the-counter (OTC) medications in managing symptoms associated with food poisoning cannot be overstated, as these medications can offer relief from discomfort while the gastrointestinal system recovers. People who have foodborne illnesses can use antiemetics, antidiarrheals and pain relievers, which are available over the counter. Even so, people should be careful, as some OTC drugs can hide symptoms that mean a more serious problem needs medical attention. Also, many people are choosing to use OTC drugs because they are easy to get and often prefer them to consulting a doctor. The implications of this behavior are significant, demanding careful consideration of educational initiatives aimed at informing the public about safe medication use, and highlighting the importance of properly managing prescriptions and OTC availability during health crises (Kilgore et al., 2010; Portzky et al., 2019) (Figure 9.15).

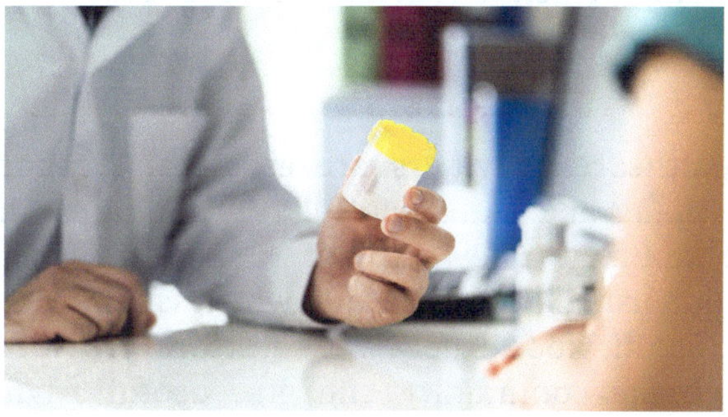

Figure 9.15. The role of over-the-counter (OTC) medications in managing symptoms associated with food poisoning cannot be overstated, as these medications can offer relief from discomfort while the gastrointestinal system recovers.

Source: https://images.ctfassets.net/4f3rgqwzdznj/4adaBuyicadydxRzhGLoA4/68bdebf555d43cbbe01ad88fd1b49d1f/closeup_urine_test_cup_1065782760.jpg.

9.3.4. Prescription Medications for Severe Cases

In severe food poisoning, rational drug prescribing is central to patient outcomes. Some of these include antibiotics in bacterial food poisoning from contaminated food. These can help to relieve symptoms and speed recovery. However, these are not to be overprescribed to prevent resistance from inappropriately prescribed antibiotics, worsening public health challenges. Secondly, drugs for the control of severe gastrointestinal symptoms, such as antiemetics, can relieve symptoms and restore hydration levels. However, practitioners have to be careful and avoid these interventions to prevent side effects. Specifically, in children, drug overdoses by mistake are frequent due to improper storage and incorrect dosing (Bright et al., 2019). Lastly, although prescription medication is effective for controlling severe food poisoning, a balanced approach that ensures effectiveness and safety should be the guiding principle (Portzky et al., 2019).

9.3.5. Role of Healthcare Providers

Healthcare providers are essential for both stopping and managing food poisoning in the community. They explain to patients what foodborne illnesses are and why it is important to handle food safely. If healthcare providers help the community and give useful advice based on research, food poisoning cases can be greatly decreased. In addition, when cases occur, their skills in identifying the specific foodborne pathogen and choosing the right treatment are very important. In light of evolving health technologies, innovative methods, such as the integration of Federated Learning in healthcare can enhance provider capabilities by allowing for the efficient analysis of patient data while safeguarding privacy (Nguyen et al., 2021). Thus, healthcare providers not only address immediate health concerns but also contribute to broader public health strategies aimed at minimizing foodborne illnesses (Perkins et al., 2021) (Figure 9.16).

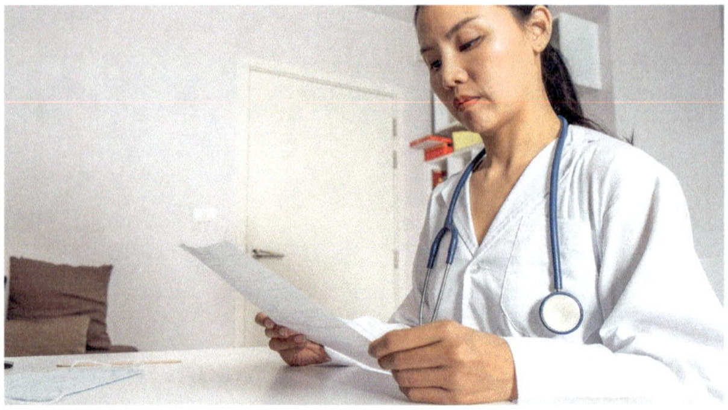

Figure 9.16. In the context of food poisoning, healthcare providers play an indispensable role in both the prevention and management of this public health concern.

Source: https://www.cdc.gov/food-safety/media/images/2024/04/GettyImages-1199201668-final.jpg

9.3.6. Monitoring for Complications

When supervising issues from food poisoning, food safety checks include both regular consumption habits and advanced technologies. Recent advancements, such as diagnostic ultrasonic technology, illustrate a proactive approach to ensuring the integrity of food products, allowing for rapid and nondestructive analysis of plant-based foods, thus enhancing food safety measures (Yan et al., 2024). Also, checking biogenic amines, such as histamine, is a key way to measure how fresh the food is and how much microbial activity it has. The insidious nature, which can remain undetected despite visible freshness, underscores the importance of employing innovative detection methods like molecularly imprinted polymers for accurate monitoring (Ahmed et al., 2024). All these technologies work together to help spot any problems in food safety, so the public remains protected from hidden risks of contaminated foods. With such monitoring, the chance of getting sick from food is greatly reduced.

9.3.7. Dietary Recommendations During Recovery

People recovering from food poisoning must be careful about their nutrition to help their health and avoid further issues. Giving fluids is important at first, since vomiting and diarrhea can result in dehydration. Drinking water, broth and electrolyte solutions are important in the first days after surgery. As patients progress, the reintroduction of easily digestible foods, such as bananas, rice, applesauce, and toast (often referred to as the BRAT diet), can help ease gastrointestinal distress. Also, slowly switching back to a balanced diet with lots of vitamins and minerals helps the immune system and supports recovery. It is also necessary to avoid spicy foods and caffeine, because they can make symptoms worse. Ultimately, understanding dietary needs during recovery not only aids in restoring health but also highlights the connection between nutrition and the body's ability to recover from illnesses, such as food poisoning, effectively (Ngudi et al., 2014; Worth et al., 2014) (Figure 9. 17).

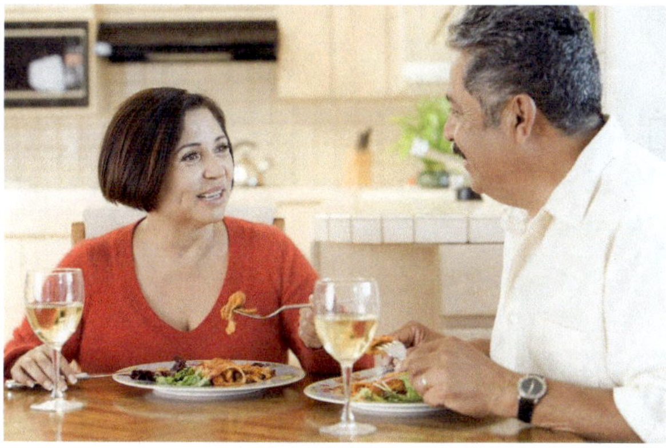

Figure 9.17. Recovery from food poisoning necessitates careful nutritional management to restore health and prevent further complications.

Source: https://www.niddk.nih.gov/-/media/Images/Health-Information/Informacion-de-la-salud/Digestivas/Elderly-Couple-Enjoying-Meal.jpg

9.3.8. Long-Term Effects of Severe Food Poisoning

Long-term effects of severe foodborne illness extend beyond acute gastrointestinal distress and often lead to chronic disease that significantly impairs the quality of life. Survivors may develop post-infectious complications, such as irritable bowel syndrome (IBS), which is a condition characterized by recurrent abdominal pain and altered bowel habits for years following the initial infection. Evidence has demonstrated that some bacterial pathogens induce autoimmune effects, whereby the body's immune system attacks its own tissues and causes disease like reactive arthritis. Psychological effects, such as depression and anxiety, have been reported, and a psychosomatic link between food poisoning trauma and resultant mental illness is implicated. Detection of these long-term effects is of paramount significance in treatment and management protocol design for affected individuals, particularly with regards to compounds, such as hydrogen sulfide, which induces neurodegeneration if exposure is severe and prolonged (Anantharam et al., 2016). The hematological effects of contaminants, such as lead, further underscore the need for cautious monitoring and potential therapeutic intervention following foodborne illness (Ghafari et al., 2007).

9.3.9. Support Resources for Affected Individuals

Having access to support resources is very important for people who have food poisoning. Various organizations provide vital assistance, including medical information hotlines and local health departments (LHDs) that offer guidance on symptoms and treatment options. Support groups in the community can be very helpful for people dealing with the emotional and psychological effects of food poisoning. Policies that help the wider community, such as those discussed in reports on poverty and inequality, can make resources more available to those who need them. For instance, Bergsten et al. (2018) illustrate how systemic issues influence health outcomes, emphasizing the need for comprehensive support frameworks. Co-management strategies in public health could also encourage individuals to speak up for their health, which would strengthen them and help them make wise decisions after an incident of foodborne illness.

A CLOSER LOOK

Diarrhea

Diarrhea is a clinical condition involving loose, watery, or frequent stools, often with accompanying abdominal pain or cramps. Diarrhea has many causes, such as infection (bacterial, viral, or parasitic), intolerance to food, drugs, gastrointestinal illness (, such as IBS or inflammatory bowel disease), or even stress. Food- and water-borne infection, such as Salmonella, E. coli, or Norovirus are common causes of diarrhea. Diarrhea will cause dehydration, especially in vulnerable populations, such as young children, elderly, and immunocompromised. Diarrhea is normally treated with rehydration, either oral rehydration therapy or intravenous fluids in severe cases, along with treatment of the underlying etiology. Diarrhea will most likely resolve on its own, but if symptoms do not abate or are worsening, it is best to consult a doctor.

SUMMARY

The multifaceted nature of food poisoning calls for an integrated response to tackle its impacts on public health. It is important to understand the various channels through, which food poisoning happens, from contaminated agrarian practices to food safety violations, as these are the building blocks of the effective prevention of food poisoning. As emphasized in recent studies, organic farming can successfully avoid exposure to some pathogens and chemical toxins, thus promoting food safety in principle (Brandt, 2007). Moreover, the health impacts of diets are more than the immediate impacts of food poisoning, as in the case of pica disorders, emphasizing the potential risks of the consumption of non-nutritive substances (Lacey et al., 1989). By creating awareness and promoting best practices in production and consumption, society can successfully guard against the risks of foodborne diseases, ensuring food is not only safe but also healthy for all.

In summarizing the major points of the understanding of food poisoning, recognition of the complexity of causes and consequences is required. Food poisoning is mainly caused by pathogens, such as bacteria, viruses, and parasites, which can originate in food at any point from farm to fork. Studies reveal that organic farming can lower some of the dangers from pathogens and toxicants in comparison with conventional farming; however, they can also pose special challenges, such as additional natural plant toxins in some cases (Brandt, 2007). The necessity for stringent controls on food safety cannot be underestimated since such controls are important in preventing outbreaks and protecting public health. Additionally, consumer education on food handling and preparation can lower food poisoning considerably. Up to now, holistic approaches to food safety are thus required in guarding individuals against the adverse health impacts linked with foodborne pathogens (Ngudi et al., 2014).

KEY TERMS FROM THIS CHAPTER

- Mercury
- Natural food toxins
- Oral rehydration solutions
- Parasitic pathogen amplification
- Quantitative standards
- Rice
- Temperature
- Toxic chemicals
- Vomiting
- Wildlife mortality
- Natural antiviral compounds
- Nausea
- Over-the-counter (OTC) medications
- Post-harvest activities
- Resource allocation
- Spicy foods
- Toast
- Toxicants
- Wildlife health

REFERENCES

1. Ackerman, D., Adelman, L., Barney, R., Beardsworth, T., British Broadcasting Association (BBC), Broad, K., Broom, D., et al. (2007). *Swimming with Captive Dolphins: Current Debates and Post-Experience Dissonance.* https://core.ac.uk/download/76897.pdf (accessed on 29 May 2025).
2. Ahmed, S., Ansari, A., Li, Z., Mazumdar, H., Siddiqui, M. A., Khan, A., Ranjan, P., et al. (2024). Point-of-care health diagnostics and food quality monitoring by molecularly imprinted polymers-based histamine sensors. *Advanced Sensor Research, 4.* https://www.semanticscholar.org/paper/220dc2528e5885608e855c92c11873aad5461c35 (accessed on 29 May 2025).
3. Anantharam, P., Poojya, A., Kanthasamy, A., Kim, D. S., Rumbeiha, W., et al. (2016). Acute hydrogen sulfide-induced neuropathology and neurological sequelae: Challenges for translational neuroprotective research. https://core.ac.uk/download/323070853.pdf.
4. Annandale, E., Clark, A. M., Craig, J., Crane, P. B., Daly, J., Dempsey, S. J., Department of Health, et al. (2005). *Women, Men and Coronary Heart Disease: A Review of The Qualitative Literature.* https://core.ac.uk/download/1393936.pdf (accessed on 29 May 2025).
5. Ayaz, M., Uddin, M. A., Sharif, Z., Mansour, A., & Aggoune, E. M. (2019). Internet-of-Things (IoT)-based smart agriculture: Toward making the fields talk. *IEEE Access, 7,* 129551–129583. https://doi.org/10.1109/ACCESS.2019.2932609.
6. Gabriel MW, Woods LW, Wengert GM, Stephenson N, Higley JM, Thompson C, et al. (2015) Patterns of Natural and Human-Caused Mortality Factors of a Rare Forest Carnivore, the Fisher (*Pekania pennanti*) in California. PLoS ONE 10(11): e0140640. https://doi.org/10.1371/journal.pone.0140640Orlando Dickson, Sam Magavern, Alyssa Bergsten, David Clayton, Chad Davenport, Melissa Kathan, Hayley Ross (2018). *Poverty in Buffalo: Causes, Impacts, Solutions.* A Report for the Truth Commission on Poverty in Western New York. https://ppgbuffalo.org/buffalo-commons/library/resource:poverty-in-buffalo-causes-impacts-solutions/#:~:text=Poverty%20in%20Buffalo%2DNiagara%20is,transit%20access%20to%20quality%20jobs. (accessed on 29 May 2025).
7. Blundell, R., & Scicluna, C. (2016). *Heavy Metal Intoxication.* https://core.ac.uk/download/46603934.pdf (accessed on 29 May 2025).
8. Ramsingh B. (2014). The emergence of international food safety standards and guidelines: understanding the current landscape through a historical approach. *Perspectives in public health, 134*(4), 206–215. https://doi.org/10.1177/1757913914536557Brandt, Dr Kirsten (2007) Organic Agriculture and Food Utilization. Paper at: Organic Agriculture and Food Security, FAO, Rome, 3-5 May. (accessed on 29 May 2025).
9. Bright, D., Gauthier, T., Rowland, M., Sanders, C., et al. (2019). *Pediatric Poisoning: Overview, Treatment, And Prevention.* https://core.ac.uk/download/231090577.pdf (accessed on 29 May 2025).
10. Broad Leib, E. M., & Pollans, M. J. (2019). *The New Food Safety.* https://core.ac.uk/download/231832064.pdf (accessed on 29 May 2025).
11. Castillo-Couch, M. (2011). *Identifying and Reducing Lead Exposure Associated with The Use of Cultural Practices in Southern Nevada Hispanic Communities* (Master's thesis, University of Nevada, Las Vegas). https://digitalscholarship.unlv.edu/cgi/viewcontent.cgi?article=2040&context=thesesdissertations (accessed on 29 May 2025).

12. Cavalieri, A. V. G., Colonius, T., Deschamps, C. J., Lajús, R., et al. (2018). *An Update on The Human and Animal Enteric Pathogen Clostridium perfringens*. https://core.ac.uk/download/pdf/196592627.pdf (accessed on 29 May 2025).
13. Ceríaco, L. M. P., Madeira, N. C., Marques, M. P., Mendes, P., et al. (2011). Folklore and traditional ecological knowledge of geckos in Southern Portugal: Implications for conservation and science. https://core.ac.uk/download/pdf/8620514.pdf.
14. Cryan, J. F., O'Riordan, K. J., Cowan, C. S. M., Sandhu, K. V., Bastiaanssen, T. F. S., Boehme, M., Codagnone, M. G., et al. (2019). The microbiota-gut-brain axis. *Physiological Reviews, 99*, 1877–2013. https://doi.org/10.1152/physrev.00018.2018.
15. Foxcroft, N., Masaka, E., & Oosthuizen, J. (2024). Prevalence trends of foodborne pathogens *Bacillus cereus*, non-STEC *Escherichia coli* and *Staphylococcus aureus* in ready-to-eat foods sourced from restaurants, cafés, catering and takeaway food premises. *International Journal of Environmental Research and Public Health, 21*. https://www.semanticscholar.org/paper/c451672e6bbadc4556d2c042b38f307acdd9470d (accessed on 29 May 2025).
16. Gauci, C., Gilles, H. M., Mamo, J., O'Brien, T., et al. (2006). Infectious intestinal disease: Do we know it all? https://core.ac.uk/download/46602090.pdf (accessed on 29 May 2025).
17. Ghafari, S., Golalipour, M. J., Kalavi, K., Kalavi, A., et al. (2007). Effect of lead intoxication and D-penicillamine treatment on hematological indices in rats. https://core.ac.uk/download/52205057.pdf (accessed on 29 May 2025).
18. Ghosh, S., Koch, M., Rao, A. N., Suresh Kumar, R., et al. (2010). Do alternative therapies have a role in autism? https://core.ac.uk/download/pdf/87427.pdf.
19. Hall, C. (2025). Consumer clusters and food safety information needs. https://core.ac.uk/download/pdf/6756806.pdf (accessed on 29 May 2025).
20. Heaviside, C., Lake, I., & Nichols, G. (2018). Climate change and water-related infectious diseases. https://core.ac.uk/download/322490318.pdf (accessed on 29 May 2025).
21. Helldén, D., Andersson, C., Skyvell Nilsson, M., Ebi, K. L., Friberg, P., & Alfvén, T. (2021). Climate change and child health: A scoping review and an expanded conceptual framework. *The Lancet Planetary Health, 5*(3), e164–e175. https://doi.org/10.1016/S2542-5196(20)30274-6.
22. Hou, Z., Xu, B., Liu, L., Yan, R., & Zhang, J. (2024). Isolation, identification, antimicrobial resistance, genotyping, and whole-genome sequencing analysis of *Salmonella Enteritidis* isolated from a food-poisoning incident. *Polish Journal of Microbiology, 73*, 69–89. https://www.semanticscholar.org/paper/8b406c76d10d4da8a4ddc205e76ae0a6896b02c1 (accessed on 29 May 2025).
23. Jaffee, S., Henson, S., Unnevehr, L. J., Grace, D., & Cassou, E. (2018). *The Safe Food Imperative: Accelerating Progress in Low- And Middle-Income Countries*. World Bank eBooks. https://doi.org/10.1596/978-1-4648-1345-0.
24. Kilgore, D., & Najm, W. (2010). Common respiratory diseases. https://core.ac.uk/download/323075715.pdf.
25. Kruk, M. E., Gage, A., Arsenault, C., Jordan, K., Leslie, H. H., Roder-DeWan, S., Adeyi, O., et al. (2018). High-quality health systems in the Sustainable Development Goals era: Time for a revolution. *The Lancet Global Health, 6*(11), e1196–e1252. https://doi.org/10.1016/s2214-109x(18)30386-3.

26. Labarta, R. A., & Swinton, S. M. (2025). Do pesticide hazards to human health and beneficial insects cause or result from IPM adoption? Mixed messages from farmer field schools in Nicaragua. https://core.ac.uk/download/pdf/6429796.pdf (accessed on 29 May 2025).

27. Labuza, T. P., Peck, J., & Szybist, L. M. (2025). Perishable refrigerated products and home practices survey. https://core.ac.uk/download/pdf/7025323.pdf.

28. Lacey, E. P. (1989). Pica: Consideration of a historical and current problem with racial ethnic/cultural overtones. https://core.ac.uk/download/130354166.pdf (accessed on 29 May 2025).

29. Landrigan, P. J., Stegeman, J. J., Fleming, L. E., Allemand, D., Anderson, D. M., Backer, L. C., Brücker-Davis, F., et al. (2020). Human health and ocean pollution. *Annals of Global Health, 86*, 151. https://doi.org/10.5334/aogh.2831.

30. LeBlanc, T. T., Chang, A., Svendsen, E., & Allwood, P. B. (2024). Perspectives on childhood lead exposure prevention: Looking back and looking ahead. *Pediatrics, 154*(Suppl 2). https://www.semanticscholar.org/paper/52277d7b5e3d6b1a1c13f968389460046db992bf (accessed on 29 May 2025).

31. Manyi-Loh, C. E., Mamphweli, S., Meyer, E. L., & Okoh, A. I. (2018). Antibiotic use in agriculture and its consequential resistance in environmental sources: Potential public health implications. *Molecules, 23*(4), 795. https://doi.org/10.3390/molecules23040795.

32. Modi, N., & Wilcox, M. H. (2001). Evidence for antibiotic induced Clostridium perfringens diarrhoea. *Journal of clinical pathology, 54*(10), 748–751. https://doi.org/10.1136/jcp.54.10.748Ncube, F., Kanda, A., Chijokwe, M., Mabaya, G., & Nyamugure, T. (2020). Food safety knowledge, attitudes and practices of restaurant food handlers in a lower-middle-income country. *Food Science & Nutrition, 8*, 1677–1687. https://doi.org/10.1002/fsn3.1454.

33. Neme, K. (2017). Assess sanitary condition and food handling practices of restaurants in Jimma Town, Ethiopia: Implication for food born infection and food intoxication. https://core.ac.uk/download/234684535.pdf (accessed on 29 May 2025).

34. Ngudi, D. D. (2014). *KONZO: The IBRO Africa Regional Committee (ARC) Organizes its first Global Advocacy Workshop for Neuroscience in Kinshasa*. https://core.ac.uk/download/55767487.pdf (accessed on 29 May 2025).

35. Nguyen, D. C., Ding, M., Pathirana, P. N., Seneviratne, A., Li, J., & Poor, H. V. (2021). Federated learning for Internet of Things: A comprehensive survey. *IEEE Communications Surveys & Tutorials, 23*(3), 1622–1658. https://doi.org/10.1109/COMST.2021.3075439.

36. Nile, S. H., Venkidasamy, B., Selvaraj, D., Nile, A., Xiao, J., & Kai, G. (2020). Nanotechnologies in food science: Applications, recent trends, and future perspectives. *Nano-Micro Letters, 12*, Article 45. https://doi.org/10.1007/s40820-020-0383-9.

37. Pandhare, S., & Urade, D. (2024). Understanding Dushi Visha: Chronic poisoning and its management in Agad Tantra. *Sanjeevani Darshan–National Journal of Ayurveda & Yoga*. https://www.semanticscholar.org/paper/1711b6ece2dc33e5560df39ab50def88579f7504 (accessed on 29 May 2025).

38. Park, M. N., Yeo, S. G., Park, J., Jung, Y., & Hwang, S. M. (2024). Usefulness and limitations of PFGE diagnosis and nucleotide sequencing method in the analysis of food poisoning pathogens found in cooking employees. *International Journal of Molecular Sciences, 25*. https://www.semanticscholar.org/paper/2d448a4c7197f6c291e6d11893ca7f18bbd1ed9a (accessed on 29 May 2025).

39. Perkins, G. D., Gräsner, J. T., Semeraro, F., Olasveengen, T. M., Soar, J., Lott, C., Van de Voorde, P., et al. (2021). European Resuscitation Council Guidelines 2021: Executive summary. *Resuscitation, 161*, 1–60. https://doi.org/10.1016/j.resuscitation.2021.02.003.
40. Pier, S. M., & Valentine, J. L. (2025). *Food Safety*. https://core.ac.uk/download/pdf/42887923.pdf (accessed on 29 May 2025).
41. Portzky, G., Rotsaert, I., Van Heeringen, C., & Vancayseele, N. (2019). Medication used in intentional drug overdose in Flanders 2008–2013. https://core.ac.uk/download/287939401.pdf (accessed on 29 May 2025).
42. Qaderi, M. M., Martel, A. B., & Strugnell, C. A. (2023). Environmental factors regulate plant secondary metabolites. *Plants, 12*(3), 447. https://doi.org/10.3390/plants12030447.
43. Qayyum, A., Qadir, J., Bilal, M., & Al-Fuqaha, A. (2020). Secure and robust machine learning for healthcare: A survey. *IEEE Reviews in Biomedical Engineering, 14*, 156–180. https://doi.org/10.1109/RBME.2020.3013489.
44. Raghu, G., Berk, M., Campochiaro, P. A., Jaeschke, H., Marenzi, G., Richeldi, L., Wen, F., et al. (2020). The multifaceted therapeutic role of N-acetylcysteine (NAC) in disorders characterized by oxidative stress. *Current Neuropharmacology, 19*, 1202–1224. https://doi.org/10.2174/1570159x19666201230144109.
45. Regina, G., Jing, L. S., & Hassan, Z. (2021). Food borne disease and the lifestyles of the students and food handlers in rural schools: A preliminary observation. https://core.ac.uk/download/480423510.pdf (accessed on 29 May 2025).
46. Resosudarmo, B. P. (2025). *The Economy-Wide Impact of The Integrated Food Crop Pest Management in Indonesia*. https://core.ac.uk/download/pdf/7010547.pdf (accessed on 29 May 2025).
47. Rogerson, M., & Parry, G. (2020). Blockchain: Case studies in food supply chain visibility. *Supply Chain Management: An International Journal, 25*, 601–614. https://doi.org/10.1108/scm-08-2019-0300.
48. Roxburgh, J. W., & Wong, R. Y. P. (2010). Lasalocid awareness and sampling in Scotland. https://core.ac.uk/download/9025118.pdf (accessed on 29 May 2025).
49. Ruíz-Capillas, C., & Herrero, A. M. (2019). Impact of biogenic amines on food quality and safety. *Foods, 8*(2), 62. https://doi.org/10.3390/foods8020062.
50. Sánchez-Bayo, F. (2021). Indirect effect of pesticides on insects and other arthropods. *Toxics, 9*(8), 177. https://doi.org/10.3390/toxics9080177.
51. Schanes, K., Dobernig, K., & Gözet, B. (2018). Food waste matters—A systematic review of household food waste practices and their policy implications. *Journal of Cleaner Production, 182*, 978–991. https://doi.org/10.1016/j.jclepro.2018.02.030.
52. Schultz, S. (2016). *International Implications of Lead Poisoning in School Aged Children*. https://core.ac.uk/download/48623405.pdf.
53. Seabela, M. D. L. (2020). *Assessment of food safety hazards among day care centres in Mbombela, Republic of South Africa* [University of Johannesburg]. https://ujcontent.uj.ac.za/esploro/outputs/graduate/Assessment-of-food-safety-hazards-among/999735407691#file-0

54. In China, T. W. C. O. T. R. O. C. H. A. D., & Hu, S. S. (2023). Report on cardiovascular health and diseases in China 2021: an updated summary. *Journal of geriatric cardiology : JGC, 20*(6), 399–430. https://doi.org/10.26599/1671-5411.2023.06.001(accessed on 29 May 2025).

55. Wilson, B. A. (2014). *Testing the Message: Making Sense of Converging Multimodal Messages in A Foodborne Illness Outbreak*. https://core.ac.uk/download/232563964.pdf (accessed on 29 May 2025).

56. Worsfold, D. (1994). *An Evaluation of Domestic Food Hygiene and Food Preparation Practices*. https://core.ac.uk/download/161771547.pdf (accessed on 29 May 2025).

57. Worth, G. (2014). *Dairy Calves' Preference for Rearing Substrate*. https://core.ac.uk/download/29202582.pdf (accessed on 29 May 2025).

58. Yan, J., Zhang, Y., Jiao, Z., Song, L., Wang, Z., Zhang, Q., Liu, Y., et al. (2024). Opportunities and challenges of ultrasonic diagnostic techniques for plant-based food monitoring: Principle, machine system, and application strategies. *Critical Reviews in Food Science and Nutrition*. https://www.semanticscholar.org/paper/807d341443dacded407ada8a1745052a84801cab (accessed on 29 May 2025).

59. Yatham, L. N., Kennedy, S. H., Parikh, S. V., Schaffer, A., Bond, D. J., Frey, B. N., Sharma, V., et al. (2018). Canadian Network for Mood and Anxiety Treatments (CANMAT) and International Society for Bipolar Disorders (ISBD) 2018 guidelines for the management of patients with bipolar disorder. *Bipolar Disorders, 20*, 97–170. https://doi.org/10.1111/bdi.12609.

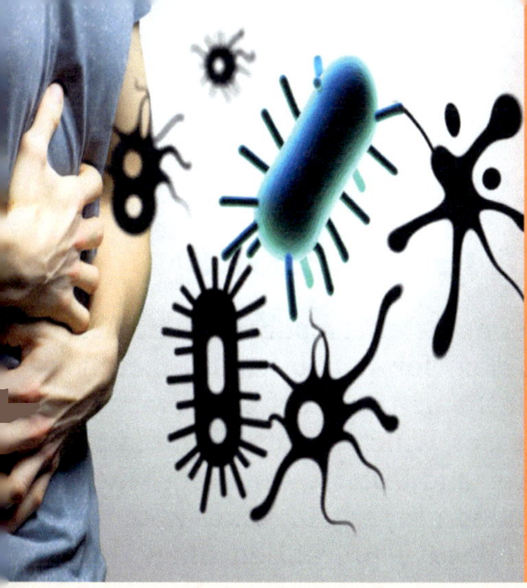

Chapter 10

BACTERIAL AND VIRAL FOODBORNE ILLNESSES

Contents

Introduction........233
10.1. Bacterial Foodborne Illnesses........234
10.2. Viral Foodborne Illnesses........238
10.3. Comparison of Bacterial and Viral Foodborne Illnesses........241
10.4. Public Health and Food Safety Measures........245
Summary........250
References........251

Introduction

Food poisoning is a significant public health risk, with millions of cases each year. These illnesses, which are largely caused by bacteria and viruses, not only worsen an individual's condition but also place a strain on healthcare and economic resources. A weak and mostly incomplete regulatory framework, adding to the complexity of food safety, is overburdened to deal with the vast array of causes for such outbreaks. Current evidence indicates that knowledge of the main causes of foodborne illness and proper prevention measures is crucial to enhancing food safety culture (Levi et al., 2008). In addition, the capacity to assign these diseases to one food vehicle is also of utmost significance; it makes it possible to have targeted interventions and prevention. Through diverse methodologies, ranging from microbial subtyping to case-control studies, scientists can identify the dynamics of foodborne disease (Batz et al., 2025). Thus, there is a call for concerted efforts towards ongoing education as well as stringent regulatory policies for fighting these pervasive health risks.

Importance of Studying Foodborne Pathogens

Foodborne pathogen research is important in ensuring public health and food security. The understanding of foodborne pathogen complexity enables researchers and policymakers to design effective interventions against bacterial and viral infections that could be caused by foodborne pathogen contamination. Analysis of mortality data on human disease caused by foodborne pathogens identifies the locales in the food production chain where intervention is necessary, thus enhancing food safety. Furthermore, with the agricultural ecosystem exposed to constantly changing natural and malicious factors, awareness of the threat of agroterrorism enhances the need for scientists, policymakers, and law enforcement agencies to cooperate to minimize the possibility of food supply chain disruption (Forrest et al., 2020). Ultimately, a holistic approach to foodborne pathogen research not only guarantees the health of the consumers but also guarantees economic security through management of the pervasive effects of foodborne disease (Figure 10.1).

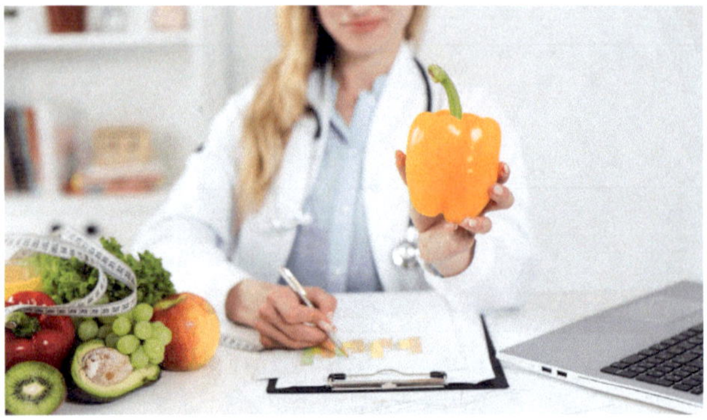

Figure 10.1. The study of foodborne pathogens is vital for safeguarding public health and ensuring food security.

Source: https://www.care-learning.com/images/blogs/detail_ page_ imageb3c0ad454d83a5b634 96cf209 366deecc 4d606fc.png.

10.1. Bacterial Foodborne Illnesses

The high number of bacterial foodborne illnesses is a major problem for public health, mainly because it is difficult to detect and manage them. Such diseases, which are often caused by Salmonella, *E. coli* and Listeria, can occur when food is not handled properly or when water is contaminated. Effective prevention hinges on robust testing and rapid detection protocols that are crucial for identifying pathogenic organisms, as highlighted in Rajapaksha et al. (2018). Also, recognizing the way bacteria can contaminate food means putting in place strong risk management plans throughout the food supply chain. Even though viruses are often in the news for causing food poisoning, bacterial threats are still very important. As food safety experts explain, more stringent control actions need to be applied, and continuous evaluation of existing practice needs to be done in order to guarantee their effectiveness in avoiding risk from bacterial pathogens (Bosch et al., 2018).

10.1.1. Common Bacterial Pathogens (e.g., Salmonella, E. coli)

Among the most prevalent bacterial pathogens responsible for foodborne disease, *Salmonella* and *E. coli* are of greatest importance because of their public health relevance. The pathogens are most likely to infect a variety of food products, such as undercooked meat, unpasteurized milk, and raw fruits and vegetables. The complexity of attributing foodborne disease to their respective causes is underscored by a series of food attribution strategies, which are required for effective intervention strategies (Batz et al., 2025). Findings from case-control studies and outbreak surveillance not only determine the incidence of these pathogens but also inform policymakers on control measures within the food supply chain. It is thus critical to know the transmission dynamics and risk factors of

Salmonella and *E. coli* to apply effective food safety interventions. Further efforts toward improving food safety databases and strategies remain critical in addressing the threats posed by these ubiquitous bacterial pathogens (Figure 10.2).

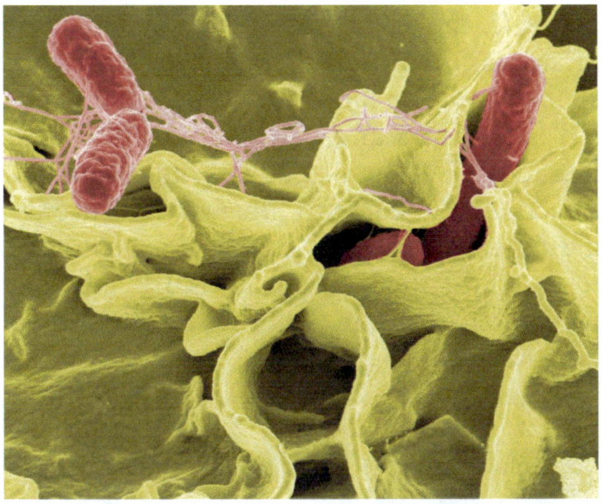

Figure 10.2. Among the most prevalent bacterial pathogens associated with foodborne illnesses, Salmonella and *E. coli* are particularly noteworthy due to their significant public health impact.

Source: https://www.worldatlas.com/r/w1200/upload/a5/a2/ce/916px-salmonellaniaid.jpg

10.1.2. Mechanisms of Bacterial Infection

It is highly important to know about how bacteria infect food because different pathogens have different mechanisms of invading the body. Pathogens, such as Shiga toxin-producing *E. coli*, which also infect fresh produce, have certain virulence factors that allow them to bind to intestinal epithelium and invade (Crowley et al., 2014). It shows how bacteria can survive in many places and also infect humans. These bacteria can remain alive in soil for long periods because of environmental factors that also affect how they enter food and end up in consumers. It is important to know about such factors in detail because food safety policymakers have stated that linking pathogen data along the food chain helps to increase prevention. Better data analysis methods prove highly useful in tracing how these infections happen and responding to them.

10.1.3. Symptoms of Bacterial Foodborne Illnesses

People may show different symptoms of bacterial foodborne illnesses and these usually appear within a few hours to a few days after eating contaminated food. Many times, diarrhea, abdominal pain and vomiting are seen, along with fever and muscle pain, which shows that the infection has spread throughout the body. Studies have found that certain pathogens are more common in the warmer months because hot weather may cause more bacteria to grow in food.

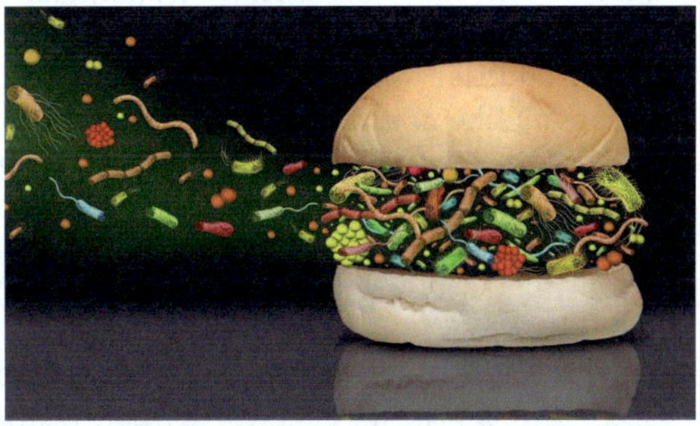

Figure 10.3. The symptoms of bacterial foodborne illnesses can vary widely, typically manifesting within hours to days after consumption of contaminated food.

Source: https://www.carygastro.com/uploads/_1200x720_crop_center-center_100_none/Food-Poisoning.jpg.

Additionally, the severity of symptoms often correlates with the specific bacterial agent involved; for instance, infections caused by Enteroaggregative *Escherichia coli* can lead to profuse diarrhea and dehydration, prompting medical attention (Monarez et al., 2025). Notably, comprehensive surveillance of these symptoms and their association with food-related events is crucial for outbreak prevention, as indicated by recent surveillance findings that emphasize bacterial predominance in cases reported to health authorities (Monarez et al., 2025) (Figure 10.3).

10.1.4. Transmission Routes of Bacterial Pathogens

The routes of transmission of bacterial pathogens are central to the understanding and control of foodborne disease. Shiga toxin-producing *Escherichia coli* (STEC), for instance, highlights the complexity of such routes, considering that the most significant sources vary significantly between regions of the globe. Beef and fresh produce account for the majority of outbreaks in the Americas, whereas contaminated fresh produce is the most significant transmission vehicle in the Western Pacific (Pires et al., 2019). In addition, the zoonotic pathogenesis of pathogens like *E. coli* O157, which is mainly shed by cattle, complicates the control of disease, and an interdisciplinary approach is required to harmonize public and veterinary health interventions (Bonfoh et al., 2013). The occurrence of super shedding events by cattle, particularly those with markers, such as stx2, shows how certain transmission dynamics are able to significantly increase human susceptibility to infection. These findings highlight the importance of focused prevention measures to neutralize the routes along, which such bacterial pathogens are transmitted and influence public health.

10.1.5. Prevention Strategies for Bacterial Infections

It is very important to use effective methods to prevent bacterial infections linked to foodborne illnesses for public health. A main strategy is to have strict food safety regulations in place for food production, processing and distribution. Use of the Hazard Analysis Critical Control Point (HACCP) system is particularly important since it seeks to identify possible hazards along the food chain and implement controls to prevent risks. In addition, public awareness is vital, educating people on how to prepare food properly, store it in the refrigerator and prevent cross-contamination. Recent data indicate a startling rise in foodborne illnesses (FBDs), and hence a need for caution and adherence to food safety procedures (Levi et al., 2008). When regulations and active public health interventions are used simultaneously, the risk of bacterial infection declines and food safety is improved. These strategies are vital in fostering an environment where foodborne pathogens pose less risk to consumers (Figure 10.4).

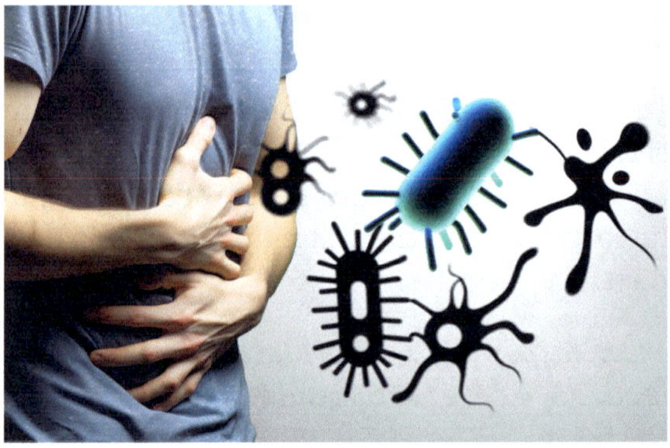

Figure 10.4. Effective prevention strategies for bacterial infections associated with foodborne illnesses are critical to safeguarding public health.

Source: https://www.huankaigroup.com/wp-content/uploads/2024/05/2024051601273414.jpeg.

10.1.6. Treatment Options for Bacterial Foodborne Illnesses

In the management of bacterial foodborne illness, treatment has come a long way to counter the growing risk of antimicrobial resistance. The classical use of antibiotics as first-line therapy has led to excessive use, creating resistant strains and making treatment more difficult, as well as creating learning in the medical community about new methods. One of the areas gaining more attention is bacteriophages, viruses that kill bacteria specifically. This is a promising area of treatment as it could solve the problem of killing bacterial pathogens without adding to the overall problem of antibiotic resistance, as indicated by recent research (Ranveer et al., 2024). Furthermore, the integration of One Health Approach strategies is expected to enhance public health by encouraging intersectoral collaboration to tackle the growing risk of antimicrobial resistance, as evidenced by the high global interest engaged (Tang et al., 2023). Such new treatments have the potential to revolutionize our treatment of bacterial foodborne illness.

10.1.7. Role of Food Safety Regulations

Food safety regulations play a vital part in reducing the risk of bacterial and viral foodborne diseases, since they require food to be produced, processed and distributed under strict health rules. By establishing frameworks for monitoring food safety, regulations promote the use of vital methods, such as microbial subtyping and source-tracking, which help in identifying pathogens and their food vehicles, thereby preventing outbreaks (Batz et al., 2025). Besides, these rules help promote One Health, which highlights how human, animal and environmental health are linked. This perspective is essential to training the next generation of food safety and security professionals because it encompasses a wide range of disciplines necessary for the design of effective foodborne pathogen countermeasures (Angelos et al., 2017). Ultimately, effective food safety regulation not only provides protection of public health but also allows food systems to be sustainable, providing a long-term safe food supply (Figure 10.5).

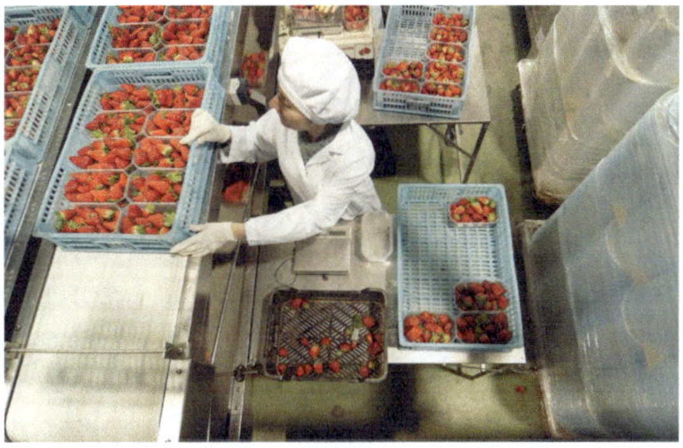

Figure 10.5. The role of food safety regulations is crucial in mitigating the risk of bacterial and viral foodborne illnesses, as these laws are designed to ensure that food production, processing, and distribution adhere to stringent health standards.

Source: https://knowhow.distrelec.com/wp-content/uploads/2024/02/image-13.jpeg.

10.1.8. Future Trends in Bacterial Foodborne Illness Research

The field of bacterial foodborne illness research is ready for major progress because of recent improvements in research techniques and data collection. Future efforts will likely stress using food attribution to identify the sources of outbreaks, which can help improve how risks are evaluated and how to respond to them. The work of the Food Safety Research Consortium highlighted in Batz et al. (2025) underscores the necessity of employing diverse analytical methods, including microbial subtyping and expert judgment, to effectively navigate this complexity. Also, it will be important for people from different fields to team up, as seen in the January 1995 conference, where policymakers and scientists looked at pathogen data from all parts of the food system and found significant gaps in connecting them. Tackling these issues allows researchers to develop policies that lessen the effects of bacterial foodborne illnesses and also make food safety better overall.

10.2. Viral Foodborne Illnesses

Viral foodborne diseases are a major public health issue, unique from those of their bacterial counterparts, with their own mode of transmission and impact. Norovirus and hepatitis A are some of the common viruses that share a common mode of transmission through contaminated water and food, with a focus on food safety from production to consumption. The 1995 food safety conference put into perspective the intricate context of interplay between foodborne pathogens and public health, calling for integrative data to assess risks posed by these viral pathogens. Integrating a One Health approach to pedagogical models can enable the unveiling of the intricate nature of food security, taking into account the environmental aspect of food production as well as health (Angelos et al., 2017). As the trend continues with an increase in the number of viral outbreaks, especially in food service facilities, the strengthening of surveillance and public awareness programs becomes imperative in reducing the risks posed by viral foodborne diseases.

10.2.1. Common Viral Pathogens (e.g., Norovirus, Hepatitis A)

Norovirus and Hepatitis A, which are viral pathogens, are now more often mentioned in talks about foodborne illnesses. Norovirus, which is responsible for many cases of gastroenteritis, is very contagious and can be spread by eating or drinking contaminated things or by touching someone who has it. Its ability to persist in the environment poses substantial public health challenges, especially in settings with high food handler turnover (Radin, 2014). Hepatitis A, on the other hand, is primarily spread through fecal-oral routes, often linked to contaminated fruits and vegetables that have been compromised at any stage of the supply chain (Dragoslava, 2012). People buying more fresh fruit and vegetables is linked to the rise in viral outbreaks, as these can be carriers of the pathogens. Consequently, understanding and mitigating these risks is crucial for effective food safety practices (Figure 10.6).

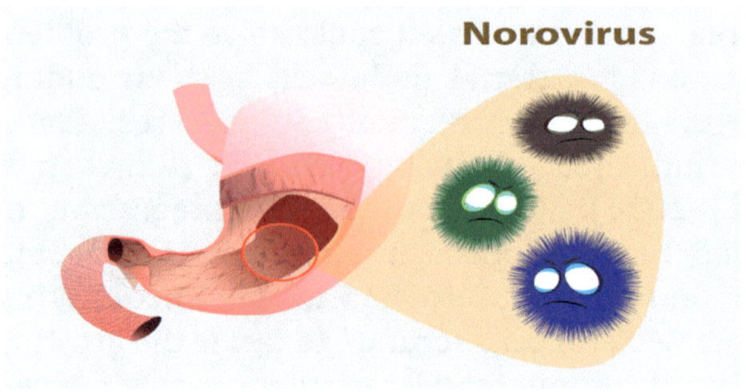

Figure 10.6. Norovirus, a leading cause of gastroenteritis, is notorious for its high contagion rates and can be transmitted through contaminated food, water, or direct contact with infected individuals.

Source: https://acko-cms.ackoassets.com/Norovirus_597df8efc2.png.

10.2.2. Mechanisms of Viral Infection

The viral infection processes are core to foodborne illness due to the presence of viruses that can contaminate food products. Viruses, such as noroviruses and hepatitis A have the ability to bind to food surfaces and resist standard washing procedures used in food service outlets. Past research has found that certain sanitation procedures are core to reducing viral contamination on fruits and vegetables, but are ineffective in a random manner. For instance, evaluations of aqueous ozone treatments have found inconsistent effectiveness in inactivating viruses, such as murine norovirus and their corresponding bacteria on surfaces, such as lettuce and stainless steel (Dawley et al., 2018). This is as much a product of the complexity of viral interaction with food matrices as the need to embrace holistic food safety standards to prevent risk in the food chain. The scientific study of such processes is most essential in delivering interventions that may reach and effectively stop viral transmission in foodborne illness.

10.2.3. Symptoms of Viral Foodborne Illnesses

Viral foodborne illness is an acute public health issue, with a variety of symptoms of varying severity. Characteristic symptoms are gastrointestinal, including nausea, vomiting, diarrhea, and abdominal pain, with fever and malaise as well. Symptoms typically progress within hours of ingesting contaminated water or food, noting the rapid onset, in contrast to certain bacterial illnesses.

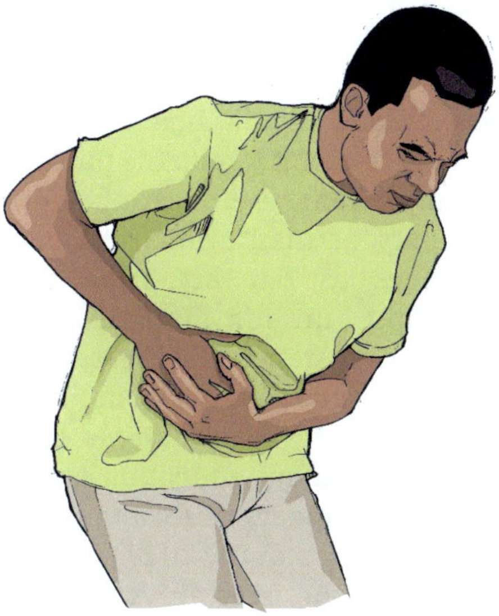

Figure 10.7. Common manifestations include gastrointestinal distress, such as nausea, vomiting, diarrhea, and abdominal cramps, often accompanied by fever and malaise.

Source: https://upload.wikimedia.org/wikipedia/commons/8/8f/Symptoms-stomach-pain.jpg

As viruses are the most frequent cause of foodborne illness in industrialized countries, detection and reporting are critical in order to be able to control the outbreaks effectively. In addition, inefficiencies within the regulatory system hinder surveillance and response to these illnesses, with under-reporting and potentially increased health effects (Levi et al., 2008). The substantial economic impact of infectious intestinal disease reinforces the need for large population-based studies to quantify these diseases and improve public health response (Gauci et al., 2006) (Figure 10.7).

10.2.4. Transmission Routes of Viral Pathogens

How viral pathogens are spread through food causes many public health problems. They can be spread through contaminated food, water and surfaces, which is why it's important to keep hygiene high throughout all food handling and eating. Notably, zoonotic pathogens contribute to this complexity, as over 60% of human pathogens have origins in animals, which amplifies the risk posed by poor sanitation and environmental management, particularly in developing regions like Laos, where evidence of foodborne contaminants is scarce (Thompson et al., 2024). Factors, such as climate change and urbanization further exacerbate these transmission routes, facilitating the emergence and spread of new viral diseases that can have devastating effects on human health, as seen with the COVID-19 pandemic, which highlights the urgent need for interdisciplinary approaches like One Health to mitigate risks associated with zoonotic transmissions (Rahman et al., 2020).

10.2.5. Prevention Strategies for Viral Infections

Stopping viral infections linked to food, including those causing foodborne illnesses, needs a combination of public health actions and personal cleanliness. Some effective steps are strict food safety rules, better cleaning at food production and handling and informing the public about how viruses are spread. For example, applying the HACCP system can greatly reduce risks during all parts of food production, from making to eating. It is also important to keep researching and collecting data to spot new viruses and study their spread in the food chain, as recent work on foodborne pathogens and data integration has stressed. Ultimately, a coordinated effort among policymakers, scientists, and the community is essential for tackling the complex landscape of viral foodborne illnesses and ensuring food safety (Levi et al., 2008) (Figure 10.8).

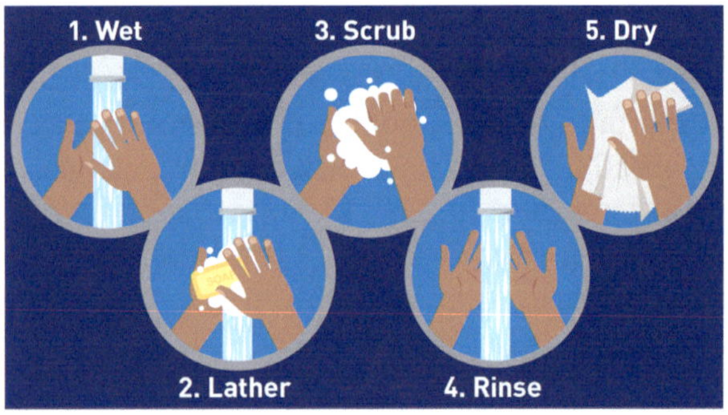

Figure 10.8. Effective measures include the implementation of stringent food safety protocols, enhanced sanitation practices in food production and handling, and robust public education campaigns promoting awareness of viral transmission.

Source: https://www.fda.gov/files/Handwashing-Food-Safety_11072023.png

10.2.6. Treatment Options for Viral Foodborne Illnesses

Proper management of viral foodborne disease is generally supportive, given that most viral infections are self-limiting. Fluid replacement is ensured by the intake of clear fluids to replenish lost fluid from vomiting or diarrhea, which are characteristic symptoms of diseases, such as norovirus infection. Even though antiviral medication is effective in controlling some viral causatives, such an application is limited in foodborne disease. Furthermore, emerging technologies, such as 3D food printing, are being explored to enhance food safety processes, such as the transfer of pathogens from food contact equipment to food products (Hamilton et al., 2024). Compliance with rigorous cleaning procedures and HACCP is now obligatory in the avoidance of viral contamination of food preparation. With food safety legislation still under development, knowledge of the treatment modalities as well as the preventive measures can be highly useful in attenuating the virulence of viral foodborne illness.

10.2.7. Role of Food Safety Regulations

Because of food safety regulations, the risk of bacterial and viral foodborne illnesses is greatly reduced, as they outline the necessary rules for food production, handling and distribution. Food regulations help companies use safe practices, which keep the public healthy. Having comprehensive educational programs on food safety at institutions can encourage food handlers to pay attention to safety, which is important for maintaining proper procedures. For instance, the Western Institute for Food Safety and Security emphasizes the importance of integrating diverse disciplines to enhance food safety education and address environmental impacts associated with food production (Angelos et al., 2017). Also, finding and focusing on the best prevention methods helps reveal where foodborne pathogens come from. Techniques, such as food attribution methodologies and outbreak analyses contribute to a proactive risk-based approach in the U.S., ultimately enhancing regulatory effectiveness (Batz et al., 2025) (Figure 10.9).

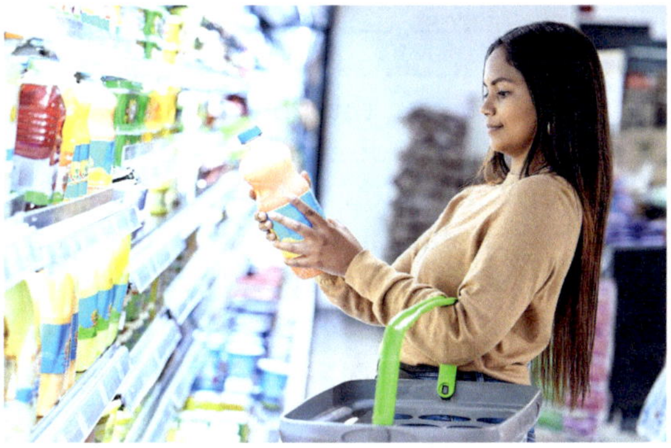

Figure 10.9. Regulations ensure that food businesses adopt best practices to limit contamination, thereby protecting public health.

Source: https://www.ficsi.in/blog/wp-content/uploads/2024/05/Blog-4-7.jpg.

10.2.8. Future Trends in Viral Foodborne Illness Research

As viral foodborne disease research continues, several significant trends are beginning to emerge that hold potential for increasing our understanding and control of these public health threats. One of the most significant research areas is the development of more sophisticated means of food attribution, which are needed to detect the specific food vehicles involved in outbreaks. These are combined microbial subtyping and source-tracking techniques that allow for more effective surveillance of foodborne viruses (Batz et al., 2025).

Along with this, an interdisciplinary approach is increasingly being demanded, as this allows for collaboration among scientists and policymakers in the study of the economic impact of changes in food production practices on the risk of disease. These collaborations can make risk assessment tools more accurate and enhance food safety approaches, directly addressing the economic impact of foodborne disease. All in all, these trends are a step toward more effective and integrated control strategies in viral foodborne disease.

10.3. Comparison of Bacterial and Viral Foodborne Illnesses

It is important to distinguish between bacterial and viral foodborne illnesses when planning food safety measures. Foods that are not handled properly can contain bacteria like Salmonella and *Escherichia coli*, which can multiply in suitable environments and cause more serious or lasting health problems. Unlike other pathogens, viruses like norovirus and hepatitis A usually need fewer of the pathogens to infect a person and they can easily spread through contaminated food or surfaces, which makes it difficult to control outbreaks. It is very important to monitor and assign foodborne illnesses to find out what pathogens are responsible and put preventative measures in place. Tools, such as outbreak surveillance and case-control studies have been employed to enhance our understanding of these pathogenic impacts across the food chain, as highlighted in discussions surrounding food attribution data (Batz et al., 2025) and the need for a multidisciplinary approach to improve data on food safety. A thorough analysis of the causes can eventually help reduce the occurrence of FBDs.

10.3.1. Differences in Pathogen Structure and Function

Differences in how bacteria and viruses are built and function must be understood when studying foodborne illnesses. Because bacteria are unicellular, they have a firm cell wall and multiply by dividing in two, which allows them to increase their numbers quickly in good conditions. Unlike bacteria, viruses do not have cells and depend on host cells for reproduction, which can damage the cells and cause disease. Because of this difference, bacteria can either release toxins or stick to host tissues to cause harm, whereas viruses get inside host cells to take over their metabolism, which affects normal cell functions. The way pathogens and agriculture interact also makes it more difficult for public health to respond effectively. For instance, agricultural intensification increases interactions between humans, animals, and pathogens, and therefore risk for zoonotic disease (Rohr et al., 2019). Such nuances point towards the importance of targeted preventive action to counter the unique challenges of bacterial and viral foodborne pathogens (Landrigan et al., 2020) (Figure 10.10).

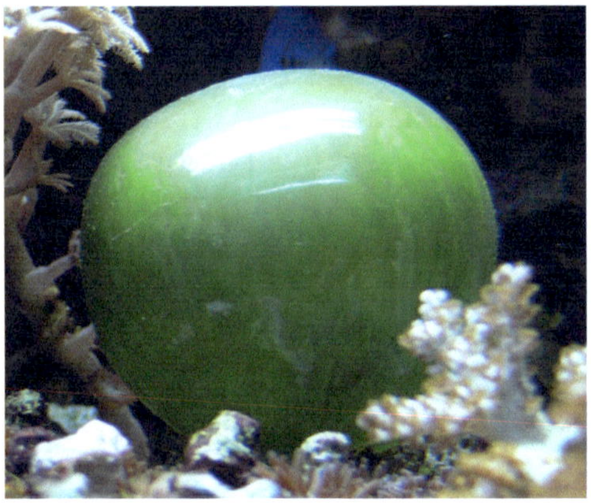

Figure 10.10. Bacteria, as unicellular organisms, possess a rigid cell wall and replicate independently through binary fission, allowing rapid population increases in favorable environments.

Source: https://upload.wikimedia.org/wikipedia/commons/3/3d/Ventricaria_ventricosa.JPG.

10.3.2. Variations in Symptoms and Severity

The variability in symptoms and severity of bacterial and viral foodborne illnesses is due to a number of different factors, such as the pathogen type, dose of exposure, and host. Such pathogens as *Coxiella burnetii*, the etiologic agent of Q fever, are a case in point, with clinical presentation ranging from mild flu-like illness to severe respiratory distress, depending on the prevailing strain and the patient's health status (Eldin et al., 2016). Moreover, the immunocompromised host has a high probability of developing a more severe infection, and therefore, the is a need for urgent and accurate diagnostics. Other bacterial pathogens can produce gastrointestinal symptoms of highly disparate intensities, which represent the dynamic interactions of the pathogens with hosts. These variations necessitate an understanding of the underlying mechanisms of each pathogen, as prevailing in guidance documents, in order to permit healthcare professionals to select the right diagnostic tests according to symptom profiles (Miller et al., 2018). An appreciation of the heterogeneity in clinical presentations is therefore critical to effective management and treatment strategies.

10.3.3. Distinct Transmission Methods

It is important to know how bacterial and viral foodborne illnesses are transmitted to handle food safety issues well. They may be spread through water that is not clean, food that is not properly handled and when food is prepared in an unsafe way. As an illustration, Norovirus is usually spread from one person to another or by using contaminated surfaces and Salmonella is commonly linked to eating poultry or eggs that have not been cooked thoroughly. Finding out these unique pathways is very important, since it helps with interventions that reduce risks. As highlighted in recent discussions surrounding food attribution methodologies, effective food safety interventions require a detailed analysis of, which specific food vehicles contribute to outbreaks (Batz et al., 2025). Moreover, the examination of data from different points in the food chain emphasizes the need for a comprehensive understanding of how pathogens propagate, facilitating the development of robust policies geared toward reducing foodborne illness (Figure 10.11).

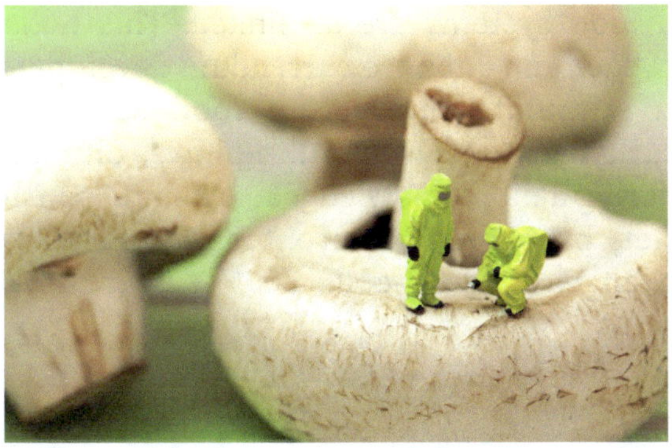

Figure 10.11. Understanding the distinct transmission methods of bacterial and viral foodborne illnesses is essential for effectively addressing food safety concerns.

Source: https://www.hawaiipacifichealth.org/media/10431/6-common-foodborne-illnesses-how-to-prevent-them-web.jpg.

10.3.4. Differences in Prevention Strategies

To bridge the gap in prevention measures for bacterial and viral foodborne illnesses, it is important to understand the various approaches employed to reduce risks associated with each category of pathogens. Bacterial pathogens are likely to demand aggressive intervention measures, such as the application of HACCP systems, which aim at identifying and controlling the critical points during food manufacturing and processing to prevent contamination. Viral foodborne illnesses, which are likely to be more challenging to monitor and attribute to food vehicles, rely on large-scale surveillance networks and outbreak studies. Case-control studies and microbial subtyping are critical in the determination of sources of viral contamination (Batz et al., 2025). The difference in these prevention measures reflects the complexity of food safety management because proper strategies need to be tailored to the specific nature of each category of pathogens in an effort to enhance public health gains.

10.3.5. Treatment Approaches for Bacterial vs. Viral Infections

Bacterial and viral infections are treated differently because they are not the same biologically. Antibiotics are usually given to fight bacterial infections by targeting certain functions or parts of the bacteria, which stops their growth or kills them. Unlike bacteria, viruses use the host's cells to replicate, so antibiotics are not effective and antiviral medicines are used to stop the virus from entering or replicating inside the host. This distinction highlights the importance of accurate diagnosis, as misapplication of antibiotics can lead to resistance, complicating treatment efforts (Rajapaksha et al., 2018). Also, zoonotic diseases, which spread from animals to humans, highlight the importance of strong surveillance systems to detect and address them quickly. As noted, the emergence of zoonotic pathogens underscores the importance of implementing comprehensive One Health strategies for effective management and prevention (Rahman et al., 2020). Each treatment modality thus reflects the necessity for tailored public health responses in combating foodborne illnesses (Figure 10.12).

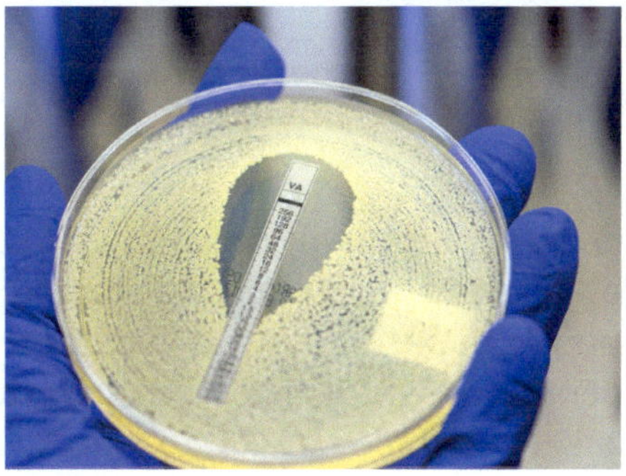

Figure 10.12. Bacterial infections are typically addressed with antibiotics, which target specific bacterial functions or structures, thereby halting their growth or killing them outright.

Source: https://static.scientificamerican.com/sciam/cache/file/D2EB299D-B8C9-45F7-A162FD6DB47FC91F_source.jpg?crop=4%3A3%2Csmart&w=1200.

10.3.6. Public Health Responses to Outbreaks

Effective public health interventions against foodborne bacterial and viral disease outbreaks are needed to control their impact on community health. Such interventions are usually backed by robust surveillance systems made up of local laboratories, which are tasked with the identification and tracing of pathogens. However, the problem is that few enteric infection cases are tested using stool sample testing, hence the need for additional laboratory practice and notification systems in order to maximize response efficiency (Gauci et al., 2007). Additionally, risk assessment tools like the Foodborne Illness Risk Ranking Model (FIRRM) can greatly help public health officials by ranking interventions in order to quantify the social burden of various foodborne pathogens. FIRRM not only gives an approximation of attributable illnesses and costs but also gives evidence-based strategies to decision-making and resource allocation in public health interventions (Batz et al. (2025). Hence, an integrated approach that combines laboratory information and risk assessment tools is needed in responding to foodborne outbreaks.

10.3.7. Role of Education in Prevention

Education is important for preventing foodborne illnesses caused by bacteria and viruses by helping people see risks and act safely. When people are informed, they can do a lot to reduce the effects of foodborne diseases, which are usually made worse by poor hygiene and incorrect food handling. As highlighted in recent findings, the current U.S. food safety regulatory system is perceived as ineffective, necessitating comprehensive educational initiatives to address the public's awareness and understanding of food safety issues (Levi et al., 2008). Also, using a One Health approach in education stresses how health, the environment and food systems are all linked. This holistic approach can enhance curriculum development and stimulate interest in food safety and security across various disciplines, ultimately fostering a more knowledgeable and responsible society prepared to confront foodborne disease challenges (Angelos et al., 2017) (Figure 10.13).

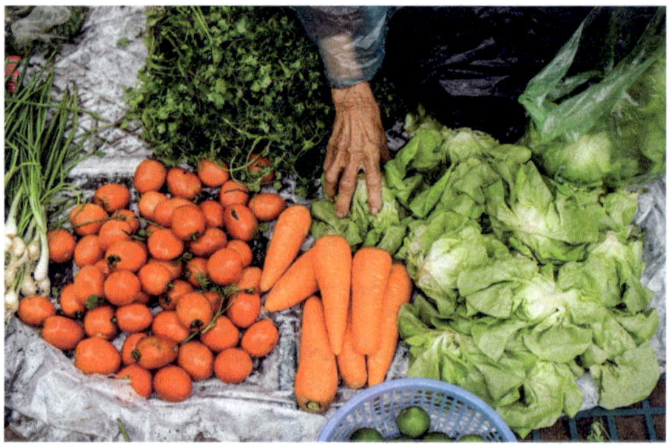

Figure 10.13. An informed populace can significantly mitigate the impact of foodborne diseases, which are often exacerbated by poor hygiene and inadequate food handling procedures.

Source: https://www.who.int/images/default-source/who-campaigns/world-food-safety-day-2021/who_061147.jpg?sfvrsn=fa8fd738_7.

10.3.8. Future Research Directions in Foodborne Illnesses

Appreciation of the complexities of foodborne disease requires a robust framework for future research agendas. At the core of the agenda is the development of novel food attribution techniques that are capable of tracing pathogens to their respective food sources, as discussed in previous arguments for policymaking and action on food safety based on precise food attribution information (Batz et al. (2025). Moreover, a multi-disciplinary framework is necessary to investigate the farm-to-plate life cycle of foodborne pathogens, with particular emphasis on filling pathogen information gaps along the food supply chain. Through an interdisciplinary partnership among scientists, policymakers, and industry leaders, future research can be optimized to drive analytical tools to examine the impact of emerging food production and consumption patterns. This strategic focus not only aims to reduce threats of bacterial and viral foodborne disease but also to enhance our general knowledge of food safety in an evolving world.

10.4. Public Health and Food Safety Measures

Dealing with public health and food safety is very important in fighting bacterial and viral foodborne illnesses since they affect health worldwide. Since FBDs affect about 600 million people every year, strict food safety measures are needed to look after consumers and support public health. Every country needs to establish complete food control systems by using strict rules, thorough checks and constant monitoring of food items. These systems are pivotal in mitigating risks associated with food contaminants, particularly in vulnerable regions, where compliance with international standards is increasingly demanded for trade (Landrigan et al., 2020). Since ocean pollution is now a major risk to marine food, understanding and controlling its health effects is very important. Pollution not only compromises food safety but also exacerbates the prevalence of harmful pathogens, further emphasizing the need for integrated public health strategies to safeguard food safety and public health (Landrigan et al., 2020).

10.4.1. Role of Government Agencies in Food Safety

The government agency's role in food safety is pivotal in decreasing the incidence of bacterial and viral foodborne diseases. Government agencies, such as the Food and Drug Administration (FDA) and the United States Department of Agriculture (USDA), have a responsibility to design regulatory systems that ensure the safety of the food supply. A flawed regulatory system has been identified as one of the most critical issues in U.S. food safety, and this results in escalated threats of FBDs, which emphasizes the necessity of stringent regulations and on-time inspections (Levi et al., 2008). Besides this, interdisciplinary collaboration between scientists and policymakers is instrumental in enhancing food safety practices. Interdisciplinary collaboration, as represented through conferences examining key data and pathogen transmission along the food supply chain, facilitates informed decision-making. Such an effort can prove instrumental in averting the spread of outbreaks, making food safety standards conform to the evolving public health needs (Figure 10.14).

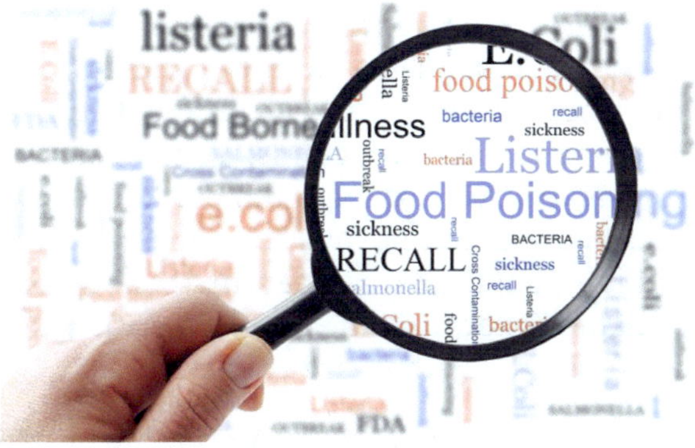

Figure 10.14. The role of government agencies in food safety is pivotal in mitigating the incidence of bacterial and viral foodborne illnesses.

Source: https://www.fda.gov/files/styles/landscape_16_9_800_x_450/public/Outbreaks%20of%20Foodborne%20Illness.jpg?itok=m1NlF8q1

10.4.2. Importance of Food Handling Practices

Proper food handling is very important for preventing illnesses caused by bacteria and viruses. Good food handling plays a big role in preventing contamination at every part of the food supply chain.

A well-regulated approach improves food safety and addresses significant public health concerns stemming from improper practices, as highlighted by Levi et al. (2008). Also, important food safety measures, such as the HACCP system encourage taking steps to prevent illness by identifying and controlling risks early. If food is not handled correctly, the risk of outbreaks rises, which can be very dangerous for people who eat the food. So, improving food safety education can greatly reduce the number of FBDs and help keep the public healthy.

10.4.3. Education and Awareness Campaigns

Spreading knowledge and awareness is very important for preventing bacterial and viral illnesses in food. They help the public learn about food safety and encourage them to take steps to stop infections. For example, a study shows that although almost half of U.S. adults know about noroviruses, many still do not understand how to prevent their spread, especially by not realizing that fecal-oral routes are the main way they are transmitted.

Even with many food safety educational resources, most only talk about bacteria and not viruses like norovirus, which shows that we need to develop educational programs that cover all types of foodborne pathogens. Additionally, research indicates that implementing policies that incorporate a One Health approach, integrating human, animal, and environmental health, can significantly strengthen awareness and response efforts to foodborne illnesses across diverse populations (Dar et al., 2016) (Figure 10.15).

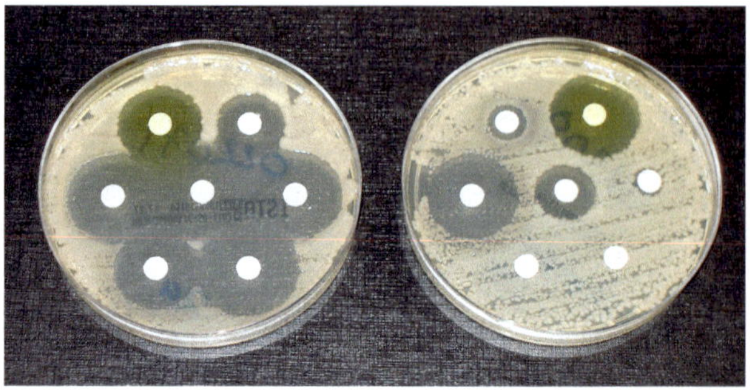

Figure 10.15. Effective education and awareness campaigns are critical components in combating bacterial and viral foodborne illnesses.

Source: https://upload.wikimedia.org/wikipedia/commons/a/ab/Antibiotic_sensitivity_and_resistance.jpg.

10.4.4. Surveillance and Monitoring of Foodborne Illnesses

Surveillance and monitoring of foodborne disease are critical components of public health interventions to minimize the impact of bacterial and viral pathogens. Development of an effective surveillance system facilitates early detection of outbreaks, a prerequisite for controlling the spread of FBDs. For instance, an integrated One Health system incorporating the interdependence of human, animal, and environmental health is increasingly promoted as an efficient approach to disease management, particularly in zoonosis, where over 60% of human pathogens have animal sources (Rahman et al., 2020). Furthermore, the evidence gathered using the National Outbreak Reporting System also confirms the necessity of monitoring drinking water quality, as evidenced by reported 2013–2014 outbreaks that emphasized the potential of contaminants to generate severe health impacts (Benedict et al., 2017). Enhanced surveillance methods not only facilitate timely public health response but also facilitate evidence-based policymaking that averts future foodborne disease outbreaks.

10.4.5. Role of Technology in Food Safety

Technology plays a bigger role now in making food safer, mainly by addressing the dangers of bacterial and viral foodborne diseases. With the use of blockchain and other advanced systems to monitor food supply chains, stakeholders can make sure there is more transparency and accountability, which helps prevent food contamination.

New technologies, for example, rapid pathogen detection kits and biosensors, allow foodborne pathogens to be identified quickly, which helps with prompt recalls and reduces the risk to public health. In addition, with more people to feed, using smart farming technologies can assist in managing resources and lower the chances of zoonotic diseases linked to food production. The interconnectedness of agro-ecosystems and human health underscores the essential role of technology in safeguarding food safety and addressing the emerging challenges posed by infectious diseases associated with food consumption (Rohr et al., 2019; Landrigan et al., 2020) (Figure 10.16).

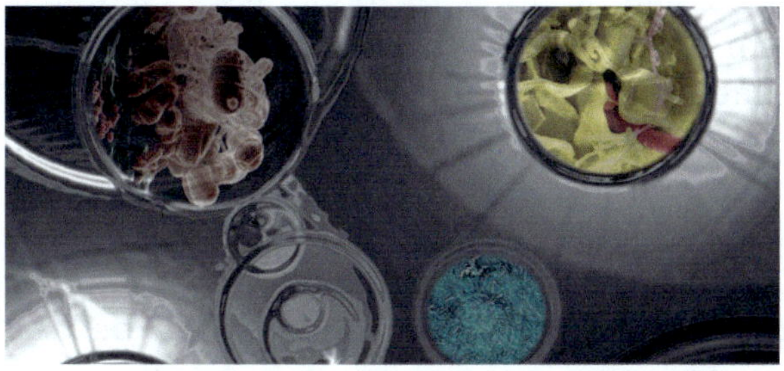

Figure 10.16. The role of technology in enhancing food safety is increasingly critical, particularly in mitigating the risks associated with bacterial and viral foodborne illnesses.

Source: https://www.food-safety.com/ext/resources/fsm/cache/file/9C34EAE8-D750-440F-8900B3039BF729C9.jpg?1611013788.

10.4.6. International Collaboration on Food Safety

International cooperation in food safety is a leading force in addressing the rising challenges of viral and bacterial foodborne disease in the world. With growing globalization, transportation of food across borders substantially increases the potential for foodborne disease outbreaks to be spread globally. To address these effectively, countries should harmonize food safety practices, improve information exchange, and facilitate capacity building in developing nations. Initiatives, such as the Food Safety Modernization Act (FSMA) clearly reflect the efficiency of interagency coordination and surveillance in the context that effective surveillance structures are essential to identification and response to FBDs. Research further confirms that more coordination can improve foodborne disease surveillance and strengthen the response system between countries (Levi et al., 2008). In summary, the creation of international cooperation not only advances food safety but also ensures public health globally.

10.4.7. Impact of Foodborne Illness on Healthcare Systems

Foodborne illnesses put a lot of strain on healthcare systems because they cause both obvious and hidden effects that make it hard for public health to function well. In the US, FBDs are responsible for a huge number of illnesses, many hospitalizations and many deaths, which greatly overwhelm healthcare services and facilities. For instance, the establishment of the event-based surveillance (EBS) system during EXPO Milan highlights the necessity for proactive measures to monitor and manage potential outbreaks, emphasizing the evolving landscape of infectious disease surveillance in response to mass gatherings (Bastiampillai et al., 2016). Furthermore, the role of specialized centers, such as the National Center for Emerging and Zoonotic Infectious Diseases (NCEZID), underscores the importance of collaboration and expertise in addressing both common and rare foodborne illnesses within the healthcare system (National Center for Emerging and Zoonotic Infectious Diseases, 2025). Consequently, the pervasive challenge of FBDs necessitates ongoing investment in prevention and education to alleviate overwhelming healthcare burdens (Figure 10.17).

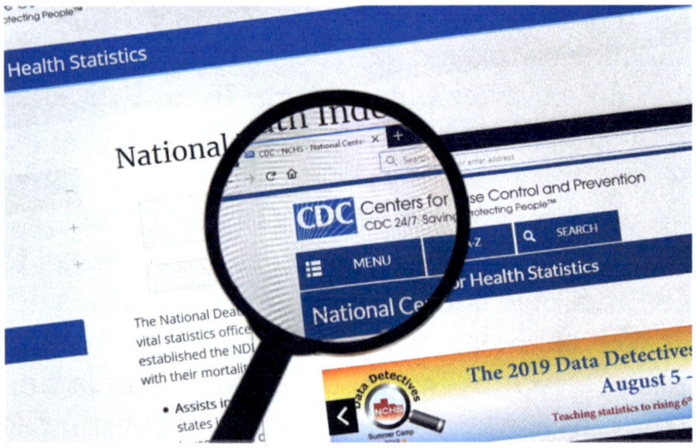

Figure 10.17. The impact of foodborne illnesses on healthcare systems is profound, encompassing both direct and indirect consequences that strain resources and challenge public health initiatives.

Source: https://www.foodpoisoningnews.com/wp-content/uploads/2024/09/usa-government-home-page-stockpack-deposit-photos-scaled.jpg.

10.4.8. Community Involvement in Food Safety

Getting communities involved in food safety efforts helps lower the number of bacterial and viral illnesses from food. Informing and motivating people in the community helps them understand how to handle food safely. It is very important to have programs that encourage communication among food producers, consumers and health experts. For example, workshops in the community can inform families about safe food storage and preparation, which lowers the risks of foodborne infections. In addition, policymakers focus on using various strategies for food safety, which can be improved by listening to the community. Besides, adding community-level information can improve the databases that follow foodborne illnesses, which can lead to better public health policies. It is important to have communities that come together and are well informed to fight FBDs.

10.4.9. Future Challenges in Public Health and Food Safety

With the growth of the world's population, future food safety and public health issues will be of prime concern, particularly in the context of bacterial and viral foodborne illness. The complexity of the food chain system, casually termed a farm-to-fork system, offers several avenues of contamination and risk that can have a significant impact on health outcomes (Ahmed et al., 2025). Smart sensor technology offers a possible solution to food safety challenges with the capacity to rapidly and accurately identify pathogens and toxins that plague much of the world, including Bangladesh. Alongside this, minimizing food waste will also be a key factor to consider, as improper disposal will magnify the potential for foodborne pathogens (Ha, 2025). Continued collaboration between policymakers, regulators, and scientists will be the solution to facilitating novel solutions that maximize food safety, minimize risks, and maximize public health in the face of emerging threats.

A CLOSER LOOK

Food Supply Disruptions

When there are problems in producing, processing, distributing or making food available, it is called a disruption in the food supply. These disruptions can occur due to various factors, including natural disasters (, such as hurricanes, floods, or droughts), pandemics (like COVID-19), economic instability, geopolitical conflicts, labor shortages, and transportation bottlenecks. Climate change is now a major issue because unusual weather patterns are affecting the amount of crops that can be grown and the food that is produced. Because of these disruptions, people may not get enough food, and food may become more expensive and essential nutrients may be less accessible, mainly for those who are most at risk. Also, when global supply chains are disrupted, there may not be enough imported foods, which can cause shortages in some places or everywhere. Governments, businesses and communities can address food supply problems by improving food systems by using different sources, boosting local production and making supply chains stronger.

SUMMARY

The increasing prevalence of bacterial and viral foodborne disease further highlights the need to address this recurring public health threat. Prevention must be multi-faceted, including stringent food safety legislation, public awareness, and good surveillance to detect and contain outbreaks. A clear understanding of the transmission dynamics, especially of zoonotic disease, is essential. More than 60% of human pathogens are zoonotic in nature, underlining the connectedness of human, animal, and environmental processes of health, as explained in Rahman et al. (2020). Additionally, significant economic and societal burdens are created through these diseases, necessitating active intervention. Through evidence-based policy interventions and multi-disciplinary coordination between stakeholders, such as policymakers and the general public, we can achieve significant reductions in the incidence of FBDs, ultimately safeguarding health while also contributing to overall economic and ecological stability, as explained in Landrigan et al. (2020).

In evaluating viral and bacterial foodborne illness, several points are made in the discussion of the importance of sound food safety practices. The first is the insufficiency of the existing regulatory framework, one too often unable to protect consumers from emerging foodborne illness hazards (Levi et al., 2008). Recent outbreaks have highlighted the need for improved tracking and control of foodborne pathogens throughout the food supply chain. Second, there is a need for a multidisciplinary solution, as seen in presentations from a 1995 conference in, which policymakers and scientists addressed food safety analytics. Effective data management, including the development of detailed databases, is a foremost key to putting a quantitative measure on the economic cost of these illnesses and implementing solutions. Overall, a good regulatory system coupled with improved analytical tools is in order to prevent the risk of bacterial and viral foodborne illness, thereby protecting public health.

KEY TERMS FROM THIS CHAPTER

- Accountability
- Agroterrorism
- Blockchain
- Complexity
- Economic security
- Environmental management
- Food attribution
- Laos
- Law enforcement agencies
- Mortality data
- Normal cell functions
- Norovirus
- Policymakers
- Poor sanitation
- Scientists

REFERENCES

1. Dar, O. A., Hasan, R., Schlundt, J., Harbarth, S., Caleo, G., Dar, F. K., Littmann, J., Rweyemamu, M., Buckley, E. J., Shahid, M., Kock, R., Li, H. L., Giha, H., Khan, M., So, A. D., Bindayna, K. M., Kessel, A., Pedersen, H. B., Permanand, G., Zumla, A., ... Heymann, D. L. (2016). Exploring the evidence base for national and regional policy interventions to combat resistance. *Lancet (London, England), 387*(10015), 285–295. https://doi.org/10.1016/S0140-6736(15)00520-6 (accessed on 29 May 2025).
2. Ahmed, M. W., & Kamruzzaman, M. (2025). Advancing food safety in Bangladesh: Challenges and the promise of smart sensor technology. *Food Safety and Health*. https://www.semanticscholar.org/paper/efcfd0fa34af694bd19feda444658c2688647fcf (accessed on 29 May 2025).
3. Angelos, J. A., Arens, A. L., Johnson, H. A., Cadriel, J. L., & Osburn, B. I. (2017). One Health in food safety and security education: Subject matter outline for a curricular framework. *One health (Amsterdam, Netherlands), 3*, 56–65. https://doi.org/10.1016/j.onehlt.2017.04.001Bastiampillai, A. J., Caporali, M. G., Costanzo, V., Declich, S., et al. (2016). *Event-Based Surveillance During Expo Milan 2015: Rationale, Tools, Procedures, And Initial Results*. https://core.ac.uk/download/84928141.pdf (accessed on 29 May 2025).
4. Batz, M., Doyle, M., Lo Fo Wong, D., Morris, J. G., et al. (2025). *Linking Illness to Food: Summary of A Workshop on Food Attribution*. https://core.ac.uk/download/pdf/6759576.pdf (accessed on 29 May 2025).
5. Batz, M., Hoffmann, S., Krupnick, A., Morris, J. G., et al. (2025). *Identifying the Most Significant Microbiological Foodborne Hazards to Public Health: A New Risk Ranking Model*. https://core.ac.uk/download/pdf/6759577.pdf (accessed on 29 May 2025).
6. Benedict, K. M., Reses, H. E., Vigar, M., Roth, D., Roberts, V. A., Mattioli, M., Cooley, L. A., et al. (2017). Surveillance for waterborne disease outbreaks associated with drinking water–United States, 2013–2014. *MMWR Morbidity and Mortality Weekly Report, 66*, 1216–1221. https://doi.org/10.15585/mmwr.mm6644a3.
7. Bonfoh, B., Chase-Topping, M., Gally, D. L., Haydon, D. T., Fisman, D., Foster, D., Fox, A., et al. (2013). *Predicting the Public Health Benefit of Vaccinating Cattle Against Escherichia coli O157*. https://core.ac.uk/download/16461478.pdf.
8. Bosch, A., Gkogka, E., Le Guyader, F. S., Loisy-Hamon, F., Lee, A., van Lieshout, L., Marthi, B., et al. (2018). Foodborne viruses: Detection, risk assessment, and control options in food processing. *International Journal of Food Microbiology, 285*, 110–128. https://doi.org/10.1016/j.ijfoodmicro.2018.06.001.
9. Crowley, D. E., Ibekwe, A. M., Johnson, A. M., Lum, A., et al. (2014). *Topological Data Analysis of Escherichia Coli O157:H7 And Non-O157 Survival in Soils*. https://core.ac.uk/download/323067727.pdf.
10. Dawley, C. (2018). *Aqueous Ozone Inactivation of Viruses and Bacteria on Biotic and Abiotic Surfaces*. https://core.ac.uk/download/215462749.pdf (accessed on 29 May 2025).
11. Pires, S. M., Majowicz, S., Gill, A., & Devleesschauwer, B. (2019). Global and regional source attribution of Shiga toxin-producing Escherichia coli infections using analysis of outbreak surveillance data. *Epidemiology and infection, 147*, e236. https://doi.org/10.1017/S095026881900116XDivyashri, G., Harini, H., Likitha, V., Mv, L., Mahima, E. D., & Shreya,

M. (2024). Traditional and novel foods as vectors for human parasitic diseases. *Journal of Biomedical Research & Environmental Sciences*. https://www.semanticscholar.org/paper/ef05d50a8259e04aa87b42d2a1aba822a3fd7599 (accessed on 29 May 2025).

12. Eldin, C., Melenotte, C., Mediannikov, O., Ghigo, É., Million, M., Edouard, S., Mège, J. L., et al. (2016). From Q fever to *Coxiella burnetii* infection: A paradigm change. *Clinical Microbiology Reviews, 30*, 115–190. https://doi.org/10.1128/cmr.00045-16.

13. Faour-Klingbeil, D., & Todd, E. C. D. (2019). Prevention and control of foodborne diseases in Middle-East North African countries: Review of national control systems. *International Journal of Environmental Research and Public Health, 17*(1), 70. https://doi.org/10.3390/ijerph17010070.

14. Forrest, A. (2020). *The Growing Threat of Agroterrorism and Strategies for Agricultural Defense*. https://core.ac.uk/download/322850909.pdf (accessed on 29 May 2025).

15. Gauci, C., Gilles, H. M., Mamo, J., O'Brien, S., et al. (2006). *Infectious Intestinal Disease: Do We Know It All?* https://core.ac.uk/download/46602090.pdf (accessed on 29 May 2025).

16. Gauci, C., Gilles, H. M., Mamo, J., O'Brien, S., et al. (2007). *Laboratory Surveillance of Communicable Diseases: Enteric Pathogens*. https://core.ac.uk/download/46602116.pdf (accessed on 29 May 2025).

17. Ha, Y. (2025). Advancements in gaseous sensor technology for ensuring food safety: A review. *International Journal of Food Science and Technology*. https://www.semanticscholar.org/paper/3d533586bbfe3847df32e35a87ec2c3567b51e02 (accessed on 29 May 2025).

18. Hamilton, A. N. (2024). *Determination of Factors Influencing Microbial Food Safety Risks of Additive Manufacturing and 3D Printing of Food*. https://core.ac.uk/download/619597376.pdf (accessed on 29 May 2025).

19. Landrigan, P. J., Stegeman, J. J., Fleming, L. E., Allemand, D., Anderson, D. M., Backer, L. C., Brücker-Davis, F., et al. (2020). Human health and ocean pollution. *Annals of Global Health, 86*, 151. https://doi.org/10.5334/aogh.2831.

20. Levi, J., Segal, L. M., & Vinter, S. (2008). *Fixing Food Safety: Protecting America's Food Supply from Farm-To-Fork*. https://core.ac.uk/download/71351319.pdf (accessed on 29 May 2025).

21. Miller, J. M., Binnicker, M. J., Campbell, S., Carroll, K. C., Chapin, K. C., Gilligan, P. H., Gonzalez, M. D., et al. (2018). A guide to utilization of the microbiology laboratory for diagnosis of infectious diseases: 2018 update by the Infectious Diseases Society of America and the American Society for Microbiology. *Clinical Infectious Diseases, 67*(1), e1–e94. https://doi.org/10.1093/cid/ciy381.

22. Monarez, S., Houry, D., Posner, S. F., Berkwits, M., Gorwitz, R., Gottardy, A. J., Leahy, M. A., et al. (2025). Contributing factors of foodborne illness outbreaks–National Outbreak Reporting System, United States, 2014–2022. *MMWR Surveillance Summaries, 74*(1), 1–12. https://www.semanticscholar.org/paper/2bcb3c0f9142e2c3612d3aac3352746dd4600fb1 (accessed on 29 May 2025).

23. National Center for Emerging and Zoonotic Infectious Diseases (U.S.). (2025). *Strategic Plan 2012–2017*. https://core.ac.uk/download/144194143.pdf (accessed on 29 May 2025).

24. Nielsen, R., Dalby, T., Emborg, H., Larsen, A., Petersen, A., Torpdahl, M., Hoffmann, S., et al. (2022). COVID-19 preventive measures coincided with a marked decline in other infectious diseases

in Denmark, spring 2020. *Epidemiology and Infection, 150*. https://www.semanticscholar.org/paper/31519e18d9730592e711c8b0eb4ccf67034d1a12 (accessed on 29 May 2025).

25. Qi, L., Zhou, S., & Gu, D. (2024). Etiology, clinical features, and epidemiological analysis of diarrhea patients visiting a gastrointestinal clinic in a comprehensive hospital in Beijing, China, in 2023. *iLABMED*. https://www.semanticscholar.org/paper/a72a80b1520800bc636bcb5357fca3468d7baab4 (accessed on 29 May 2025).
26. Radin, D. (2012). *Human Norovirus Transmission Due To Contaminated Fresh Fruit and Vegetables*. https://core.ac.uk/download/pdf/27035486.pdf (accessed on 29 May 2025).
27. Radin, D. (2014). *New Trends in Food- And Waterborne Viral Outbreaks*. https://core.ac.uk/download/489560576.pdf (accessed on 29 May 2025).
28. Rahman, M. T., Sobur, M. A., Islam, M. S., Ievy, S., Hossain, M. J., El Zowalaty, M. E., Rahman, A. T., et al. (2020). Zoonotic diseases: Etiology, impact, and control. *Microorganisms, 8*, 1405. https://doi.org/10.3390/microorganisms8091405.
29. Rajapaksha, P., Elbourne, A., Gangadoo, S., Brown, R. R., Cozzolino, D., & Chapman, J. (2018). A review of methods for the detection of pathogenic microorganisms. *The Analyst, 144*(2), 396–411. https://doi.org/10.1039/c8an01488d.
30. Ranveer, S., Dasriya, V., Ahmad, M. F., Dhillon, H. S., Samtiya, M., Shama, E., Anand, T., et al. (2024). Positive and negative aspects of bacteriophages and their immense role in the food chain. *npj Science of Food, 8*, Article 2. https://doi.org/10.1038/s41538-023-00245-8.
31. Roberts, T., & Steahr, T. E. (2025). *Microbial Foodborne Disease: Hospitalizations, Medical Costs and Potential Demand for Safer Food*. https://core.ac.uk/download/pdf/6253554.pdf (accessed on 29 May 2025).
32. Rohr, J. R., Barrett, C. B., Civitello, D. J., Craft, M. E., Delius, B. K., De Leo, G. A., Hudson, P. J., et al. (2019). Emerging human infectious diseases and the links to global food production. *Nature Sustainability, 2*, 445–456. https://doi.org/10.1038/s41893-019-0293-3.
33. Tang, K. W. K., Millar, B. C., & Moore, J. E. (2023). Antimicrobial resistance (AMR). *British Journal of Biomedical Science, 80*. https://doi.org/10.3389/bjbs.2023.11387.
34. Thompson, L., Sipes, P., Ebner, P., Soukhavong, S., & Shively, G. (2024). Food safety in Laos: Status, current challenges and opportunities. *International Journal of Food Science & Technology, 59*, 7727–7738. https://doi.org/10.1111/ijfs.17193.

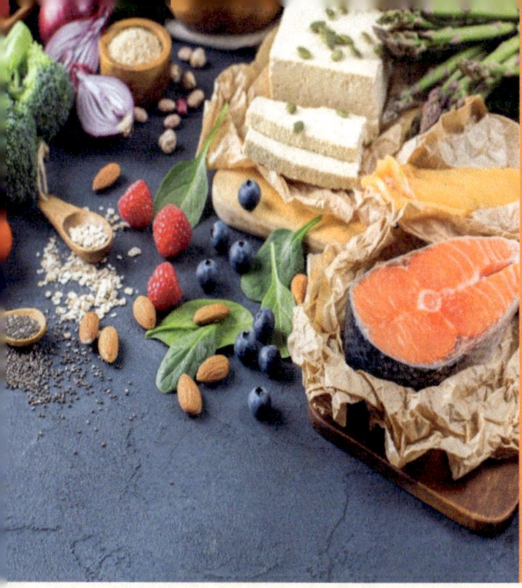

Chapter 11

POISONING FROM CHEMICALS AND NATURAL TOXINS

Contents

Introduction 255

11.1. Types of Chemicals Causing Food Poisoning 256

11.2. Natural Toxins in Food 260

11.3. Prevention and Control Measures 263

Summary 269

References 270

Introduction

Food poisoning, a public health concern, is caused by the consumption of contaminated food and is caused by various chemicals and naturally occurring toxins. Understanding the sources and effects of toxic substances is vital in ensuring consumer protection against health hazards. Chemical contaminants , such as pesticides, have been linked to severe health consequences, ranging from acute poisoning to chronic illness , such as Parkinson's disease, particularly among farm workers who handle chemical substances (Brandt, 2007). Moreover, natural toxins, which are naturally present in certain plant and animal foods, exert their risks irrespective of the presence of some of the compounds with positive attributes at low levels. For instance, although organic foods contain higher levels of natural plant toxins, such toxins are generally safe and could even benefit human health (Brandt, 2007). Once again, the risk posed by microbial contamination from the growth of bacteria in poorly processed foods underscores the importance of thorough safety screening, particularly in the dairy industry.

Understanding these determinants is vital in effectively controlling foodborne diseases.

Overview of Chemicals and Natural Toxins

It is important to know about chemicals and natural toxins to reduce food poisoning risks. They may come from farming, food processing or from contamination that happens when handling. Bacteria from the *genera Sporosarcina* and *Bacillus* can survive pasteurization , which allows them to form biofilms that contain microorganisms that spoil dairy products. This not only poses a quality control issue but contributes to a cycle of contamination that threatens consumer safety (Gopal et al., 2015).

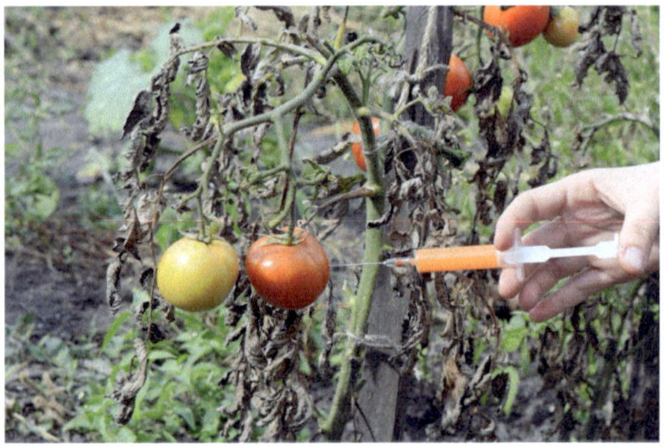

Figure 11.1. Understanding the nature of chemicals and natural toxins is vital for addressing food poisoning risks.

Source: https://www.thestatesman.com/wp-content/uploads/2020/09/food.jpg.

Also, since these pathogens are common, the food industry must have strong systems in place to prevent foodborne illnesses. Consequently, implementing effective cleaning protocols and utilizing chemical biocides become essential components of assuring food quality and safety amidst the complex interplay of chemicals and natural toxins impacting food products (Panel E on Contaminants in the EFSA Panel on Contaminants in the Food Chain (CONTAM), 2017). These insights emphasize the importance of vigilance in food safety management (Figure 11.1).

11.1. Types of Chemicals Causing Food Poisoning

Food poisoning is often caused by heavy metals , such as lead and mercury found in food , which can be very harmful to people's health. Such toxic elements usually come from polluted air and water, waste from factories and soil used in farming that is polluted. Upon ingestion, heavy metals accumulate in human tissues and can lead to serious health issues and oxidative stress, as indicated by their ability to induce reactive oxygen species within the body (Bandyopadhyay et al., 2016).

Furthermore, the ingestion of marine organisms, which are known to bioaccumulate these heavy metals, underscores the critical connection between marine ecosystem health and human health outcomes (Baden et al., 2018). Because people are becoming more aware of these dangers, it is necessary to put in place effective monitoring and strict regulations to reduce the risk of chemical contamination in food.

11.1.1. Pesticides and Herbicides

The widespread use of pesticides and herbicides in modern agriculture has been a primary cause of food poisoning from chemical contamination. The chemicals used to poison pests and weeds tend to leave residues in the very environment they are intended to eliminate. These residues enter the food chain unintentionally and, on consumption, cause acute symptoms of poisoning in the consumers, thus posing public health hazards.

Additionally, studies have shown that dependence on pesticides disproportionately affects organic forms of production and has a tendency to increase environmental pollution, thus affecting not just human health but also the agroecosystems on , which the very survival of agriculture is based (Azeez et al., 2001). Food science studies have shown intricate interactions between food and these chemicals, and regulation and monitoring of pesticide use have been the need of the hour (Dave et al., 2021). It is in the absence of regulation that consumers and the environment are exposed to a high level of risk from these poisonous chemicals (Figure 11.2).

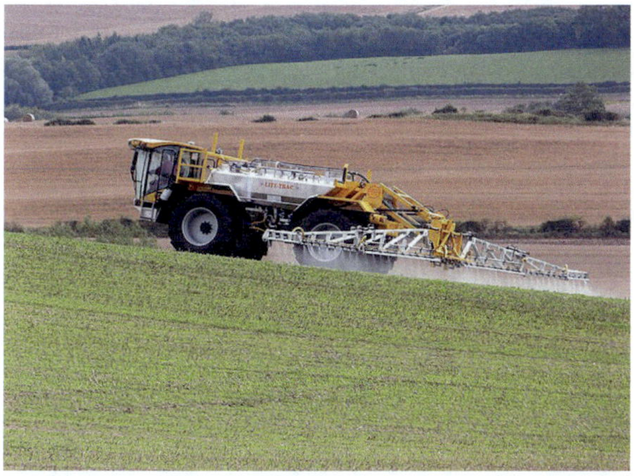

Figure 11.2. The widespread use of pesticides and herbicides in modern agriculture plays a significant role in the incidence of food poisoning linked to chemical contaminants.

Source: https://upload.wikimedia.org/wikipedia/commons/thumb/d/df/Lite-Trac_Crop_Sprayer.jpg/640px-Lite-Trac_Crop_Sprayer.jpg

11.1.2. Heavy Metals (e.g., Lead, Mercury)

The presence of heavy metals , such as lead and mercury in food significantly contributes to the phenomenon of food poisoning, with negative acute and chronic health implications for consumers. Such toxic agents typically appear due to environmental pollution, industrial effluent disposal, and farm use of polluted water or soil. In the human body, when ingested, heavy metals have a tendency to bioaccumulate in body tissues and can lead to serious health implications and oxidative stress, as evidenced by their ability to produce reactive oxygen species in the body (Bandyopadhyay et al., 2016). Furthermore, the consumption of sea life, having a tendency to bioaccumulate such heavy metals, brings into prominence the crucial relationship between the health of sea ecosystems and human health implications (Baden et al., 2018). With increased awareness of such hazards, there is an imperative need for stringent monitoring and regulatory control in order to prevent exposure to such toxic agents in food items in the long term, safeguarding the public from the hazards of chemical contamination.

11.1.3. Food Additives and Preservatives

Because people now want food that is both convenient and lasts longer, more additives and preservatives are being used. While they are meant to improve flavor, texture and how long food lasts, they may expose people to chemicals that can harm their health. For instance, the presence of toxic contaminants and artificial components in food products can trigger a range of health issues over time, as highlighted by the concept of food pollution, which includes various adulterants and the harmful effects of pesticides and heavy metals present in our food supply (Kumari et al., 2021).

Furthermore, the extensive list of over 1000 approved food additives documented by the FDA raises concern, particularly since the potential side effects of many of these substances remain inadequately described and understood, underscoring the need for greater scrutiny in their usage (Kumar et al., 2023) (Figure 11.3).

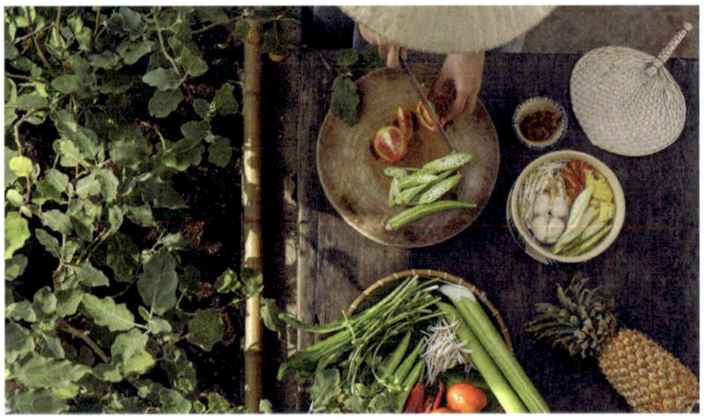

Figure 11.3. As the demand for convenience and prolonged shelf-life in food products has surged, so too has the incorporation of various food additives and preservatives.

Source: https://restaurantindia.s3.ap-south-1.amazonaws.com/s3fs-public/2025-04/Seasonal%20Menu.jpg.

11.1.4. Industrial Chemicals (e.g., PCBs)

Industrial chemicals, and in particular polychlorinated biphenyls (PCBs), are a severe threat to food safety and public health. The synthetic chemicals were heavily utilized in electrical appliances and other industrial processes before their banning due to their ability to persist in the environment and bioaccumulate in the food chain. Excessive PCB contamination has been linked to various health diseases, from cancer to reproductive health. As seen from studies , such as the Exposure Investigation in Mossville, Louisiana, where dioxin levels are high among residents due to local industrial plants, the impacts of such chemical exposure are not only confined to short-term health ailments but also long-term environmental impacts with adverse effects on aquatic food supply and, in turn, human consumers (Subra, 2007). Additionally, the discovery of how marine ecosystem health is interrelated with human wellness justifies the need for sound monitoring and prevention measures to mitigate such risks (Baden et al., 2018).

11.1.5. Contaminants from Packaging Materials

The safety of food is greatly affected by packaging materials when it comes to food poisoning from chemicals and natural toxins. Some packaging materials, for example, plastic and cardboard, can let harmful chemicals into food , which can be dangerous to eat. These contaminants, which may include bisphenol A (BPA) and phthalates, have been associated with adverse health effects, including hormonal disruptions and increased risk of chronic diseases. Also, some pollutants can remain in packaging , which can be harmful if the packaging touches food. The complexity of food contamination underscores the necessity for vigilant assessment of packaging safety, particularly as foodborne disease outbreaks linked to contaminants gain international recognition (Njue et al., 2022). The interplay between contamination during processing and packaging highlights a critical area for regulatory scrutiny and public health initiatives aimed at mitigating risks associated with food consumption (Brandt, 2007) (Figure 11.4).

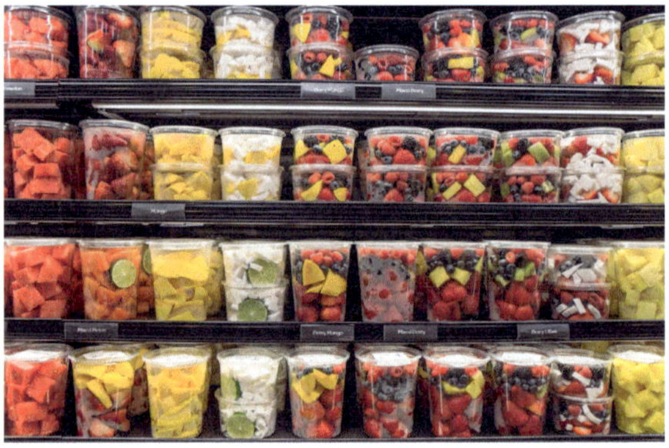

Figure 11.4. Contaminants can leach from various packaging types, including plastic and cardboard, into food products, introducing harmful substances into the human diet.

Source: https://foodprint.org/wp-content/uploads/2019/11/food-packaging-report.jpg.

11.1.6. Chemical Residues in Processed Foods

The presence of chemical residues in processed food is a critical food safety and public health issue, particularly with respect to chemical food poisoning and natural toxins. Organic and conventional products both contain pesticide residues, which are health-hazardous in origin; however, studies have indicated that residues in organic products are always lower, potentially minimizing harm to consumers (Brandt, 2007). Moreover, the prevalence of unidentified chemical residues in processed food products across the board highlights the need for stringent regulatory measures and rigorous examination to prevent outbreaks of contamination with health-damaging consequences. The debate that has plagued the safety of organic versus conventional foods illustrates the complexity of food production systems and suggests organic farming systems can be a more reliable pathway to chemical reduction (Azeez et al., 2001). Lastly, greater insight into these residues is necessary in developing effective measures for public health protection.

11.1.7. Role of Food Processing in Chemical Exposure

Food processing plays a key part in how chemicals affect the safety of our food. How harmful substances are handled can either help or worsen their presence in food. Even though processing helps lower some harmful substances, it can introduce chemicals from pesticides and other additives meant to improve taste and freshness. Studies indicate that pesticide residues are notably higher in conventionally processed foods compared to organic options, suggesting a significant disparity in exposure levels (Brandt, 2007). Furthermore, the acute consequences of pesticide poisoning highlight the importance of examining the systems through , which food is produced and processed (Brandt, 2007). Ultimately, a thorough assessment of food processing practices is essential to safeguard consumer health and minimize the risk of foodborne illnesses stemming from chemical exposure (Figure 11.5).

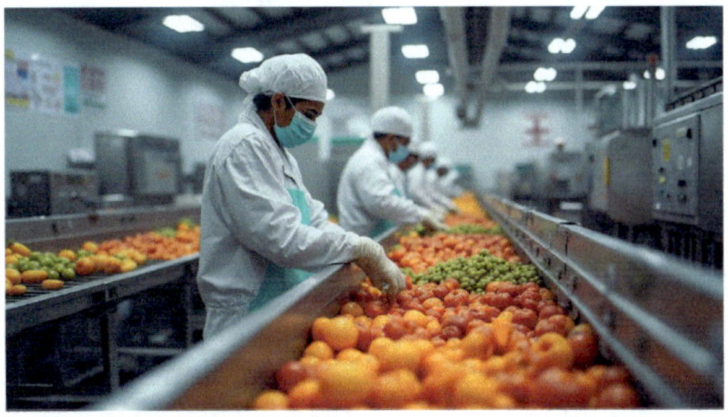

Figure 11.5. The role of food processing in chemical exposure is a critical factor in understanding the safety of our food supply.

Source: https://prathameshe.co.in/uploads/2025/01/understanding-the-risks-in-food-processing-safety-and-health-concerns.webp.

11.1.8. Regulatory Standards for Chemical Use

Regulatory norms in chemical use are a fundamental part of protecting public health and preventing foodborne illness. The norms are intended to minimize hazards posed by exposure to pesticides, which have been shown to cause severe health complications, , such as acute poisoning and long-term diseases like Parkinson's disease, to farmers (Brandt, 2007). Second, as is evident from environmental case histories, , such as the Mossville, Louisiana case, failure by regulatory agencies to regulate the release of toxic chemicals has been found to compound public health crises, particularly those caused by dioxins, which have been found to have no safe level of exposure (Subra, 2007). A comprehensive regulatory framework that includes strict controls on toxic chemicals and emphasis on openness to the use of chemicals is required in a way that will increase food safety and protect vulnerable groups from the adverse consequences of toxic exposure. By plugging these regulatory loopholes, we can offer enhanced food system integrity and public health protection.

11.2. Natural Toxins in Food

Having natural toxins in food is a major issue in food safety and public health, especially regarding food poisoning. Some plants produce these chemicals to protect themselves from being eaten or attacked by diseases, so their amounts may change depending on the environment and how they are grown. Notably, research indicates that organic plants may contain 10 to 50% higher levels of certain natural toxins compared to conventionally grown counterparts, although these levels often remain below toxic thresholds and may even confer health benefits (Brandt, 2007). Additionally, natural contaminants, , such as bacterial spores discovered in dairy products, underscore the challenge of maintaining food safety despite the inherent advantages of organic farming systems (Gopal et al., 2015). So, a clear grasp of the dangers and positive effects of natural toxins is required to help create safe food rules and practices.

11.2.1. Mycotoxins From Mold

The presence of mycotoxins, toxic compounds that are produced by some molds, represents a serious threat in the field of food safety, primarily for food poisoning caused by natural toxins. Mycotoxins are present widely in a wide range of farm products, including grains, nuts, and seeds, which have a tendency to accumulate while in growth, the harvesting process, or storage.

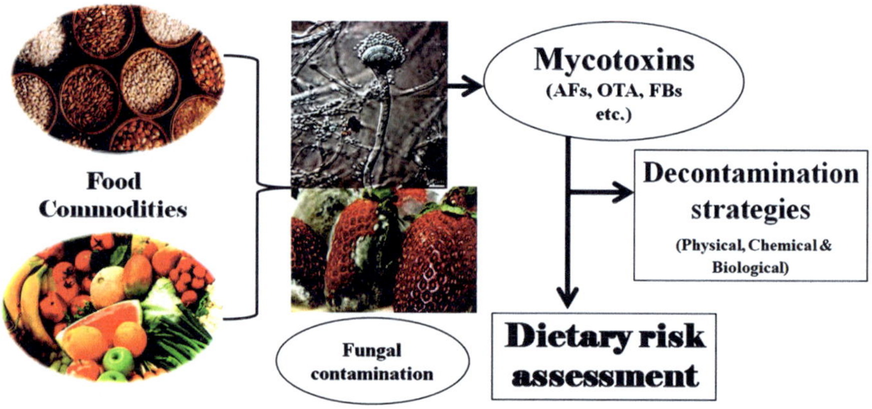

Figure 11.6. The presence of mycotoxins, toxic compounds produced by various molds, poses a significant risk in the realm of food safety, particularly concerning food poisoning caused by natural toxins.

Source: Pandey AK, Samota MK, Kumar A, Silva AS and Dubey NK (2023) Fungal mycotoxins in food commodities: present status and future concerns. Front. Sustain. Food Syst. 7:1162595. doi: 10.3389/fsufs.2023.1162595

Their presence depends directly on environmental conditions, particularly hot and humid weather under , which fungi develop, leading to heavy contamination in the concerned food. It has been found from research that mycotoxins are not only potent mutagens and carcinogens but also cause chronic diseases like liver, kidney, and immune system diseases, particularly in developing countries where food sources are localized in vulnerable crops. The diversity of these toxins, as indicated by their various chemical structures and toxicological properties, emphasizes the serious need for strict food safety measures to minimize risks of exposure to these natural toxins (Paulraj et al., 2002) (Figure 11.6).

11.2.2. Plant Toxins (e.g., Solanine in Potatoes)

Many foods , such as potatoes containing solanine, have plant toxins that are not always noticed when thinking about food safety. Solanine, a glycoalkaloid concentrated primarily in the skin and sprouts of green potatoes, can induce toxic symptoms when ingested in large amounts; adult humans may experience adverse effects from doses as low as 200–400 mg, while children are more susceptible at 20–40 mg per exposure (Caroline et al., 2022). The average commercially available potato contains less than 0.2 mg of glycoalkaloids, highlighting the effectiveness of regulatory measures implemented by agencies like the US Food and Drug Administration (FDA) to mitigate consumer risk (Anthoni et al., 2010). Still, the risk of toxicity is there, mainly when people eat large amounts or handle spoiled potatoes that could contain more solanine. It is important to understand these risks to support food safety and make people more aware.

11.2.3. Marine Toxins (e.g., Ciguatera, Scombroid)

The situation with marine toxins, , such as ciguatera and scombroid poisoning, is the classic illustration of an root cause in foodborne illness due to naturally occurring toxins. Ciguatera, which is primarily associated with the consumption of reef fish, results from the bioaccumulation of toxins produced by marine microalgae, which induce neurological and gastrointestinal symptoms in the human body. Such poisoning is most prevalent in the tropics and, as such, is of public health concern. Scombroid poisoning, on the other hand, is due to improper storage of tuna and mackerel and other fish, which facilitates the growth of histamine, a toxin that can induce severe allergic reactions. Such marine toxins are a testament to the intersection of issues in the environment and food safety and that food poisoning may result from chemical contamination and natural biological processes as well, as seen in various food safety research studies, especially in regions where such toxins are endemic (Malangu, 2016) (Figure 11.7).

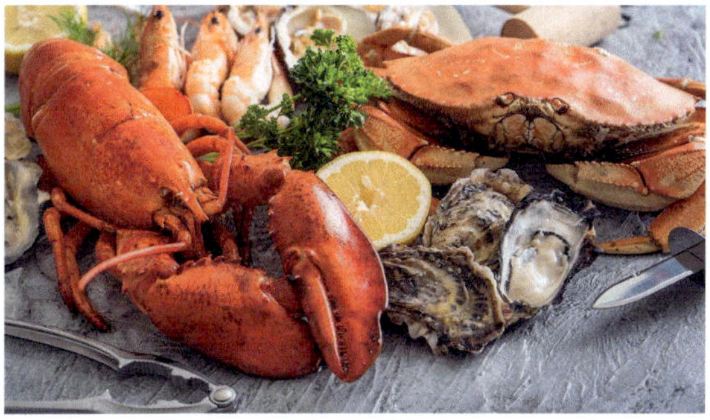

Figure 11.7. The phenomenon of marine toxins, particularly ciguatera and scombroid poisoning, exemplifies a critical aspect of foodborne illnesses stemming from natural toxins.

Source: https://world.dan.org/wp-content/uploads/2020/07/seafood-poisonings-1149620933-DAN-1200x700-1.jpg.

11.2.4. Bacterial Toxins (e.g., Botulinum Toxin)

Bacterial toxins, prominently exemplified by botulinum toxin, pose a significant threat in the context of food poisoning, specifically within the realm of foodborne diseases (FBDs). The toxin made by *Clostridium botulinum* , which is very harmful to the nervous system, may appear in foods that are not preserved properly. As noted, FBDs caused by such toxins result in severe health complications, including debilitating infections and gastrointestinal disturbances that can lead to life-threatening conditions , such as dehydration and toxic shock syndrome (Castro-Escarpulli et al., 2017).

In this regard, the role of pathogenic microorganisms becomes crucial, as some can release toxins during food colonization or within the gastrointestinal tract after ingestion (Castro-Escarpulli et al., 2017). Moreover, examining honey and other foods has found that natural toxins can be dangerous for consumers , which can affect how safe traditional foods are seen. As a result, knowing how these toxins affect us is very important for both food safety and public health.

11.2.5. Animal Toxins (e.g., Pufferfish Poison)

Eating animal toxins, mainly pufferfish poison, is a major health issue in relation to food poisoning caused by chemicals and natural toxins. Pufferfish contain tetrodotoxin, a potent neurotoxin that has been linked to numerous cases of intoxication, with over 430 reported incidents and 52 fatalities in recent years (Carrascosa et al., 2015).

When pufferfish migrate to new places, the chance of encountering the toxin goes up , which makes it important to have strong monitoring systems. Even though many people are attracted to pufferfish for its taste, its legal and health issues must not be ignored. In regions , such as those along the Indian Ocean and Red Sea, there is a notable lack of specific monitoring for marine toxins, which can exacerbate cases of poisoning and hinder public health efforts (Silva et al., 2019). Therefore, regulatory measures are crucial to mitigate the risks associated with these hazardous dietary choices (Figure 11.8).

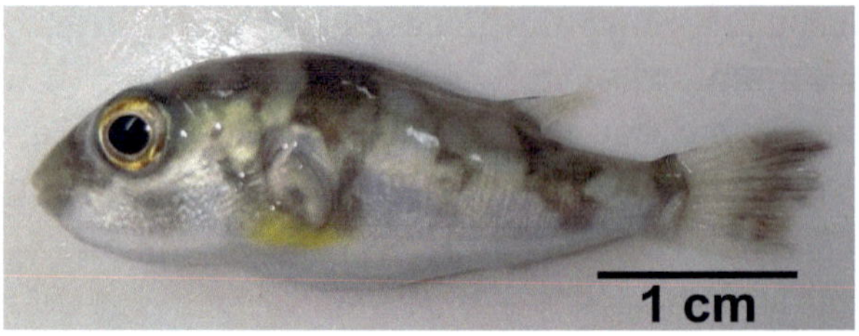

Figure 11.8. The consumption of animal toxins, particularly pufferfish poison, raises significant public health concerns within the broader context of food poisoning from chemicals and natural toxins.

Source: Zhu H, Sakai T, Doi H, Yamaguchi K, Yamada A, Takatani T, Arakawa O. Tetrodotoxin/Saxitoxin Accumulation Profile in the Euryhaline Marine Pufferfish *Chelonodontops patoca*. *Toxins*. 2024; 16(1):18. https://doi.org/10.3390/toxins16010018

11.2.6. Fungal Toxins in Grains

Fungal toxins in cereals pose a serious issue in the field of food safety, in chemical and natural toxin food poisoning. Fungi like Aspergillus, Fusarium, and Penicillium infect cereal crops like maize, rice, and sorghum and produce toxic mycotoxins that are harmful to human and animal health. Mycotoxins like aflatoxins, deoxynivalenol, and ochratoxin cause serious adverse health effects ranging from immunosuppression to cancer based on the level and duration of exposure. Inadequate agricultural and storage practices enhance the risk, favoring the development of fungi and hence mycotoxin production (Blaney et al., 2013). Good management measures are thus vital, as described in available literature, since they reduce the risk of contamination and ensure the safety of public health. Combined interventions through good agricultural practice and regulation are required to ensure food safety and consumer health (Blaney et al., 2013).

11.2.7. Risk Factors for Natural Toxin Exposure

Exposure to natural toxins in food can be very risky for safety, especially in farming. Farming practices play a key role; organic farming methods can help reduce the use of chemicals and pathogens , which is better than what conventional farming offers. However, a noteworthy concern is that certain natural plant toxins may be present in higher concentrations in organically grown plants, which may reach levels that, while not acutely toxic, warrant attention for their long-term health implications (EFSA Panel on Contaminants in the Food Chain (CONTAM), 2017). In addition, things like the environment, the crops grown and poor storage methods can make the risk of toxins in food even higher. The complexity of managing these risks highlights the need for continuous monitoring and education about safe agricultural practices to mitigate the potential hazards of natural toxins in our food systems, thereby enhancing public health and safety in the realm of food consumption (EFSA Panel on Contaminants in the Food Chain (CONTAM), 2017) (Figure 11.9).

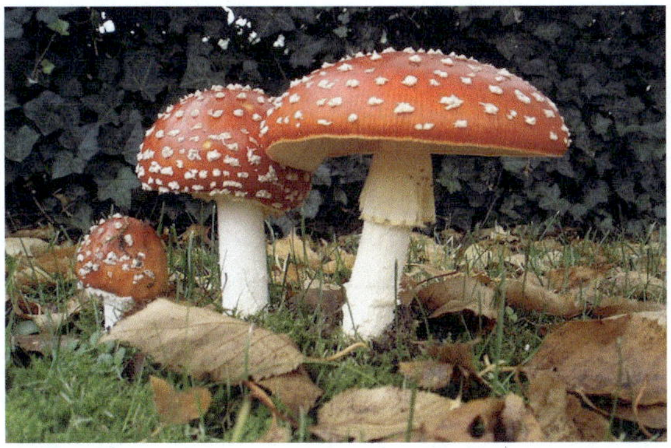

Figure 11.9. Natural toxin exposure presents significant risk factors that can compromise food safety, particularly in agricultural practices.

Source: https://upload.wikimedia.org/wikipedia/commons/7/7d/Amanita-muscaria-mushroom20151014-1336-ex6cst.jpg

11.2.8. Identification and Testing of Natural Toxins

Finding and checking natural toxins is very important for preventing food poisoning caused by toxic plants and fungi. For instance, the analysis of mushrooms like those from the Cortinarius genus reveals significant challenges in diagnosing orrellanine (OR) poisoning, as it traditionally relies on patient history and histopathological examination of biopsies. The development of high-performance liquid chromatography (HPLC) and liquid chromatography-tandem mass spectrometry (LC-MS/MS) has enhanced the ability to detect OR in tissue samples, providing a crucial diagnostic tool that increases the sensitivity and specificity of testing methods. Moreover, as noted in recent studies, improved methods can lead to a better understanding of OR-induced pathology, which is vital for advancing treatment protocols (Anantharam et al., 2016). Simultaneously, awareness regarding the presence of toxic materials in collections, , such as those found in museums, emphasizes the need for proper documentation and safety plans (Slocum et al., 2018). All these actions highlight the importance of keeping strong identification and testing systems to defend public health from natural toxins.

11.3. Prevention and Control Measures

It is very important to prevent and control risks by using effective measures for food poisoning from chemicals and natural toxins. These steps involve closely checking how pesticides are used and the crops that might be affected by natural toxins. Organic farming has demonstrated clear advantages in reducing exposure to chemical residues, as it typically results in lower pesticide levels compared to conventional methods, decreasing the likelihood of toxicity (Brandt, 2007). Moreover, enhancing food safety protocols, , such as improving the quality of drinking water and sewage disposal systems, is critical in curbing waterborne diseases linked to food safety (Heaviside et al., 2018). This way of working , which includes both sustainable farming and strong food safety rules, helps to improve the quality of food and also lowers the number of food poisoning cases, thus supporting public health in many ways.

11.3.1. Safe Food Handling Practices

One of the most important elements of preventing food poisoning risks due to chemicals and natural toxins is safe food handling practices. These practices constitute a series of actions that avoid contaminating food through the food chain, from production to consumption.

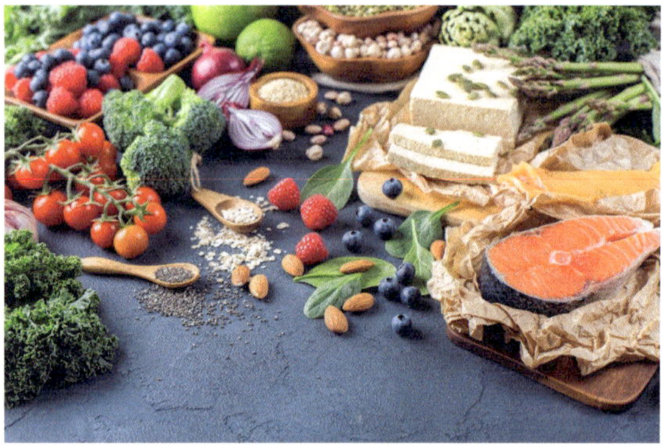

Figure 11.10. A critical aspect of mitigating food poisoning risks from chemicals and natural toxins is the implementation of safe food handling practices.

Source: https://cdn2.hubspot.net/hubfs/559937/assortment%20of%20food.jpg.

Food safety, according to the Codex Alimentarius Commission, ensures food freedom from harm upon consumption when consumed in the manner in , which it is prepared, emphasizing hygiene and prevention of contact with pathogens (Uçar et al., 2016). Food safety can yet be enhanced with the application of organic farming practices, which reduce the exposure to chemical contaminants due to their reduced pesticide residue compared to conventional practices (Brandt, 2007). Application of safe handling procedures, , such as cooking heat and food hygiene controls, can by the consumer significantly decrease the risk of foodborne disease, safeguarding individual and public health. Lastly, these practices are a major line of defense against the risks of both natural toxins and industrial contaminants (Figure 11.10).

11.3.2. Importance of Cooking Temperatures

The importance of cooking temperatures cannot be overrated, particularly in minimizing the threats posed by both chemical contaminants and natural toxins in foodborne diseases. Proper cooking temperatures are crucial in eliminating pathogenic bacteria that cause food poisoning, like *Bacillus cereus*, which tends to infect starchy foods like rice. Recent studies suggest that food handling and low temperatures in cooking result in the excessive proliferation of *B. cereus* and toxin production, with probable severe gastrointestinal symptoms (Woh et al., 2024). Additionally, a shift in climatic patterns exacerbates the threat of food safety by favoring the proliferation of harmful microorganisms and food quality alterations. Temperature conditions lead to increased food infection and bacterial development, particularly in seafood and crops (Heidari et al., 2023). Hence, the application of proper cooking temperatures is not only relevant to safety but also food integrity, and it demands the adoption of strict food safety protocols immediately.

11.3.3. Proper Food Storage Techniques

Properly storing food prevents chemicals and natural toxins from causing food poisoning. Keeping food in the right way reduces the chances of microorganisms growing and chemicals contaminating the food. For instance, maintaining appropriate refrigeration temperatures can significantly reduce the likelihood of mycotoxin production, as fungi known to produce these toxins thrive in warm, moist environments (Awuchi et al., 2021). When you use airtight containers, you stop food from touching other products and being exposed to things that might harm it. Therefore, it is crucial to regularly review and adhere to good manufacturing practices (GMP) and standardized procedures , such as Hazard Analysis Critical Control Point (HACCP) to enhance food safety. Properly executed storage techniques collectively safeguard public health against the pervasive threats posed by food-borne pathogens and toxins (Abebe et al., 2020) (Figure 11.11).

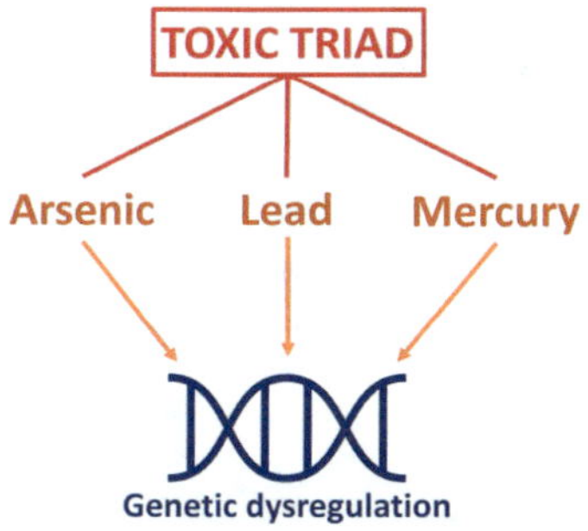

Figure 11.11. Effective food storage practices not only slow down the proliferation of harmful microorganisms but also minimize the chances of chemical contamination from improperly stored items.

Source: Ellwanger JH, Ziliotto M, Chies JAB. Toxicogenomics of Arsenic, Lead and Mercury: The Toxic Triad. *Pollutants*. 2025; 5(3):18. https://doi.org/10.3390/pollutants5030018

11.3.4. Role of Food Safety Education

Successful food safety education has been instrumental in the reduction of food poisoning risks through chemicals and natural toxins by ensuring that the consumer is informed on proper food handling practices, detection of possible hazards, and the importance of hygiene. Through the provision of such information, educational programs can contribute significantly to the prevention of foodborne illness. Moreover, with a changing food system in the world influenced by health concerns, it is imperative that education programs also change and address the complexity of the food supply. For instance, information on how farming practices influence contaminant levels in food commodities is essential in informing consumers in the making of decisions between organic and conventional food (Azeez et al., 2001). Integrated food safety education that interfaces health, nutrition, and food policy can empower individuals to make informed decisions, resulting in an enhanced population in health and food systems that are more resilient (Pinstrup-Andersen, 2025). The contribution of food safety education cannot be overstated in maintaining public health and safety.

11.3.5. Government Regulations and Inspections

Laws and inspections by the government are important in controlling the risks of food poisoning from chemicals and natural toxins. In the United States, regulatory agencies , such as the FDA and the Environmental Protection Agency (EPA) are tasked with establishing safety standards for food production and processing. Nonetheless, there are doubts about how well these rules work, mainly in dealing with new chemical dangers. Research indicates a pressing need for enhancements in regulatory practices to ensure comprehensive oversight of chemical management in the food industry, as highlighted by studies analyzing the current legal framework's efficacy (Khoat, 2024). Moreover, such initiatives can help by raising awareness and providing financial support for research on dangerous exposures , which supports the recommendations for better safety standards.

Strengthening these governmental frameworks is essential for safeguarding public health against potential foodborne hazards (Figure 11.12).

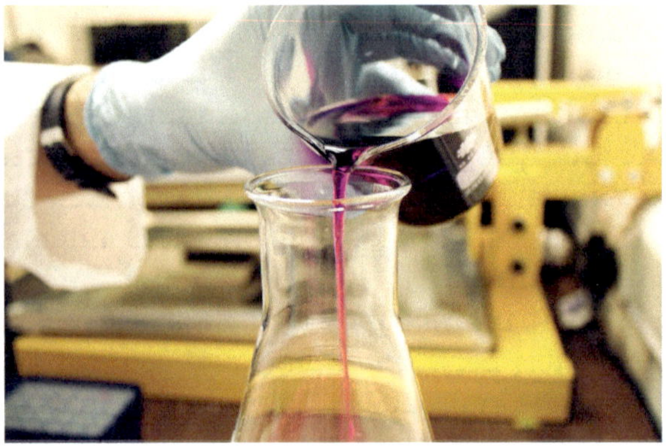

Figure 11.12. Government regulations and inspections play a pivotal role in mitigating the risks associated with food poisoning from chemicals and natural toxins.

Source: https://www.deskera.com/blog/content/images/2023/03/louis-reed-JeInkKlI2Po-unsplash.jpg.

11.3.6. Consumer Awareness and Labeling

Strong labeling and knowledge are at the core of public health protection in contemporary consumer societies, particularly with regard to chemical and natural toxin-induced food poisoning. Strong labeling is a powerful instrument that educates individuals to make informed choices, allowing them to be able to read and comprehend potential dangers from various foods. Most consumers, however, have no information regarding the poisonous substances that may be included in foods, partly because of weak labeling. The presence of poisonous substances in museum collections, for instance, indicates a broader failure of unawareness and documentation, which can also be applied to food labeling (Slocum et al., 2018). The absence of transparency not only creates individual health hazards but also economic effects, as seen in ongoing public health challenges and the cost imposed by industries like fishing (Kazmierczak et al., 2025). The effectiveness of labeling and consumer education regarding toxins therefore, needs to be enhanced to ensure safety and confidence in the food supply.

11.3.7. Innovations in Food Safety Technology

Because foodborne illnesses are still a big problem, new technologies in food safety are now necessary to reduce the risks caused by both chemical and natural toxins. Advanced methods , such as systems that detect microbes in real time and use blockchain for supply chain monitoring, help quickly find the source of contamination , which improves food safety.

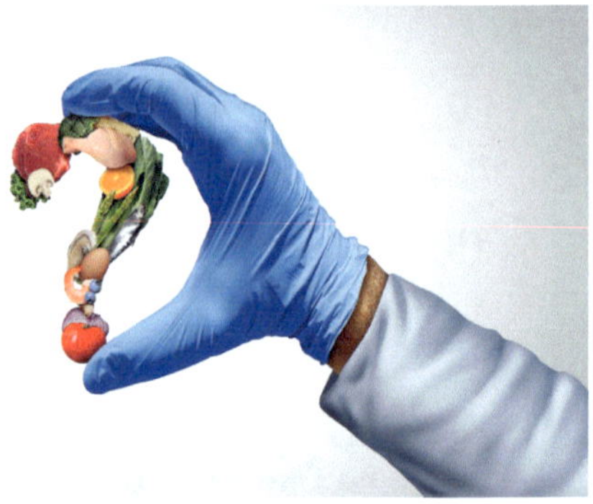

Figure 11.13. As the prevalence of foodborne illnesses continues to impact public health, innovations in food safety technology have emerged as essential tools for mitigating risks associated with chemical and natural toxins.

Source: https://www.foodsafetynews.com/files/2024/02/fighting-foodborne-illnesses-question.jpg.

For instance, digital solutions for seafood supply chains aim to address the complexities of ciguatera poisoning, a prominent non-bacterial seafood-related illness caused by toxic fish consumption, which can lead to severe health consequences in affected communities (Bodi et al., 2021). Furthermore, the examination of organic food production processes challenges misleading claims about food safety, underscoring the importance of evidence-based practices in agriculture (Azeez et al., 2001). By leveraging cutting-edge technologies, the food industry can better protect consumers and promote a safer food environment, ultimately reducing the incidence of food poisoning from harmful substances (Figure 11.13).

11.3.8. Community Initiatives for Food Safety

The importance of food safety programs within communities cannot be exaggerated, especially in cases of chemical- and natural toxin-induced food poisoning. Such programs allow local communities to recognize and control foodborne disease risks, promoting a prevention and awareness culture. By integrating best practices in food preparation and handling, communities can prevent food poisoning, which disproportionately affects vulnerable populations, , such as women, who are several times at the crossroads of food production and distribution. This interdependence between food safety and environmental health is observed in collaborations that seek to address overarching issues of environmental contamination, , such as noted by the Environmental Justice/ Reproductive Justice (EJ/RJ) Collaborative, in recommending collective advocacy for stronger communities (Khan, 2009). In addition, in areas like Africa, where food poisoning is a chronic health issue, community-specific interventions are critical in addressing unique risk factors and enhancing overall public health outcomes (Malangu, 2016).

11.3.9. Global Efforts to Combat Food Poisoning

Many countries now realize the importance of dealing with food poisoning, mainly because of chemicals and natural toxins. Organizations , such as the Food and Agriculture Organization (FAO) and the World Health Organization (WHO) have collaborated since the early 1960s to establish standards and guidelines aimed at ensuring food safety. The Codex Alimentarius , which was developed by them together, sets important standards for food hygiene around the world. Particularly notable is the work of the Codex Committee on Food Hygiene (CCFH), which continues to shape microbial hygiene standards despite ongoing debates regarding its qualitative versus quantitative approaches to food safety (Ramsingh, 2014). Thanks to Rachel Carson and others, the discussion about environmental health risks due to contaminants in our food has gained more attention. Her seminal work brought to light the dangers posed by toxic chemicals, thus emphasizing the necessity of stringent safety measures to protect public health from both chemical and natural toxins (Aragonès et al., 2012).

A CLOSER LOOK

Pesticides

Pesticides are materials used to stop, control or get rid of pests that might harm crops, animals or other agricultural items. These include insects, weeds, fungi, rodents, and microorganisms. Farmers use pesticides to get more crops, shield plants from illnesses and make food production more efficient. They are categorized into different types based on their target, , such as insecticides (for insects), herbicides (for weeds), fungicides (for fungi), and rodenticides (for rodents). Using pesticides properly and in limited amounts helps with pest management and guarantees food security, but using them too much or incorrectly can cause environmental damage, make pests resistant to pesticides and endanger the health of humans, animals and bees. Many times, IPM strategies are used to manage pests , which rely on biological, mechanical and chemical methods to achieve sustainability.

SUMMARY

The complexity of natural and chemical toxin food poisoning highlights the need for rigorous food safety protocols and critical assessment of agricultural production. The blending of organic and synthetic agriculture has unique strengths and weaknesses; organic agriculture can minimize exposure to toxic residues of pesticides and respond to consumer needs for health and environmental purity, but it is not hazard-free for natural toxin risk inherent in plants, , which, on occasion, occur in higher concentrations than in conventional crops (Brandt, 2007). Organic food consumers have been shown to likely have better health status, implying a potential health-protective effect against certain diseases (Brandt, 2007). Balanced perception must be utilized, however, in that food system safety relies on judicious management practices that control chemical and biological hazards, ultimately delivering society the nutritional and health value of our food supply.

Finally, the universal issue of chemical and natural toxin food poisoning highlights the necessity of enhanced food safety controls and consumer education. In this chapter, a number of salient points have been clarified, , such as the extensive range of sources of such toxins from farm pesticides to naturally occurring products in some foods and fish. The mechanism of action through , which such toxins lead to disease is greatly diverse, often leading to both acute and chronic adverse health effects, with a heavy burden on healthcare facilities. Moreover, the existing systems of regulation excluding such hazards, although necessary, must be reviewed continuously to encompass the evolving methods of food production. The overlap of consumer education and stringent enforcement of food safety controls is necessary to prevent foodborne disease based on such hazards. Lastly, preventive control can efficiently reduce the risk of food poisoning due to chemicals and natural toxins (Malik et al., 2011).

KEY TERMS FROM THIS CHAPTER

- Aflatoxins
- Aspergillus
- Bioaccumulate
- Bisphenol A (BPA)
- Body tissues
- Chemical contamination
- Chronic health implications
- Ciguatera
- Deoxynivalenol
- Effluent disposal
- Environmental pollution
- Fusarium
- Good manufacturing practices (GMP)
- Human health
- Lead

REFERENCES

1. Abamecha, N. (2022). *Health Impacts of Foodborne Mycotoxins and Factors Affecting Occurrence of Toxigenic Fungi and Their Toxins in Stored Foods.* https://core.ac.uk/download/543639083.pdf (accessed on 29 May 2025).
2. Abdul Malik, & Grohmann, E. (2011). *Environmental Protection Strategies for Sustainable Development.* Springer Science & Business Media. https://play.google.com/store/books/details?id=OELoLmZLdPsC&source=gbs_api (accessed on 29 May 2025).
3. Abebe, E., Gugsa, G., & Ahmed, M. (2020). Review on major food-borne zoonotic bacterial pathogens. *Journal of Tropical Medicine, 2020*, 1–19. https://doi.org/10.1155/2020/4674235.
4. Anantharam, P., Shao, D., Imerman, P. M., Burrough, E., Schrunk, D., Sedkhuu, T., Tang, S., & Rumbeiha, W. (2016). Improved Tissue-Based Analytical Test Methods for Orellanine, a Biomarker of Cortinarius Mushroom Intoxication. *Toxins, 8*(5), 158. https://doi.org/10.3390/toxins8050158Anthoni, A., Arneson, A., Ascherio, A., Ashwood-Smith, M., Bailey, B., Bannister, L., et al. (2010). *Naturally Occurring Food Toxins.* https://core.ac.uk/download/pdf/8605174.pdf.
5. Awuchi, C. G., Ondari, E. N., Ogbonna, C. U., Upadhyay, A. K., Baran, K., Okpala, C. O. R., & Korzeniowska, M. (2021). Mycotoxins affecting animals, foods, humans, and plants: Types, occurrence, toxicities, action mechanisms, prevention, and detoxification strategies—A revisit. *Foods, 10*(6), 1279. https://doi.org/10.3390/foods10061279.
6. Azeez, M. G. (2001). *Myth and Reality: Organic vs Non-organic.* https://core.ac.uk/download/10924622.pdf (accessed on 29 May 2025).
7. Backer, L. C., Faustman, E. M., Fleming, L. E., Gast, R., et al. (2008). *Linking The Oceans to Public Health: Current Efforts and Future Directions.* https://core.ac.uk/download/4167146.pdf (accessed on 29 May 2025).
8. Baden, D., Bowen, R. E., Depledge, M., Dewailly, É., et al. (2018). *Indicators of Ocean Health and Human Health: Developing A Research and Monitoring Framework.* https://core.ac.uk/download/144580390.pdf (accessed on 29 May 2025).
9. Bandyopadhyay, D., D. Ghosh, A. Chattopadhyay, and E. Mitra. "CURRY LEAVES AS ALTERNATIVE MEDICINE IN HEAVY METAL INDUCED OCCUPATIONAL HEALTH HAZARDS". *International Journal of Pharmacy and Pharmaceutical Sciences*, vol. 8, no. 8, Aug. 2016, pp. 8-20, https://journals.innovareacademics.in/index.php/ijpps/article/view/11694.(accessed on 29 May 2025).
10. Gopal, N., Hill, C., Ross, P. R., Beresford, T. P., Fenelon, M. A., & Cotter, P. D. (2015). The Prevalence and Control of Bacillus and Related Spore-Forming Bacteria in the Dairy Industry. *Frontiers in microbiology, 6*, 1418. https://doi.org/10.3389/fmicb.2015.01418 (accessed on 29 May 2025).
11. Bhat, R. V., & Vasanthi, S. (2025). *Mycotoxin Food Safety Risk in Developing Countries.* https://core.ac.uk/download/pdf/6289224.pdf (accessed on 29 May 2025).
12. Blaney, B. J., Cook, L. G., Klim, E., & MacLachlan, D. J. (2013). *A Review of Potential Contaminants in Australian Livestock Feeds and Proposed Guidance Levels for Feed.* https://core.ac.uk/download/77135913.pdf.
13. Bodi, D., Friedemann, M., Kappenstein, O., Loeffler, C. R., Spielmeyer, A., & Tartaglione, L. (2021). *Ciguatera Mini Review: 21st Century Environmental Challenges and The Interdisciplinary Research Efforts Rising to Meet Them.* https://core.ac.uk/download/541687914.pdf (accessed on 29 May 2025).

14. Ramsingh B. (2014). The emergence of international food safety standards and guidelines: understanding the current landscape through a historical approach. *Perspectives in public health, 134*(4), 206–215. https://doi.org/10.1177/1757913914536557Brandt, Dr Kirsten (2007) Organic Agriculture and Food Utilization. Paper at: Organic Agriculture and Food Security, FAO, Rome, 3-5 May.(accessed on 29 May 2025).

15. Brooks, P. M., Miller, C. J., & Roheim, C. A. (2025). *Toxic Algae Contamination and Demand for Shellfish: A Case Study of Demand for Mussels in Montreal.* https://core.ac.uk/download/pdf/6553825.pdf (accessed on 29 May 2025).

16. Caroline, A., Francis, A., & Bhuvaneshwari. (2022). *Development of a Machine and Detection of Glycoalkaloids in Potato Using Image Processing Technique.* https://core.ac.uk/download/622609451.pdf (accessed on 29 May 2025).

17. Carrascosa, C., Jaber, J. R., Panão, I., & Raposo, A. (2015). *Puffer Fish and Its Consumption: To Eat or Not to Eat?* https://core.ac.uk/download/62698836.pdf (accessed on 29 May 2025).

18. Castro-Escarpulli, G., Gonzalez-Avila, L. U., Guerrero-Mandujano, A., & Hernández-Cortez, C. (2017). *Food Poisoning Caused by Bacteria (Food Toxins).* https://core.ac.uk/download/322432394.pdf (accessed on 29 May 2025).

19. Dave, P., & Dutta, G. (2021). *Detection of Pesticides in Food by CDs Blue Luminescent Material with The Help of Fluorescence Quenching Study.* https://core.ac.uk/download/595875514.pdf (accessed on 29 May 2025).

20. Heaviside, C., Lake, I., & Nichols, G. (2018). *Climate Change and Water-Related Infectious Diseases.* https://core.ac.uk/download/322490318.pdf (accessed on 29 May 2025).

21. Heidari, T., Sadighara, P., Oskoei, V., & Zeinali, T. (2023). Significance of climate change in food safety and hygiene. *Jundishapur Journal of Health Sciences.* https://www.semanticscholar.org/paper/05e5fd8937755d15610e7599f1f5c9b28cf2712d (accessed on 29 May 2025).

22. Kazmierczak, R. F., Jr., & Willson, T. M. (2025). *The Public Health and Economic Impacts of Persistent, Bio Accumulative, and Toxic (PBT) Contaminants on U.S. Fisheries.* https://core.ac.uk/download/pdf/6546529.pdf (accessed on 29 May 2025).

23. Khan, S. (2009). *Climate of Opportunity: Gender and Movement Building at The Intersection of Reproductive Justice and Environmental Justice.* https://core.ac.uk/download/75784987.pdf (accessed on 29 May 2025).

24. Khoat, N. V. (2024). *Crimes Related to Toxic Chemicals Use in Vietnam: The Cases and Recommendations.* https://core.ac.uk/download/640070155.pdf (accessed on 29 May 2025).

25. Praveen Kumar, Anita, Neha Joshi, Are the Food Additives, Safe or Harmful? - A Review. J Ayu Int Med Sci. 2023;8(5):140-144.

26. Available From

27. https://jaims.in/jaims/article/view/2487Kumari, A., Negi, D., Thakur, K., & Joshi, R. (2021). *Effects of Food Pollution on Human Health and Its Management Through Panchakarma.* https://core.ac.uk/download/478522120.pdf (accessed on 29 May 2025).

28. Malangu, N. (2016). Risk Factors and Outcomes of Food Poisoning in Africa. InTech. doi: 10.5772/62274

29. Miglas, H. (2025). *Review on the Hidden Potential Health Risks of Natural Toxins in Honey Bees (Apis mellifera) "Honey" in Tigray, Ethiopia*. https://core.ac.uk/download/654538509.pdf (accessed on 29 May 2025).

30. Njue, L. G., & Wanjiru, J. W. (2022). *Food Safety Issues Across the Food Chain and The Contaminants Involved*. https://core.ac.uk/download/543639317.pdf (accessed on 29 May 2025).

31. Paulraj, R. (2002). Mycotoxins in feeds and their impact on fish and shrimp. In *Winter School on Recent Advances in Diagnosis and Management of Diseases in Mariculture* (Course Manual, 7th–27th November 2002). https://core.ac.uk/download/33015553.pdf (accessed on 29 May 2025).

32. Pinstrup-Andersen, P. (2025). *Agricultural Research and Policy for Better Health and Nutrition in Developing Countries: A Food Systems Approach*. https://core.ac.uk/download/pdf/7055873.pdf (accessed on 29 May 2025).

33. Ros I Aragonès, J. (2012). *Rachel Carson, Sensitive and Perceptive Interpreter of Nature*. https://core.ac.uk/download/39027317.pdf (accessed on 29 May 2025).

34. Silva, M., Tamele, I., & Vasconcelos, V. (2019). The incidence of marine toxins and the associated seafood poisoning episodes in the African countries of the Indian Ocean and the Red Sea. https://core.ac.uk/download/344682171.pdf (accessed on 29 May 2025).

35. Slocum, N. (2018). *Toxins in the Collection: Museum Awareness and Protection*. https://core.ac.uk/download/230759598.pdf (accessed on 29 May 2025).

36. Subra, W. (2007). *Industrial Sources of Dioxin Poisoning in Mossville, Louisiana: A Report Based on The Government's Own Data*. https://core.ac.uk/download/71345911.pdf (accessed on 29 May 2025).

37. Uçar, A., Yilmaz, M. V., & Çakıroğlu, F. P. (2016). *Food Safety–Problems and Solutions*. https://core.ac.uk/download/322426193.pdf.

38. Woh, P. Y., & Ng, C. (2024). *Bacillus cereus* in rice: A review on food poisoning, antimicrobial resistance, and control measures. *Tropical Biomedicine, 41*(3), 298–309. https://www.semanticscholar.org/paper/a316fcf46b486a01f40431f67ec1bd6ab6c31f88 (accessed on 29 May 2025).

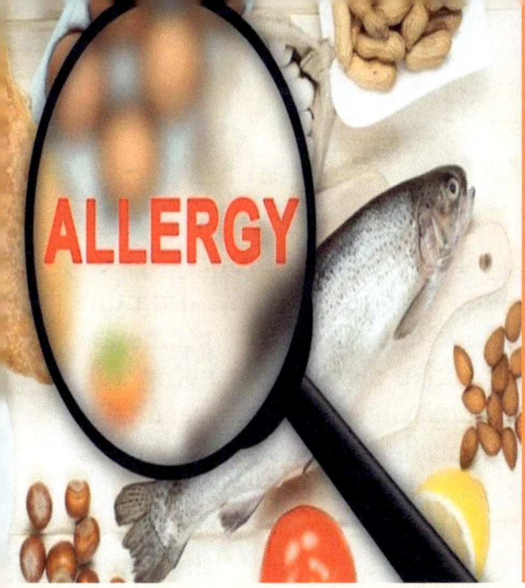

Chapter 12

FOOD ALLERGIES AND INTOLERANCES

Contents

Introduction...273
12.1. Types of Food Allergies 276
12.2. Types of Food Intolerances 280
12.3. Management and Treatment 284
12.4. Societal and Economic Impact...288
Summary 294
References 295

Introduction

Food allergies are a public health concern, particularly in the context of an increasingly diverse food environment. Their increasing prevalence has been consistently reported, with 18% reported increments between 1997 and 2007, suggesting that more research and education are is necessary (Centers for Disease Control and Prevention, 2013). This is also the case in certain populations, such as college students, who are typically responsible for providing allergen-friendly options through campus food systems, a demonstration of the intersection of food allergies and accessibility (Food Allergy Research & Education, 2014). Additionally, while reporting of food allergies among pregnant women reflects established trends among the adult population as a whole, the potential impact on maternal and infant health remains unknown (Seita, 2013). As such, it is necessary to grasp the complexities involved with food allergies and intolerances to the development of effective management strategies and the encouragement of healthier communities.

Definition of Food Allergies

When the body mistakes some proteins in food for threats, it leads to an immune response , which is called a food allergy. When this happens, symptoms may be as simple as hives or as serious as anaphylaxis , which can be dangerous. The prevalence of food allergies has notably increased in Western countries, particularly among young children, leading researchers to investigate the underlying causes and risk factors associated with this phenomenon (Seita, 2013). While previous studies have concentrated largely on childhood allergies, there remains a significant gap in understanding their prevalence among adults and expectant mothers (Seita, 2013). It is also necessary to tell apart food allergies from food intolerances , which are not related to the immune system and can cause problems like stomach upset. This distinction is crucial for effective diagnosis and management of dietary reactions (Figure 12.1).

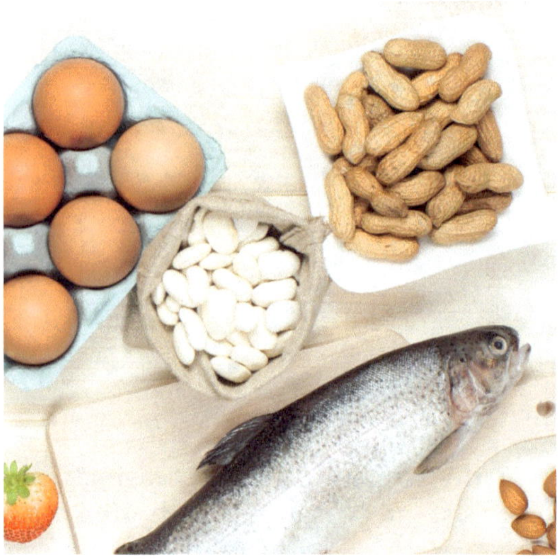

Figure 12.1. Food allergies are defined as adverse immune system reactions that occur when the body misidentifies certain proteins in food as harmful, prompting an immune response.

Source: https://foodallergycanada.ca/wp-content/uploads/what-is-food-allergy-2.jpg.

Definition of Food Intolerances

Food intolerances , which are not the same as food allergies, involve a different physical reaction that does not involve the immune system. Most of the time, these symptoms are caused by the digestive system not being able to handle some substances , which results in bloating, gas and diarrhea. Unlike food allergies, intolerances are usually not as dangerous, but they can still have a big influence on someone's daily life. Many people struggle with lactose intolerance, where they are missing the enzyme needed to handle lactose and gluten sensitivity , which may cause distress but is not linked to the immune issues of celiac disease. Because more people are aware of food intolerances, there are now more talks about modifying diets and managing them. As highlighted in various studies, addressing food intolerances involves understanding individual triggers and may also intersect with broader dietary trends, such as the misguided perception linking grains to adverse reactions (Seita, 2013; Dunn, 2020).

Prevalence of Food Allergies and Intolerances

The increasing incidence of food allergies and intolerances has also attracted significant attention from researchers and health experts, with evidence of alarming trends, predominantly in children. The most recent evidence indicates that food allergies have emerged as the second most common type of allergic disorder in Western countries, with dramatic increases in the United States over the past decades, particularly in children (Seita, 2013). Alarming, almost half of boy children and about 40% of girl children exhibit signs of food hypersensitivity, such as food allergies and intolerances (Patel, 2020). The evidence suggests the urgent need for increased awareness and regulation of food allergies, especially in maternal health and infant outcomes. It is required to identify the determinants of increasing numbers to evidence-based policy-making and intervention to manage the related risks of food allergies and intolerances in children and adults (Figure 12.2).

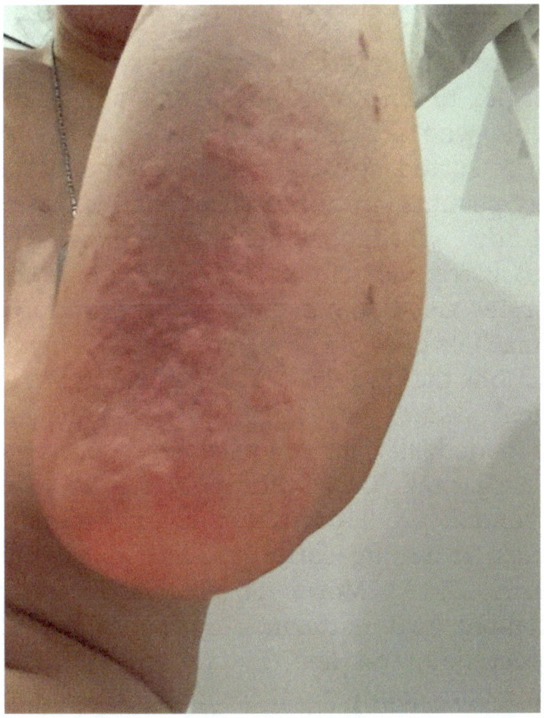

Figure 12.2. The increasing prevalence of food allergies and intolerances has garnered significant attention from researchers and health professionals alike, revealing alarming trends, particularly among young populations.

Source: https://blogger.googleusercontent.com/img/b/R29vZ2xl/AVvXsEhSaFQ-CbZsTCzYQWmM8dmpW50guQOlD_oyRvyBCfpLv0cLgsm7-bFWUuTh0Azov-6N2B3wJIBD4jvZaxBh-W-R2rqHZrhsule6GAySEgte2e_RoFYGYLXxakgrzxumraZAgVmAj-4mxqFlvhyphenhyphen9mtkPEEWucSk8pkHUOXVAXx8mMLOTI_zDLtC43afWPiQ/s1024/51535730081_1b6042d1dc_b.jpg.

Overview of Symptoms and Reactions

The expression of food intolerance and allergies is also extremely varied, affecting people in countless ways through their specific physiological mechanisms. For food allergies, the body reacts to proteins in food, and allergic reactions manifest within a few minutes to hours after ingestion. The symptoms may vary from the least severe presentations, including hives and gastrointestinal discomfort, to complete, life-threatening anaphylaxis, which manifests as difficulty in breathing and a drop in blood pressure.

For food intolerances, not an immune system issue, usually manifests as gastrointestinal discomfort in the form of bloating, diarrhea, and gas, indicating that they are less immediately life-threatening but no less intensely unpleasant. The rising prevalence of these conditions has been well-documented, with food allergies increasing by 18% between 1997 and 2007, showing the need for education and awareness of effective management of such reactions (Brummel et al., 2019; Seita, 2013).

Impact on Daily Life and Health

Daily life and health can be affected by food allergies and intolerances , which influence both meals and moods. Individuals often experience heightened food anxiety, which can detract from social interactions and family activities, as highlighted in studies measuring health-related quality of life (HRQL) among affected individuals and their families (Dean et al., 2015). Having to avoid allergens can make people feel cut off from others and always watchful , which makes everyday eating a challenge. Also, it is very important to have clear nutritional information, as can be seen by efforts to redesign restaurant nutrition labels. These measures aim to empower consumers so that they can make informed choices and may mitigate risks through unhealthy diets, which are linked to larger health problems like obesity (Lages et al., 2013). These issues being overcome through education and improved resources can hence enhance the welfare of the affected (Figure 12.3).

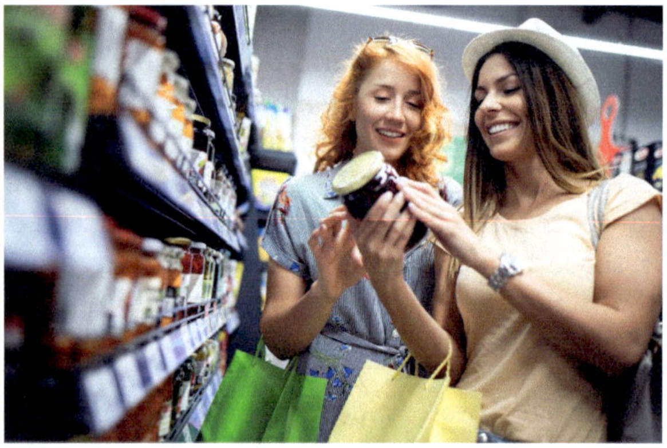

Figure 12.3. Food allergies and intolerances can significantly impact daily life and overall health, influencing not only dietary choices but also emotional well-being.

Source: https://www.julienutrition.com/wp-content/uploads/2024/12/Factors-that-Influence-Food-Choices-JM-Nutrition.jpg.

Food intolerance and food allergy management through diet is predominantly dietary since there are no cures. People diagnosed with food allergies are typically instructed to avoid foods to , which they are allergic completely, and learning about this takes a lot of education on ingredient labeling and cross-contamination risk. In the same way, food intolerance patients can also be treated through the elimination diet technique, where they isolate and methodically eliminate culprit foods from their diets to monitor symptomatic responses. The lifestyle changes involved have great repercussions, however, which can lead to eating disorders, particularly among vulnerable groups like students. The eating disorders arise from heightened awareness of dietary restrictions, which impact mental health and social relationships (Burns, 2025). Moreover, the lack of availability of allergen-free food products, especially among poor populations, makes dietary control even harder (Parmely et al., 2017). Hence, ongoing education and support systems are necessary for individuals experiencing these dietary challenges.

12.1. Types of Food Allergies

It is very important to learn the types of food allergies to help prevent and manage them in people who are affected. Most food allergies can be sorted into eight main allergens: milk, eggs, peanuts, tree nuts, fish, shellfish, wheat and soy , which together are responsible for most allergic reactions. The symptoms of these allergies may be mild , such as hives and upset stomach or they can be severe, like anaphylactic reactions that require quick medical treatment. Recent studies have also noted a concerning rise in food allergies among children, prompting investigations into underlying causes , such as genetic predisposition and environmental factors, including early exposure to allergens (Burns, 2019). Moreover, emerging research indicates that maternal food allergies may impact neonatal health outcomes, although significant connections remain inadequately explored (Seita, 2013). When we know more about allergies, we can improve the ways we diagnose and manage them in the future.

12.1.1. Common Food Allergens (e.g., Peanuts, Tree Nuts)

Food allergy is a public health concern, with children especially being affected, and peanuts and tree nuts being significant allergens. As the incidence of these allergies has increased, especially in Western populations, the etiology of sensitization and the role of diet have been the subject of study. It has been demonstrated that early allergenic food introduction, e.g., peanuts and tree nuts, can have a significant influence on the development of allergy; for instance, 63% of infants exposed to the allergens before 12 months had an allergy, while 33% had an allergy when exposed later (Shaw et al., 2017). Maternal food allergy has also been labeled as a concern, with these being reported to be consistent with national averages, with the implication that diet during pregnancy influences infant health outcomes (Seita, 2013). These are aspects that need to be considered when crafting appropriate prevention measures and formulating guidelines on infant allergenic food introduction (Figure 12.4).

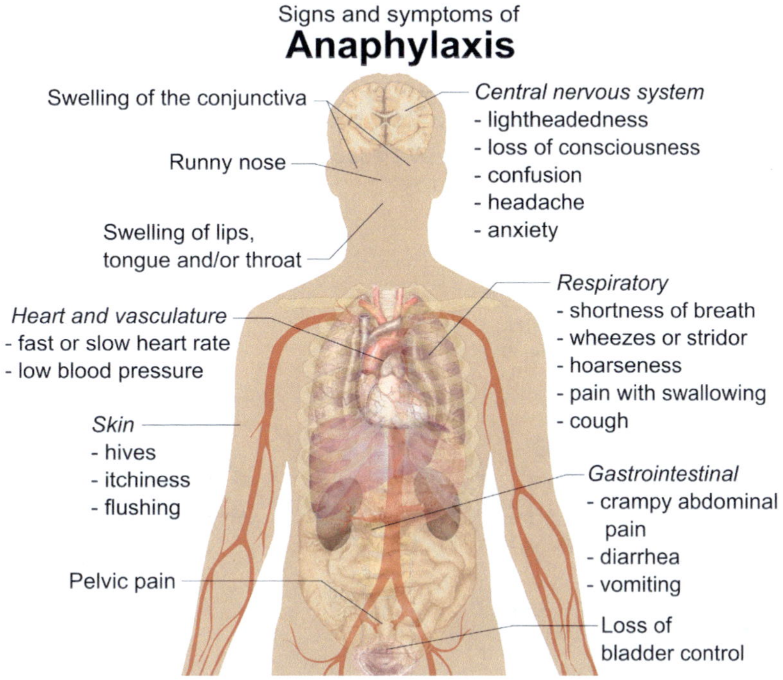

Figure 12.4. Food allergies represent a significant public health concern, particularly among children, with common allergens including peanuts and tree nuts.

Source: By Mikael Häggström - Own work, CC0, https://commons.wikimedia.org/w/index.php?curid=17700391

12.1.2. Less Common Food Allergens (e.g., Shellfish, Soy)

There has been more focus on food allergies lately, mainly because of allergies to shellfish and soy. Although most people know about peanuts and tree nuts, new studies show that some other allergens can cause serious allergy symptoms in certain individuals. Many adults have shellfish allergies that can cause mild to highly severe reactions and therefore, it is crucial to study why these hypersensitivities occur. Knowing the factors leading to these hypersensitivities, including inherited tendency and exposure, will help establish successful management plans (Burns, 2019). Additionally, the hygiene hypothesis also suggests that reduced exposure to different microbial environments may be held responsible for the increasing incidence of food allergies, including allergies from less common allergens like soy and shellfish (Candreva et al., 2016). Therefore, additional study is needed in order to enhance the diagnosis and management of patients.

12.1.3. IgE-Mediated vs. Non-IgE-Mediated Allergies

It is very important to tell IgE-mediated allergies apart from non-IgE-mediated allergies to better understand food allergies. An IgE-mediated response happens when the immune system produces immunoglobulin E antibodies after eating certain food proteins and this often leads to immediate hypersensitivity reactions. Hives, anaphylaxis or stomach problems may appear a short time after contact with the allergen. In contrast, allergies that do not involve IgE antibodies usually cause reactions that happen later. As a result, these reactions might appear as long-lasting stomach or skin problems , which makes it hard to diagnose them. A recent study indicated that food allergies are rising, especially among expectant mothers, yet it remains unclear how these allergies may affect maternal and infant health outcomes (Seita, 2013). In addition, the same dichotomy is found in veterinary medicine since the non-IgE-mediated reactions can also have a significant effect on canine health, illustrating the broader context of these allergic reactions beyond human situations (Dunn, 2020) (Figure 12.5).

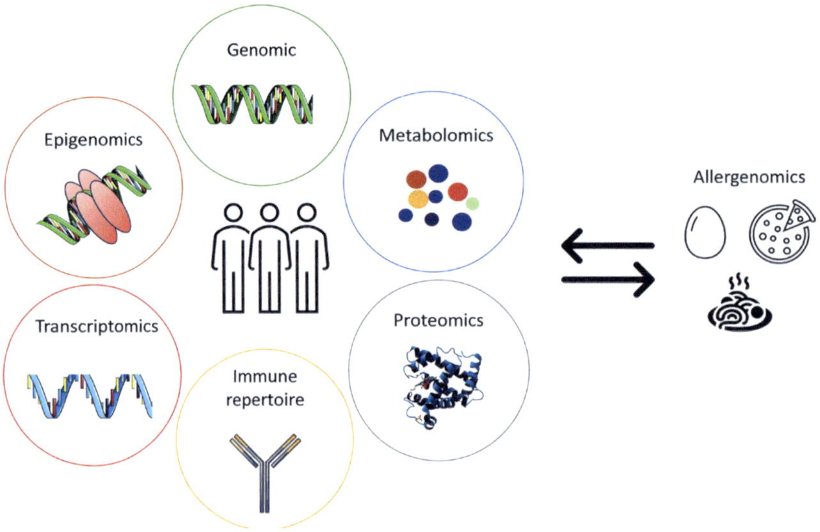

Figure 12.5. The distinction between IgE-mediated and non-IgE-mediated allergies is crucial in understanding the complex nature of food allergies.

Source: https://www.immunology.theclinics.com/cms/10.1016/j.iac.2021.01.003/asset/44efcedb-ff18-42ef-9cf4-887b6035a053/main.assets/gr3_lrg.jpg.

12.1.4. Cross-Reactivity Among Allergens

It is difficult to understand food allergies and intolerances because allergens can react with each other. The immune system can confuse proteins in one food with those in another , which can cause allergies. As an example, those allergic to nuts could also react to foods that have similar proteins , which makes it harder to manage their diet. It is very important to understand cross-reactivity because it affects both the diagnosis and the treatment and strategies for avoiding allergens should consider these interactions. Furthermore, misconceptions about food allergens can exacerbate the problem; for example, the prevalent belief that grains are the primary culprits in allergic reactions has resulted in dietary changes that may not address the underlying issues, as highlighted by the growing awareness of food reactions among dogs with elimination diets (Dunn, 2020). Addressing cross-reactivity requires a more refined approach that considers individual responses and the broader spectrum of allergens, reminiscent of the epidemiological challenges faced in Africa regarding allergies (Adams et al., 2010).

12.1.5. Anaphylaxis and Its Implications

Anaphylaxis, a condition of severe allergic reaction and life-threatening in nature, is prevalent in people with food allergy, and hence the extreme significance of awareness and preparedness in the treatment of food allergies. Documented increases, particularly in children, in food allergy have been reported, with both environmental and genetic factors significantly playing a contributory role towards their development (Seita, 2013).

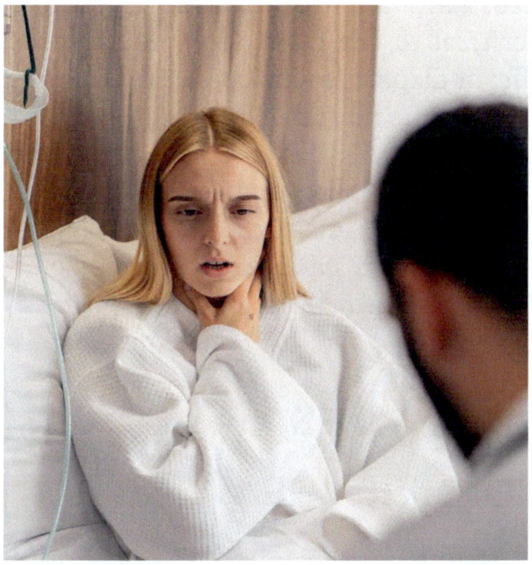

Figure 12.6. Anaphylaxis, a severe and potentially life-threatening allergic reaction, often occurs in individuals with food allergies, highlighting the critical need for awareness and preparedness in managing such conditions.

Source: https://keepsmilin4abbie.org/wp-content/uploads/2024/06/allergic-reaction-anaphylaxis-treatment-and-prevention-e1720019483735.jpg.

Anaphylaxis develops very rapidly, and immediate action with epinephrine must be initiated to avert severe health repercussions, and hence, education toward the identification of symptoms is the very essence of those involved and their families. Aside from this, individuals might take restrictive diets to prevent exposure to allergens, which can have the consequence of inducing disordered eating behavior and nutrition insufficiencies (Burns, 2025). Appreciation of the implications of anaphylaxis, therefore, not only emphasizes the significance of preparedness in emergencies but also demands cautious planning concerning dietary management to ensure security and overall health for food-allergic individuals (Figure 12.6).

12.1.6. Diagnosis Methods for Food Allergies

A healthcare provider uses both evaluation and various tests to diagnose food allergies. Elimination diets are seen as the best approach, where patients remove possible allergy-causing foods, then add them back one by one to spot the triggers. Even though this approach takes time, it gives valuable knowledge about what affects a person. Also, new ways to diagnose allergies , such as serum antibody tests and skin prick testing, are being used more often. They are used to check the immune system's reaction to possible allergens, but they do not give a definitive answer for everyone. Studies done lately point out that correct diagnosis is very important, especially because there are many false beliefs about food allergens , such as the belief that grains can cause food reactions. Specifically, research in Ireland highlighted that almost half of male children experience food hypersensitivity, underscoring the pressing need for effective diagnosis and management in the pediatric population (Dunn, 2020; Patel, 2020).

12.1.7. Role of Genetic Factors in Food Allergies

The way genes work together is a major reason why food allergies are more common in children. Several studies point out that children with family members who have atopy are more likely to develop food allergies. It is crucial because it points out the need to study better how the immune system causes hypersensitivity reactions. According to recent research, one's genetic composition can identify whether an individual's immune system can differentiate between harmful and harmless entities, and consequently, the level of susceptibility to various allergens (Burns, 2019). Moreover, the increase in food allergies over the last few decades suggests that environmental factors could mix with genetic makeup, strengthening their effect (Seita, 2013). Thus, unraveling the genetic underpinnings of food allergy is important in developing targeted interventions and enhancing clinical outcomes (Figure 12.7).

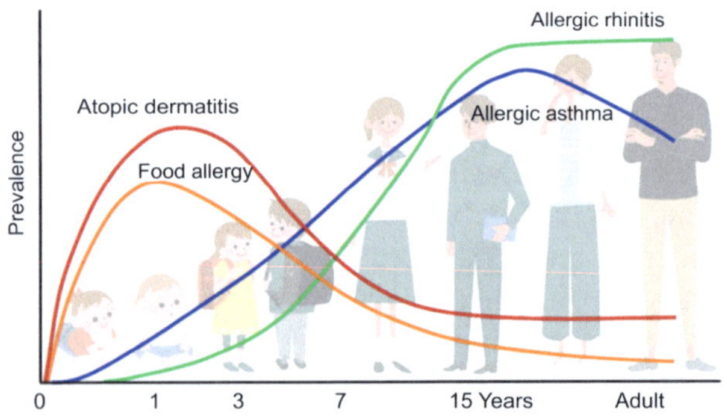

Figure 12.7. Multiple studies have indicated that a strong hereditary component exists in allergies, where children with a family history of atopy are at a heightened risk for food sensitivities.

Source: Tsuge M, Ikeda M, Matsumoto N, Yorifuji T, Tsukahara H. Current Insights into Atopic March. *Children*. 2021; 8(11):1067. https://doi.org/10.3390/children8111067

12.1.8. Environmental Factors Contributing to Allergies

The heightened occurrence of food intolerance and allergy has been linked to a number of environmental factors that complicate the health outcomes of the population. Urban lifestyles and high levels of exposure to some pollutants, such as pesticides and industrial emissions, have been found to play a significant role in raising the incidence of allergic diseases, particularly among children. Studies have established that children exposed to urban environments report increased food hypersensitivity, suggesting a link between environmental stresses and immune response abnormalities. For instance, a recent study postulated that almost half of male children in some areas have reported food hypersensitivity, which calls for further studies on how environmental exposure affects this population (Patel, 2020). Access to healthcare services and allergen-free food products is also critical to the control of the diseases, but significant disparities in access exist, particularly for low-income households, which suggests that socio-economic factors complicate the influence of environmental allergens (Parmely et al., 2017). This intersection of environmental and socio-economic factors calls for a multidisciplinary approach to controlling food allergies.

12.2. Types of Food Intolerances

It is essential to realize the various food intolerances within the broader framework of food allergies and intolerances. Food intolerances normally stem from the body's inability to digest some substances properly, usually because of a deficiency in digestive enzymes, such as the case of lactose intolerance, where the absence of lactase results in the body's inability to digest lactose in milk products. Gluten intolerance is another significant form that results in discomfort and fatigue, but not celiac disease-based immune response. The prevalence of food intolerances, particularly within the framework of child allergies, also makes it evident that there is an immense need for research. For instance, whereas genetic and environmental factors are the cause of food sensitivities among children, the cause of these intolerances remains under researched (Burns, 2019). In addition, epidemiological research proves that a lot more adults are also affected by the same intolerances, necessitating the need to differentiate various sensitivities to food (Seita, 2013).

12.2.1. Common Food Intolerances (e.g., Lactose, Gluten)

Trouble with lactose and gluten in food is a major concern for many people when they try to manage their diet. If the body does not make enough lactase enzyme, eating dairy products causes gastrointestinal problems.

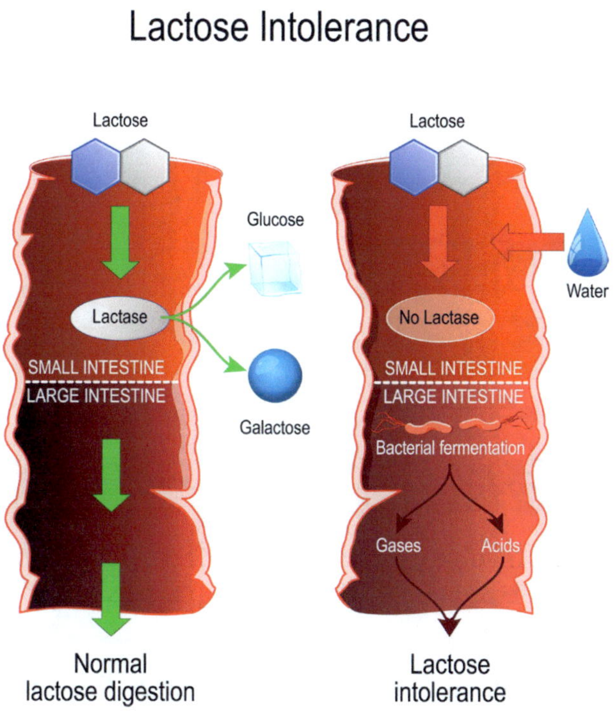

Figure 12.8. Lactose intolerance, caused by the insufficient production of lactase enzyme, leads to gastrointestinal distress upon the consumption of dairy products.

Source: https://media.islamicity.org/wp-content/uploads/2020/11/Infographic-lactose-scaled.jpg.

In the same way, gluten intolerance , which is often linked to celiac disease, causes problems when someone consumes foods with gluten. Research indicates that food hypersensitivities are prevalent, particularly among children; a study found that nearly half of male children and about 40% of female children experience various forms of food hypersensitivity, including food intolerances like lactose and gluten (Patel, 2020). Along with this, as increased emphasis is being placed on food labeling and allergens, the baking industry is evolving to accommodate special diets around these common intolerances (BC Cook Articulation Committee, 2015). It is critical to comprehend these issues in an effort to create better health outcomes and reach culinary satisfaction on the part of those involved (Figure 12.8).

12.2.2. Symptoms of Food Intolerances

Understanding the symptoms of food intolerances is important in differentiating them from food allergies, which are immune-mediated. Food intolerances seem to present with gastrointestinal symptoms, including bloating, gas, diarrhea, and abdominal pain, especially after the consumption of problem foods , such as dairy or gluten (Bevan et al., 2020). Such discomfort can be explained by the body's inability to digest certain substances normally, resulting in malabsorption and consequent symptoms. In contrast to allergies, which can elicit more serious, systemic symptoms, intolerances are more likely to elicit milder, chronic symptoms that do not necessarily occur immediately following the consumption of the offending food (Kumar, 2019). While food allergies can elicit life-threatening reactions, food intolerances will more likely necessitate a low-key management strategy, with dietary adjustments to alleviate unpleasant symptoms. Understanding and awareness of such reactions enable individuals to make informed dietary choices, ultimately supporting their overall health and quality of life.

12.2.3. Mechanisms Behind Food Intolerances

Food intolerances are different from allergies because the digestive system is unable to process some substances. Food allergies happen right away, but intolerances usually cause problems later , such as discomfort, bloating and similar issues. Intolerances can be caused by a lack of the needed enzyme, for example, lactose intolerance is due to not having enough lactase or they may be related to sensitivity to gluten or additives. Such intolerances can compel individuals to eliminate specific foods, often resulting in disordered eating patterns, as indicated in recent studies that correlate dietary restrictions with adverse emotional and social outcomes (Burns, 2025). As pediatric allergies and intolerances have gained heightened attention in research, understanding the underlying mechanisms, including genetic predispositions and environmental factors, has become crucial in developing effective interventions for affected populations (Burns, 2019) (Figure 12.9).

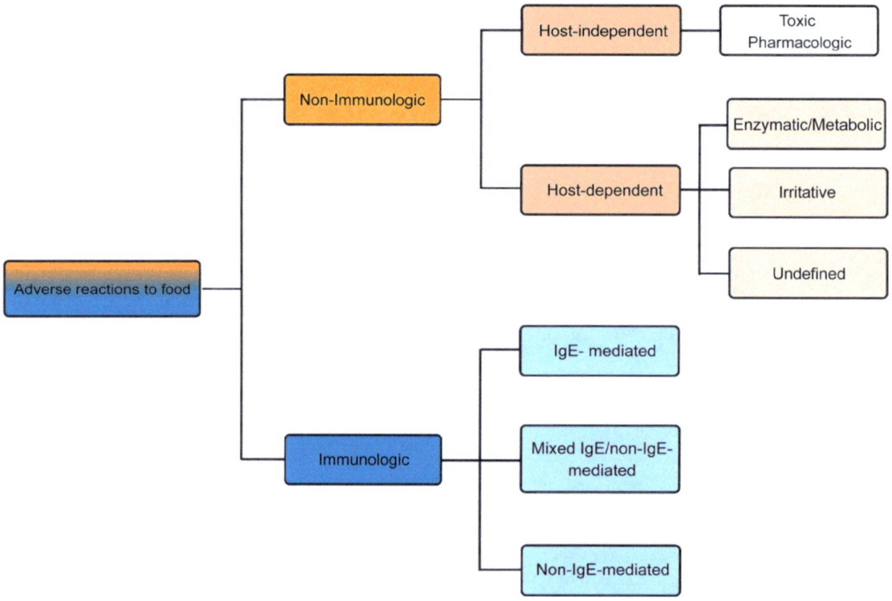

Figure 12.9. Food intolerances are complex phenomena that involve various physiological mechanisms distinct from allergies, primarily concerning the digestive system's inability to process certain substances.

Source: Gargano D, Appanna R, Santonicola A, De Bartolomeis F, Stellato C, Cianferoni A, Casolaro V, Iovino P. Food Allergy and Intolerance: A Narrative Review on Nutritional Concerns. *Nutrients*. 2021; 13(5):1638. https://doi.org/10.3390/nu13051638

12.2.4. Diagnosis Methods for Food Intolerances

Finding better ways to diagnose food intolerances is still a major concern in the overall study of food allergies and intolerances. Usually, the first step in diagnosing is to review the patient's medical history and check how symptoms relate to their diet. Certain laboratory tests , such as specific IgG antibodies, are often carried out, but their usefulness is questionable. Avoiding certain foods, then reintroducing them gradually, allows the patient to recognize the food that is causing symptoms in them. Recent studies have indicated an increasing realization of food intolerances amongst certain groups, and this acts to reinforce the requirement for properly developed and standardized diagnostic techniques (Seita, 2013). Besides, understanding the mechanisms of hypersensitivity reactions will offer avenues to enhance diagnostic and therapeutic strategies and is hence a viable area for future research in the management of food intolerance (Burns, 2019).

12.2.5. Role of Gut Health in Food Intolerances

The role of gut health in food intolerances has been a major area of research with implications for prevalence and management. The gut microbiome, a complex microbial ecosystem that resides in the gastrointestinal tract, regulates the digestion of food and the immune response to potential allergens.

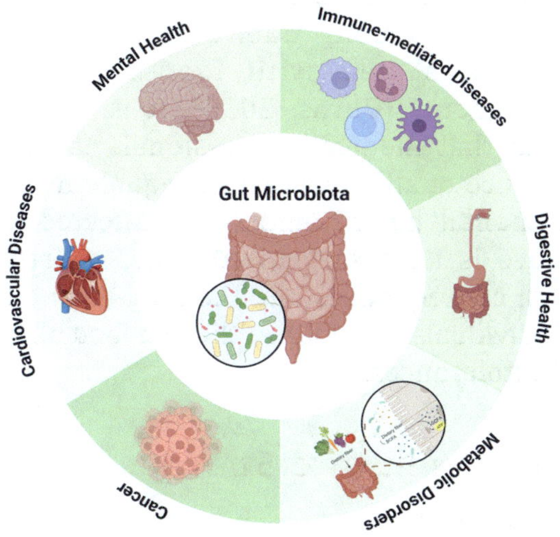

Figure 12.10. The role of gut health in food intolerances has emerged as a critical area of research, given its implications for both prevalence and management.

Source: Yaqub MO, Jain A, Joseph CE, Edison LK. Microbiome-Driven Therapeutics: From Gut Health to Precision Medicine. *Gastrointestinal Disorders*. 2025; 7(1):7. https://doi.org/10.3390/gidisord7010007

Deviations from gut health result in increased intestinal permeability, or leaky gut, allowing undigested food material to pass into the bloodstream and potentially trigger intolerances and hypersensitivity reactions. Current evidence indicates diet, antibiotic exposure, and environmental exposures are major determinants of the makeup of gut microbiota, which may be associated with the prevalence of food intolerances in children. , such as associations are central to developing effective interventions that restore gut health, providing a mechanism for the prevention of rising rates of food allergies and intolerances, as demonstrated by findings of studies of children with food sensitivities (Burns, 2019; Patel, 2020) (Figure 12.10).

12.2.6. Impact of Food Intolerances on Nutrition

Food intolerances can seriously affect nutrition, because many people must remove entire food groups from their diets to avoid problems. A vegan diet may not supply all the necessary nutrients, especially when the main sources of those nutrients are the foods that are excluded. Avoiding dairy may not give you enough calcium and vitamin D , which are important for your bones. Furthermore, as noted in research, food intolerances have been linked to disordered eating patterns among affected individuals, exacerbating the situation by potentially promoting unhealthy dietary habits (Burns, 2025).

Additionally, socio-economic factors influence access to allergen-free foods and nutritional guidance, further complicating the health landscape for those with food intolerances (Parmely et al., 2017). When there are not enough resources and proper nutrition management, people may have a hard time maintaining healthy eating , which stresses the importance of strong support systems.

12.2.7. Psychological Effects of Food Intolerances

The psychological effect of food intolerances is increasingly becoming universally accepted as a prominent factor, particularly in adolescents and young adults. Individuals with food intolerances indicate heightened levels of anxiety and stress in having to be constantly vigilant with the avoidance of the offending foods. Such avoidance diets result in social withdrawal and loss, as such individuals will not engage in social events centered on food, a socialized activity. According to research, food avoidance has been identified as a predictor of disordered eating behavior, indicating that the psychological effect of dealing with food intolerances can be manifested as maladaptive eating behavior (Burns, 2025).

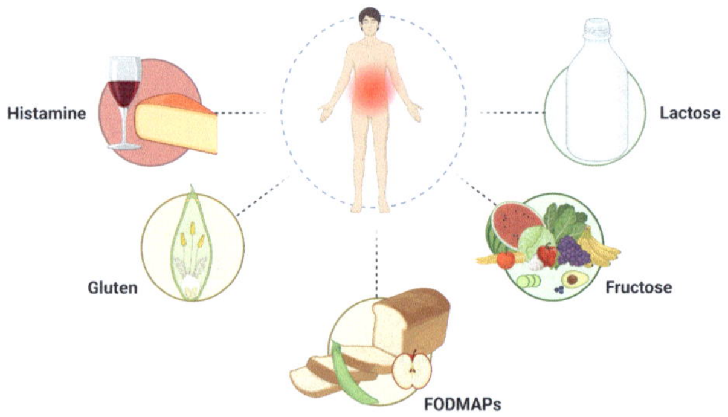

Figure 12.11. The psychological effects of food intolerances are increasingly recognized as significant, particularly among adolescents and young adults.

Source: Zingone F, Bertin L, Maniero D, Palo M, Lorenzon G, Barberio B, Ciacci C, Savarino EV. Myths and Facts about Food Intolerance: A Narrative Review. *Nutrients*. 2023; 15(23):4969. https://doi.org/10.3390/nu15234969

Research has also documented high levels of food hypersensitivity in children, and implications for their psychological health in coping with their social lives and avoidance diets (Patel, 2020). It is thus critical to comprehend these psychological factors for the development of effective support systems for individuals who must persevere with food intolerances (Figure 12.11).

12.3. Management and Treatment

Managing and treating food allergies and intolerances requires teaching patients, adjusting their diets and continuing research on the causes. Strictly avoiding known allergens is usually the first step in management, since even a tiny amount can cause a severe reaction in children who have just been diagnosed. Also, awareness of risk factors for pediatric allergy, such as genetic susceptibility and environment, can inform prevention and intervention (Burns, 2019). While dietary avoidance is common, it carries the potential to increase the risk of developing disordered eating behavior, particularly among adolescents and young adults presented with food-based social environments (Burns, 2025). It is, therefore, crucial that medical professionals tackle the avoidance of allergens with adequate nutrition and mental health among the affected. Such a move is necessary to curb the short-term health consequences and the long-term effects on individuals' mental health from food allergies and intolerances.

12.3.1. Avoidance Strategies for Allergens

The rising prevalence of food allergy has necessitated effective avoidance strategies as a primary management approach in vulnerable individuals. Strict diet avoidance is generally the first line of defense, where patient and carer rely on careful reading of food labels and awareness of food preparation cross-contamination hazards is expected (Burns, 2019). This is especially necessary in settings , such as schools and restaurants where allergen exposure may inadvertently occur. Apart from dietary intervention, allergen immunotherapy (AIT) has been shown to be an innovative treatment approach, particularly in children, as the potential of modulating the immune system and decreasing sensitivity over time (Arasi et al., 2018). Although avoidance is the primary concern, AIT offers some form of intervention that can decrease the risk of future allergic reactions. Education regarding avoidance strategies and new therapies is crucial in patients with food allergy, in the end, to minimize the risk of exposure and enhance quality of life (Figure 12.12).

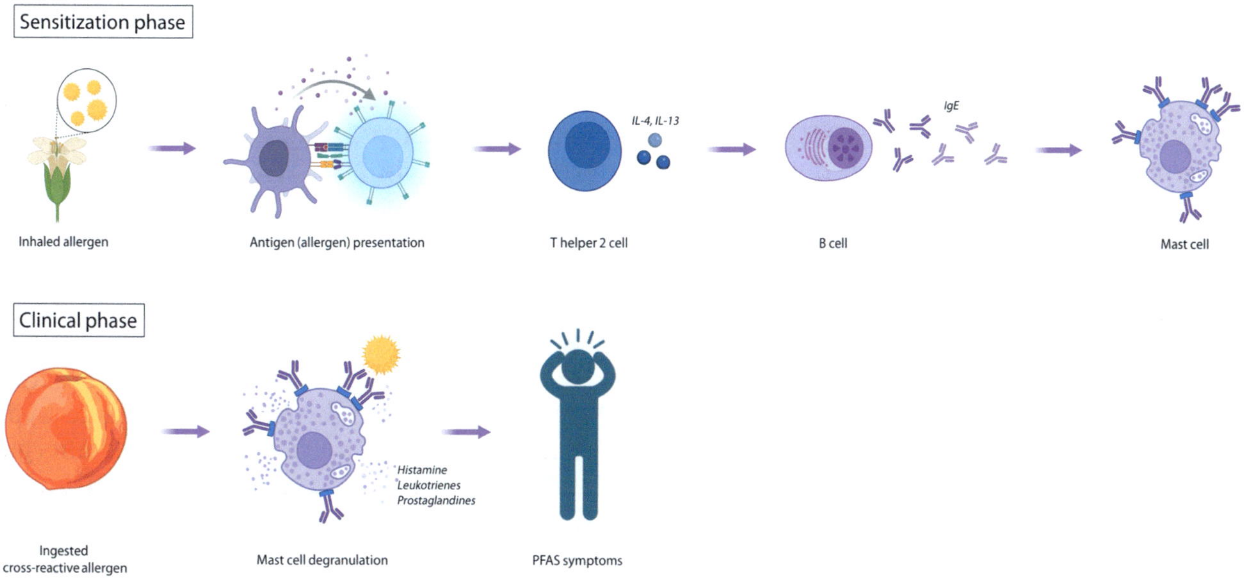

Figure 12.12. The rising prevalence of food allergies has necessitated the development of effective avoidance strategies as a critical management approach for individuals at risk.

Source: Haidar L, Bănărescu CF, Uța C, Moldovan SI, Zimbru E-L, Zimbru R-I, Ciurariu E, Georgescu M, Panaitescu C. Pollen–Food Allergy Syndrome: Allergens, Clinical Insights, Diagnostic and Therapeutic Challenges. *Applied Sciences*. 2025; 15(1):66. https://doi.org/10.3390/app15010066

12.3.2. Dietary Modifications for Intolerances

The increasing prevalence of food intolerances has provided the impetus for dietary changes to accommodate individual sensitivity without reducing nutrition. The most frequent of these changes are the exclusion of foods or food groups, which can lead to a degree of nutritional deficiency if well monitored. An unsettling association with food avoidance and the onset of disordered eating patterns in individuals, especially college students (Burns, 2025), has been reported. Also, dietary changes to minimize inflammatory reactions have been found to have significant health effects, with amelioration of inflammatory markers and body composition (Hoppensteadt et al., 2015). Such findings highlight the need for using evidence-based diet regimens that not only provide relief from the symptoms of food intolerances but also enable an overall approach to nutrition, enabling individuals to ensure balanced intake despite individual dietary restrictions.

12.3.3. Use of Medications (e.g., Antihistamines, Epinephrine)

Understanding how to use antihistamines and epinephrine is very important for managing food allergies. Antihistamines are commonly taken to control mild allergic reactions and ease itching, hives and other symptoms in one area. In cases where the reaction is very severe , such as anaphylaxis, epinephrine should be used as the first treatment. A study indicated that only 34% of severe allergic reactions were treated with epinephrine, despite a high likelihood of anaphylaxis in many cases, illustrating a critical gap in awareness and response among caregivers and healthcare professionals (Green et al., 2012). Also, including antihistamines and epinephrine in a patient's overall care plan , which should include emergency action plans and visits to an allergist, is very important. Challenges in accessibility to allergy specialists and medications further complicate treatment efforts, emphasizing the need for educational initiatives to enhance recognition and appropriate responses to food allergies (Al-Shilaly et al., 2025) (Figure 12.13).

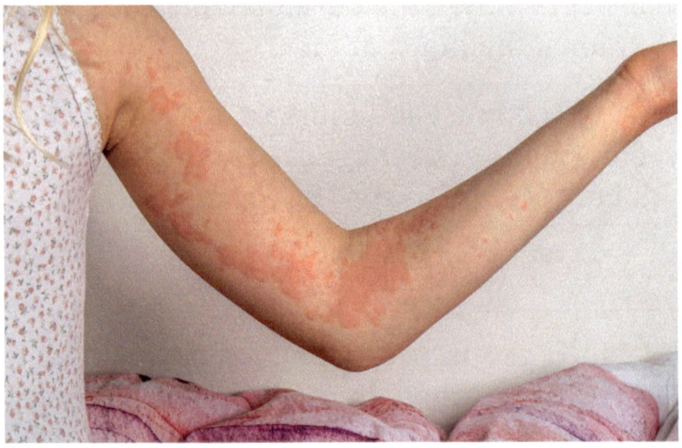

Figure 12.13. Antihistamines are often utilized to mitigate mild allergic reactions, providing symptomatic relief from itching, hives, and other localized symptoms.

Source: https://www.inquirer.com/resizer/NRmOkK4bh4wRqscsf5V0PTLPPV0=/arc-anglerfish-arc2-prod-pmn/public/5NLVPOCR3JEBVOOKF73XMJ4UOM.jpg.

12.3.4. Importance of Reading Food Labels

It is very important for anyone with food allergies or intolerances to understand the meaning of reading food labels. Food labels tell consumers what ingredients are present, so they can avoid things they are allergic to. Since more people have food allergies and intolerances, reading labels is now very important for staying healthy and safe. Research indicates that clear nutritional information can guide healthier eating habits, particularly in environments where food choices are abundant, such as restaurants (Lages et al., 2013). Moreover, access barriers to allergen-free options point to the necessity for food labeling to enable choice-making since individuals' information about products available varies significantly (Parmely et al., 2017). Through careful reading of food packets, individuals are able to avoid risks of health compromise through allergies and their overall health, another indicator of their relevance in solving food allergies and intolerances.

12.3.5. Role of Allergists and Dietitians

Allergists and dietitians are central to managing food allergy and intolerance due to the specialist knowledge they offer that is needed for appropriate treatment and meal preparation. Allergists are central to diagnosis, using clinical evaluation and skin tests to determine individual allergens, which informs patients regarding their sensitivities and avoidance of hazardous reactions. Dietitians, on the other hand, are central to using these medical results to devise practical dietary advice, so patients receive appropriate nutrition without sacrificing their allergen-free needs. With the increasing prevalence of food allergies, as indicated by an 18% increase from 1997 to 2007 (Brummel et al., 2019), access to educated healthcare professionals becomes increasingly necessary.

Additionally, research identifies healthcare access disparities, especially for those with lower incomes, as an indication of the necessity of collaborative strategies among allergists, dietitians, and community care to treat food allergy and intolerance sufferers (Parmely et al., 2017) (Figure 12.14).

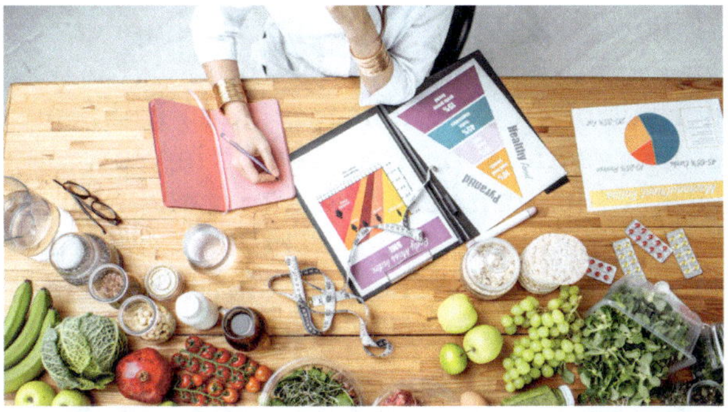

Figure 12.14. The roles of allergists and dietitians are integral in managing food allergies and intolerances, as they provide specialized expertise essential for effective treatment and dietary planning.

Source: https://s3.amazonaws.com/contents.newzenler.com/23021/blog/blog-post/18830/data/thumb/l-9.jpg.

12.3.6. Emergency Action Plans for Severe Reactions

The increasing prevalence of food allergies necessitates the development of holistic emergency action plans to address severe reactions efficiently. Emergency action plans are critical for food hypersensitive individuals, which form a majority of the population, as recent studies have shown that nearly half of male children and about 40% of female children experience food hypersensitivity (Patel, 2020). A good emergency action plan should involve the determination of allergens, staff training on identification of anaphylaxis signs, and immediate availability of emergency medical interventions , such as epinephrine injection. Access to healthcare and support systems within the community, however, may be variable, particularly among marginalized populations, as studies have revealed that there are wide variations in access to food intolerance and allergy management services (Parmely et al., 2017). Individualized emergency action plans must therefore be developed to address not only individual requirements but also the broader socioeconomic variables determining access to primary healthcare services.

12.3.7. Support Groups and Resources for Individuals

Facing food allergies and intolerances is not easy , which is why support groups and easy-to-find resources play a key role. They support members emotionally and also teach them ways to handle their diet and deal with stigma. Moreover, the increase in food intolerance diagnoses has illuminated gaps in healthcare access and dietary education, particularly for low-income individuals, as emphasized in the findings of Parmely et al. (2017).

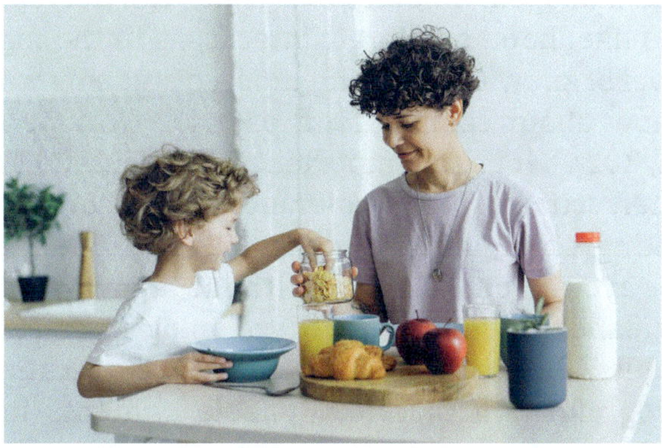

Figure 12.15. Navigating the challenges posed by food allergies and intolerances can be daunting, underscoring the importance of support groups and accessible resources for affected individuals.

Source: https://www.attis.in/wp-content/uploads/2024/08/vitaly-gariev-1WQjGYX0P1s-unsplash.jpg.

Inaccessibility leads to higher isolation and makes it difficult for a person to adopt the right diet. Additionally, the connection between food elimination and disordered eating behaviors suggests the need for social support to prevent adverse psychological consequences, as discussed by Scholma et al. (2025). Thus, creating robust support networks and accessibility to resources is imperative to improve the overall quality of life in people exposed to these complex dietary problems (Figure 12.15).

12.3.8. Education and Awareness Initiatives

Education and awareness programs are important in the management of food intolerances and allergies, especially in college, where students are most likely to face new dietary challenges. By encouraging better understanding of these health conditions through specific programs, the institution can enable students to make intelligent dietary decisions. For example, awareness programs regarding the symptoms and management of food allergies can decrease the likelihood of allergic attacks, as in the high level of knowledge among exposed students who know about campus food pantries (Aktepe et al., 2024). It is also important to understand the intersection of food intolerances and disordered eating since most students have a tendency to avoid some foods without appropriate guidance, unconsciously developing unhealthy habits (Burns, 2025). Comprehensive education programs can therefore enable students not only to adapt to their dietary limitations but also to build a healthy relationship with food, promoting overall health.

12.4. Societal and Economic Impact

Food allergies and intolerances have a major and varied impact on people and society as a whole. Because of food allergies, people often need to visit doctors, use emergency services and continue their treatment , which increases the cost of healthcare. For instance, students facing food insecurity, with around 41.6% of California State University students affected, may struggle to access allergy-friendly foods, exacerbating financial and health disparities (Aktepe et al., 2024). Socially, the implications extend beyond health, as those with food allergies often experience isolation from social eating practices, particularly during formative years, which can severely impact their quality of life (Ell et al., 2024). The fact that many people with food allergies suffer from both economic problems and social isolation shows that we need better food allergen labeling, more education and support for them everywhere.

12.4.1. Economic Burden of Food Allergies and Intolerances

Food intolerance and allergy cost families and society exorbitantly and in so many different ways. The more people experience these unwanted reactions, the higher the cost of medical bills to families through extra medical costs, money for substitute foods and the likelihood of not going to work when an allergic reaction appears. Such economic burdens are compounded in settings like college campuses, where students may have difficulty accessing food that is free from allergens and thus result in expensive modifications to their diets and reduced quality of life (Brummel et al., 2019). Furthermore, the crosslink between food allergies and eating disorders further shows a despicable trend whereby food restrictions can result in even extreme physical and mental consequences further complicating economic consequences (Burns, 2025). Economic solutions to these consequences have been necessary in order to better the lives of those who have food allergies and intolerance (Figure 12.16).

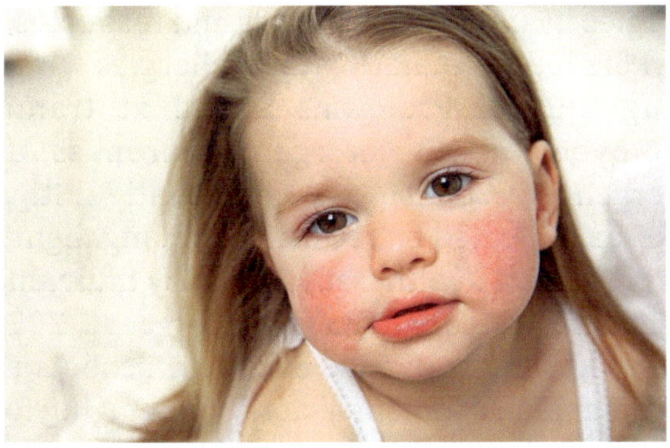

Figure 12.16. The economic burden of food allergies and intolerances is significant and multifaceted, affecting individuals and society at large.

Source: https://d2jx2rerrg6sh3.cloudfront.net/images/news/ImageForNews_730353_16678795683218948.jpg.

12.4.2. Impact on Food Industry and Labeling Practices

The growing prevalence of food intolerance and allergy has had a considerable influence on food industry practice, not least labeling and consumer communication policy. With heightened sensitivities to the problem of their health, companies are under pressure to adopt more stringent labeling practice to guarantee consumer protection and compliance with regulation. The Commission of the European Communities has identified nutritional labeling as essential in promoting healthier food choice and particularly in the food service sector (Lages et al., 2013). Also, poor allergen labeling generates increased population anxiety, resulting in higher demands on clearer regulation and staff training in the food service sector (Ell et al., 2024). This trend not only demonstrates a commitment to consumer protection but also represents alignment with wider public health policy in preventing the increase in obesity and related medical problems. It is therefore important that food companies and restaurateurs adopt open and consistent labeling policies to promote consumer confidence and enable informed dietary choice.

12.4.3. Social Implications for Affected Individuals

Food allergies and intolerances not only limit what people can eat; they also have a major effect on their general health. Because their food restrictions can keep them from joining in with others, people with food allergies often feel cut off from social events. This lifestyle alteration can manifest in disordered eating patterns, as individuals may avoid specific foods to the detriment of their nutritional health, potentially correlating with mental health issues , such as anxiety and depression (Burns, 2025).

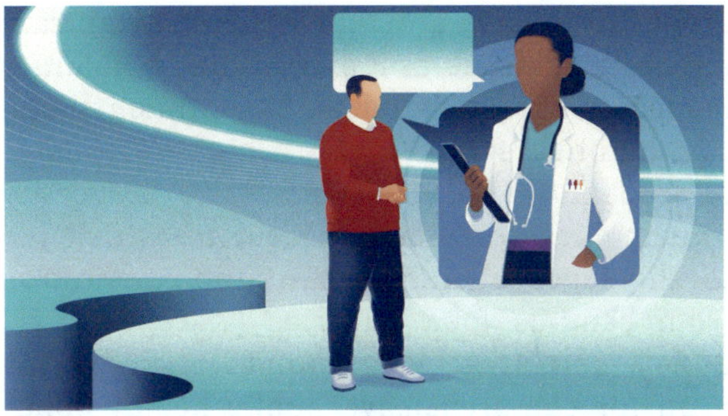

Figure 12.17. The social implications of food allergies and intolerances extend beyond mere dietary restrictions; they significantly impact the well-being of affected individuals.

Source: https://www.empr.com/wp-content/uploads/sites/7/2024/06/Care_Compass_Counseling_Curriculum_HCP_F.jpg.

Moreover, cultural and social influences contribute to the complexities of culinary preferences among affected individuals, revealing how shared dining experiences are shaped by the interplay of social expectations and personal health conditions (Coughlan et al., 2018). Ultimately, these factors illustrate the pressing need for greater awareness and understanding within communities to foster inclusive environments for individuals managing food allergies and intolerances (Figure 12.17).

12.4.4. Public Health Policies Regarding Food Allergies

Public policies for managing food allergies have become increasingly vital with the rising cases of food intolerances, and a need for strategic intervention calls for action. The policies target enhancing access to healthcare and allergen-free foods, particularly among marginalized communities, i.e., low-income individuals. The evidence indicates that patients with food allergies are facing significant barriers in accessing adequate healthcare services, particularly dietetic services, and allergen-free resources (Parmely et al., 2017). Moreover, food insecurity is also a health issue of significant public health issue, as it exacerbates difficulties in accessing safe food among students and communities. For instance, a high percentage of students at the California State University system indicated food insecurity, which led to shortages of nutritional supplementation from campus food pantries (Aktepe et al., 2024). Combined, these points highlight the need for comprehensive public health policy that addresses not only allergy control but also interventions to enhance access to food in an equitable manner.

12.4.5. Role of Schools and Workplaces in Management

Both schools and workplaces are very important in ensuring that food allergies and intolerances are handled safely and addressed. It is important for schools to put in place detailed policies that teach students, staff and parents about allergens and encourage all students to be accepting. By being proactive, people with food allergies feel less anxious and their friends learn important things about allergies. In the same way, companies should focus on managing food allergies by offering clear rules and resources, so workers feel safe sharing their allergies without being judged. Programs aimed at training employees about allergen awareness and emergency response can significantly mitigate risks, as indicated by recent studies highlighting the persistent health issues faced by individuals in adverse environments (Hyvönen et al., 2022). Therefore, the collective efforts of schools and workplaces are indispensable in managing food allergies effectively (Figure 12.18).

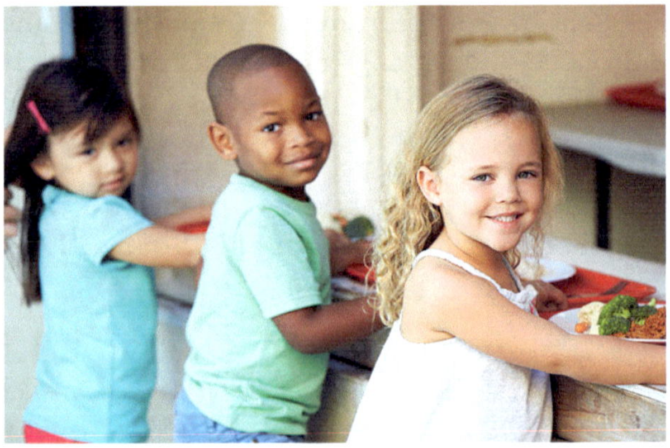

Figure 12.18. In managing food allergies and intolerances, both schools and workplaces play critical roles in fostering an environment conducive to safety and awareness.

Source: https://townsquare.media/site/385/files/2017/08/RS14487_178095373.jpg?w=780&q=75.

12.4.6. Cultural Attitudes Towards Food Allergies

Cultural beliefs regarding food allergy contribute significantly to influenceing how individuals respond and navigate dietary restrictions. Food, in most cultures, is not just sustenance but also an essential part of cultural heritage and social ceremonies, and this complicates the lives of individuals with food allergies. For instance, social stigma of food allergy can lead to social exclusion or enforced adherence to group food ways, directly affecting one's relationship with food. Further, studies have demonstrated that food allergy awareness and knowledge may vary significantly across populations, affecting food adherence and health perceptions. These variations show that cultural context is at the core of how people view and manage food allergy, which is key to the success of health policy implementation. The intersection between food allergy and nutritional knowledge is core, as depicted by the relationship between food intake and medical condition among various groups (Cardoso et al., 2018; Burns, 2025).

12.4.7. Media Representation of Food Allergies

The media greatly influences the way food allergies are perceived, often telling stories that show how society feels about this health issue. Food allergies have become more noticeable and the way they are presented can strongly influence both personal and government views. Research indicates that the framing of food allergies within various media outlets can contribute to heightened risk perceptions among the public, thereby reinforcing anxiety around food consumption and safety (Harrington et al., 2011).

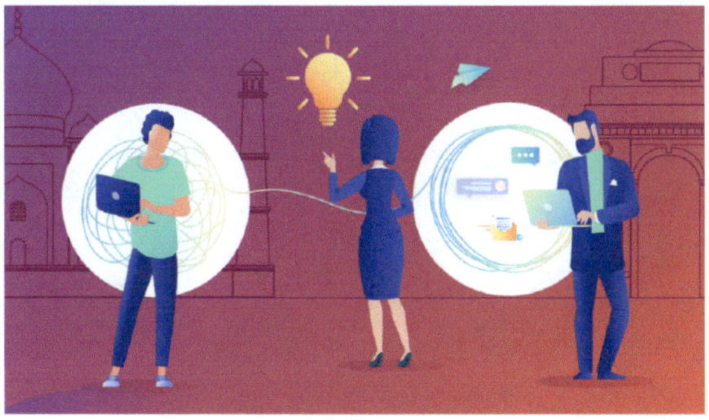

Figure 12.19. The media plays a pivotal role in shaping public perceptions of food allergies, often constructing narratives that reflect societal attitudes toward this emerging health concern.

Source: https://indian-retailer.s3.ap-south-1.amazonaws.com/s3fs-public/2022-06/1.PNG.

The problem is especially serious because explaining food allergies is not easy and sensational news may take away focus from the need to manage risks wisely instead of panicking. Additionally, exploring the relationship between such media portrayals and urban lifestyles reveals that misconceptions about allergens can proliferate without adequate scientific guidance (Salbitano et al., 2021). Ultimately, understanding these representations is vital for fostering a more nuanced public dialogue around food allergies (Figure 12.19).

12.4.8. Advocacy and Legislation Efforts

Advocating and making laws are important for helping people with food allergies and intolerances. Since advocacy groups like the Anaphylaxis Campaign were formed in 1994, there has been a major impact on public policy and the food industry because of increased awareness of food allergies. They carry out studies and encourage community support, influencing efforts to improve food labeling and allergen rules in the industry. Also, by joining forces, advocacy groups and regulators can make sure that food businesses have clear guidelines to prevent risks and inform consumers about allergens. Effective advocacy not only raises awareness but also cultivates trust between stakeholders, allowing for the development of tailored regulations that reflect the complexities of food allergies and enhance the quality of life for affected individuals (Barnett et al., 2020; Gowland, 2025).

12.4.9. Global Perspectives on Food Allergies and Intolerances

The growing prevalence of food allergies and intolerances in various heterogeneous populations highlights the need for a comprehensive understanding of these conditions worldwide. New research indicates a dramatic increase in diagnosis associated with beyond-personal health challenges to encompass social and economic consequences (Parmely et al., 2017). The right medicine and food without allergens are essential for the said population; nevertheless, disparities are present, particularly within poor populations, making it challenging for them to control these conditions effectively. Further, research has found that HRQL in food hypersensitivity may greatly be impaired, affecting social interactions and family function (Dean et al., 2015). Therefore, the treatment of food intolerance and allergies has to be a multi-faceted approach that not only includes greater medical access and resources but also greater understanding of the social implications of these increasingly common conditions.

A CLOSER LOOK

Nutritional Deficiencies

Deficiency of nutrients is when the body fails to get necessary nutrients to undergo normal growth, development, and overall well-being. The deficiencies could be due to insufficient or unbalanced consumption, impaired absorption of nutrients, or increased nutritional need for certain medical conditions. These include some of the most common deficiencies , such as deficiency in vitamin D, causing brittle bones; iron deficiency, resulting in anemia and fatigue; and vitamin B12 deficiency, causing neurological disorders and fatigue, particularly among vegetarians and vegans. Deficiency in calcium, iodine, and folate can further lead to serious health conditions like osteoporosis, thyroid disorder, and congenital defects, respectively. Nutrient deficiency can be prevented or cured with a healthy, diversified diet, and in some instances, with supplements. However, proper diagnosis and treatment through medical consultation need to be accessed to avoid long-term damage.

SUMMARY

In examining the key issues regarding food intolerances and allergies, one should consider their significant impact on eating habits as well as public health. Food allergies, tending to involve the immune system, can lead to severe reactions that necessitate increased sensitization among food service industry employees, for example, the need for catering staff to understand some of the most prevalent allergenic foods (Jarrett, 2011). By contrast, food intolerance, not immunologically reacting, still poses a problem for subjects, particularly in social meal contexts. The relevance of labeling in talk regarding intuitive food choice, an initiative aimed to prevent obesity and overweight related to out-of-home eating (Lages et al., 2013), is highlighted. Through the encouragement of wide comprehension about these issues, buyers and sellers of food can make more informed decisions, ultimately improving the health condition and welfare of the people with dietary restrictions.

KEY TERMS FROM THIS CHAPTER

- Allergen immunotherapy (AIT)
- Allergens
- Childhood allergies
- Food hypersensitivity
- Food proteins
- Gluten sensitivity
- Immunoglobulin E antibodies
- Non-IgE-mediated allergies
- Allergen-free food products
- Anaphylaxis
- Commission of the European Communities
- Food intolerances
- Genetic predisposition
- Health-related quality of life (HRQL)
- Industrial emissions
- Nutritional information

REFERENCES

1. Adams, A., Araujo, A., Araujo, A., Asmah, A., Breman, J., Brugman, G., Butler, D., et al. (2010). *Allergic disorders in Africa and Africans: Is it Primarily a Priority?* https://core.ac.uk/download/pdf/18410775.pdf (accessed on 29 May 2025).
2. Aktepe, B. (2024). *Factors Affecting the Use of Food Pantries by California State University Students.* https://core.ac.uk/download/603654313.pdf (accessed on 29 May 2025).
3. Al-Shilaly, H. I., Alonazi, A. S., Mahdi, R. H., Muazen, R., et al. (2025). *Children Allergies in Saudi Arabia: The Situation and Challenges–Narrative Review.* https://core.ac.uk/download/646092815.pdf (accessed on 29 May 2025).
4. Arasi, S., Corsello, G., Pajno, G. B., & Villani, A. (2018). *The Future Outlook on Allergen Immunotherapy in Children: 2018 and beyond.* https://core.ac.uk/download/286528686.pdf (accessed on 29 May 2025).
5. Barnett, J., Lucas, J. S., & Vasileiou, K. (2020). *Conversations About Food Allergy Risk with Restaurant Staff When Eating Out: A Customer Perspective.* https://core.ac.uk/download/334409935.pdf (accessed on 29 May 2025).
6. Bevan, S., Israelsen, A., & Savoie-Roskos, M. R. (2020). *Preventing Allergies in Infants: What Foods to Introduce and When.* https://core.ac.uk/download/342065311.pdf (accessed on 29 May 2025).
7. BC Cook Articulation Committee. (2015). *Food Safety, Sanitation, and Personal Hygiene.* Victoria, B.C.: BCcampus. Retrieved from https://opentextbc.ca/foodsafety/.Brummel, A. (2019). *The Relationship Between Food Allergy Reporting and Allergen Friendly Food Availability in A University Foodservice.* https://core.ac.uk/download/387593443.pdf (accessed on 29 May 2025).
8. Burns, Heather, "The Development of Hypersensitivity Reactions in the Pediatric Population: A Review" (2019). *Senior Honors Theses.* 897. https://digitalcommons.liberty.edu/honors/897(accessed on 29 May 2025).
9. Candreva, A. M., Curciarello, R., Docena, G., Smaldini, P., et al. (2016). *Allergenic Milk Proteins. Friend or Foe Nutritional Proteins?* https://core.ac.uk/download/322426561.pdf (accessed on 29 May 2025).
10. Canello, S., Di Cerbo, A., & Guidetti, G. (2017). *Nutrition: From the First Medicine to The First Poison.* https://core.ac.uk/download/322433006.pdf (accessed on 29 May 2025).
11. Cardoso, A. P., Correia, P., Duarte, J., Ferreira, M., et al. (2018). *Perceptions Towards a Healthy Diet Among a Sample of University People in Portugal.* https://core.ac.uk/download/160796135.pdf (accessed on 29 May 2025).
12. Coughlan, L. M., & Saayman, M. (2018). *The Importance of Different Culinary Aspects When Travelling–The Case of International Tourists to South Africa.* https://core.ac.uk/download/222967827.pdf (accessed on 29 May 2025).
13. Dean, T., Glasbey, G., Grundy, J., Moonesinghe, H., et al. (2015). *Health-Related Quality of Life in Children with Perceived and Diagnosed Food Hypersensitivity.* https://core.ac.uk/download/29589188.pdf (accessed on 29 May 2025).

14. Dunn, Savannah, "Development and Management of Canine Adverse Food Reactions and its Connections to the Grain-Free Dog Food Movement" (2020). *Senior Honors Theses*. 947. https://digitalcommons.liberty.edu/honors/947Ell, A. (2024). *The Increase of Allergies in Developed Countries: A Comparison of The Quality of Life and Psychosocial Burden of Individuals with Food Allergies in Switzerland and the United States of America*. https://core.ac.uk/download/619721873.pdf (accessed on 29 May 2025).
15. Gowland, M. (2025). *Food Allergy: Innovation in Advocacy, Research and Training to Support and Protect Those at Risk*. https://core.ac.uk/download/190362500.pdf (accessed on 29 May 2025).
16. Harrington, D. W. (2011). *Newly Emerging Environmental Health Risks in A Risk Society: A Case Study of The Public Perception of Food Allergies*. https://core.ac.uk/download/639160355.pdf (accessed on 29 May 2025).
17. Holgersen, R. (2013). *Prototyping a Decision Support System Based on Semantic Web Technologies to Aid Consumers with Food Sensitivities in Their Assessment of Product Safety*. https://core.ac.uk/download/636683255.pdf (accessed on 29 May 2025).
18. Hoppensteadt, J. M. (2015). *Effects of Food Elimination, Based on Alcat Testing, on Inflammatory Markers, Body Composition, and Medical Symptoms*. https://core.ac.uk/download/643697260.pdf (accessed on 29 May 2025).
19. Hyvönen, S. (2022). *Persistent Respiratory Problems, Neurologic, Cardiac, Muscle and Joint Symptoms of Occupants in Water and Microbe Damaged Buildings*. https://core.ac.uk/download/521287942.pdf (accessed on 29 May 2025).
20. Jarrett, P. (2011). *Food Allergies and Intolerances*. https://core.ac.uk/download/33473245.pdf (accessed on 29 May 2025).
21. Kohut, D. (2014). *Integrative and Functional Nutrition Practices and Use of The Integrative and Functional Medical Nutrition Therapy Radial Among Registered Dietitians*. https://core.ac.uk/download/215700092.pdf (accessed on 29 May 2025).
22. Kuta, E. (2016). *Food Allergies and Eating Disorders: A Review of Current Literature*. https://core.ac.uk/download/210605666.pdf (accessed on 29 May 2025).
23. Lages, C. C. D. (2013). *The Design of Nutrition Labels*. https://core.ac.uk/download/70687569.pdf (accessed on 29 May 2025).
24. Parmely, R. (2017). *Accessibility to Food Intolerance and Food Allergy Resources in Mclean County, Illinois: An Interdisciplinary Pilot Study*. https://core.ac.uk/download/84884454.pdf (accessed on 29 May 2025).
25. Patel, R. (2020). *An investigation into the prevalence of food hypersensitivity amongst children in the early years service in Ireland. Masters dissertation. Technological University Dublin. doi:10.21427/s57a-g581*(accessed on 29 May 2025).
26. Saint Raphael Healthcare System. (1999). *1999: A Community Report* (Inside Saint Raphael's Better Health Magazine). https://core.ac.uk/download/571283223.pdf (accessed on 29 May 2025).
27. Salbitano, F., & Speak, A. F. (2021). Thermal comfort and perceptions of the ecosystem services and disservices of urban trees in Florence. https://core.ac.uk/download/483690786.pdf (accessed on 29 May 2025).

28. Sankala, M., & Bhatt, V. (2019). *Anti-Allergic Drugs: A Review.* https://core.ac.uk/download/229502780.pdf (accessed on 29 May 2025).

29. Scholma, L. M. (2025). The Relationship Between Food Allergies and Intolerances and the Development of Disordered Eating Patterns. *Human Nutrition and Hospitality Management Undergraduate Honors Theses* Retrieved from https://scholarworks.uark.edu/hnhiuht/36(accessed on 29 May 2025).

30. Seita, H. M. (2013). *Food Allergies in Pregnant Women: A Study of Prevalence in Expecting Mothers and Association with Neonatal Outcomes* [Master's thesis, Boston University]. https://open.bu.edu/bitstream/2144/12219/6/Seita_Helene_2013.pdf (accessed on 29 May 2025).

31. Shaw, J. A. (2017). *The Influence of Dietary Factors on Child Food Allergies* [Master's thesis]. https://core.ac.uk/download/215508142.pdf (accessed on 29 May 2025).

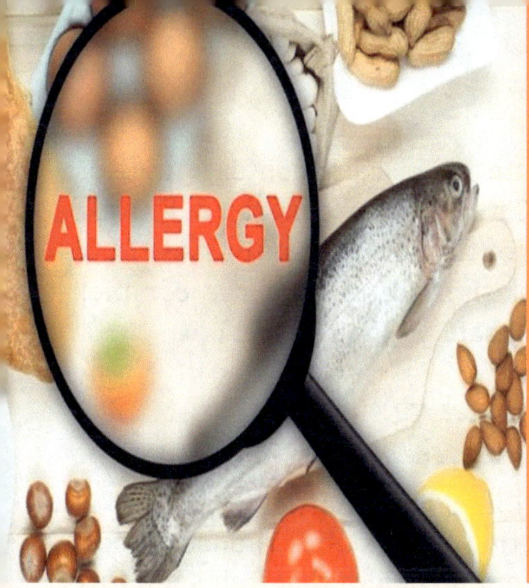

Chapter 13

FOODBORNE OUTBREAK INVESTIGATION

Contents

Introduction ... 299
13.1. Identifying Foodborne Outbreaks ... 301
13.2. Investigation Process ... 305
13.3. Source Identification ... 309
13.4. Prevention and Control Measures ... 313
Summary ... 319
References ... 320

Introduction

Foodborne illnesses remain a leading public health issue globally and often result in high morbidity and mortality. Accurate investigation of foodborne outbreaks is required to identify the pathogens, explain modes of transmission, and implement effective preventive interventions. For example, the emergence of hybrid strains of diarrhoeagenic *Escherichia coli*, i.e., those that carry both Shiga toxin and heat-stable toxin, shows the complexity of tracking and controlling such pathogens, as evident from recent findings of hybrid Shiga toxin-producing *E. coli*/enterotoxigenic *E. coli* in the UK with escalated health hazard (Rodwell et al., 2025). Similarly, the presence of non-typhoidal *Salmonella enterica* in abattoirs points towards the risk of antibiotic resistance, adding to the complexities of outbreak investigations and eventually necessitating broader genomic surveillance to monitor such risks (Aworh et al., 2024). Integrating microbiological and epidemiological information, foodborne outbreak investigations can readily mitigate the impact of such illnesses on public health.

Definition of Foodborne Outbreaks

Foodborne outbreaks are instances where two or more individuals fall ill due to illnesses caused by the consumption of the same infected food or beverage. The event typically results from pathogenic microorganisms like bacteria, viruses, and parasites that intrude into the food supply through one of over a dozen pathways, including environmental, handling, or processing improperness. Identification of foodborne outbreaks is significant to public health due to the capacity of timely and effective responses to restrict extensive sickness and death. Techniques, such as whole-genome sequencing (WGS) have revolutionized outbreak investigations by providing more precise identification of related cases, revealing previously unknown clusters of illness that are possibly geographically distinct (Dallman et al., 2015).

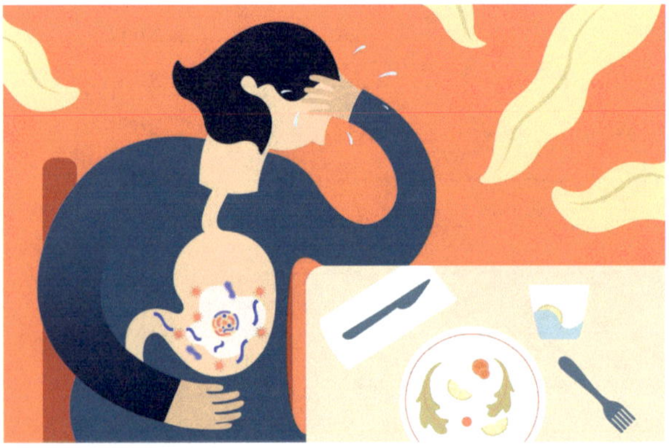

Figure 13.1. Foodborne outbreaks are defined as incidents in, which two or more individuals experience similar illnesses after consuming the same contaminated food or beverage.

Source: https://obesitydoctor.in/img/galleryuploads/food%20borne%20diseases_81292485961a377c2a7fa9.jpg

Besides, there is a need to understand the interface of environmental elements and food safety from a multidisciplinary point of view, as emphasized in educational frameworks that consider the broader implications of food safety precautions in the One Health context (Angelos et al., 2017). Therefore, a general definition of foodborne outbreaks encompasses both epidemiological significance and the complex systems of food safety (Figure 13.1).

Importance of Investigating Foodborne Outbreaks

The investigation of foodborne outbreaks is not something that occurs after the fact; it is a critical part of public health that helps identify sources, minimize risk, and implement preventive measures. By analyzing these outbreaks in a detailed manner, health authorities can trace the origin of pathogens, thereby leading both to inform public health policy and consumer protection. For instance, knowledge of the specific food sources associated with STEC infections can inform interventions, as highlighted by studies that have shown wide regional variations in sources of foodborne illness, including beef and vegetables (Pires et al., 2019). Aside from this, collaboration among federal, state, and local governments is required for a successful and coordinated response, highlighting the need for systemic reforms to facilitate outbreak control (Taylor & David, 2009). Lastly, the importance of foodborne outbreak investigation is because of its potential to provide assurance of public health protection and construct more effective food safety systems worldwide.

Role of Government Agencies in Investigations

Government agencies' role in investigating foodborne outbreaks cannot be substituted since these agencies have the sole responsibility to safeguard public health through effective surveillance and response strategies. Local governments must conduct routine inspection of food hygiene, and it is essential for the detection of potential threats and prevention of outbreaks As noted, budget constraints have significantly impacted the capacity of such agencies; a reduction in food safety expenditures is associated with steep declines in staff numbers and the volume of high-priority interventions conducted per facility (Murrell et al., 2025). Moreover, integration of advances in technology, such as whole genome sequencing (WGS), is a manifestation of the evolving environment of outbreak investigations. WGS provides precise identification of pathogen strains and virulence factors, enhancing the effectiveness of public health interventions (Emílio Gomes et al., 2025). Hence, collaborative efforts on the part of government agencies ensure prevention of threats by foodborne disease and ensure public safety (Figure 13.2).

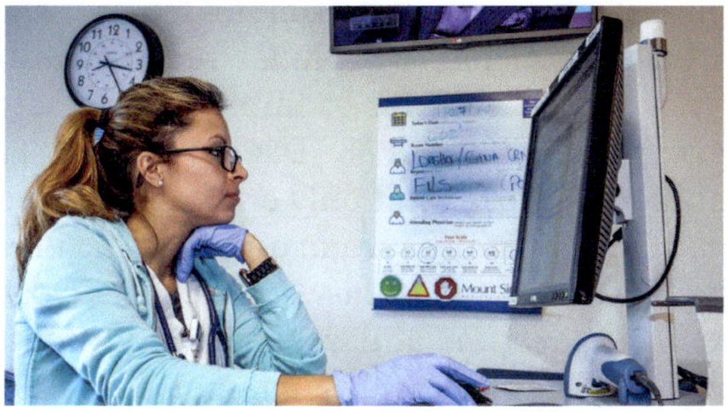

Figure 13.2. The role of government agencies in foodborne outbreak investigations is indispensable, as they are primarily responsible for safeguarding public health through effective surveillance and response mechanisms.

Source: https://www.pewtrusts.org/-/media/post-launch-images/2024/12/gettyimages671217564jpgmaster/16x9_m.jpg.

13.1. Identifying Foodborne Outbreaks

Identification of foodborne outbreaks is a major component of public health strategies to minimize the impact of foodborne disease. Effective outbreak investigations depend on the identification of a causative pathogen and its attribution to specific food sources. A series of food attribution techniques, including case-control studies and microbial subtyping, are engaged in the process, and therefore, there is a significance of robust data analysis strategies (Batz et al., 2025). For instance, a survey of Shiga toxin-producing *Escherichia coli* (STEC) infection reveals that infection sources may vary significantly across different regions and that beef has been identified as the dominant source in the Americas, while fresh produce has been rated highest in the Western Pacific (Pires et al., 2019).

These findings not only confirm regional variation in causing foodborne illness but also indicate that intervention measures must be modulated and addressed to the respective food consumption behavior and conditions prevailing in each region. By proper identification procedures, foodborne disease outbreaks may be prevented and controlled more efficiently.

13.1.1. Definition of an Outbreak

The term outbreak in foodborne disease refers to the sudden occurrence of two or more instances of a similar illness resulting from the consumption of a shared food or drink. An outbreak not only indicates a rise in cases of illness but also alerts public health authorities to investigate potential causes and means of spread. For instance, an outbreak investigation of psittacosis in workers at a wildlife rescue facility highlighted the importance of zoonotic transmission and of poor biosecurity practice, stating that environmental and operational controls can make a huge difference to disease occurrence. Similarly, identification of Salmonella Enteritidis as the etiologic agent in a cheese-associated outbreak illustrated how raw milk dairy foods have the potential to pose a significant health risk when contaminated (Napoleoni et al., 2021). Knowing the definition and implications of outbreaks is critical to develop efficient control strategies and ensure public health safety against foodborne pathogens (Figure 13.3).

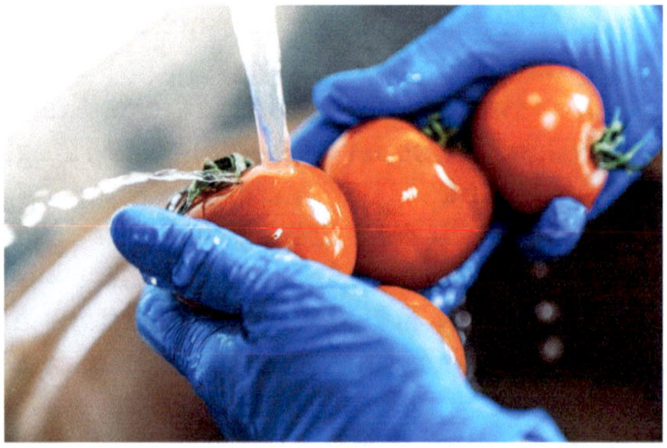

Figure 13.3. The term outbreak in the context of foodborne illness refers to the occurrence of two or more cases of a similar illness resulting from the ingestion of a common food or drink.

Source: https://d2jx2rerrg6sh3.cloudfront.net/images/news/ImageForNews_804795_17419147486146146.jpg.

13.1.2. Symptoms and Signs of Foodborne Illnesses

Recognition of the signs and symptoms of foodborne diseases ensures prevention of delays in management and intervention of an outbreak. The infected individuals may present a range of signs and symptoms, including dizziness, nausea, vomiting, diarrhea, abdominal cramps, fever, and malaise, each showing the body's response to foodborne agents. The following case study is applicable to this dynamic: following the consumption of contaminated snacks in an elementary school, an outbreak was encountered with 150 students participating, the most frequent symptoms being dizziness, vomiting, and nausea (Aryanto et al., 2024). Diagnosis of such signs is timely for health care providers, who are stakeholders in the reporting of suspected outbreaks to public health institutions, thus enabling quick investigation and control. Detection and surveillance of such signals not only allow for early diagnosis and treatment but also increase the general level of food safety management in society.

13.1.3. Surveillance Systems for Detecting Outbreaks

Surveillance systems for foodborne outbreaks are crucial in the detection of outbreaks, enabling rapid response and identification of potential health hazards. By integrating advanced molecular detection techniques, such systems enhance epidemiologic surveillance and provide valuable insights on the dynamics of transmission of enteric viruses, as indicated in the inter-European collaborative research program to harmonize data collection and analysis in an effort to better understand foodborne illness (Brown et al., 2003). Success of such surveillance efforts relies to a greater extent upon coordination among federal, state, and local agencies, who must reconcile their varying responsibilities to improve food safety interventions (Taylor & David, 2009). This combined approach not only encourages a more robust early warning system of foodborne illness but also calls for system-wide reforms closing gaps in inspection and regulation, ultimately protecting public health against the linked nature of an increasingly globalized food supply chain (Figure 13.4).

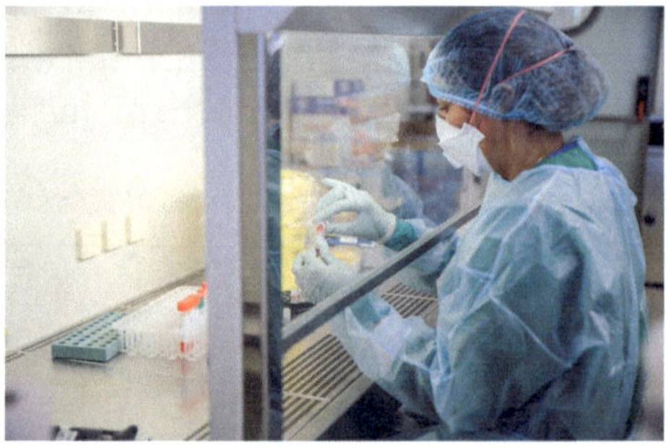

Figure 13.4. Surveillance systems play a crucial role in detecting foodborne outbreaks, facilitating rapid identification and response to potential health threats.

Source: https://www.who.int/images/default-source/departments/genomic-surveillance/lab_technician_mixes_mpox_samples.jpeg?sfvrsn=23f978e2_13

13.1.4. Role of Healthcare Providers in Reporting

It is very important for healthcare providers to report foodborne illnesses to help control outbreaks and keep the public safe. Gastroenterologists are usually the first medical team patients see when they experience foodborne illness symptoms. Because of this, they are expected to notice signs of disease and quickly inform the public health authorities. The results of their studies can play a big role in how public health responds quickly to stop the spread of the disease. In instances where healthcare providers encounter challenges—, such as burnout or inadequate organizational support, reporting may be compromised, potentially delaying outbreak responses (D'Alessandro-Lowe et al., 2024). Furthermore, robust surveillance systems must rely on accurate and complete data reporting by healthcare providers to identify trends and prevent endemic patterns, as seen in various investigations of infectious diseases (Githinji et al., 2024). Improving how providers are trained and supported is necessary for good foodborne illness reporting.

13.1.5. Importance of Epidemiological Data

Epidemiological data are central to outbreak investigations of foodborne illness, upon, which optimal public health responses are founded. With the proper application of accurate subtyping methods, such as whole genome sequencing (WGS), it is then simple to quickly identify and link cases in a geographically distant food system, enhancing overall outbreak response.

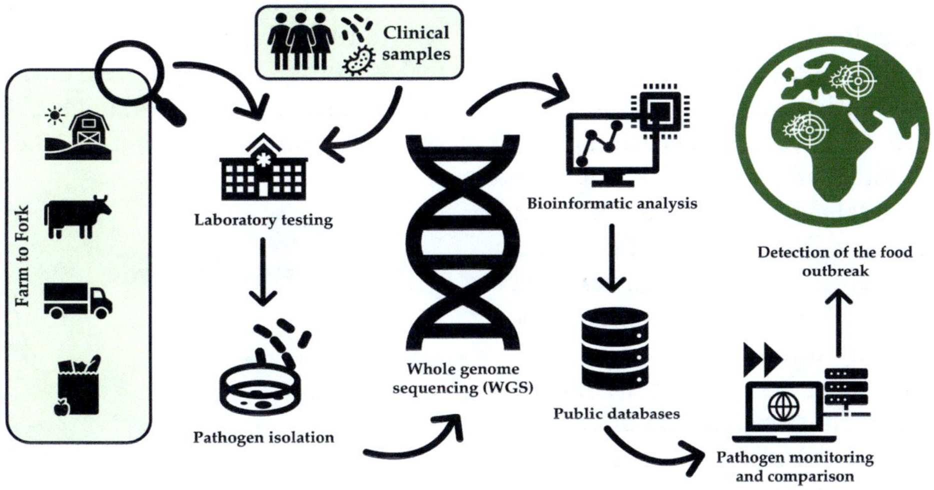

Figure 13.5. Epidemiological data play a pivotal role in foodborne outbreak investigations, serving as a cornerstone for effective public health interventions.

Source: Gomes E, Araújo D, Nogueira T, Oliveira R, Silva S, Oliveira LVN, Azevedo NF, Almeida C and Castro J (2025) Advances in whole genome sequencing for foodborne pathogens: implications for clinical infectious disease surveillance and public health. Front. Cell. Infect. Microbiol. 15:1593219. doi: 10.3389/fcimb.2025.1593219

For instance, studies have shown that WGS not only improves the identification of clusters that are related but also provides real-time data that other methods may not capture, significantly contributing to the containment of outbreaks (Dallman et al., 2015). For instance, studies have shown that WGS not only improves the identification of clusters that are related but also provides real-time insights that traditional methodologies may overlook, significantly enhancing outbreak containment strategies (Dallman et al., 2015). Furthermore, correct identification of the source of an outbreak is also crucial in the prediction of future outbreaks; in a notable investigation of Salmonella outbreaks, SNP-based analysis confirmed both the occurrence of outbreaks and the contaminated food source involved (Mohammed et al., 2020). Robust epidemiological evidence is thus critical not only for the identification of the causative pathogens but also to guide corresponding public health interventions and policy (Figure 13.5).

13.1.6. Case Definitions and Criteria

In investigations for foodborne outbreaks, clearly defined case definitions and criteria are needed for the proper identification and analysis of affected populations. These models also specify not just the boundary of an outbreak but what constitutes individuals who meet the criteria to be classified as cases. Definition of this sort is crucial in effective epidemiological surveillance and planning for response. For instance, food handlers may greatly add to the transmission of viral infection, which also has a tendency to contaminate food during preparation or serving (Brown et al., 2003). Additionally, molecular surveillance also underscored the significance of integrating genetic data in order to complement traditional epidemiological approaches. Through such integration, tracing of pathogens is made more accurate, hence allowing rapid outbreak and source identification (Dufour et al., 2015). Lastly, well-defined case definitions enable public health responses to be coordinated such that interventions are effective and focused.

13.1.7. Use of Laboratory Testing in Identification

Lab testing for identification is currently the core aspect of foodborne outbreak management. The advancement of molecular technologies, such as next-generation sequencing (NGS), has put public health officials in a better position to demystify the dynamics of pathogen transmission. NGS has demonstrated its potential in the case of outbreaks, enabling source tracing, early detection, and interpretation of transmission patterns, thereby bridging the gap with traditional methods of identification (Boon et al., 2019). Besides, intense research in many European nations is highlighting increasing awareness of viral foodborne illness and advocating for harmonized surveillance networks with strict laboratory diagnosis (Brown et al., 2003). Such a framework helps us follow foodborne pathogens more accurately and allows us to take action more quickly, which reduces the risk to the public. Together, these advancements in laboratory testing are essential for effective identification and control in foodborne outbreak investigation efforts (Figure 13.6).

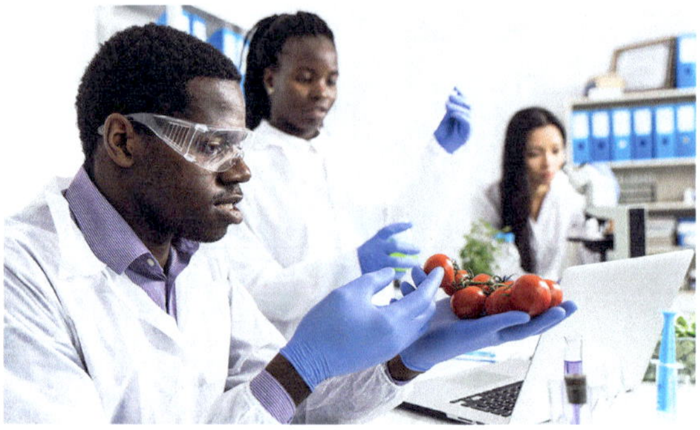

Figure 13.6. The use of laboratory testing in identification has become a cornerstone in managing foodborne outbreak investigations.

Source: https://www.food-safety.com/ext/resources/Images/2022/Oct_Nov/RegRep-900.jpg?height=635&t=1665520165&width=1200.

13.1.8. Challenges in Outbreak Identification

Spotting foodborne outbreaks is not easy, which makes it harder to manage risks to public health. Among the prominent issues is the heterogeneity of foodborne pathogens, which vary in their adaptability and transmission dynamics; microorganisms can infiltrate the food chain at multiple stages, complicating pinpointing the source of contamination (Boon et al., 2019). Also, using NGS and other advanced genomic methods in regular monitoring has shown both positive and negative aspects. Although NGS enhances outbreak detection and provides superior resolution for transmission tracing, its application requires high-quality contextual data and interdisciplinary collaboration (Boon et al., 2019). Besides, some regions have fewer resources and different public health systems, which can make it hard to deal with threats quickly. Consequently, addressing these challenges necessitates innovative risk assessment methodologies and robust communication among stakeholders in the food safety landscape (Brul et al., 2025).

13.1.9. Examples of Recent Outbreaks

Recent foodborne outbreak cases reflect the pressing challenges in maintaining food safety in the highly globalized food system. For instance, the emergence of STEC has initiated numerous outbreaks, which also reflected not only the difficulty in tracing such infections but also the inability of conventional surveillance systems. One recent analysis of 510 clinical STEC isolates proved that while pulsed-field gel electrophoresis (PFGE) has been conventional for the detection of outbreaks, whole-genome sequencing (WGS) offers more genetic resolution that allows superior outbreak cluster detection (Blankenship et al., 2023). Additionally, issues with the cold chain system have also been discovered to contribute to the occurrence of cold-tolerant pathogens, which are capable of thriving even under temperature measures aimed at repressing microbial dangers. This highlights the imperative need to develop and strengthen existing food safety practices in the cold chain to avert future outbreaks (Liu et al., 2024) (Figure 13.7).

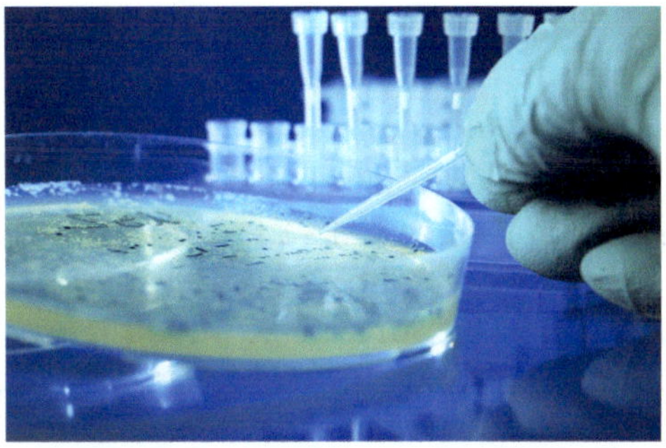

Figure 13.7. Shiga toxin-producing *Escherichia coli* (STEC).

Source: https://www.cidrap.umn.edu/sites/default/files/styles/article_detail/public/images/news/bacteriaculture.jpg?itok=PLQ7mrl0.

13.2. Investigation Process

The investigation process is crucial in foodborne outbreak control as it involves a systematic approach to identifying the cause of contamination and implementing effective interventions. Initial measures typically include the collection and analysis of data regarding reported cases of illness, as well as the use of case-control studies and microbial subtyping techniques for the identification of the causative pathogen. Effective food attribution practices are important as they can assist in linking specific food vehicles to disease cases, thus informing priority-setting in interventions (Batz et al., 2025). Moreover, advances in molecular techniques and epidemiological monitoring provide increased sensitivity and ability to detect and respond to outbreaks in real-time, facilitating increased source tracing of contamination (Brul et al., 2025). Overall, a consistent process of investigation informs risk management plans, affords public health protection, and ultimately assists in alleviating the foodborne disease burden in communities.3

13.2.1. Initial Response to an Outbreak

How a foodborne outbreak is handled at the start helps to reduce risks to people and restore trust in the food supply. After an outbreak is found, it is important to investigate right away and communicate to identify the source and stop the outbreak from spreading. Local health departments (LHDs) play a central role in coordinating these efforts, as evidenced by their historical involvement in managing emergencies, including foodborne illness cases. A decline in emergency preparedness among LHDs underscores the critical need for sustained funding and strategic planning to effectively address such outbreaks (Shah, 2014).

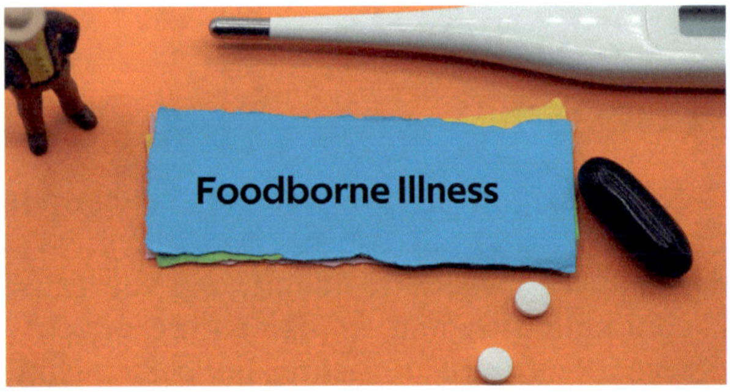

Figure 13.8. The initial response to a foodborne outbreak is crucial for mitigating public health risks and restoring consumer confidence.

Source: https://acko-cms.ackoassets.com/First_Aid_Guide_Foodborne_illness_4966641b46.png.

Also, it is clear that good information sharing during the response phase is crucial because of the way public perception and incident management are linked. For instance, the negative impact of a product recall can diminish over time if the response is appropriately managed, showcasing that effective communication can significantly influence consumer behavior regarding affected products (Bakhtavoryan et al., 2014). Thus, a robust initial response is imperative for both public safety and the stability of the food industry (Figure 13.8).

13.2.2. Formation of an Investigation Team

Formation of an investigation team is a vital process in the effective management of foodborne outbreaks, as it brings together differing expertise essential to a thorough investigation. A central role within the team is a multidisciplinary nature through the incorporation of specialists from different fields, including epidemiology, microbiology, public health, and food safety regulation. Such heterogeneity facilitates achieving comprehensive knowledge of the causes behind outbreaks and assists in the development of effective interventions. Additionally, as noted by the Western Institute for Food Safety and Security, cross-disciplinary training enhances team members' competence to manage the complexities of food production and its environmental implications (Angelos et al., 2017). Along with an organized team management, the establishment of a Food Safety Administration has been proposed to unify regulation and heighten the effectiveness of investigations, further ensuring consistency and strictness in policies and enforcement. A capable investigation team is therefore essential to safeguard public health in the case of foodborne outbreaks.

13.2.3. Data Collection Methods

Collecting data in the right way is important for foodborne outbreak investigations because it allows researchers to spot trends and the sources of contamination. They usually rely on both primary and secondary data, which includes interviews, laboratory tests and a look at epidemiological records. For instance, systematic documentation of outbreak characteristics, such as environmental factors and outbreak size, significantly influences the likelihood of pinpointing a food vehicle responsible for illness (Gould et al., 2015).

Furthermore, the integration of geographic information systems (GIS) enhances the visualization of outbreak data, allowing for better identification of affected regions and contaminated food sources. In a global context, variability in food sources associated with outbreaks has been highlighted, with beef and produce being predominant in different world regions (Pires et al., 2019). By applying comprehensive data collection techniques, public health officials can effectively manage response strategies and prevent future outbreaks, ultimately improving public health outcomes (Figure 13.9).

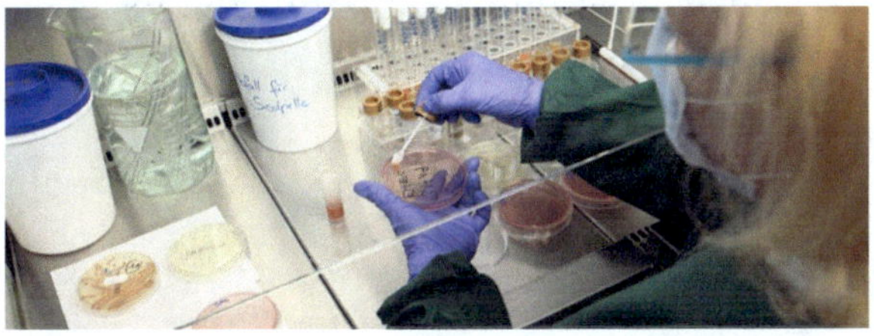

Figure 13.9. Effective data collection methods are essential in foodborne outbreak investigations, as they enable researchers to identify trends and sources of contamination.

Source: https://ncceh.ca/sites/default/files/foodborne%20outbreak%20cropped.jpg.

13.2.4. Interviews with Affected Individuals

Interviewing those affected by food poisoning is essential in investigations, since it helps explain the outbreak and find the possible sources of contamination. To investigate a foodborne outbreak, interviews were held with every one of all 140 people who had diarrhea and abdominal pain after eating chicken from the public health center. This active case finding revealed that 68 individuals fell ill, with data collection supplemented by e-questionnaires to ensure a comprehensive understanding (Iskandar et al., 2025). Similarly, an investigation into a norovirus outbreak at a daycare center emphasized the significance of gathering firsthand accounts from staff and children to assess potential transmission pathways and risk factors (Lee et al., 2025). Interviews with affected individuals allow investigators to build a clear timeline and recognize, which foods were exposed, which helps set up steps to prevent future outbreaks of the same type.

13.2.5. Environmental Assessments

Environmental surveys are a valuable element of foodborne outbreak investigations since they provide an all-inclusive method of gaining insight into environmental contributions to food safety threats. By evaluating factors, such as farming practices, water quality, and sanitary waste disposal systems, environmental surveys can be beneficial towards the identification of suspected source points of contamination for certain outbreaks.

For instance, effective pathogen attribution methods, including case-control studies and microbial subtyping, are grounded on accurate environmental data for tracking the source of foodborne disease back to its food vehicle (Batz et al.). Additionally, adopting a One Health strategy to food safety education enhances the interconnectedness of human, animal, and environmental health, guiding researchers and policymakers in developing strategies that ensure food security and preserve natural resources (Angelos et al., 2017). Environmental assessments are hence extremely important in the creation of effective interventions that reduce the risk of FBDs and support sustainable food systems (Figure 13.10).

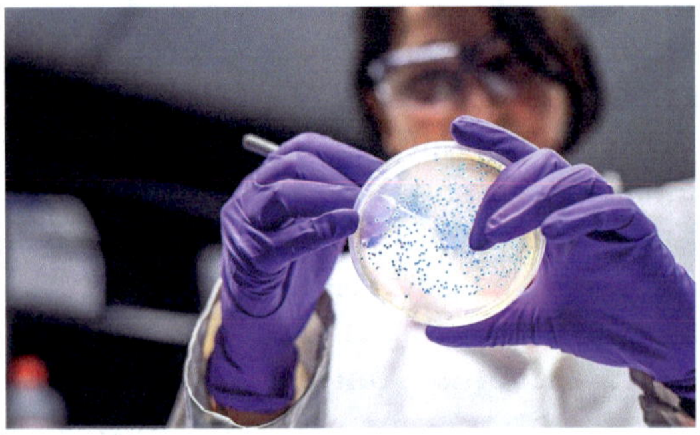

Figure 13.10. Environmental assessments play a crucial role in the investigation of foodborne outbreaks.

Source: https://www.food-safety.com/ext/resources/Images/2024/Apr_May/FSI-0424-900-Img1.jpg?1712951557.

13.2.6. Laboratory Analysis of Food Samples

In foodborne outbreak investigations, laboratory analysis of food samples is central to the identification and prevention of contamination-causing pathogens. Rapidity and accuracy are essential as traditional epidemiological measures are prone to errors and slow in action. Molecular techniques, such as pulsed field gel electrophoresis (PFGE) and novel CRISPR-based technologies offer significant improvements in the subtyping of outbreak-causing bacterial strains of higher resolution than traditional methods (Nadin-Davis et al., 2022). Metagenomics is also an extremely powerful method that enables the simultaneous detection and typing of multiple foodborne pathogens without previous growth, thereby enhancing investigation speed (Jützke et al., 2019). Sample handling and data analysis challenges should, however, be overcome to ensure the accuracy of outcomes. The development of such laboratory procedures not only raises response speed in the face of outbreaks but also increases credibility in source detection, ultimately bringing security to public health.

13.2.7. Timeline of the Investigation

The order in, which events happen in a foodborne outbreak investigation helps explain how the contamination occurred and what actions were taken. In most cases, the investigation begins when healthcare professionals or patients report new illness cases and then the team collects data to see if there are any links between the cases. As data accumulates, investigators employ methods, such as adaptive sampling and metagenomic sequencing to rapidly identify pathogens without relying on traditional culture enrichment techniques (Buytaers et al., 2024). Reviewing old outbreaks helps researchers find patterns that guide their present work. Statistical analyses and predictive modeling are utilized to ascertain the relationships between food sources and pathogens, leading to timely interventions that mitigate further risk (Tao et al., 2023). This systematic approach ensures a comprehensive understanding of outbreak dynamics, which is essential for enhancing food safety measures and protecting public health (Figure 13.11).

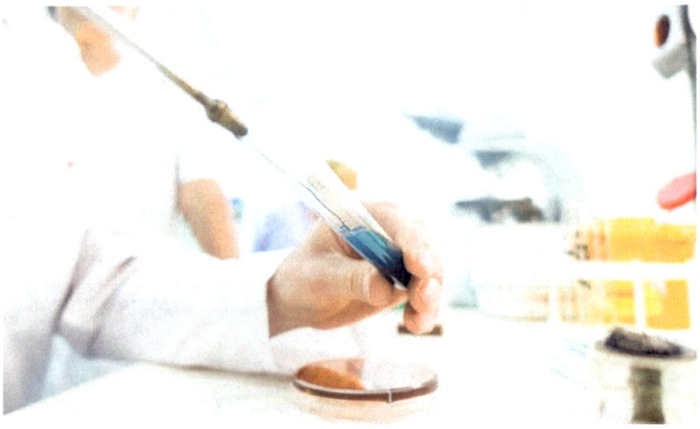

Figure 13.11. The timeline of the investigation into foodborne outbreaks is critical for understanding the sequence of events leading to contamination and subsequent public health responses.

Source: https://www.foodengineeringmag.com/ext/resources/Issues/2018/09-September/FE0918-pathogen01-pathogen-testing.jpg?height=635&t=1536948986&width=1200.

13.2.8. Collaboration with Local Health Departments (LHDs)

It is very important to collaborate with LHDs in the investigation of foodborne outbreaks to ensure a good public health response. Local agencies are responsible for finding and reporting foodborne illness cases as soon as they are detected. Because they understand the health trends in the community, they can react and control health problems quickly. In addition, working together with federal and state agencies helps LHDs improve the way food safety regulations are monitored. As noted, there is a pressing need for systemwide reforms that bolster state and local roles in improving outbreak response and regulation, which can drastically impact surveillance effectiveness (Taylor & David, 2009). Additionally, the evaluation of state preparedness to handle emergencies, such as bioterrorism, underscores the need for adequate funding and restructuring to strengthen LHDs (Levi et al., 2008). As a result, the public health system becomes more able to handle challenges.

13.2.9. Communication with the Public

Effective communication with the public plays a crucial role in the coordination of foodborne outbreak investigations. The timely provision of authentic and clear information during emergencies has the ability to minimize health risk effectively, as reported by a recent epidemic in Bantul District, where the health authorities responded promptly in covering widespread illness following consumption of contaminated chicken (Iskandar et al., 2025). Public health officials are entrusted with the duty to tailor messages to various groups based on established best practices informed by large-scale studies, emphasizing building public trust and utilizing media outlets effectively (Mucevi et al., 2025). Through establishing openness and applying the appropriate communication channels, such officials have been able to effectively inform and educate the public on potential risks, prevention strategies, and health details. Finally, an active public communication strategy not only enhances community resilience but also becomes a determinant driver of bringing the outbreak to an end and ensuring public health (Figure 13.12).

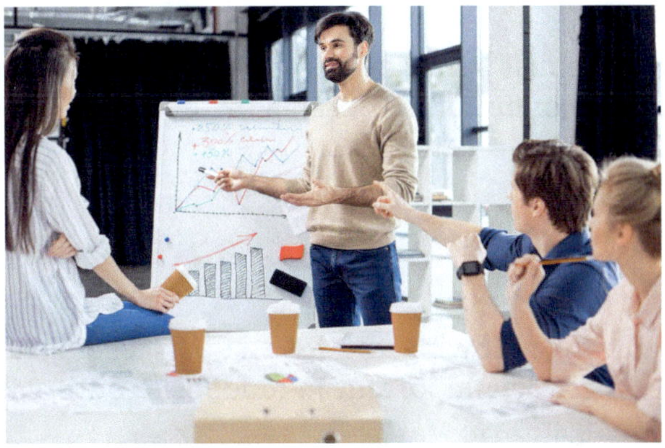

Figure 13.12. Effective communication with the public plays a critical role in the management of foodborne outbreak investigations.

Source: https://www.foodpoisoningnews.com/wp-content/uploads/2024/09/business-people-on-meeting-stockpack-deposit-photos-scaled.jpg.

13.3. Source Identification

In the foodborne outbreak setting, successful source identification is critical for successful public health action and prevention in the future. New technologies like WGS provide increased resolution for distinguishing between very similar strains of pathogens, followed by correct species identification. Such technological advances are even more necessary with increasing foodborne disease epidemiology complexity and the inability of traditional detection methods, such as culture-based systems and serotyping, to keep pace with the demands of outbreak resolution (Gomes et al., 2025). Moreover, as characterized in previous studies, contamination source tracking is complex and requires epidemiologic methods with several dimensions, especially in healthcare settings where drug diversion could complicate outbreak investigations (Pierce et al., 2025). As such, adopting WGS as a routine tool for food safety surveillance not only increases source tracking ability but also constructs a more robust public health infrastructure that is capable of better addressing the evolving issue of foodborne pathogens.

13.3.1. Tracing the Food Supply Chain

Recently, following the food supply chain has become very important in foodborne outbreak investigations.

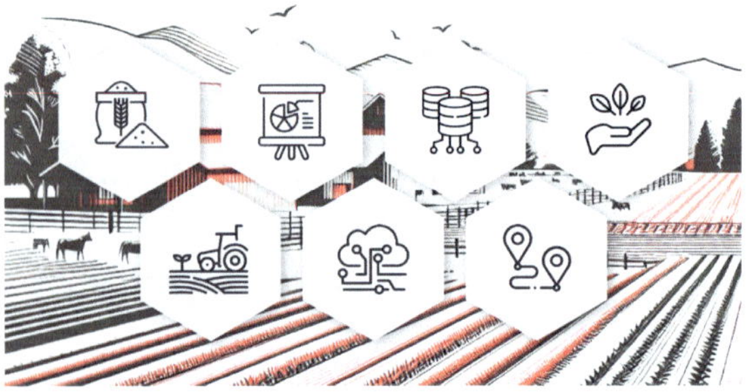

Figure 13.13. In recent years, tracing the food supply chain has become a critical focus in the realm of foodborne outbreak investigation.

Source: https://blaize.tech/wp-content/uploads/2023/12/pic2-2-1.png.

The combination of WGS and better data-sharing systems helps quickly find where food contamination occurs, which boosts public health responses to foodborne illnesses. For instance, the European surveillance system has highlighted significant outbreaks, such as the *E. coli* outbreak linked to sprouted seeds in 2011, revealing the urgency for comprehensive tracing methods that link public health, agricultural practices, and food production processes (Pezzutto et al., 2021). Furthermore, the case of Salmonella enteritidis contamination in eggs underscores how lapses in food safety can have devastating consequences, raising awareness of the need for stringent tracing protocols to prevent future outbreaks (Bousquet et al., 2019). As such, developing robust supply chain tracing mechanisms is vital for minimizing public health risks and ensuring food safety (Figure 13.13).

13.3.2. Role of Traceback Investigations

Traceback studies are very crucial in the control and management of foodborne outbreak incidents, particularly in the identification of contaminated food sources. Traceback studies allow systematic tracing of foods from the consumer to the origin, and they help determine the linkage between specific foods and reported illnesses. For instance, during outbreak investigations associated with Shiga toxin-producing *E. coli* linked with romaine lettuce, traceback activities found severe limitations, such as inordinate delay in starting the process and poor product-identifying information along the chain. Utilization of sophisticated technology and enhanced traceability systems should eliminate these hindrances, hence making it easier for investigations and public health actions. Because foodborne illness is the originator of millions of cases annually in the United States, traceback investigations that are successful not only bring definiteness to food safety issues but also enhance the ability to prevent outbreaks in the future.

13.3.3. Identifying Potential Sources of Contamination

Finding out where contamination may have come from is very important in investigating foodborne outbreaks, according to recent studies. As an example, when students at an elementary school reported illness, researchers examined what food was eaten before the symptoms appeared. In one study, "Egg Macaroni" was significantly associated with illness, pointing to the importance of food handler hygiene and proper food handling practices, as evidenced by the presence of Bacillus cereus in laboratory tests (Handika et al., 2024). Similarly, another outbreak was linked to meatballs, identified through a retrospective cohort study that revealed improper storage and reheating as potential risk factors (Iskandar et al., 2024). These findings underscore the necessity for thorough investigations that analyze not only the foods consumed but also the practices surrounding their preparation, storage, and serving, to effectively mitigate future outbreaks (Figure 13.14).

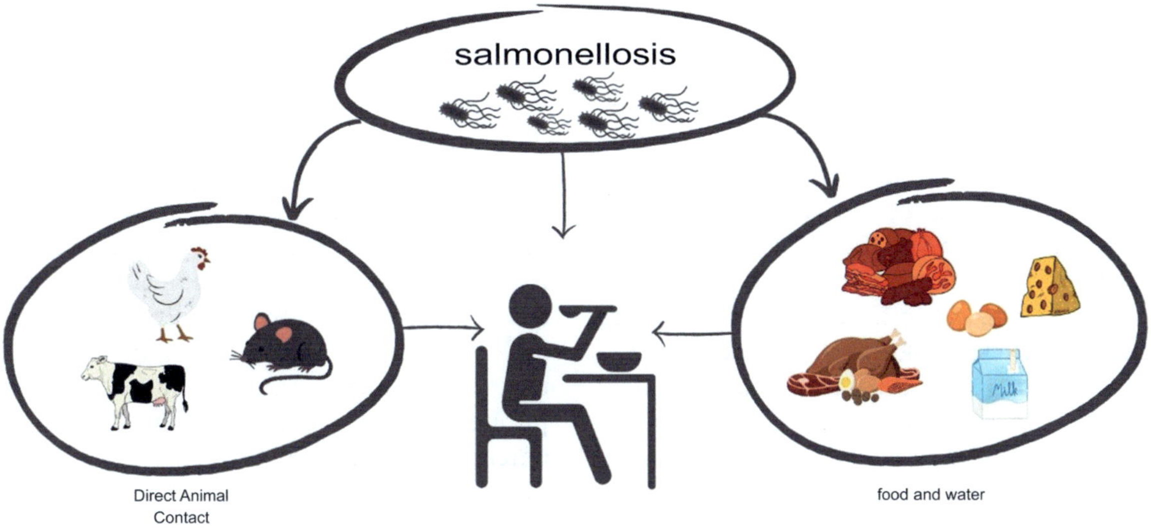

Figure 13.14. Identifying potential sources of contamination is a critical component in the investigation of foodborne outbreaks, as demonstrated in recent epidemiological studies.

Source: https://microbiologyjournal.org/wp-content/uploads/2025/05/fg02-3.jpg.

13.3.4. Common Food Vehicles in Outbreaks

It is very important to find out what foods are linked to foodborne outbreaks to guide public health actions and stop more incidents. Often, foods that are not processed much or served raw, such as leafy greens, fruits and dairy products, have been associated with outbreaks. For instance, outbreak investigations often utilize a variety of methods to attribute illnesses to specific food items, leveraging data from microbial subtyping and case-control studies, as noted in the discussions surrounding food attribution approaches (Batz et al., 2025). Moreover, the advent of whole-genome sequencing (WGS) has significantly enhanced the resolve of outbreak investigations, allowing for the precise identification of linked cases within widespread food distribution networks (Dallman et al., 2015). Because of this technology, food vehicles can be identified more accurately, which helps in promptly carrying out public health actions and lessens the effects of foodborne illnesses on the public.

13.3.5. Environmental Factors Contributing to Outbreaks

Understanding the environmental causes of foodborne outbreaks is critical to minimizing the risk to public health. A critical review of United States reported outbreaks between 2014 and 2022 indicates that contamination, growth, and survival of foodborne pathogens during food preparation are central to outbreak causes. For instance, microbial pathogen contamination of food in the pre-final preparation stage typically results from improper control in the environment, such as animal and environmental contamination sources, which increased from 22.2% to 32.3% throughout the three periods considered (Monarez et al., 2025). Besides, environmental factors in their most favorable conditions, such as temperature and humidity, can promote the growth of pathogens, as recorded in outbreaks resulting from substandard cooling methods (Monarez et al., 2025). At the same time, the same environmental drivers can intensify vector-borne diseases, such as chikungunya, where mosquito breeding sites correlate with high levels of outbreak risk. The treatment of such environmental determinants is the key to effective prevention and control of outbreaks (Figure 13.15).

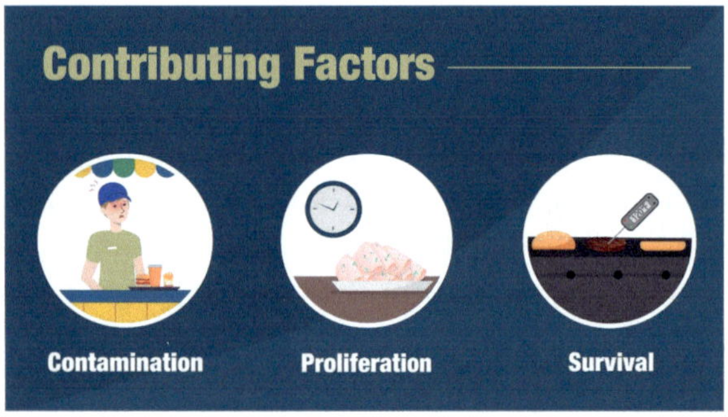

Figure 13.15. Understanding the environmental factors contributing to foodborne outbreaks is crucial for mitigating public health risks.

Source: https://www.cdc.gov/restaurant-food-safety/media/images/Contributing-factors.jpg.

13.3.6. Use of Technology in Source Identification

The use of technology underpins the improvement of source identification during investigations of foodborne outbreaks. Advanced data mining techniques enable researchers to deconstruct complicated patterns in historical outbreak data, from, which they can have a significant impact on public health interventions. For instance, statistical modeling identifies informative associations among various outbreak parameters and food vehicles so that epidemiologists can generate more accurate predictions of contamination sources. Techniques, such as support vector machines and logistic regression models have proved beneficial in etiology estimation from food vehicles to make the identification process easier under real-time conditions. A wedding in Kyrgyzstan is a good case in point for the use, where incorporation of food sampling and public health surveillance proved contaminated chicken as the likely causative factor in the disease of the guests (Dautov et al., 2023). Finally, these advances in technology not only speed up the process of investigation but also feed into proactive efforts that can ensure future foodborne illness outbreaks are avoided (Tao et al., 2023).

13.3.7. Challenges in Pinpointing Sources

Finding the sources of foodborne outbreaks is very difficult, which makes it hard to respond and prevent them effectively. In regions with insufficient surveillance systems, such as those represented in studies from Jinhua city, Zhejiang province, the majority of outbreaks are connected to unidentified pathogens, complicating containment measures (Yang et al., 2025). Furthermore, in Central America and the Caribbean, systemic issues like inadequate resources and inconsistent reporting practices hamper the ability to trace pathogens (Severino et al., 2025). Not having complete data prevents us from acting promptly and also from planning for the future of public health and safety. Because the food distribution is complex and there are various kinds of pathogens, it is not possible to identify where a food poisoning outbreak has started. Thus, there is a need to establish cooperation among governmental agencies, food industries, and health professionals for the advancement of surveillance capacity and accuracy of source attribution in foodborne outbreak investigations (Figure 13.16).

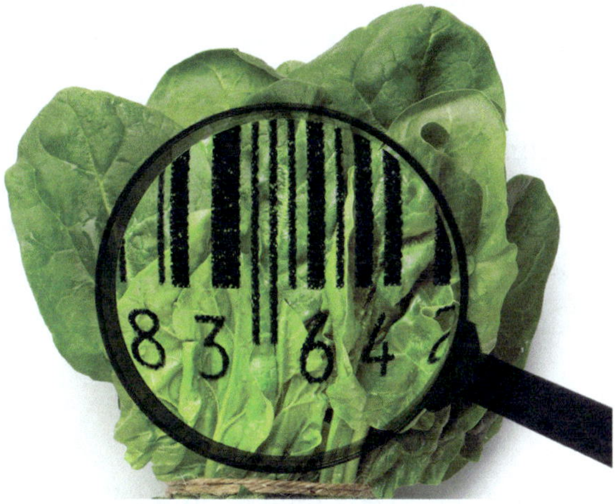

Figure 13.16. Identifying the sources of foodborne outbreaks presents significant challenges that complicate effective response and prevention efforts.

Source: https://assets.farmjournal.com/dims4/default/63042c6/2147483647/strip/false/crop/1200x857+0+0/resize/1200x857!/quality/90/?url=https%3A%2F%2Ffj-corp-pub.s3.us-east-2.amazonaws.com%2Fs3fs-public%2F2024-03%2Ffoodsafety1.png.

13.3.8. Importance of Rapid Identification

Rapidly finding out what caused a foodborne outbreak is very important because it helps to reduce the impact of foodborne illnesses. Recognizing the pathogens quickly enables health officials to take steps to stop the infection and reduce the number of sick and dead. Because global food systems are more complex and can carry contaminated food across borders, it is now more important to identify problems quickly. For instance, collaborative efforts across multiple laboratories can significantly enhance surveillance capabilities, providing essential data on enteric viruses and their transmission pathways (Brown et al., 2003). Besides, advances in molecular detection technology enable quicker response rates and more effective source attribution, as detailed in contemporary food safety approaches (Brul et al., 2025). Therefore, using quick methods of detecting foodborne disease can contain the outbreak instantly and promote food safety in the future.

13.4. Prevention and Control Measures

Effective prevention and control are the critical factors in curbing the impact of foodborne outbreaks, particularly in the context of a multi-agency complex system. The CIFOR guidelines emphasize inclusive procedures that can be applied by agencies in order to enhance their capacity to respond to outbreaks. These regulations provide a formal structure to outbreak control, from preparation and detection to investigation and control, with well-defined roles at the state, local, and federal levels. Better communication and coordination among these agencies are needed, since this facilitates an easy opportunity for a unified response to multijurisdictional outbreaks and provides food-safety infrastructure (Taylor & David, 2009). In offering procedures and measures of performance to provision agencies, CIFOR guidelines aim to bridge gaps that now confront the requirements of food safety and ultimately lead to more effective prevention and control against FBDs.

13.4.1. Public Health Recommendations

Public health policy is of greatest significance in the regulation of foodborne outbreak risk, as proven by several studies pinpointing sources and control means. A wedding reception outbreak in Kyrgyzstan, where chicken is suspected to have caused disease since it was contaminated, prompted the regulation of restaurant conformity to food protection procedures (Dautov et al., 2023). These actions are vital in the improvement of gastrointestinal disease diagnostic testing to efficiently identify and treat disease during epidemic times. Besides, as far as the general public health concerns, the Community-based Outbreak Investigation and Response (COIR) approach is an essential policy. By empowering the local health authorities to conduct effective disease surveillance and coordinate a response, COIR enables the communities' confidence and ensures fair health practices (Oza et al., 2023). Therefore, embracing these recommendations is crucial in strengthening food safety controls and predicting future outbreaks (Figure 13.17).

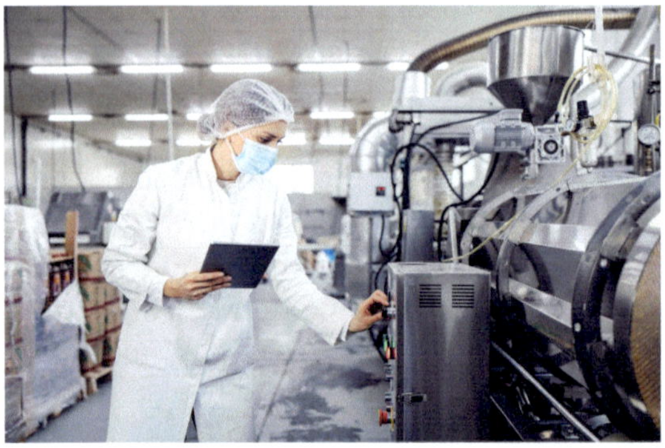

Figure 13.17. Public health recommendations play a crucial role in mitigating the risks associated with foodborne outbreaks, as evidenced by various investigative studies that pinpoint the sources and necessary preventative measures.

Source: https://knowhow.distrelec.com/wp-content/uploads/2024/02/GettyImages-1377412499.jpg.

13.4.2. Role of Food Safety Regulations

The rules for food safety help to lower the risks of foodborne diseases, which impact many people around the world. They set rules for creating, shipping and using food so that it is not contaminated by harmful substances. As highlighted, the presence of pathogenic microorganisms, such as *Listeria monocytogenes* and *Salmonella enterica* in the food supply can lead to severe health complications, including hospitalization and even death, particularly among vulnerable populations like children and the elderly (Gali et al., 2018). Moreover, as the food sector grows, the need for new food safety interventions is evident, with rapid detection methods for pathogens becoming increasingly important (Fung et al., 2018). Strong enforcement of food safety policies keeps people healthy and enables consumers to trust what they eat.

13.4.3. Importance of Proper Food Handling

Adopting appropriate food handling is of prime concern since it is directly related to not getting foodborne illness and foodborne outbreaks. Foodborne pathogens, such as Salmonella and *E. coli* are very dangerous to health, so both consumers and food industry personnel should learn and implement meticulous food safety practices. Research indicates that the foodborne pathogens cause an approximate 47.8 million illnesses per year in the U.S., where during manufacturing and preparation, improper handling is one of the major causes of these outbreaks (Wang et al., 2024). Also, the identification of new pathogens along with issues involving antimicrobial resistance indicates the evolving problem in food safety prevention along the supply chain (Hassan et al., 2023). To combat such risks, appropriate food handling procedures like storage, cooking, and hygiene need to be practiced to ensure public health and minimize the risks of consuming foods (Figure 13.18).

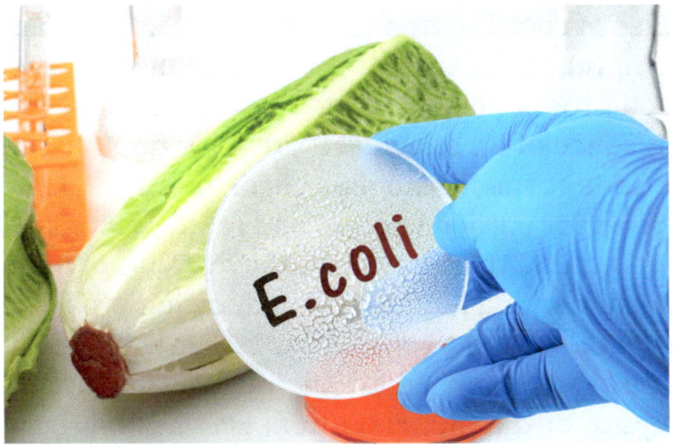

Figure 13.18. With foodborne pathogens, such as Salmonella and *E. coli* posing significant health risks, understanding and implementing meticulous food safety practices is essential for both consumers and food industry professionals.

Source: https://www.nemistech.com/wp-content/uploads/2024/07/shutterstock_1258412335.jpg.

13.4.4. Education and Training for Food Industry Workers

Training and education of food industry personnel play a crucial role in the prevention of foodborne illness outbreaks, as attested to by recent food safety failure investigations. For instance, Company A's study of contaminated ekiben meal production found glaring shortcomings in hygiene training and work practices, an immediate reason for FBD outbreaks among consumers (Eita et al., 2025). With this, a study conducted in Dhaka, Bangladesh, among food handlers identified gaps in awareness of key practices, such as cross-contamination prevention and temperature control. Although the majority of the workers were aware of basic hygiene, male workers were informed of fewer food safety facts than female workers, which requires certain education programs (Rahman et al., 2025). These disclosures highlight the necessity for extensive training programs and adherence to proper health and safety measures as a measure of providing the learning and knowledge required for food industry personnel to diminish the risk of foodborne illness.

13.4.5. Implementation of Hazard Analysis Critical Control Point (HACCP)

Implementation of the Hazard Analysis Critical Control Point (HACCP) system is a milestone in food safety management, particularly in foodborne outbreak investigation. By determining CCPs in food production, HACCP avoids pathogens from contaminating and spreading and surviving, which avoids outbreaks from taking place.

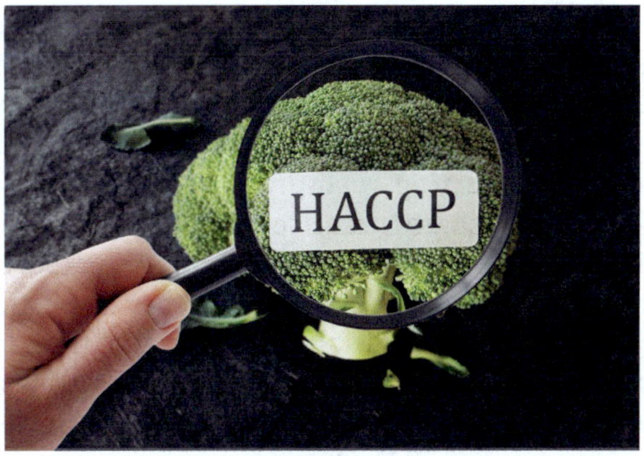

Figure 13.19. The implementation of the Hazard Analysis Critical Control Point (HACCP) system represents a pivotal advancement in food safety management, particularly in the context of foodborne outbreak investigation.

Source: https://cdn.prod.website-files.com/65afd8dc16873da38e2b5ecb/6601737c8a7924cf0be4aafd_2022_12_Picture3.jpeg.

Following high-profile foodborne illness incidents, including the 1993 outbreak of Jack-in-the-Box, regulatory bodies mandated federally inspected meat and poultry facilities to use HACCP, identifying its use in protecting public health (Murano et al., 2018). This systemic approach permits action to be proactive, not reactive; instead of trying to control outbreaks once they happen, HACCP promotes continuous monitoring of food safety routines and customs, as evident from data collected in outbreak investigations, which identify factors contributing towards foodborne disease (Monarez et al., 2025). Ultimately, proper implementation of HACCP can successfully put a stop to the existence of FBDs (Figure 13.19).

13.4.6. Role of Consumer Awareness

Consumer education is a key factor in reducing the risks of foodborne diseases, especially in high-risk outlets like fast-food restaurants. While the occurrence of pathogenic bacteria outbreaks like *E. coli* increases, consumers need to be well-educated about proper handling of food and hygiene to follow. Research has illustrated that higher consumer knowledge leads to more informed buying behaviors, for example, selecting restaurants that take food hygiene and safety practices into consideration (Ajekiigbe et al., 2025). Furthermore, research indicates that socio-demographic characteristics greatly influence food safety attitudes, with more educated consumers having better knowledge of foodborne pathogens and methods of prevention (Hridoy et al., 2025). Through such a culture of awareness, not only can consumers of healthy food make an effort to protect their own health, but also push food providers to have a better standard. This eventually translates into public health and reduces the occurrence of FBDs.

13.4.7. Strategies for Outbreak Prevention

Effective strategies for outbreak prevention are central to preventing the public health threat that accompanies foodborne disease. Regulation of food safety is one such strategy that can potentially play a major role in protecting the food supply from contamination. Establishment of a distinct Food Safety Administration, as has been proposed in reform suggestions, would establish policy, inspection, and enforcement roles in coordination to provide consistency and comprehensiveness across the various phases of food production and distribution. Moreover, the presence of an effective system for the tracking of foodborne pathogens through surveillance allows for early detection and rapid response to potential outbreaks before they get out of hand. Consumer and food handler education programs have the ability to encourage better hygiene and food safety knowledge and practices that are the keys to outbreak prevention. Last but not least, integrating these complex programs is essential to an ongoing foodborne outbreak investigation and prevention program (International Conference on Emerging Infectious Diseases, 2008) (Figure 13.20).

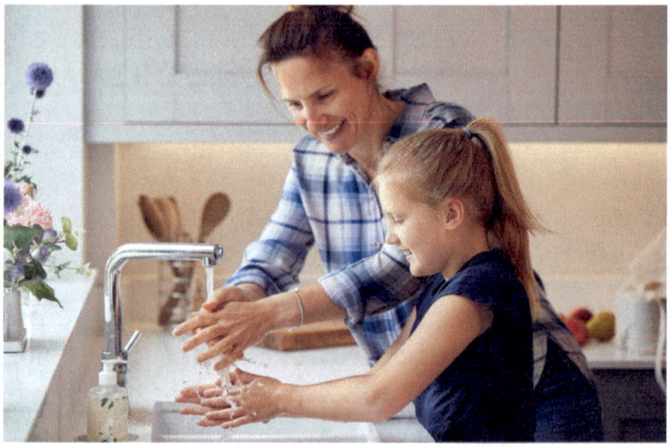

Figure 13.20. Effective strategies for outbreak prevention are integral to mitigating the public health risks associated with foodborne illnesses.

Source: https://www.fsis.usda.gov/sites/default/files/2024-09/2024%20Handwashing.jpg.

13.4.8. Importance of Ongoing Research

More research is essential in simplifying methodologies and frameworks in foodborne outbreak investigation. With mutations of the pathogens, traditional surveillance methods will be unreliable, giving rise to the integration of innovative techniques, such as NGS. NGS has been promising in public health applications through the ability to provide increased resolution for tracing sources of contaminants and for detecting outbreaks early, as underscored in a series of studies that point to its strength in demystifying transmission dynamics and tracing drug resistance (Boon et al., 2019). Moreover, addressing the complexities of food safety also requires collaboration between federal, state, and local levels to address existing issues in regulatory systems, inspection systems, and outbreak response systems (Taylor & David, 2009). With a continued advancement of studies on foodborne illness measurement and response activities, public health systems are better able to control and contain risks, thus leading to improved food safety outcomes for the population.

A CLOSER LOOK

Norovirus

Norovirus can easily spread and lead to gastrointestinal illness, which is sometimes called stomach flu. It is a main reason for acute gastroenteritis, which often causes nausea, vomiting, diarrhea, stomach pain and sometimes fever or headache. Norovirus can be transmitted by eating or drinking something contaminated, by touching infected people or things or by being close to them. It can also be spread in areas where many people are together, such as on cruise ships, in hospitals, schools and nursing homes.

It can easily spread, causing many cases and remains contagious on surfaces for days, which makes it hard to prevent. Good hygiene habits, such as regular handwashing, are the best ways to avoid getting norovirus. Thoroughly cooking shellfish and washing fruits and vegetables will help keep the food safe. Norovirus is treated by resting and drinking plenty of fluids. Most people recover in just 1 to 3 days, but in some groups, the illness can lead to dehydration, which could be dangerous and may require help from a doctor.

SUMMARY

Foodborne outbreak studies are crucial in public health, and therefore, there is a critical need to comprehend food source attribution and mechanisms of pathogen transmission. The health authorities can identify the principal food sources of infection, thus allowing interventions to be targeted in order to decrease risks, as demonstrated by studies conducted on STEC and non-typhoidal Salmonella outbreaks. For instance, STEC data further found outbreak source heterogeneity among regions, and prevention measures had to be adapted to respective cooking practices and types of pathogens in individual regions (Pires et al., 2019). Moreover, WGS improvements have revolutionized the traceability and attribution of source outbreaks so that it is possible to attain unparalleled accuracy in detecting singular contamination events (Mohammed et al., 2020). Lastly, there is a need to improve response strategies and investigative practices towards stopping outbreak occurrence, as well as protecting global public health.

An accurate understanding of foodborne outbreak investigations necessitates a critical analysis of the main issues that impact public health and safety. Federal, state, and local authorities play different roles in food safety and have strengths and weaknesses (Taylor & David, 2009). Good surveillance and response systems are essential in the prevention of outbreaks as they provide timely intervention and regulatory compliance. Also, epidemiology of foodborne pathogens, such as STEC, indicates the necessity of determining the source of the food for the disease. Data compiled across 27 countries reveals to report striking variations in the leading sources of STEC infection across regions, with beef and produce being common in Europe and the Americas, yet produce as the leading source in the Western Pacific (Pires et al., 2019). This data is important in order to design particular interventions to control the incidence of foodborne illnesses worldwide.

KEY TERMS FROM THIS CHAPTER

- Accurate subtyping methods
- CRISPR-based technologies
- Dizziness
- Elementary school
- Foodborne agents
- Heterogeneity
- Local agencies
- Malaise
- Psittacosis
- Pulsed-field gel electrophoresis (PFGE)
- Contaminated snacks
- Data collection
- Egg Macaroni
- Environmental factors
- Geographic information systems (GIS)
- Likelihood
- Local health departments (LHDs)
- Next-generation sequencing (NGS)
- Public health institutions
- Surveillance systems

REFERENCES

1. Dallman, T. J., Byrne, L., Ashton, P. M., Cowley, L. A., Perry, N. T., Adak, G., Petrovska, L., Ellis, R. J., Elson, R., Underwood, A., Green, J., Hanage, W. P., Jenkins, C., Grant, K., & Wain, J. (2015). Whole-genome sequencing for national surveillance of Shiga toxin-producing Escherichia coli O157. *Clinical infectious diseases : an official publication of the Infectious Diseases Society of America*, *61*(3), 305–312. https://doi.org/10.1093/cid/civ318 (accessed on 29 May 2025).
2. Ajekiigbe, V., Ogieuhi, I., Anthony, C. S., Bakare, I. S., Anyacho, S., Ogunleke, P., Fatokun, D. I., et al. (2025). Consumer behavior and its role in *E. coli* outbreaks: The impact of fast-food preparation practices and hygiene awareness. *Tropical Medicine and Health, 53*. https://www.semanticscholar.org/paper/f0dcc4105d349fe365289c1ea7bc179c1d7d2a80 (accessed on 29 May 2025).
3. Ali Hassan, M. K. I., Summaia, F., Ali Hasan, S., Khalid, S., Naeem, M., & Usman, A. (2023). *Emerging Foodborne Pathogens: Challenges and Strategies for Ensuring Food Safety*. The 2nd International Electronic Conference on Microbiology. https://www.semanticscholar.org/paper/6a16bb6260f4adef56ca5dc1b0bf53ef04d85aa2 (accessed on 29 May 2025).
4. Angelos, J. A., Arens, A. L., Johnson, H. A., Cadriel, J. L., & Osburn, B. I. (2017). One Health in food safety and security education: Subject matter outline for a curricular framework. *One health (Amsterdam, Netherlands), 3*, 56–65. https://doi.org/10.1016/j.onehlt.2017.04.001Aryanto, S., Iskandar, S. I., Janah, M., Wiratama, M., et al. (2024). *Foodborne Outbreak Investigation in Elementary School Students in Bantul, Yogyakarta, 2023*. https://core.ac.uk/download/624327674.pdf (accessed on 29 May 2025).
5. Aworh, M., Nilsson, P., Egyir, B., Owusu, F., & Hendriksen, R. S. (2024). Rare serovars of non-typhoidal *Salmonella enterica* isolated from humans, beef cattle and abattoir environments in Nigeria. *PLOS ONE, 19*. https://www.semanticscholar.org/paper/031d586634c90df0cca7f9c3b60c2b0c803bb75e (accessed on 29 May 2025).
6. Bakhtavoryan, R., Capps, O., & Salin, V. (2014). Dynamics of consumer response to food contamination: The 2007 peanut butter recall. *Journal of Food Distribution Research, 45*, 66–81. https://www.semanticscholar.org/paper/1408b89e7841e948651c3dc2328941e92ff5f622 (accessed on 29 May 2025).
7. Basome, S., & Mwangi, P. N. (2024). The social-economic implications of COVID-19 pandemic on parents' income and pupils learning in Iganga District, Uganda. *Journal of Research Innovation and Implications in Education*. https://www.semanticscholar.org/paper/917270f66db21862f4e47f927b3f9c0ee8fdb4d7 (accessed on 29 May 2025).
8. Batz, M., Doyle, M., Lo Fo Wong, D., Morris, G., et al. (2025). *Linking Illness to Food: Summary of a Workshop on Food Attribution*. https://core.ac.uk/download/pdf/6759576.pdf (accessed on 29 May 2025).
9. Blankenship, H., Dietrich, S., Burgess, E., Wholehan, J. M., Soehnlen, M., & Manning, S. (2023). Whole-genome sequencing of Shiga toxin-producing *Escherichia coli* for characterization and outbreak investigation. *Microorganisms, 11*. https://www.semanticscholar.org/paper/c5170cdd88f3dad9d4bbd0c6fd2caad584472321 (accessed on 29 May 2025).
10. Boon, N. A. M., Descamps, T., Devleesschauwer, B., Robert, A., et al. (2019). *Status and Potential of Bacterial Genomics for Public Health Practice: A Scoping Review*. https://core.ac.uk/download/227041617.pdf (accessed on 29 May 2025).

11. Bousquet, K. (2019). *A Meticulous Food Safety Plan Today Avoids Handcuffs Tomorrow*. https://core.ac.uk/download/223094004.pdf (accessed on 29 May 2025).

12. Brown, D., European Consortium on Foodborne Viruses, Heersma, H., Koopmans, M., et al. (2003). *Early Identification of Common-Source Foodborne Virus Outbreaks in Europe*. https://core.ac.uk/download/13102801.pdf (accessed on 29 May 2025).

13. Brul, S., Havelaar, A. H., de Jong, A. E. I., et al. (2025). *Future Challenges to Microbial Food Safety*. https://core.ac.uk/download/pdf/29244275.pdf (accessed on 29 May 2025).

14. Buytaers, F., Verhaegen, B., Van Nieuwenhuysen, T., Roosens, N., Vanneste, K., Marchal, K., & De Keersmaecker, S. D. (2024). Strain-level characterization of foodborne pathogens without culture enrichment for outbreak investigation using shotgun metagenomics facilitated with nanopore adaptive sampling. *Frontiers in Microbiology, 15*. https://www.semanticscholar.org/paper/3b738e05957d36d28869c06d8a49e53d6c39970b (accessed on 29 May 2025).

15. D'Alessandro-Lowe, A. M., Brown, A., Sullo, E., Pichtikova, M., Karram, M., Mirabelli, J., McCabe, R., et al. (2024). Why are healthcare providers leaving their jobs? A convergent mixed-methods investigation of turnover intention among Canadian healthcare providers during the COVID-19 pandemic. *Nursing Reports, 14*, 2030–2060. https://www.semanticscholar.org/paper/03a03be7b794329aa65817d4b23dab09c8b4bb38 (accessed on 29 May 2025).

16. Dautov, T., Kemelbek, N., Malisheva, M., Otorbaeva, D., Horth, R., & Nabirova, D. (2023). 652. Foodborne outbreak investigation at a wedding event–Batken, Kyrgyzstan, June 2022. *Open Forum Infectious Diseases, 10*. https://www.semanticscholar.org/paper/9436a1bfdd4f6536df2a65e783e0e20c686c100a (accessed on 29 May 2025).

17. Pires, S. M., Majowicz, S., Gill, A., & Devleesschauwer, B. (2019). Global and regional source attribution of Shiga toxin-producing Escherichia coli infections using analysis of outbreak surveillance data. *Epidemiology and infection, 147*, e236. https://doi.org/10.1017/S095026881900116X (accessed on 29 May 2025).

18. Dufour, S., Muellner, P., Stärk, K. D. C., Zadoks, R. N., et al. (2015). 'Next-generation' surveillance: An epidemiologists' perspective on the use of molecular information in food safety and animal health decision-making. https://core.ac.uk/download/46567794.pdf (accessed on 29 May 2025).

19. Eita, M., Yahata, Y., Nakamura, N., Fujita, K., Saito, M., Matsukura, K., Takagi, H., et al. (2025). P-1313. Large outbreak of *Staphylococcus aureus* and *Bacillus cereus* caused by ready-to-eat meals in Aomori, Japan. *Open Forum Infectious Diseases, 12*. https://www.semanticscholar.org/paper/53a58430eb5cdb58ca18a4ef33eb3058edd76b96 (accessed on 29 May 2025).

20. Emílio Gomes, Araújo, D., Nogueira, T., Oliveira, R., Silva, S., Oliveira, L. V. N., Azevedo, N. F., et al. (2025). Advances in whole genome sequencing for foodborne pathogens: Implications for clinical infectious disease surveillance and public health. *Frontiers in Cellular and Infection Microbiology, 15*. https://www.semanticscholar.org/paper/e95a6350e489a4d5698ed41598480ee981460080 (accessed on 29 May 2025).

21. Fung, F., Wang, H. S., & Menon, S. (2018). Food safety in the 21st century. *Biomedical Journal, 41*, 88–95. https://doi.org/10.1016/j.bj.2018.03.003.

22. Galié, S., García-Gutiérrez, C., Miguélez, E. M., Villar, C. J., & Lombó, F. (2018). Biofilms in the food industry: Health aspects and control methods. *Frontiers in Microbiology, 9*. https://doi.org/10.3389/fmicb.2018.00898.

23. Githinji, G. K., Odhiambo, F., Andala, C. M., Chepkwony, D., Sang, J., Owiny, M., Ruto, J., et al. (2024). Role of surveillance data in detecting malaria outbreaks in an epidemic-prone region in Kenya: Findings from an investigation of a suspected outbreak in Nandi County. *Malaria Journal, 23*. https://www.semanticscholar.org/paper/f3c7eaf66a252e1d61ab5d96efa9f28e32fbc77a (accessed on 29 May 2025).

24. Gould, L. H., Mecher, T., & Stauber, C. E. (2015). Contributing factors in a successful foodborne outbreak investigation: An analysis of data collected by the Foodborne Diseases Active Surveillance Network (FoodNet), 2003–2010. https://core.ac.uk/download/71426707.pdf (accessed on 29 May 2025).

25. Grützke, J., Malorny, B., Hammerl, J., Busch, A., Tausch, S. H., Tomaso, H., & Deneke, C. (2019). Fishing in the soup–Pathogen detection in food safety using metabarcoding and metagenomic sequencing. *Frontiers in Microbiology, 10*. https://www.semanticscholar.org/paper/bc797361c7e451abac0a8164b56e6f86601409de (accessed on 29 May 2025).

26. Hamaideh, S., Olaimat, A., Al-Holy, M., Ababneh, A., Shahbaz, H., Abughoush, M. H., Al-Nabulsi, A., et al. (2024). The influence of technological shifts in the food chain on the emergence of foodborne pathogens: An overview. *Applied Microbiology*. https://www.semanticscholar.org/paper/47fda0f5169645f73dbd7e26c833eeca0ff9e057 (accessed on 29 May 2025).

27. Handika, D. O., Utama, M. I., Ananda, D. R., Maula, A. W., Ahmad, R. A., & Sukoco, S. H. (2024). Foodborne outbreak investigation in elementary school, Gunungkidul District, January 2024: A cohort retrospective study design. *BIO Web of Conferences*. https://www.semanticscholar.org/paper/f37cb307a3e552f1c4a3a8d68abb3d09795845c4 (accessed on 29 May 2025).

28. Hridoy, M., Islam, Md., Masood, A., Sa'adi, Z., Bohora, N., Islam, Md., Lima, M., et al. (2025). Investigating the role of socio-demographic factors in shaping consumer attitudes towards food safety in Bangladesh: A cross-sectional study. *World Journal of Public Health*. https://www.semanticscholar.org/paper/00965f3d1d193c2e53e14abbd9a4d5e49fc16f1b (accessed on 29 May 2025).

29. International Conference on Emerging Infectious Diseases (2008: Atlanta, GA). (2025). *Emerging Infectious Diseases*. https://core.ac.uk/download/144197853.pdf (accessed on 29 May 2025).

30. Iskandar, S. I., Hertanto, D. A., Aryanto, S., & Wiratama, B. S. (2025). *E. coli*-caused foodborne outbreak in Bantul Regency, Indonesia, 2023: A retrospective cohort study. *The Open Public Health Journal*. https://www.semanticscholar.org/paper/819e87af1d4597b59a6069c46987d3dddfebf493 (accessed on 29 May 2025).

31. Lee, S. J., Jang, J., & Lee, K. (2025). An epidemiologic investigation for an outbreak of norovirus infection in a daycare center in Gyeonggi-Do, Republic of Korea, 2023. *Children, 12*. https://www.semanticscholar.org/paper/4b0cc6f5196161d9866223b5f33447dba2940be9 (accessed on 29 May 2025).

32. Levi, J., Segal, L. M., St. Laurent, R., & Vinter, S. (2008). *Ready or not? Protecting the Public's Health from Diseases, Disasters, and Bioterrorism, 2008*. https://core.ac.uk/download/71354212.pdf (accessed on 29 May 2025).

33. Liu, M., Ding, Y., Ye, Q., Wu, S., Gu, Q., Chen, L., Zhang, Y., et al. (2024). Cold-tolerance mechanisms in foodborne pathogens: *Escherichia coli* and *Listeria monocytogenes* as examples. *Critical Reviews in Food Science and Nutrition*. https://www.semanticscholar.org/paper/7188ace28

51cf4b19a451663a1c69d35121bdaa4 (accessed on 29 May 2025).

34. Mohammed, M., Mohammed, M., Thapa, S., et al. (2020). *Evaluation of WGS-Subtyping Methods for Epidemiological Surveillance of Foodborne Salmonellosis*. https://core.ac.uk/download/323057421.pdf (accessed on 29 May 2025).

35. Monarez, S., Houry, D., Posner, S. F., Berkwits, M., Gorwitz, R., Gottardy, A. J., Leahy, M. A., et al. (2025). Contributing factors of foodborne illness outbreaks–National Outbreak Reporting System, United States, 2014–2022. *MMWR Surveillance Summaries, 74*(1), 1–12. https://www.semanticscholar.org/paper/2bcb3c0f9142e2c3612d3aac3352746dd4600fb1 (accessed on 29 May 2025).

36. Mucević, H., McWhirter, J., Macleod, J., Shereefdeen, H., MacKay, M., Cheng, L., Phypers, M., et al. (2025). Best practices in public risk communication during enteric illness outbreak investigations: A scoping review. *Frontiers in Communication*. https://www.semanticscholar.org/paper/ce4c468a84223d563d91ebad494b8a913684a636 (accessed on 29 May 2025).

37. Murano, E., Cross, H., & Riggs, P. (2018). The outbreak that changed meat and poultry inspection systems worldwide. *Animal Frontiers: The Review Magazine of Animal Agriculture, 8*, 4–8. https://www.semanticscholar.org/paper/d57acacf785295e7554943902260f21e12c27cf2 (accessed on 29 May 2025).

38. Murrell, L., Clough, H., Gibb, R., Zhang, X., Green, M., Buchan, I., Barr, B., et al. (2025). Understanding the impacts of reductions in local government expenditure on food safety services, England 2009/10–2019/20. https://www.semanticscholar.org/paper/4135bcc8d9f871f0e05f32bb3e485a78f32ff0f9 (accessed on 29 May 2025).

39. Nadin-Davis, S., Pope, L., Devenish, J., Allain, R., & Ogunremi, D. (2022). Evaluation of the use of CRISPR loci for discrimination of *Salmonella enterica* subsp. *enterica* serovar Enteritidis strains recovered in Canada and comparison with other subtyping methods. *AIMS Microbiology, 8*, 300–317. https://www.semanticscholar.org/paper/8a498a4b2654128f3973ccec3b55c4ad83278c38 (accessed on 29 May 2025).

40. Nannapaneni, V. P., Rameshbabu, M., Sundaramoorthy, S., & Sethuraman, G. (2025). Source identification and clinical outcomes of *Ralstonia* outbreaks in a neonatal intensive care unit: A case series from a tertiary care center. *Tropical Doctor, 55*, 113–120. https://www.semanticscholar.org/paper/e8e435e2567340bc2953e4d3186f9d18fd70eb43 (accessed on 29 May 2025).

41. Napoleoni, M., Villa, L., Barco, L., Busani, L., Cibin, V., Lucarelli, C., Tiengo, A., et al. (2021). A strong evidence outbreak of *Salmonella Enteritidis* in Central Italy linked to the consumption of contaminated raw sheep milk cheese. *Microorganisms, 9*. https://www.semanticscholar.org/paper/a61d4f679419a8abf9165d5a768d0a38e964ea06 (accessed on 29 May 2025).

42. Oza, S., Chen, F., Selser, V., Clougherty, M. M., Dale, K. D., Johnson, J. I., Brock-Fisher, T., et al. (2023). Community-based outbreak investigation and response: Enhancing preparedness, public health capacity, and equity. *Health Affairs, 42*(3), 349–356. https://www.semanticscholar.org/paper/47faa333a4a8b2222785027c648e2e4e8103e19a (accessed on 29 May 2025).

43. Pezzutto, D., Sarno, E., Liebana, E., Rossi, M., & Rizzi, V. (2021). *A Review of Significant European Foodborne Outbreaks in The Last Decade*. https://core.ac.uk/download/589953126.pdf (accessed on 29 May 2025).

44. Pierce, R., Vazquez Deida, A. A., Perz, J., & Perkins, K. (2025). P-374. Bacterial outbreak investigations associated with drug diversion by U.S. healthcare personnel, 1990–2023. *Open Forum Infectious Diseases, 12*. https://www.semanticscholar.org/paper/a5854ec704cf471f71ecdcd1882ac04a83440d86 (accessed on 29 May 2025).

45. Rahman, S., Hossain, Md. S., & Pulok, F. H. (2025). Analysis of food safety knowledge and practices among food handlers in restaurants and street food markets in Dhaka, Bangladesh: A cross-sectional study. *International Journal of Food Science, 2025*. https://www.semanticscholar.org/paper/42e85a90a09416fe02d354c6a0797dbfe8ad73c9 (accessed on 29 May 2025).

46. Rodwell, E. V., Greig, D., Gokool, S., Olonade, I., Swift, C., Chan, Y. W., & Jenkins, C. (2025). Hybrid strains of enterotoxigenic/Shiga toxin-producing *Escherichia coli*, United Kingdom, 2014–2023. *Journal of Medical Microbiology, 74*. https://www.semanticscholar.org/paper/fa483554721add137b29a330ea4d0d49559db6a9 (accessed on 29 May 2025).

47. Roghani, I., Ashfaq, M., Sharif, M. J. H., Khan, Q., & Taj, N. (2024). The Chikungunya fever surveillance, outbreak investigation, response and its determinants factors in Peshawar, Pakistan: A descriptive and unmatched case-control study. *Journal of Ayub Medical College Abbottabad*. https://www.semanticscholar.org/paper/78a80fd8620b852b016166bc8aba5882f9aca252 (accessed on 29 May 2025).

48. Severino, N., Reyes, C., Fernandez, Y., Azevedo, V., De Francisco, L. E., Ramos, R. T., Maroto-Martín, L. O., et al. (2025). Bacterial foodborne diseases in Central America and the Caribbean: A systematic review. *Microbiology Research*. https://www.semanticscholar.org/paper/4b40ec38057cf8f6cc346fc5e358c6773dadea7f (accessed on 29 May 2025).

49. Shah, G. (2014). Editorial comment: Temporal trends in preparedness capacity. *Frontiers in Public Health, 3*, 4. https://www.semanticscholar.org/paper/6f2f9eeaf03f67a8cb281b8164d0ee48721e0a0a (accessed on 29 May 2025).

50. Tao, D., Zhang, D., Hu, R., Rundensteiner, E. A., & Feng, H. (2023). Epidemiological data mining for assisting with foodborne outbreak investigation. *Foods, 12*. https://www.semanticscholar.org/paper/869e30ae893c51c8947de844e33b014ee8800c9a (accessed on 29 May 2025).

51. Taylor, M. R., & David, S. D. (2009). *Stronger Partnerships for Safer Food: An Agenda for Strengthening State and Local Roles in The Nation's Food Safety System*.A project of Department of Health Policy School of Public Health and Health Services The George Washington University. https://core.ac.uk/download/71355283.pdf (accessed on 29 May 2025).

52. Wang, A. T., Tang, L., Gao, A., Zhang, E., Huang, G., Shen, J., Jia, Q., et al. (2024). Investigation of the antimicrobial resistance of important pathogens isolated from poultry from 2015 to 2023 in the United States. *Pathogens, 13*. https://www.semanticscholar.org/paper/8c5d37c8e42d0793e491a497bff79ebead8d5c2f (accessed on 29 May 2025).

53. Yang, Y., Xu, F. R., Zhou, Y. B., Hu, L. Q., Lu, W., Zhang, S. H., Hu, H., et al. (2025). Epidemiological characteristics of foodborne disease outbreaks in a hospital: A 5-year retrospective study. *International Journal of General Medicine, 18*, 1529–1542. https://www.semanticscholar.org/paper/a7720688b4f5e56814b86ccda6d43bf75841fc82 (accessed on 29 May 2025).

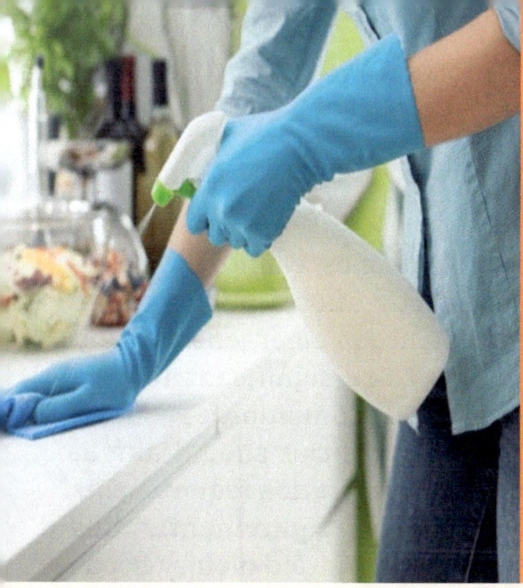

Chapter 14

EMERGENCY FOOD SAFETY MEASURES

Contents

Introduction 325

14.1. Types of Emergencies Affecting Food Safety 328

14.2. Key Emergency Food Safety Practices 332

14.3. Government and Organizational Roles in Food Safety 336

14.4. Community Involvement and Education 340

Summary 346

References 347

Introduction

In the world of globalization, the importance of effective emergency food safety control cannot be overstated. Pandemics, natural calamities, and other unforeseen events have a tendency to disorient food chains, with the likely ability to form health crises. Those crises call for vigilance and cooperation among all the parties in food production and protection. There is a requirement to educate the next generation regarding the complexities of food safety. According to Angelos et al. (2017), an integrated curriculum that encompasses the One Health approach forms a multi-faceted conceptualization of the extremely complex nature of food security. Further, discussion from (Helbing & Mukerji, 2012) of crowd catastrophes indicates that system failure and lack of preparation may lead to catastrophic outcomes. Through the integration of knowledge regarding emergency response and food safety education, policymakers and educators may come up with an agenda that provides not only safety to the public's health but also facilitates sustainable resource management during an emergency.

Definition of Emergency Food Safety Measures

An emergency can cause major issues in food systems , which is why strong food safety steps are required to reduce health risks. Emergency food safety measures cover different ways to keep food safe for use when there are natural disasters, pandemics or problems with the supply chain. Such actions involve a fast review of food safety risks, use of effective ways to inform the public and strict rules for handling and keeping food in emergencies. Coordination among government agencies, food service providers and others is necessary to handle food supplies and responses well. From observations of previous risk appraisal models, as highlighted by the authors in the instance of major chemical exposure, it is possible to appreciate the adaptability and need of current methodologies at times of crisis (Brown et al., 1990). In addition, evidence from responses to emerging food safety concerns indicates there is still a need for strategic advice in order to inform emergency responses (Advisory Council on the Misuse of Drugs, 2011) (Figure 14.1).

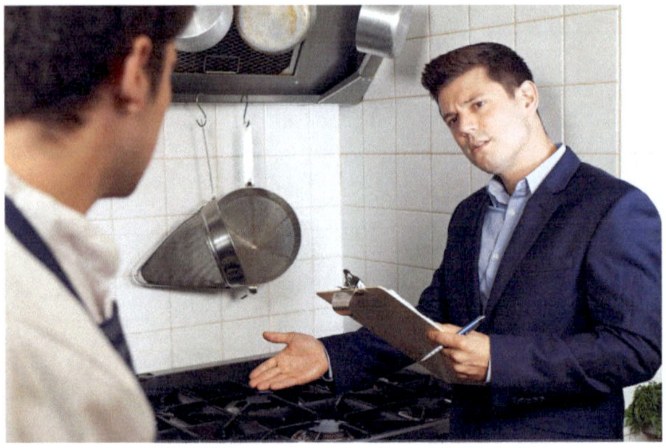

Figure 14.1. Emergencies can disrupt food systems significantly, mandating robust food safety measures to mitigate health risks.

Source: https://www.fooddocs.com/hs-fs/hubfs/food%20safety%20inspection.jpg.

Importance of Food Safety in Emergencies

Food safety in emergencies cannot be overstressed since it directly affects public health and community resilience in emergencies. Food safety and availability are significant for the management of affected communities. Short- and long-term food aid policies should aim at utilizing foods with low preparation requirements and adequate nutritional requirements, thus addressing short-term caloric and dietary needs of affected individuals. Additionally, according to Bakirova et al. (2023), controlling water quality in emergency situations is crucial because low-quality water can significantly contribute to diseases. Finally, traditional food markets, by providing low-cost and culturally appropriate food for vulnerable populations, also contribute substantially to the crisis. These markets not only facilitate economic resilience but also social cohesion in the community, underscoring the importance of robust food safety measures in safeguarding public health as well as supporting recovery efforts in times of crisis (Cook et al., 2024).

Overview of Common Emergencies Affecting Food Safety

Safety of food is at risk due to emergencies that may result from natural disasters, contamination and bioterrorism. Some common emergencies are floods, earthquakes and accidents at industrial sites and these can both interrupt the delivery of food and endanger its safety. Moreover, climatic changes exacerbate these risks by altering agricultural conditions, leading to potential crop shortages and increased pest outbreaks (de la Fuente, 2025). Also, when bioterrorism is used to contaminate, it creates special problems since there must be fast detection and immediate actions to safeguard public health. Measuring preparedness by the state to respond to such threats is crucial; studies quantify the preparedness by using indicators related to federal and hospital response, where reforming and funding areas are specified (Levi et al., 2008). Knowing these emergencies provides an opportunity to design effective emergency food safety responses, ultimately safeguarding public health during crises (Figure 14.2).

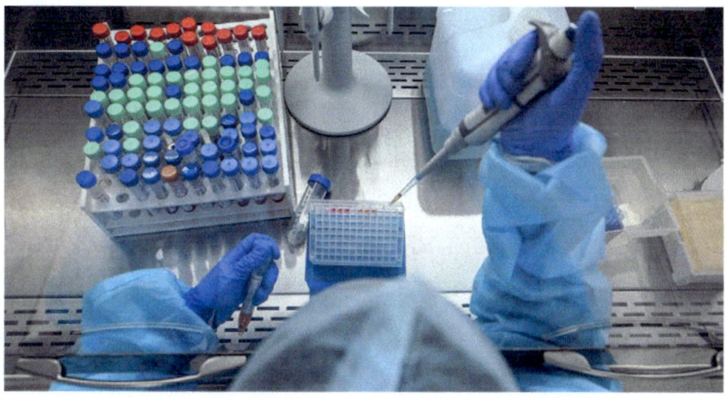

Figure 14.2. Food safety is critically impacted by various emergencies that can arise from natural disasters, contamination, and bioterrorism threats.

Source: https://carnegieendowment.org/static/media/images/GettyImages-1228545815edit-1.jpg.

Historical Context of Food Safety Measures

The history of food safety controls reflects a constant development on the basis of evolving threats, natural or man-made. Public health has been protected with measures by societies for a long time, but increasing complexity in food systems has necessitated more sophisticated approaches. It has moved into a directing role to safeguard the public health, particularly in the face of potential bioterrorism. This mission, characterized by action with the aim of enhancing national security, is a politically contentious arena where food safety law may compromise personal liberties for the sake of collective security (Gostin et al., 2003). Furthermore, global warming and its influence on supply chains for food have also prompted a re-examination of existing safety procedures in operation and emergency planning frameworks, as in the case with many studies on such timely issues (Aryal & Gadema, 2008). The fact from these historical observations is that food safety protocols will only continue to improve as new challenges arise.

Current Trends in Food Safety During Emergencies

As crises like natural disasters and outbreaks of infectious diseases are on the rise, technology use in food safety has become essential. Real-time communication platforms like FIREGUIDE use advanced features like Natural Language Processing to provide immediate guidance during periods of crises, enhance situational awareness, and aid effective decision-making by affected populations (Nangalia, 2025). At the same time, new studies have shown that food safety legislation does not consistently remain firm during times of crises.

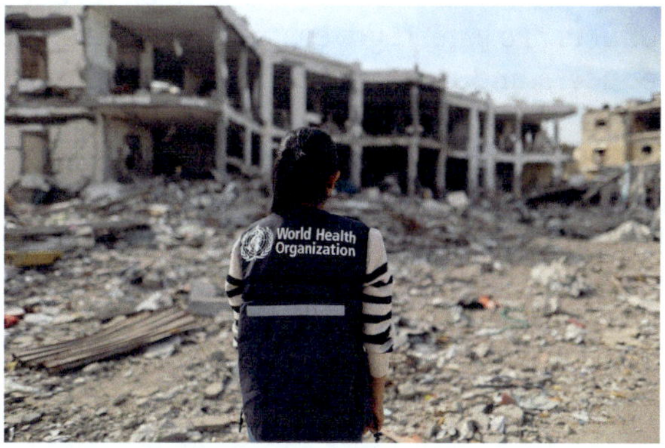

Figure 14.3. As emergencies , such as natural disasters and disease outbreaks become increasingly prevalent, the integration of technology into food safety measures has emerged as a pivotal trend.

Source: https://cdn.who.int/media/images/default-source/products/results-report/2025/148a0506.jpg?sfvrsn=1be9525f_3.

The findings reiterate the need for robust systems of compliance to withstand pressures during crisis, aligning with the call for strict monitoring and preventive measures to guarantee prevention from foodborne illness (Onyeibor et al., 2025). Emphasizing a multi-layered approach , which includes the use of technology, regulatory innovation, and community resilience, is key towards augmenting food safety practices that protect public health during crises, making it prepared as well as efficient response mechanisms (Figure 14.3).

Call to Action for Improved Food Safety Practices

Because of the challenges in the global food system, there is now a strong need to improve food safety. The volatility of food prices, as highlighted by recent analyses, adversely impacts not only the economic stability of nations but also the health of consumers worldwide (Ngongi et al., 2025). Because of this, food safety guidelines in supply chains must be reconsidered and should focus on taking steps to ensure food products are safe. If government agencies, food producers and consumers join forces, they can develop a culture where everyone is accountable for reducing the risks of foodborne illnesses. Furthermore, as evidenced by the examination of labor rights and conditions in global workplaces, similar attention must be directed towards improving food safety practices to protect not only public health but also the livelihoods of workers involved (Taylor & David, 2009). These joined efforts will form the base for a strong food system.

14.1. Types of Emergencies Affecting Food Safety

It is vital to comprehend the various types of emergencies that could impact food safety in preparation for effective response methods under the Emergency Food Safety Measures framework. Natural disasters , such as floods and earthquakes, have a tendency to destroy food supply systems and could result in food products being contaminated with poisonous substances. Moreover, bioterrorism is a deliberate threat where the damaging organisms are introduced into the food chain, necessitating improved state preparedness in identifying and ameliorating threats (Levi et al., 2008). Moreover, the use of safety nets in dealing with the implications of such a crisis is critical to enable quick recovery to prevent food insecurity (Braunholz et al., 2025). By identifying such critical emergencies, stakeholders can establish combined protocols that enhance public health response to enhance public safety of the food during and after the crisis, as well as maintain community resilience

14.1.1. Natural Disasters (Hurricanes, Floods, Earthquakes)

Natural disasters , such as hurricanes, floods, and earthquakes pose food security with tremendous risk and typically have catastrophic effects on the vulnerable population. Climate change that leads to frequency and intensity of such events makes high hazard risk convergence with social vulnerability even harder. In the last decade, natural disasters have claimed roughly 79,000 lives annually and affected more than 200 million individuals, with resulting damages amounting to US$70 billion annually (de Haen and Hemrich, 2025). Effective emergency food safety management strategies must therefore involve resilience-enhancing measures for countering the vulnerability resulting from disasters. The Disaster Management cycle of response, recovery, mitigation, and preparedness is required in order to establish an integrated strategy in safeguarding food systems against emergencies (Ameratunga et al., 2010). By highlighting the evaluation of risk, upgrading agricultural infrastructure, and the development of long-term plans for adaptability, we can promote food security in affected areas, preserving lives in addition to livelihoods (Figure 14.4).

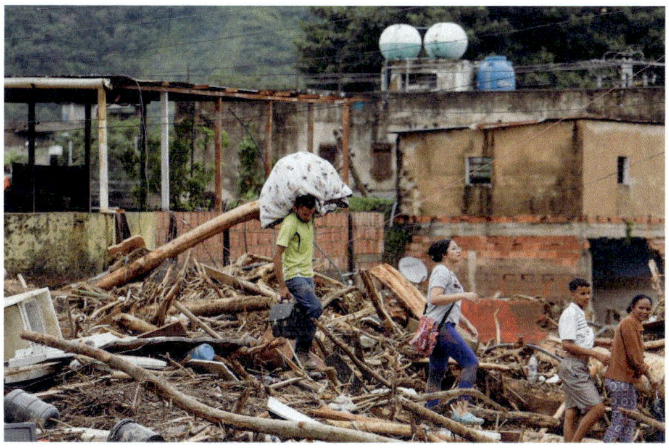

Figure 14.4. Natural disasters, , such as hurricanes, floods, and earthquakes, represent a significant challenge to food security, often leading to devastating consequences for vulnerable populations.

Source: https://dialogue.earth/content/uploads/2022/11/Loss-and-damage-COP27-Venezuela-floods_Leonardo-Fernandez_Alamy_2K5PRBX-scaled.jpg.

14.1.2. Man-Made Disasters (Chemical Spills, Terrorist Attacks)

Chemical spills and terrorist attacks , which are man-made disasters, can seriously impact food safety, so it is important to be well prepared for emergencies. They may contaminate food for a wide area , which can harm public health and safety. Disaster management helps a lot in reducing the effects of such events, especially by increasing the public's ability to handle emergencies. Risk analysis and the setting up of emergency plans allow organizations to respond better and protect themselves from food supply disruptions. Empirical evidence indicates that organization presence of a specialized risk manager is positively linked with the occurrence of necessary risk-alleviating measures, meaning the importance of well-coordinated preparedness efforts in the absence of expected threats (Graham et al., 2014). Further, the need for adequate coordination and public awareness during crises underscores the importance of appropriate coordination among governments and societies, ensuring food safety as well as wider public health (Gligorov et al., 2008).

14.1.3. Public Health Emergencies (Pandemics, Outbreaks)

When public health emergencies happen , such as the COVID-19 pandemic, they strongly affect food safety measures everywhere. Such crises expose weaknesses in supplying food and in rules , which makes it hard to guarantee safety and security of food for people at crucial moments. For instance, the COVID-19 pandemic has highlighted deficiencies in disease surveillance systems that should monitor foodborne illnesses and outbreaks amidst widespread public health risks (Morgan et al., 2021).

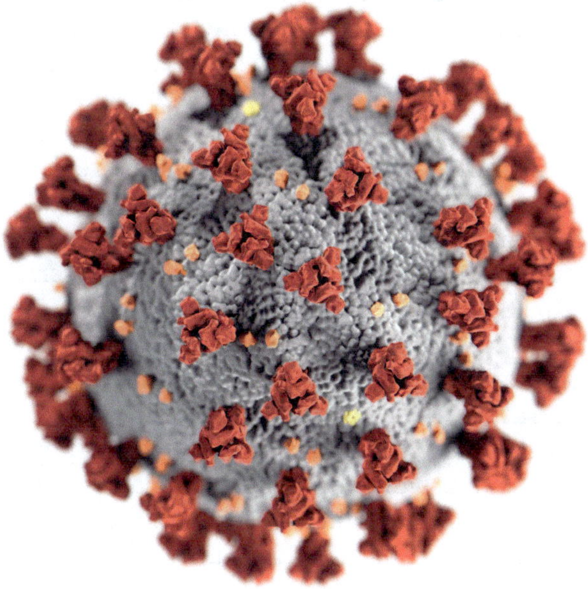

Figure 14.5. The onset of public health emergencies, particularly pandemics , such as COVID-19, profoundly impacts food safety measures worldwide.

Source: https://en.m.wikipedia.org/wiki/File:SARS-CoV-2_without_background.png

The disruption of normal food distribution channels can lead to increased risks of contamination and spoilage, exacerbating food insecurity in vulnerable communities (Rousseau et al., 2020). While communities adjust, it is necessary to set up emergency food safety measures with increased monitoring, clear communication and teamwork between public health and food officials. This proactive approach not only safeguards food quality but also reinforces public trust during emergencies, ultimately contributing to community resilience (Figure 14.5).

14.1.4. Power Outages and Their Impact on Food Storage

Losing electricity can be very dangerous for food safety, mainly for households that keep perishable items in the fridge. If electricity goes out, the temperature in refrigerators and freezers can increase fast , which helps bacteria to grow. Food safety rules state that food left at temperatures above 40°F for over two hours might not be safe and should be watched closely during power outages. Moreover, there is an elevated risk of food spoilage, which can lead to economic losses for families already burdened by rising costs of living amid an energy crisis (Tsagkaris et al., 2023). So, emergency plans should account for maintaining food safety when there is no electricity. People can buy small generators or keep their food in coolers full of ice packs when there is a long-term power outage. It is very important to manage food storage properly when there is no power, as this affects the health and safety of people in emergencies.

14.1.5. Transportation Disruptions Affecting Food Supply

The complex interrelationship between transport disruption and food supply chains has been particularly heightened by recent global crises. The COVID-19 pandemic and the enhancement of the effects of climate change have resulted in enormous logistics disruption in sea and air transport, which are both critical for food delivery within timely perspectives. Studies highlight that this convergence of disruptions has particularly challenged food safety procedures, highlighting the importance of effective safety procedures during transportation in the event of a crisis (Rizaldy et al., 2024). Besides, the disruptions have a considerable socioeconomic effect since, in the case of vulnerable populations whose access to food was severely affected when transport infrastructure broke down, it resulted in other food insecurity (Cortés et al., 2024). Such needs underscore the imperative role of including emergency preparation planning in transport planning for ensuring food system supply resiliency and safety in the face of emergencies (Figure 14.6).

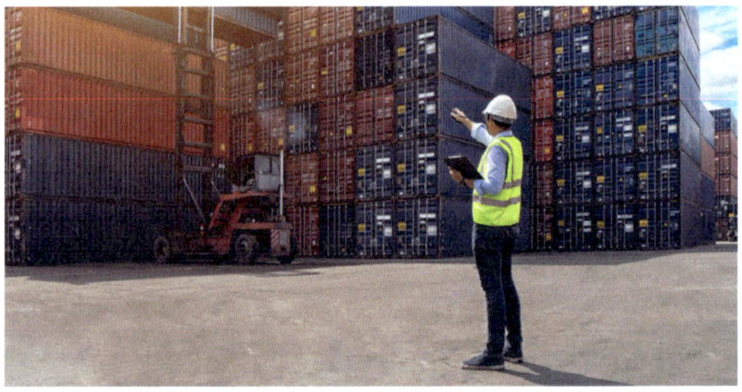

Figure 14.6. The intricate relationship between transportation disruptions and food supply chains has become especially pronounced in the context of recent global crises.

Source: https://arc-group.com/wp-content/uploads/2025/04/supply-chain-resilience-1776A.jpg.

14.1.6. Economic Crises Leading to Food Scarcity

In economic crises, food scarcity is usually among the cold hard facts, and this serves to reinforce the fragility of food production chains and farm systems. Global crises , such as the COVID-19 pandemic have precipitated the vulnerability of food security, particularly in developing nations where agriculture is a source of livelihood and economic support (Workie et al., 2020). It not only stops food production but also interferes with the availability of important inputs, further enhancing deeply entrenched inequalities. Besides this, climate change presently also threatens farm production, and the necessity for immediate and effective measures to ensure food security and safety is now essentially critical (Dwivedi et al., 2021). With shrinking economies, international trade integration becomes increasingly apparent, illustrating how economic breakdown is capable of generating food supply crises. Thus, costly mitigation strategies like investment in sustainable agriculture and adaptive technological measures have to function as shock absorbers and guarantee access to nutrition for the vulnerable groups.

14.1.7. Climate Change and Its Effects on Food Safety

Because of the link between climate change and food safety, there are major problems that must be addressed quickly. Changes in temperature and rainfall can lead to more foodborne pathogens , which can make farming products more likely to become contaminated. For example, higher temperatures can help dangerous microbes grow faster , which may result in foodborne illnesses. Furthermore, as highlighted in discussions at the UK–South Asia Young Scientists and Practitioners Seminar on Climate Change and Disaster Impact Reduction held at Kathmandu, Nepal on 5-6 June 2008 (Aryal & Gadema, 2008), vulnerable populations may face heightened food insecurity as climates change. This deterioration in food security can be seen in the slow progress towards meeting Millennium Development Goals related to hunger reduction, where climate change, along with rising food prices and the competition for bioenergy, poses a multifaceted threat to nutritional safety and access (Thompson & Cohen, 2012). Therefore, implementing emergency food safety measures becomes essential in mitigating these risks (Figure 14.7).

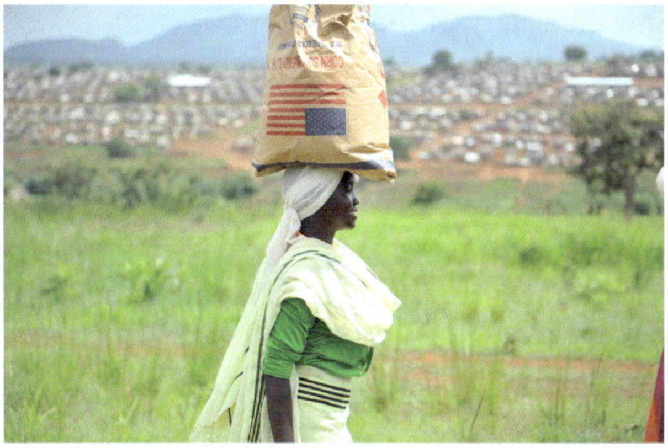

Figure 14.7. The interplay between climate change and food safety presents significant challenges that necessitate urgent attention and action.

Source: https://i0.wp.com/councilonstrategicrisks.org/wp-content/uploads/2023/08/22028292156_2746c544aa_o.jpg?resize=4256%2C2832&ssl=1.

14.1.8. Technological Failures in Food Production

Issues with technology in the food industry cause consequences that go beyond just stopping operations. Such failures usually point out important weaknesses in our food systems , which are made worse by a new emphasis on protecting the environment and ensuring enough food. As noted, the relationship between technological production methods and equitable distribution is a crucial area of discussion, underscoring the necessity for robust emergency food safety measures (Dowler et al., 2011). Moreover, the examination of workplace health hazards within food production environments highlights the need for effective regulatory actions and innovative solutions to mitigate risks associated with technological shortcomings

(Kriebel et al., 2011). These case studies teach us useful things that can be applied in the future to make food production more resilient. All of these insights underline the need to handle technological problems to ensure food safety and the safety of the public.

14.1.9. Community-Level Emergencies and Their Implications

Emergency incidents at the community level, , such as natural disasters or public health crises, significantly impact food safety and access to resources.

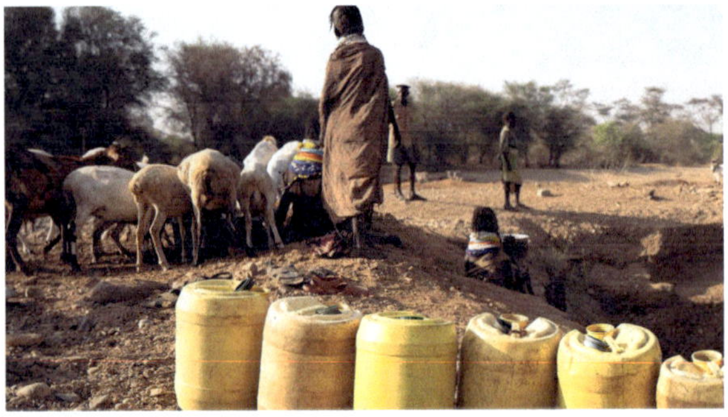

Figure 14.8. Community-level emergencies, , such as natural disasters or public health crises, significantly impact food safety and the availability of essential resources.

Source: https://dgap.org/sites/default/files/styles/dgap_content_large/public/Climate%20Change%20MENA.jpg?itok=mQd8G150.

These types of incidents can disrupt supply chains, compromise food quality, and exacerbate vulnerabilities for the most vulnerable populations. Over recent years, studies have identified how state and local preparedness programs experience federal reductions in budget, which could compromise a successful response to such emergencies. Furthermore, the role of safety nets is also brought to the center at such times because they help offset the adverse effects of disasters on societies. Safety nets not only help in controlling ex ante risks but also provide support ex post to recover from shocks, and hence, effective systems are required to deal with the unique challenges posed by different types of hazards (Braunholz et al., 2025). Finally, enhancing community resilience through effective food safety interventions is essential to sustain public health during disasters (Figure 14.8).

14.2. Key Emergency Food Safety Practices

Functional emergency food safety systems are critical in averting foodborne disease risk in emergencies. The convergence of information between emergency managers and environmental health and food safety professionals offers a coordinated approach towards enhancing food safety resilience. Empirical knowledge generates a broad gap in continuous preparedness training for EHFSPs, which undermines their ability to deal adequately with incidents of malicious contamination (Mack et al., 2019). This necessitates that policymakers demand improved training programs that merge food safety practices with emergency management techniques. In addition, anti-hunger programs , such as Pennsylvania's State Food Purchase Program (SFPP) and The Emergency Food Assistance Program (TEFAP) are great models of measures to guarantee food security during emergencies. As a result, by combining improved training with effective hunger prevention, the overall resiliency of the food safety system can be improved considerably.

14.2.1. Proper Food Storage Techniques During Emergencies

When there is an emergency, appropriate storage of food guarantees that the food is safe and of high quality. Proper food storage dramatically lowers the chances of foodborne illness and its preservation of nutrients. It is essential that it is stored at a consistent temperature; food needs to be stored at or below 40°F so bacteria will not form. Additionally, hermetically closed containers may help preserve food from insects and environmental influences that cause air and water-borne spoilage. It is also important to understand the danger contributed by mycotoxins because, in case food is stored without proper care, it favors the development of fungi responsible for producing such harmful compounds, risking public health (Saravanan et al., 2024). Education on such practices is crucial, as research shows that people who have positive food safety attitudes tend to use correct storage practices, hence enhancing overall food security in times of crisis (Zamora et al., 2024) (Figure 14.9).

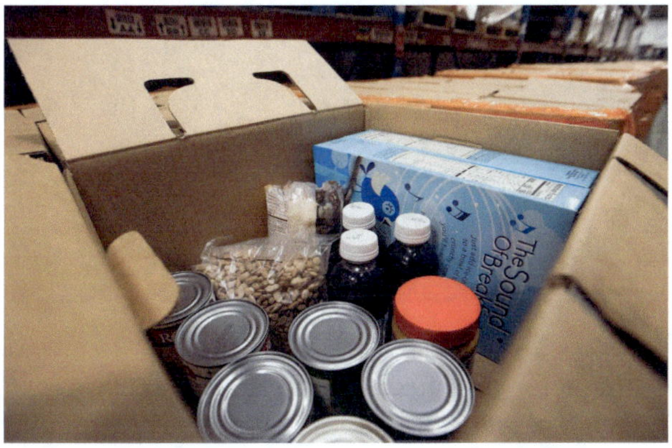

Figure 14.9. During emergencies, proper food storage techniques are essential to ensure the safety and quality of food supplies.

Source: https://extension.oregonstate.edu/sites/extd8/files/styles/full/public/images/2021-08/credit-usda.jpg?itok=O-U6eY-S.

14.2.2. Safe Food Handling Practices

In emergency food safety, how food is handled is extremely important. Handling food properly is very important to reduce the chances of getting sick from food, especially when resources are scarce. Washing your hands well before and after handling food, using different cutting boards for raw and cooked foods and ensuring that food is cooked correctly are some safe practices. The implementation of these practices becomes even more critical in various contexts, as highlighted in discussions surrounding globalization and labor rights (Fair Labor Association, 2003). Being aware of the link between safe food and employee safety makes it clear that education and training are very important in food safety during emergencies. Food safety rules should always be followed to keep the public healthy and the emergency food safe to eat.

14.2.3. Importance of Food Temperature Control

The significance of food temperature control must not be exaggerated when describing emergency food safety procedures. Food temperature control is essential to preventing the spread of unsafe pathogens that lead to foodborne illness. If food is kept within the range of 40°F and 140°F, the risk of bacterial growth becomes astronomically higher.

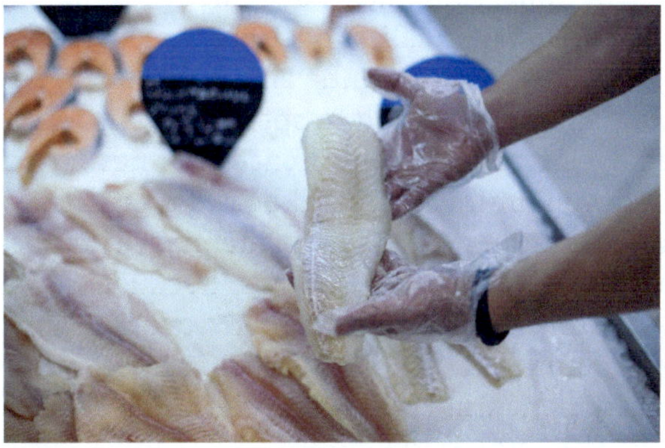

Figure 14.10. The significance of food temperature control cannot be overstated in the context of emergency food safety measures.

Source: https://www.foodsafety.gov/sites/default/files/2021-09/safe-selection-handling-of-fish.jpg.

This is echoed by the shift towards preventive safety measures, as seen in such regulatory guidelines as HACCP, which stresses maintaining

CCPs in food manufacturing in check (Aalberts et al., 2003). Moreover, integration of adequate temperature monitoring systems is pivotal towards ensuring compliance with food safety regulations, even as temporary transient failures would result in lethal health consequences. So, proper training in temperature control is required for food handlers during crises, both to fulfill existing safety standards and to maintain public health matters in the long term (Figure 14.10) (Fair Labor Association, 2003).

14.2.4. Guidelines for Food Preservation Methods

Good food preservation methods are crucial to ensure the safety and shelf life of perishables, especially during emergencies. Freezing, drying, and canning are some methods employed to ensure that food is not contaminated and that pathogens are avoided from flourishing in foods and undermining their safety. Sterilization under appropriate heat and pressure, for instance, can destroy dangerous microbes, hence guaranteeing food safety and quality for a long time. Freezing also preserves nutrients and halts enzymatic reactions that can lead to spoilage. Dehydration removes water content, hence it is not a good environment for mold and bacteria growth. An understanding of these principles is critical to individuals and societies because it has the potential to enhance food security under emergency conditions by securing resources for efficient utilization and minimizing health risk. This integrative approach to preservation methods finally results in sustainability and food supply system resilience.

14.2.5. Use of Safe Water Sources for Food Preparation

If there is an emergency, using safe water for cooking is very important to avoid foodborne illnesses, since cleanliness may not be possible. If water contains pathogens, it can be very dangerous for your health, so it is necessary to use water from treated municipal sources or bottled water. During emergencies, there is a higher risk of cross-contamination , which means special rules are needed for using water to rinse, cook and prepare food. In addition, using clean water for food preparation follows both food safety rules and helps protect people who are more susceptible to getting sick. Therefore, prioritizing safe water sources can significantly mitigate health threats during emergencies, emphasizing its critical role in effective food safety management strategies (Fair Labor Association, 2003) (Figure 14.11).

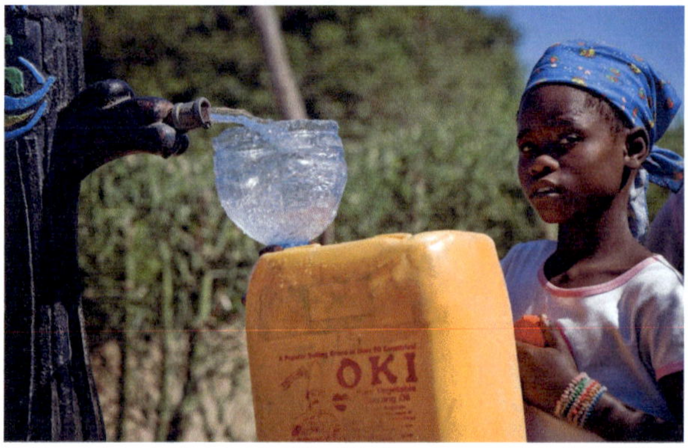

Figure 14.11. Water contaminated with pathogens can lead to severe health risks, making it essential to source water from reliable and safe supplies , such as treated municipal systems or bottled water.

Source: https://www.who.int/images/default-source/departments/wash/10665623274-56e7b3f2e3-k.jpg?sfvrsn=63e594ad_13.

14.2.6. Emergency Food Supply Planning

Effective emergency food supply planning guarantees public health and safety in emergencies , such as natural disasters or pandemics. Planning involves analyzing the food needs of the community, having reliable sources of emergency food, and maintaining the capability to distribute despite disruption. A scan of state readiness reveals tremendous gaps, as highlighted in recent reviews, showing the impact of budget cuts on public health readiness programs.

These fiscal reductions undermine the ability to create inclusive emergency food plans, since most of those programs that increase food security are at risk of being cancelled or cut significantly. In addition, the lack of infrastructure to respond to emergency response in the food supply accentuates the need for an effective response mechanism so that short- and long-term requirements can be met (Levi et al., 2008). Strengthening these programs not only promotes community resilience but also ensures equity in the response to emergency food insecurity.

14.2.7. Role of Food Safety Education and Training

Emergency food safety measures depend greatly on food safety education and training, since it prepares individuals and groups to deal with risks from foodborne diseases. Emphasizing how to maintain hygiene, handle food correctly and be aware of dangers, especially in an emergency, should be a main part of any effective training program. Promoting safety in the community, food safety education helps people and organizations respond well during emergencies. This is in agreement with evidence that public health law can enable essential health functions, including food safety, through proper education systems (Cabrera et al., 2017).

Furthermore, rigorous training programs are vital in assessing state readiness to manage public health crises, as they enhance preparedness across sectors like hospitals and municipalities (Levi et al., 2008). Regular food safety education is hence a prime determinant of effective emergency responses (Figure 14.12).

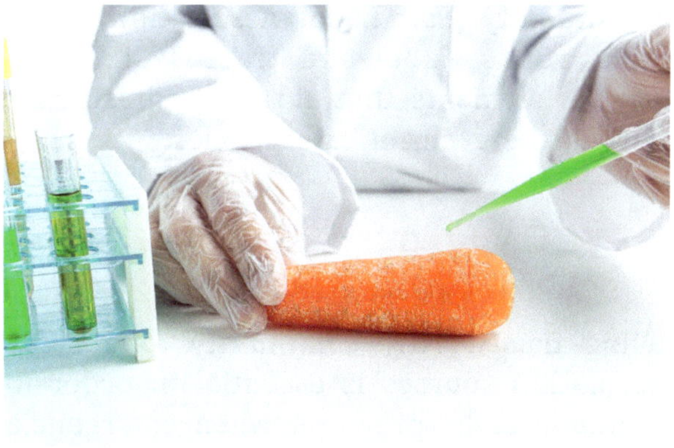

Figure 14.12. The role of food safety education and training is paramount in the framework of emergency food safety measures, as it equips individuals and organizations with critical knowledge and skills to mitigate risks associated with foodborne illnesses.

Source: https://smsla.global/wp-content/uploads/2023/04/front-view-carrot-injected-with-chemicals-scaled.jpg.

14.2.8. Importance of Labeling and Tracking Food Supplies

From the perspective of emergency food safety interventions, the importance of tracing and labeling food supplies cannot be overstated. Adequate labeling plays a crucial role in marking food products as necessary, allowing for the rapid and efficient response needed under emergency circumstances. Labeling provides consumers and food handlers with convenient access to essential details , such as expiration dates and origin sources of ingredients, critical in preventing foodborne disease. Additionally, tracking systems enable authorities to maintain food inventories in a proper order and ensure that the commodities are of reasonable standards, particularly during food shortages or crises. Coupled tracking technologies can enhance transparency to the fullest; for instance, when looking at labor rights and labor conditions in food supply chains, data based on such systems can spot potential ethical issues and impose accountability (Fair Labor Association, 2003). Hence, robust label and trace systems are essential elements that aid public health and safety in the event of emergencies.

14.2.9. Community Resources for Food Safety Information

Having trustworthy community food safety information sources is essential in order for the public to be prepared when emergencies occur. LHDs often are major sources of advice, providing information on food handling securely, particularly whenever there are breaks in food supply chains. The departments use various strategies, including workshops, leaflets, and websites, to advise the population on potential foodborne hazards (Levi et al., 2008).

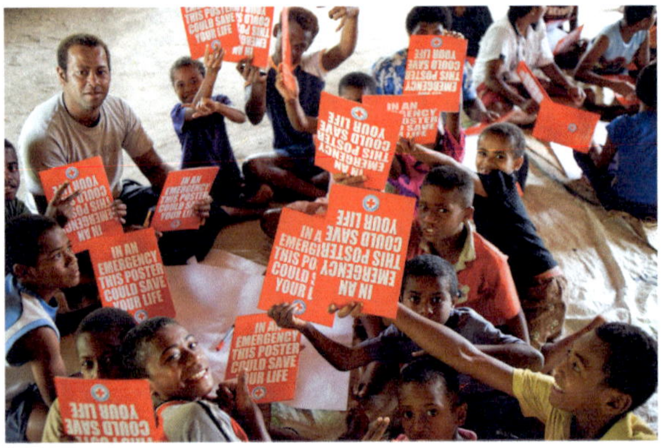

Figure 14.13. Access to reliable community resources for food safety information is essential in ensuring public awareness and preparedness during emergencies.

Source: https://preparecenter.org/wp-content/uploads/2013/10/p-FJI0005_jpg-scaled.jpg.

Furthermore, community groups are instrumental in getting food safety messages across through hosting events and offering resources to those in the greatest need. Still, when budgets for public health are cut, it can be difficult for these efforts, as shown in studies that talk about the risk of losing important preparedness programs. Therefore, maintaining and enhancing community resources is critical to bolstering food safety awareness and ensuring the public can effectively respond to emergencies involving food safety issues (Figure 14.13).

14.3. Government and Organizational Roles in Food Safety

Appropriate management of food safety is an integrated activity that falls within the ambit of both governmental and organizational authorities. Federal, state, and local regulatory agencies all have various roles to play in the monitoring and implementation of food safety measures. Their spheres of operation encompass surveillance, outbreak response, regulation, and inspection of foods that are initiated during emergencies when public health is threatened. However, a significant study reveals that such systems are prone to challenges, including shortages of resources and coordination failures, and have consequently faced demands for system-wide reform aimed at enhancing state and local leadership in food safety, as emphasized by Taylor & David (2009). Besides, interaction between government regulation and organizational activities can shape food safety behavior within the supply chain, ultimately influencing responses by communities to food safety crises, particularly among vulnerable groups, supporting findings reached in Whittingham et al. (2010).

14.3.1. Federal Regulations and Guidelines for Food Safety

With more people worried about foodborne illnesses, federal rules and guidelines are very important for food safety, especially in emergency situations. The Food Safety and Inspection Service (FSIS) and the Food and Drug Administration (FDA) establish standards that dictate how food should be produced, stored, and handled to minimize risks. They cover many different actions, for example, labeling, controlling temperatures and maintaining cleanliness. Following these guidelines in an emergency helps stop outbreaks that might occur because of contaminated food. Also, carrying out federal policies well can boost public health measures and build trust among consumers in the food industry. By ensuring compliance with these regulations, agencies can mitigate the adverse impacts of emergencies on food safety, ultimately saving lives and protecting community health (Maududi et al., 2024; Kooli, 2025) (Figure 14.14).

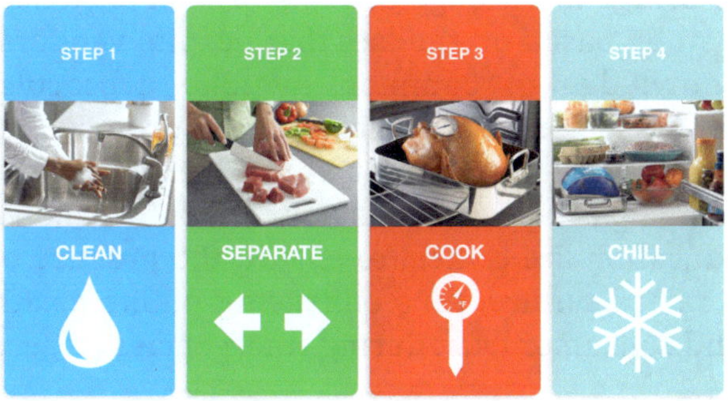

Figure 14.14. The Food Safety and Inspection Service (FSIS) and the Food and Drug Administration (FDA) establish standards that dictate how food should be produced, stored, and handled to minimize risks.

Source: https://www.fda.gov/files/SafeFoodHandling_11072023.png.

14.3.2. Role of Local Health Departments (LHDs) in Emergencies

LHDs play a critical function in managing food safety during emergencies since they are the frontline action-takers during times of public health crisis. Their functions involve monitoring the food supply chains, implementing health legislations, and facilitating rapid response mechanisms to prevent food-borne risks from contaminated food sources. As observed from recent assessments, these agencies have suffered from funding cuts that undermine their readiness programs, in turn capable of inhibiting them from effectively responding to food safety threats.

In addition, state and national readiness reviews have documented improvements and persistent issues in funding and accountability, particularly in the context of how responsive they are to outbreaks , such as H1N1, yet again emphasizing the importance of good local health infrastructure in times of crisis. Hence, LHD competence is essential to ensuring effective emergency food safety interventions and public health protection.

14.3.3. Collaboration between Government and NGOs

Effective emergency food safety measures necessitate a robust collaboration between government agencies and non-governmental organizations (NGOs). Although governments are usually considered the main leaders in disaster management, their work can be improved by partnering with NGOs , which have special skills and resources. As noted, "governments need to be supported by NGOs because NGOs have abilities , which governments don't have" (Safril et al., 2013).

In this way of working, both parties have to resolve issues that may arise, for example, misunderstandings about what each partner does. Developing guidelines for teamwork helps everyone respond more smoothly and increases the effectiveness of disaster governance. Also, encouraging continuous dialogue through training and capacity-building projects can help governments and NGOs work better together to handle food safety during emergencies. Such synergy is essential for safeguarding public health and ensuring food security in times of crisis (Figure 14.15).

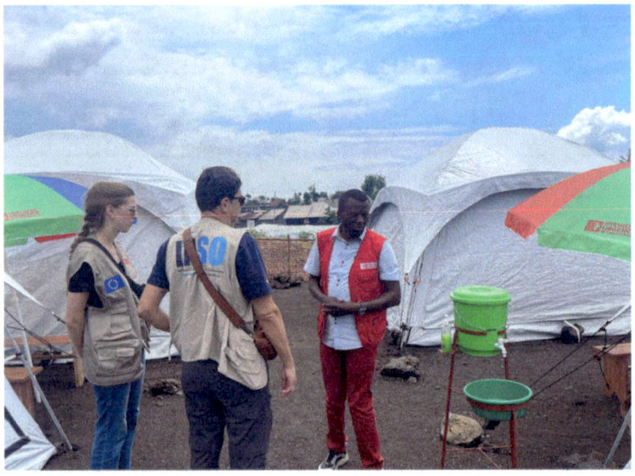

Figure 14.15. Effective emergency food safety measures necessitate a robust collaboration between government agencies and non-governmental organizations (NGOs).

Source: https://insowebsite.blob.core.windows.net/uploads/2024/04/image-scaled.jpg.

14.3.4. Emergency Response Plans for Food Safety

In the framework of food safety, emergency response plans serve as an important tool to reduce exposure to contamination and public health hazards. They not only define how foodborne illness outbreaks are to be handled but also include strategic components to reduce large-scale health effects in the event of an emergency. For instance, during a nuclear incident, emergency readiness regulations may involve bans on locally-grown food sales to prevent exposure, as has been brought up in discussions on nuclear readiness (Ashley et al., 2017). Furthermore, assessments of state readiness for bioterrorism response and public health crises have highlighted the importance of effective emergency systems with the capability to link finance and efficient mobilization of resources (Levi et al., 2008). Lastly, the development and constant revision of food safety emergency response plans are of highest significance to promote community resilience and safeguard public health during emergencies.

14.3.5. Public Awareness Campaigns on Food Safety

Public campaigns on food safety play an important role in deterring unhealthy behavior and preventing foodborne illnesses, especially in times of crisis. They inform consumers on how to handle, prepare, and store foods properly, which is crucial in minimizing the risk of contaminated food. Specifically, Portugal's NIMCP is a well-organised approach that hinges on stakeholder engagement and compliance with standard safety protocols (Rodrigues et al., 2025). For those sectors still under the dominance of high-risk food customs, like street vendors, public awareness campaigns are able to bridge knowledge-action gaps. For instance, a study based on the fact that despite vendors' knowledge of common hygiene protocols, the inclusion of advanced safety protocols is still lacking (Ibrahim et al., 2024). Therefore, campaigns aimed at consumer and food handler education are critical to ensure the practice of a safety culture, thus enhancing public health and consumer trust during emergencies (Figure 14.16).

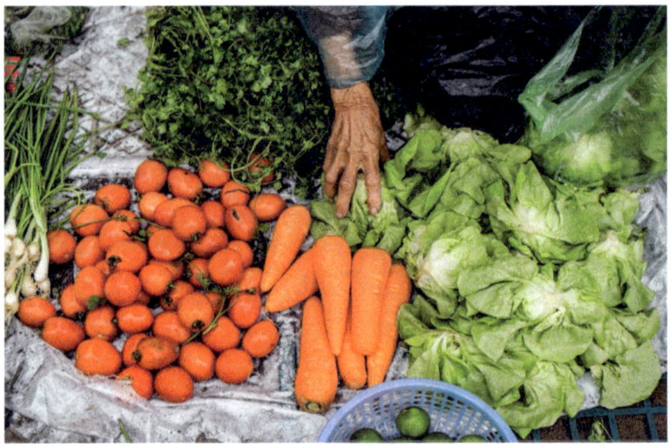

Figure 14.16. Public awareness campaigns on food safety play a vital role in promoting healthy practices and preventing foodborne illnesses, especially during emergencies.

Source: https://www.who.int/images/default-source/who-campaigns/world-food-safety-day-2021/who_061147.jpg?sfvrsn=fa8fd738_7.

14.3.6. Funding and Resources for Food Safety Initiatives

In emergency food safety interventions, resource availability and availability of adequate finances remain pivotal in ensuring proper implementation and sustainability of food safety interventions. Without proper financing, measures to enhance food safety handling will frequently fail since this could compromise resilience against emergencies , such as pandemics or disasters. For instance, investment in climate-resilient agriculture and intensified water management is essential in minimizing climate-based food security risks in nations like Bangladesh, where agricultural productivity is particularly susceptible (Farah et al., 2025). Secondly, the organization of cooperative networks between government, academic, and civil institutions enhances resource organization and competence in the successful control of food safety concerns (Bino, 2024). These concerted efforts are necessary not only for effective response in time, but also for maintaining long-term food system resiliency, which in turn assures public health and enables food availability during emergencies.

14.3.7. International Cooperation in Food Safety Measures

Because of the intricate nature of global food safety, nations must come together, especially when there is a crisis. Because the world is globalized, foodborne risks can travel around the world and national actions alone cannot safeguard human beings. When nations act globally, they shall be in a position to share important practices, the latest research and regulations that benefit all in responding to food safety matters. In particular, Disaster Studies constructs emphasize the need to address the multidimensionality of food governance, underlining the importance of both qualitative and quantitative indicators of food safety and security in shaping responsive action (Burger et al., 2025). Moreover, understanding the interaction between food systems and vulnerable groups is important, since individuals depending on food resources might respond differently to safety interventions, as noted in reef ecosystem evaluations and their impact on poor livelihoods (Whittingham et al., 2010). Thus, it is important to build international collaboration to achieve resilient food safety systems that are responsive to emerging problems (Figure 14.17).

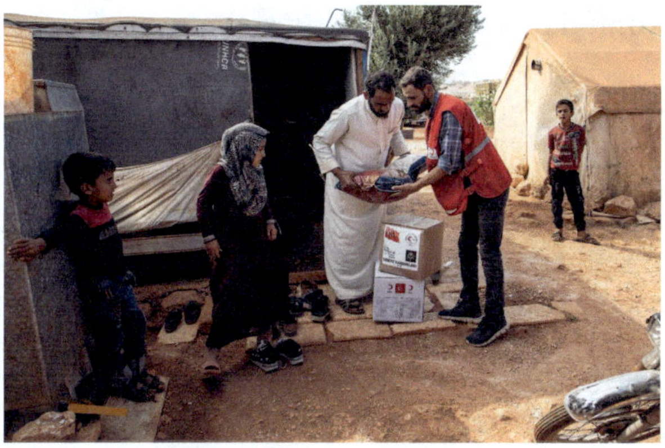

Figure 14.17. As global interconnectedness increases, foodborne risks transcend borders, making unilateral national measures insufficient to safeguard public health.

Source: https://production-tcf.imgix.net/app/uploads/2021/06/04090023/GettyImages-1175914400-scaled.jpg.

14.3.8. Case Studies of Successful Government Interventions

Successful government reactions to emergency food safety interventions are typically founded on inclusive approaches that intervene both on immediate needs and underlying vulnerabilities. A clear example is the implementation of social protection programs in Somalia, which has seen decades of humanitarian emergencies prompting a transition from reactive to sustainable interventions. The study carried out on behalf of a group of agencies like Save the Children and Adeso centers around this paradigm shift by advocating for long-term social protection systems that both cut hunger and also build resilience against possible future shocks (Brewin et al., 2014). Through regional social protection systems, the report highlights the need to integrate food safety interventions into development targets, particularly in regions with climate change-induced problems and political instability (de la Fuente, 2025). These systems reveal the way government interventions can conclusively prevent food insecurity while promoting socio-economic stability.

14.3.9. Challenges Faced by Organizations in Food Safety

Food safety agencies are confronted with a complication of issues that complicate their attempt to protect public health. At the top of these are those concerning governance and coordination, particularly following crises that ignite the demand for effective food safety measures.

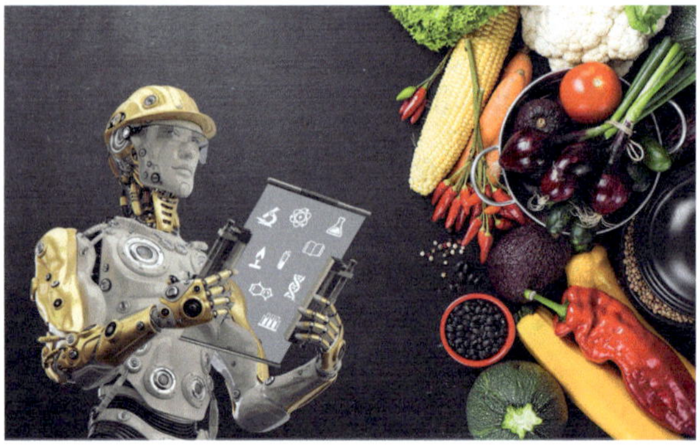

Figure 14.18. Organizations involved in food safety encounter a myriad of challenges that complicate their efforts to guarantee public health.

Source: https://www.digicomply.com/hubfs/ai%20in%20food%20safety%20%281%29.png.

As noted, the risk of creating complex systems with cross-incentives often occurs when expanding safety net programs, and uncertainty in the choice of beneficiaries ensues along with decreased accountability (Giannozzi and Khan, 2025). Furthermore, global trading regimes like that of the World Trade Organization have the ability to place countries under restrictions on technical measures limiting countries from being able to effectively deal with legitimate food safety priorities in a manner that settles trade interests and public health (Josling et al., 2025). The issues underscore the need for better cooperation and open institutions of governance to guarantee effective food safety procedures to safeguard the consumer against potential health risks (Figure 14.18).

14.4. Community Involvement and Education

Community education and participation serve pivotal roles in enhancing emergency food safety measures, raising local population awareness and preparedness. The training of community residents through educational programs can inform citizens with the knowledge necessary to properly handle food during emergencies. The activities of Iowa's community action network highlight, for instance, the power of locally focused education to significantly enhance the prevention of foodborne disease outbreaks during emergencies.

Through the deployment of comprehensive training programs intended for the appropriate handling, storage, and sanitation of food, communities are able to foster a better-educated populace. In addition, government-public partnerships amongst governmental organizations and community organizations can amplify the coverage of these education efforts, as seen in the Agency Performance Plan of its successful strategies for reaching the public.

Long-term, creating a safety culture by engaging the public not only enhances individual welfare but also the public health resilience during emergencies.

14.4.1. Importance of Community Engagement in Food Safety

Involvement of the community in food safety is particularly important at times of crisis when swift communication and collective response can minimize health risks. By actively engaging in food safety campaigns, the members of the community enhance awareness and a culture of accountability in food handling and preparation activities.

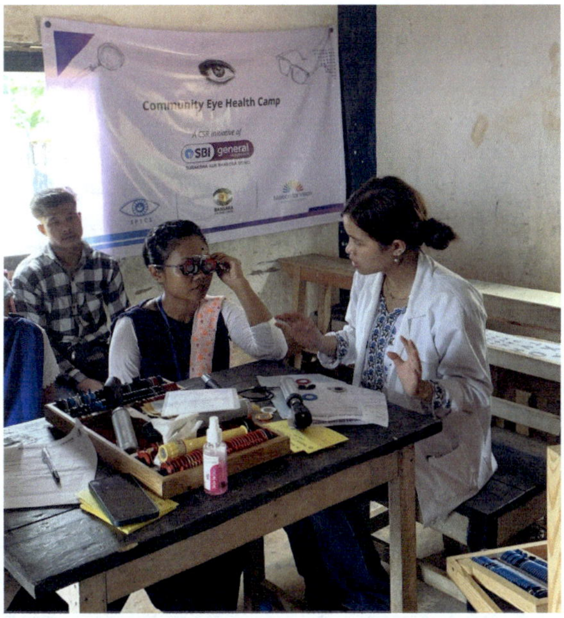

Figure 14.19. Community engagement in food safety is vital, particularly in emergency situations where swift communication and collective action can mitigate health risks.

Source: https://www.csrmandate.org/wp-content/uploads/2024/12/Eye-Checkup-in-Meghalaya_2-scaled-e1733481560426.jpeg.

By concerted action, not only is the individual made strong, but there is also a collective responsibility created that can be translated into more efficient food safety action. For instance, the community members can provide valuable information about common foodborne diseases and assist in sensitization outreach programs among vulnerable populations.

Public engagement can further facilitate a quick response in case of food safety emergencies through rapid dissemination of life-saving information. Lastly, professionalism and community resource mobilization together can optimize the effectiveness of food safety emergency work to make a safer food environment for all parties involved (Davies et al., 2018) (Figure 14.19).

14.4.2. Training Programs for Local Volunteers

Local volunteer training initiatives are significant elements in establishing emergency community preparedness, particularly in food safety procedures. Preparation of volunteers to deal with and guarantee food safety through effective handling and safety practices enables communities to minimize foodborne disease outbreak threats during emergencies. Volunteer training programs are crucial not only during direct disaster responses but also in establishing sustained readiness in public health.

Research has indicated that preparedness programs are facing real threats due to potential budget cuts, requiring stable funding and support for volunteer training. In addition, deliberate evaluation of public health responsiveness underscores the importance of local volunteers in achieving emergency responses effectively (Levi et al., 2008). Lacking correctly trained volunteers, efforts towards ensuring food safety during times of crisis become precarious, requiring constant investment in training programs so that effective local reactions may be sustained in times of disaster.

14.4.3. Role of Schools in Promoting Food Safety Education

Schools are the basis of food safety education, which offers the platform for the transmission of relevant information and procedures at an early age among children. With the addition of extensive food safety curriculum based on safe handling of food, practices of hygiene, and sensitivity towards the effects of foodborne illnesses, schools can successfully avert risks concerning unsafe consumption of food. Besides, schools can engage children through experiential experiences like school gardening and cooking school that facilitate healthy eating habits as well as advocate for a healthy eating mentality. Effective food safety programs are capable of empowering students to express themselves in speaking up for themselves and their family's health, ultimately leading to community awareness. As illustrated in recent studies, establishing robust frameworks in schools with regards to food safety knowledge is not only attuned to legal health mandates but also advocates for equality of access to safe food practices, and thus shapes the development of healthier generations in the future (Birnbaum et al., 2011; Cabrera et al., 2017) (Figure 14.20).

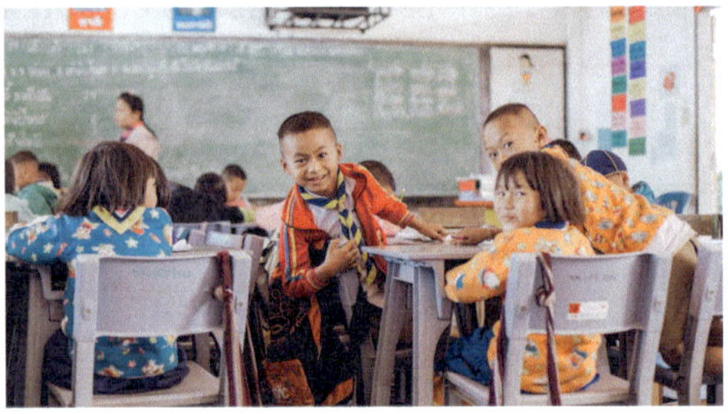

Figure 14.20. Schools play a pivotal role in promoting food safety education, serving as a foundation for instilling critical knowledge and practices in students from an early age.

Source: https://images.squarespace-cdn.com/content/v1/63064607eb816a4d50027fd1/bb35408d-4ab1-4076-a5fc-4312b4778aed/image-asset.jpg.

14.4.4. Community Workshops on Emergency Preparedness

Effective community-based training in disaster preparedness is key to increasing public awareness and building the capacity of individuals with the competencies and capabilities needed to manage emergencies, particularly in food safety during emergencies. Such workshops can effectively provide key training on the handling of food in a safe manner so that people in communities learn to store, prepare, and consume food safely in emergencies. Through making programs sensitive to local weaknesses, like natural disasters or human-made crises, workshops can strengthen community resilience that would otherwise lack it. Further, lessons from past disasters direct towards meticulous planning that includes rapid response and recovery plans, as indicated in disaster management dynamics research across the world. Thus, community-driven programs not only empower the inhabitants but also drive a more robust system capable of averting the adverse effects of emergencies towards food safety (Alinden et al., 2010; Cohen et al., 2011).

14.4.5. Building Local Food Safety Networks

For enhancing emergency food safety interventions, setting up local food safety networks is crucial in ensuring effective risk management and response activities. The networks facilitate cooperation among LHDs, food manufacturers, and community groups, enabling an instant exchange of information and resources during foodborne disease outbreaks. Such connections foster resilience at the community level by blending real-time and big data with traditional surveillance methods, as demonstrated through current frameworks applying big data and machine learning to risk communication and assessment (Zhuang et al., 2022). Apart from that, the Food Safety Modernization Act considers coordinated response at all government levels and the significance of multistakeholder participation at the local level during multistate foodborne illness investigations (Seelman et al., 2021). These local-level networks give communities more of a collective and adaptable form of food safety in the end, which eventually ensures public health protection during emergencies (Figure 14.21).

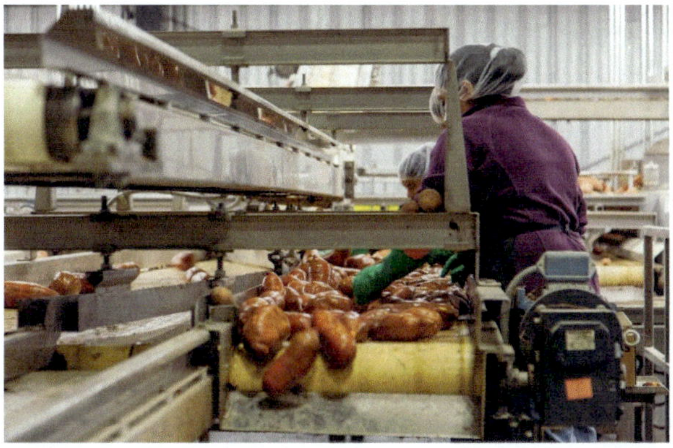

Figure 14.21. In the context of enhancing emergency food safety measures, building local food safety networks plays a critical role in effective risk management and response strategies.

Source: https://www.theauditoronline.com/wp-content/uploads/2023/10/food-safety.jpg.

14.4.6. Utilizing Social Media for Food Safety Awareness

In addressing the immediate need for food safety information during emergencies, the strategic use of social media provides an effective tool for conveying important information within a limited time frame. Social media platforms like Twitter, Facebook, and Instagram provide government agencies and health departments with the ability to communicate with varying demographics with up-to-date news, preventive measures, and food handling and storage safety information. Under social media's internal virality, the organizations are then capable of educating the consumer on best practices, , such as food preparation and food sickness symptom identification. Furthermore, social media is a good interactive platform for questioning and sharing experiences, thereby inducing community engagement and mutual education. Such an active process is critical, especially in the context of evidence that underscores the significance of information communities in alleviating the impacts of crises (Bai, 2020) as well as coping with the psychological trauma of such emergencies (Sasangohar et al., 2020). Ultimately, social media use not only enhances awareness but also cultivates resilience when confronted with food safety challenges.

14.4.7. Encouraging Local Food Production and Sustainability

The assistance of local food production takes a pivotal role in enhancing the sustainability, and particularly in emergency food safety programs. Through encouraging domestic agriculture in communities, we can decrease dependence on global supply chains, thus avoiding threats of food shortages during emergencies. Besides, local foods allow better control of sourcing and supply management, which is crucial in maintaining food safety levels.

Projects based on the principles articulated in the International Guidelines for Securing Sustainable Small-scale Fisheries aim to mainstream sustainability into local operations to ensure that food production is aligned to ecological harmony and conducive to meeting community needs. Further, the focus of working through host country systems as outlined in the USAID Water and Development Strategy highlights the importance of local involvement and management of resources towards constructing resilient food systems. Lastly, encouraging local food production not only favors sustainability but also guarantees enhanced food safety in times of crisis (Figure 14.22).

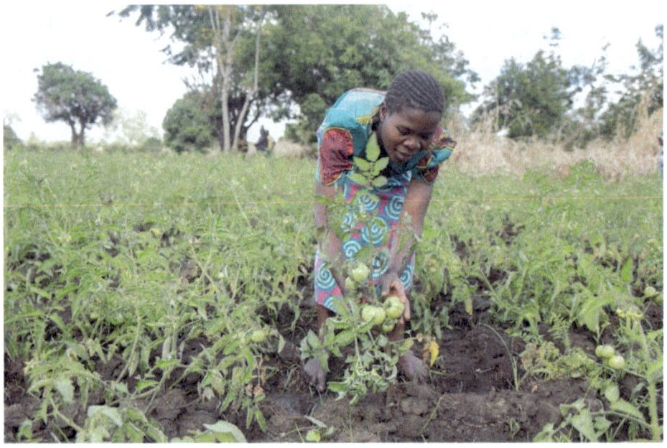

Figure 14.22. The promotion of local food production plays a critical role in enhancing sustainability, particularly in the context of emergency food safety measures.

Source: https://e3az4yc7762.exactdn.com/wp-content/uploads/2021/10/Food-Security-Agriculture-New-Header-Image.jpg?strip=all&lossy=1&ssl=1.

14.4.8. Involving Local Businesses in Food Safety Initiatives

Involving local businesses in food safety activities is essential for establishing community resilience and making sure plans for the response operate efficiently in times of crisis. Local businesses are partners in disseminating food safety awareness and practices to their employees and customers, which fosters a culture of safety in the community. As stipulated in the Sandy Regional Assembly Recovery Agenda, local involvement can play a key function in determining local resiliency priorities, enhance the capacity of vulnerable populations, and reduce public health hazards. Furthermore, engagement with local businesses is in accordance with policy frameworks for enhancing food safety and quality (as stipulated in European Union legislation that emphasizes collaborative action along food value chains) (Barling et al., 2019). Through the inclusion of local businesses in food safety programs, communities are able to tap into customized solutions that draw on local knowledge and resources, ultimately making more effective emergency food safety responses overall.

14.4.9. Evaluating Community Food Safety Programs

Evaluating community food safety programs helps guarantee that they serve the nutrition and health of those who are most at risk, especially during emergencies. Often, such evaluations depend on extensive indicators that check both the initial response and the lasting effectiveness of food safety actions. For instance, insights derived from federal preparedness assessments highlight the need for systemic reforms to enhance community resilience and response times in times of crisis (Levi et al., 2008). Furthermore, the World Bank's extensive involvement in various countries demonstrates a growing recognition of the importance of safety nets and food assistance in public health policy (Grosh and Milazzo, 2025). After studying these frameworks, communities can find weaknesses in their food safety procedures, take targeted steps to fix them and be better prepared for emergencies , which can lead to better health for at-risk people.

A CLOSER LOOK

Bioterrorism Through Food Supply

Food supply bioterrorism is the intentional food or water contamination with poisonous biological agents, , such as bacteria, viruses, or toxins, to make individuals sick, panic, and have an economic effect. The goal of an attack is typically to impair public health, undermine the faith in the food chain, and create widespread fear. A few of the most frequent biological agents that can be used in food-based bioterrorism are *Salmonella*, *E. coli*, *Botulinum toxin*, and *Anthrax spores*. Such toxins can be introduced into food at the production, processing, distribution, or preparation stage, rendering them difficult to track and likely to cause large-scale foodborne illness outbreaks.

The effects of bioterrorism through the food supply chain can be devastating, ranging from severe illness or death in the individuals who are infected to widespread economic damage to the agriculture and food industries. The effects may also include loss of public faith in the safety of food and increased regulatory control. Preventive measures to combat this threat are improved vigilance, enhanced security at food production and distribution facilities, surveillance for unusual patterns of illness, and contingency plans for rapid response in case of an outbreak. Public health agencies and food safety authorities collaborate to have food supply systems in place to detect, contain, and respond to possible bioterrorism threats effectively.

SUMMARY

Its enforcement is at the heart of ensuring public health, particularly with rising food insecurity in both developed and developing nations. With more complex food supply chains, law systems like the Good Samaritan Act play a crucial role in recovering surplus food, converting potential wastage into active resources available to vulnerable communities (Planchenstainer et al., 2013). This paradigm shift not only addresses short-term hunger concerns but also promotes sustained practices in food distribution systems. Besides, constant innovation in these safety nets ensures the quality of food is ensured even in the event of a crisis, improving overall food security. As highlighted, the coming together of all-inclusive policies and public engagement is required to foster resilience to food crises, corroborating the assertion that good food safety must adapt along with our continually evolving societal needs (Cornet et al., 2017).

In investigating the conditions critical to emergency food safety measures, several key points emerge that demonstrate their role in protecting public health amidst crisis. Most paramount among them is the imperative for mechanisms for rapid response; these are pivotal in effecting food safety in the face of natural disasters or pandemics, which tend to skew supply chains and compromise the integrity of foodstuff. For example, research in Napier City highlights the necessity for vulnerable groups to be part of effective evacuation and disaster preparedness, foregrounding the need for ready access to reliable food supplies following the emergency (Becker et al., 2019). Additionally, public health legislation has a significant responsibility to provide an appropriate response, and sound public health legislation is imperative to ensure that everyone gets access to healthy and safe food, thus ensuring the right to health (Cabrera et al., 2017). In summary, there is a necessity for all-rounded planning with the above factors in place for effective emergency food safety management.

KEY TERMS FROM THIS CHAPTER

- Chemical spills
- Earthquakes
- Globalization
- Hurricanes
- Natural calamities
- Natural Language Processing
- Real-time communication
- Social vulnerability
- Vulnerable population
- Disorient food chains
- Floods
- Health crises
- Man-made disasters
- Natural disasters
- Pandemics
- Risk analysis
- Terrorist attacks

REFERENCES

1. Aalberts, C. H. J. (2003). *HACCP Plan Fresh Fish Processing Martina*. https://core.ac.uk/download/pdf/29294826.pdf (accessed on 29 May 2025).
2. Brian Thompson, Marc J. Cohen (2012). *Impact of Climate Change and Bioenergy on Nutrition*. https://doi.org/10.1007/978-94-007-0110-6 (accessed on 29 May 2025).
3. Advisory Council on the Misuse of Drugs. (2011). *Consideration of the Novel Psychoactive Substances ('Legal Highs')*. https://core.ac.uk/download/1643031.pdf (accessed on 29 May 2025).
4. Al Maududi, A., Fanani, E., Marji, M., & Kustono, D. (2024). Assessment of emergency exit pathways and fire safety measures in Football Stadium X: An examination following Indonesian guidelines. *Prevention: The Indonesian Journal of Public Health*. https://www.semanticscholar.org/paper/eda9d8c7a1f3c60b40ff52e9bb766cb9f5df96dc (accessed on 29 May 2025).
5. Alinden, C. M., Amaratunga, R. D. G., & Perera, S. M. V. C. (2010). *Investigating the Status of Disaster Management Within a World-Wide Context: A Case Study Analysis*. https://core.ac.uk/download/1661695.pdf.
6. Ameratunga, D., McAlinden, C., & Perera, S. (2010). *Investigating the Status of Disaster Management Within a World-Wide Context: A Case Study Analysis*. https://core.ac.uk/download/17298863.pdf (accessed on 29 May 2025).
7. Angelos, J. A., Arens, A. L., Johnson, H. A., Cadriel, J. L., & Osburn, B. I. (2017). One Health in food safety and security education: Subject matter outline for a curricular framework. *One health (Amsterdam, Netherlands)*, *3*, 56–65. https://doi.org/10.1016/j.onehlt.2017.04.001Aryal, K., & Gadema, Z. (2008). *Climate Change and Disaster Impact Reduction*. https://core.ac.uk/download/9304445.pdf (accessed on 29 May 2025).
8. Ashley, S. F., Higgins, N. A., Nuttall, W. J., Thomas, P. J., et al. (2017). *Predicting the Cost of The Consequences of a Large Nuclear Accident in the UK*. https://core.ac.uk/download/132155683.pdf (accessed on 29 May 2025).
9. Bai, H. M. (2020). The socio-economic implications of the coronavirus pandemic (COVID-19): A review. *ComFin Research*, *8*, 8–17. https://doi.org/10.34293/commerce.v8i4.3293.
10. Bakirova, L., Murzalimova, A., & Imamova, B. (2023). Provision of food in emergency situations. *Bulletin of Shakarim University. Technical Sciences*. https://www.semanticscholar.org/paper/7e0f8fd0ed4a97020d3bb49d87332d0774491b4b (accessed on 29 May 2025).
11. Barling, D., Sharpe, R., Gresham, J., Mylona, K. (2018). Characterisation framework of key policy, regulatory and governance dynamics and impacts upon European food value chains: Fairer trading practices, food integrity, and sustainability collaborations. The VALUMICS project "Understanding Food Value Chains and Network Dynamics" funded by EU Horizon 2020 G.A. No 727243. Deliverable D3.3, University of Hertfordshire, UK, 416 pages.Becker, J., Kaiser, L., & Payne, B. (2019). *Understanding Residents' Capacities to Support Evacuated Populations: A Study of Earthquake and Tsunami Evacuation for Napier Hill, Napier, Aotearoa New Zealand*. https://core.ac.uk/download/304655507.pdf (accessed on 29 May 2025).
12. Bino, S. (2024). Partnerships and public health. In *Proceedings of the International Congress Public Health–Achievements and Challenges–zbornik radova*. https://www.semanticscholar.org/paper/b45825371888959e1f399e9288d3f20cfd8387a3 (accessed on 29 May 2025).

13. Birnbaum, N., Masterson, E., & Schoomaker, H. (2011). *State of Health Equity Movement, 2011 Update Part C: Compendium of Recommendations (DRA Project Report No. 11-03)*. https://core.ac.uk/download/pdf/18491812.pdf (accessed on 29 May 2025).

14. Braunholz, T., Clay, E., & Pelham, L. (2025). *Natural Disasters: What Is the Role for Social Safety Nets?* https://core.ac.uk/download/pdf/6224449.pdf (accessed on 29 May 2025).

15. Brewin, M., & Dunn, S. (2014). *Feasibility Study: Social Protection in South Central Somalia*. https://core.ac.uk/download/75778511.pdf (accessed on 29 May 2025).

16. Brown, H. S., & Goble, R. L. (1990). *The Role of Scientists in Risk Assessment*. https://core.ac.uk/download/72056967.pdf (accessed on 29 May 2025).

17. Burger, C. P. J., Derix, E., & Warner, J. F. (2025). *Governance of the World Food System and Crisis Prevention*. https://core.ac.uk/download/pdf/29238936.pdf (accessed on 29 May 2025).

18. Cabrera, O. A., Gostin, L. O., Magnusson, R., Nygren-Krug, H., et al. (2017). *Advancing the Right to Health: The Vital Role of Law*. https://core.ac.uk/download/83109641.pdf (accessed on 29 May 2025).

19. Cohen, S. (2011). *Haiti Earthquake January 2010: What Actions and Policies can the Government of Haiti Implement to Improve Emergency Management Response*. https://core.ac.uk/download/70408175.pdf (accessed on 29 May 2025).

20. Cook, B., Trevenen-Jones, A., & Sivasubramanian, B. (2024). Nutritional, economic, social, and governance implications of traditional food markets for vulnerable populations in sub-Saharan Africa: A systematic narrative review. *Frontiers in Sustainable Food Systems*. https://www.semanticscholar.org/paper/485d77f91fd13c072ff28f66d3a8943bba86fe96 (accessed on 29 May 2025).

21. Cornet, R., McCowan, C., Peek, N., Scott, P., et al. (2017). *Addendum to Informatics for Health 2017: Advancing Both Science and Practice*. https://core.ac.uk/download/132585011.pdf.

22. Cortés, D. E., Zack, R. M., Odayar, V. S., Moyer, M., Kumar, A., Libardi Maia, J., Bronico, J. V., et al. (2024). The impact of the COVID-19 pandemic on food access: Insights from first-person accounts in a safety-net health care system. *Journal of Health Care for the Poor and Underserved, 35*, 37–54. https://www.semanticscholar.org/paper/0c7cf8bda3e1fe758e9a1913c0cc63e875905ea3 (accessed on 29 May 2025).

23. Davies, M. J., D'Alessio, D. A., Fradkin, J., Kernan, W. N., Mathieu, C., Mingrone, G., Rossing, P., et al. (2018). Management of hyperglycemia in type 2 diabetes, 2018: A consensus report by the American Diabetes Association (ADA) and the European Association for the Study of Diabetes (EASD). *Diabetes Care, 41*, 2669–2701. https://doi.org/10.2337/dci18-0033.

24. de Haen, H., & Hemrich, G. (2025). *The Economics of Natural Disasters: Implications and Challenges for Food Security*. https://core.ac.uk/download/pdf/6653435.pdf (accessed on 29 May 2025).

25. de la Fuente, A. (2025). *Private and Public Responses to Climate Shocks*. https://core.ac.uk/download/pdf/6248750.pdf (accessed on 29 May 2025).

26. Dowler, E., & MacMillan, T. (2011). *Just and Sustainable? Examining The Rhetoric and Potential Realities of Uk Food Security*. https://core.ac.uk/download/1386268.pdf (accessed on 29 May 2025).

27. Dwivedi, Y. K., Hughes, L., Kar, A. K., Baabdullah, A. M., Grover, P., Abbas, R., Andreini, D., et al. (2021). Climate change and COP26: Are digital technologies and information management part of the problem or the solution? An editorial reflection and call to action. *International Journal of Information Management, 63*, 102456. https://doi.org/10.1016/j.ijinfomgt.2021.102456.

28. Fair Labor Association. (2003). *Tracking Chart 2003 Adidas Salomon, Malaysia 01024678B*. https://core.ac.uk/download/33596849.pdf (accessed on 29 May 2025).

29. Farah, F. A., Nur, A. H., Ibrahim, A. A., Warsame, A. A., Mohamed, A. A., & Ahmed, S. M. (2025). Impacts of drought on food security in Bangladesh. *East African Scholars Journal of Agriculture and Life Sciences*. https://www.semanticscholar.org/paper/117a4746c7498c63c3d6626e457d07d316b20610 (accessed on 29 May 2025).

30. Giannozzi, S., & Khan, A. (2025). *Strengthening Governance of Social Safety Nets in East Asia*. https://core.ac.uk/download/pdf/6266154.pdf (accessed on 29 May 2025).

31. Gligorov, I., Lazarevski, P., & Stikova, E. (2008). *Global Public Health Threats and Disaster Management*. https://core.ac.uk/download/333548437.pdf.

32. Gostin, L. O. (2003). *When Terrorism Threatens Health: How Far Are Limitations on Personal and Economic Liberties Justified?* https://core.ac.uk/download/70375715.pdf (accessed on 29 May 2025).

33. Graham, J. D., & Sadiq, A. A. (2014). Organizational risk perception of disasters: Do risk manager's matter? https://core.ac.uk/download/46958563.pdf (accessed on 29 May 2025).

34. Grosh, M., & Milazzo, A. (2025). *Social Safety Nets in World Bank Lending and Analytical Work: FY2002–2007*. https://core.ac.uk/download/pdf/6314176.pdf (accessed on 29 May 2025).

35. Helbing, D., & Mukerji, P. (2012). *Crowd Disasters as Systemic Failures: Analysis of The Love Parade Disaster*. https://core.ac.uk/download/pdf/81267648.pdf (accessed on 29 May 2025).

36. Ibrahim, H., & Adeola, S. (2024). Assessing food safety awareness and practices among street food vendors in Katsina State, North Western Nigeria. *FUDMA Journal of Agriculture and Agricultural Technology*. https://www.semanticscholar.org/paper/9b2183aad7e86f238c30ad30bd6a606c1ec56845 (accessed on 29 May 2025).

37. Josling, T. E., Orden, D., & Roberts, D. (2025). *Food Regulation and Trade: Toward A Safe and Open Global System—An Overview and Synopsis*. https://core.ac.uk/download/pdf/6679030.pdf (accessed on 29 May 2025).

38. Kooli, C. (2025). Ethical and safety implications of medical emergency landing exploitations: A call for policy action. *Global Journal on Quality and Safety in Healthcare, 8*, 89–92. https://www.semanticscholar.org/paper/dac61402bffb5eddd30c874bad0e7aa20e931c6f (accessed on 29 May 2025).

39. Kriebel, D., Tickner, J., Jacobs, M., & Markkanen, P. (2011). *Lessons Learned: Solutions For Workplace Safety and Health*. https://core.ac.uk/download/71352756.pdf (accessed on 29 May 2025).

40. Levi, J., Segal, L. M., St. Laurent, R., & Vinter, S. (2008). *Ready or not? Protecting the Public's Health from Diseases, Disasters, And Bioterrorism, 2008*. https://core.ac.uk/download/71354212.pdf (accessed on 29 May 2025).

41. Mack, J. C. (2019). *Policy Implications of Intentional Contamination of The Retail Food Chain*. https://core.ac.uk/download/217235980.pdf (accessed on 29 May 2025).

42. Morgan, O., Aguilera, X., Ammon, A., Amuasi, J., Fall, I. S., Frieden, T. R., Heymann, D., et al. (2021). Disease surveillance for the COVID-19 era: Time for bold changes. *The Lancet, 397*, 2317–2319. https://doi.org/10.1016/s0140-6736(21)01096-5.
43. Nangalia, R. (2025). FIREGUIDE–An advanced emergency response platform integrating chatbot assistance, path finder, and alert systems for enhanced fire safety. *International Journal of Scientific Research in Engineering and Management*. https://www.semanticscholar.org/paper/db657e86bf80302a2c420649ce391fe81dd26c04 (accessed on 29 May 2025).
44. Ngongi, N., Sheeran, J., & von Braun, J. (2025). *Responding to the Global Food Crisis–Three Perspectives: IFPRI 2007–2008 Annual Report Essay*. https://core.ac.uk/download/pdf/6289095.pdf (accessed on 29 May 2025).
45. Onyeibor, C. I., Chukwukelu, S., Onwe, I., & Ekanem, C. E. (2025). Strengthening regulatory compliance in the U.S. food industry to support health system resilience and public health preparedness. *International Medical Science Research Journal*. https://www.semanticscholar.org/paper/269c007f694db62ca0a03597ba6b813a40d7dc82 (accessed on 29 May 2025).
46. Planchenstainer, F. (2013). "They collected what was left of the scraps": Food surplus as an opportunity and its legal incentives. https://core.ac.uk/download/11830470.pdf (accessed on 29 May 2025).
47. Rizaldy, W., Suparman, A., Octaviani, R., Mulyawan, A., Ricardianto, P., Sugiyanto, S., & Endri, E. (2024). Integrated safety for sea and air transportation during the COVID-19 pandemic. *Corporate Governance and Organizational Behavior Review*. https://www.semanticscholar.org/paper/8945f439ecd2bc8df17212c6ed3e5bae2f865eab (accessed on 29 May 2025).
48. Rodrigues, J., Saraiva, C., García-Díez, J., Castro, J., & Esteves, A. (2025). Evaluating the effectiveness of food safety policies in Portugal: A stakeholder-based analysis of challenges and opportunities for food safety governance. *Foods*. https://www.semanticscholar.org/paper/b1df547681ccc4885a901e85764e79a6a17eb456 (accessed on 29 May 2025).
49. Rousseau, C., & Miconi, D. (2020). Protecting youth mental health during the COVID-19 pandemic: A challenging engagement and learning process. *Journal of the American Academy of Child & Adolescent Psychiatry, 59*, 1203–1207. https://doi.org/10.1016/j.jaac.2020.08.007.
50. Safril, A. M. (2013). *Government and NGOs Collaboration in Disaster Governance: The Indonesian Experience*. https://core.ac.uk/download/12219496.pdf (accessed on 29 May 2025).
51. Saravanan, V. O., Theradimani, M., Paranidharan, V., Kavitha, P. A., Mohamed, J. J., Juliet, H. S., & Kokila, D. E. (2024). Extenuating mycotoxin contamination in spices: Detection, regulatory frameworks and preventive strategies. *Plant Science Today*. https://www.semanticscholar.org/paper/5af1f7a1849a1aaefd1718b4af47c6e4ae7eae9d (accessed on 29 May 2025).
52. Sasangohar, F., Jones, S. L., Masud, F., Vahidy, F., & Kash, B. A. (2020). Provider burnout and fatigue during the COVID-19 pandemic: Lessons learned from a high-volume intensive care unit. *Anesthesia & Analgesia, 131*, 106–111. https://doi.org/10.1213/ane.0000000000004866.
53. Seelman, S., Viazis, S., Pack Merriweather, S., et al. (2021). Integrating the Food and Drug Administration Office of the Coordinated Outbreak Response and Evaluation Network's foodborne illness outbreak surveillance and response activities with principles of the National Incident Management System. *Journal of Emergency Management, 19*(2), 131–141. https://www.semanticscholar.org/paper/6f4ecbbfced02e48a6d900f1ddac4e07017792f2 (accessed on 29 May 2025).

54. Taylor, M. R., & David, S. D. (2009). *Stronger Partnerships for Safer Food: An Agenda for Strengthening State and Local Roles in The Nation's Food Safety System*. A project of Department of Health Policy School of Public Health and Health Services The George Washington University. https://core.ac.uk/download/71355283.pdf (accessed on 29 May 2025).

55. Tsagkaris, C., Laubsher, L., Matiashova, L., Lin, L. C., & Isayeva, A. (2023). The impact of energy shortages on health and healthcare in Europe. *Health Science Reports, 6*. https://doi.org/10.1002/hsr2.1075.

56. Whittingham, E., Campbell, J., & Townsley, P. (2010). *APFIC/FAO Regional Consultative Workshop: Securing Sustainable Small-Scale Fisheries: Bringing Together Responsible Fisheries and Social Development, Windsor Suites Hotel, Bangkok, Thailand, 6–8 October 2010*. https://core.ac.uk/download/75777521.pdf (accessed on 29 May 2025).

57. Workie, E., Mackolil, J., Nyika, J., & Sendhil, R. (2020). Deciphering the impact of COVID-19 pandemic on food security, agriculture, and livelihoods: A review of the evidence from developing countries. *Current Research in Environmental Sustainability, 2*, 100014. https://doi.org/10.1016/j.crsust.2020.100014.

58. Zamora, G., Tayco, R., & Rizada, M. L. P. (2024). Influence of consumers' sanitary practices on purchasing and dining-out amidst the COVID-19 pandemic. *Journal of Interdisciplinary Perspectives*. https://www.semanticscholar.org/paper/034385f55093c4a1811208a50f74a3d02aba71b5 (accessed on 29 May 2025).

59. Zhuang, J., Wang, C., & Lambert, J. (2022). Machine learning and other information analyses for risk in social networks. *Risk Analysis, 42*. https://www.semanticscholar.org/paper/62acb21062da0e72b1501f217b36bacea4603cfc (accessed on 29 May 2025).

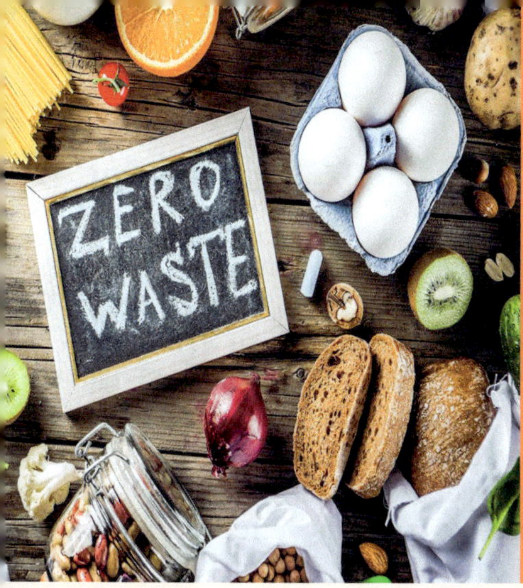

Chapter 15

WASTE MANAGEMENT IN FOOD INDUSTRY

Contents

Introduction ... 353
15.1. Types of Waste in the Food Industry ... 356
15.2. Waste Management Strategies ... 360
15.3. Regulatory and Policy Framework ... 364
15.4. Economic Impact of Food Waste ... 369
Summary ... 374
References ... 375

Introduction

Industrial food waste has now gained universal acceptance as an urgent concern that overlaps with economic sustainability, public health, and environmental integrity. With all this incredibly high level of food production and processing culminating in unimaginable amounts of waste, the implication on food security and human health is catastrophically under threat. Following Obioma et al. (2024), inefficient means of waste disposal will enhance public health risks and reduce food security, particularly in the world's developing communities where expertise and means of proper waste management are scarce. Secondly, the rate of technological development in every sector, including food industries, has accelerated the production of waste, which contributes to other environmental issues. The need for intelligent waste management arises when businesses are trying to cap the unwanted impacts of food waste and, in the process, convert drawbacks into opportunities. Such issues being addressed through sustainable approaches not only ensure the health of the population but also build a stronger food system in the event of increased world demand.

Definition of Waste Management

The purpose of waste management is to collect, move, process and dispose of waste, so it does not harm the environment or people's health. It is very important in the food industry, since there is a lot of waste created at every stage from making to delivering the food. The definition of waste in this context becomes particularly complex, as what one entity considers refuse may be deemed a resource by another, reflecting the subjective nature of waste classification (Ebikapade & Baird, 2016). The U.S. spends a huge amount, $218 billion every year, on food that ends up being wasted in the food industry. Because society is becoming more aware of the environmental damage from food waste, proper waste management is needed to save money and promote sustainable food systems that also help the environment and society. Thus, a clear understanding of waste management is critical for addressing these pressing challenges (Figure 15.1).

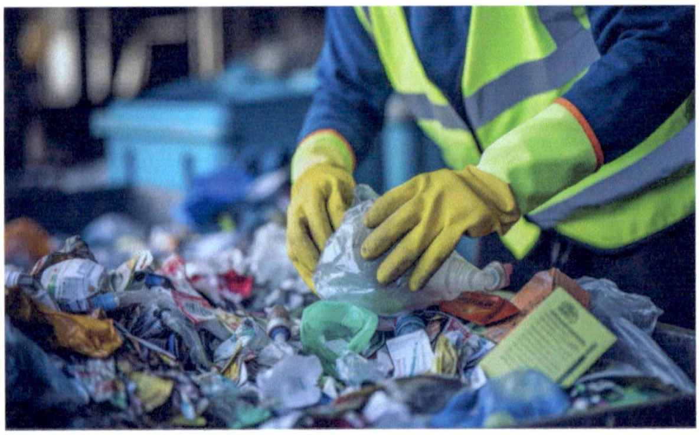

Figure 15.1. Waste management encompasses the collection, transportation, processing, and disposal of waste materials, aiming to mitigate their impact on the environment and public health.

Source: https://uffizio.com/wp-content/uploads/2024/01/ADAS-25-1-2.jpg.

Importance of Waste Management in the Food Industry

Rationally handling food waste within the food sector is relevant not merely from a financial perspective but also from the aspect of environmental conservation. The food processing sector is among the largest generators of waste, particularly at the levels of production, processing, and distribution channels; therefore, adopting effective waste management is imminent. For instance, the implementation of Lean Thinking, a management philosophy of efficiency-orientation to remove waste and create inefficiency, has resulted in significant cost savings across various industries, such as the red meat industry, where 2-3% cost savings have been realized at various levels of the value chain (Simons and Zokaei, 2025). In addition, waste reclamation principles focus on the critical relationship between pig farming and agricultural practices so that maximum transfer of waste can maximize soil fertility while reducing environmental degradation (Gonzalez-Soria et al., 2012). Through prior scheduling of waste management strategies, the food industry can not only decrease its environmental footprint but also increase financial robustness in an emerging marketplace.

Wet waste and Dry Waste

Food production creates many types of waste that have a big effect on the environment. Out of these, organic waste made up of uneaten food, spoiled products and agricultural leftovers forms a big part of the total waste stream. Also, during processing and manufacturing, items like packaging are produced and many of these are not recycled, causing landfills to fill up. Identifying and grouping these wastes can give useful guidance for reducing them, especially when seen from an industrial ecology angle. Using frameworks to look at waste flows allows us to spot similarities in the food supply chain and find chances to recycle and recover resources. They are needed because they follow the European waste hierarchy, which puts more emphasis on minimizing waste and recycling than on landfilling. Ultimately, fostering collaboration within the food industry can help mitigate waste and advance towards a more sustainable production paradigm, as emphasized in Batista et al. (2015) and Davies et al. (2025) (Figure 15.2).

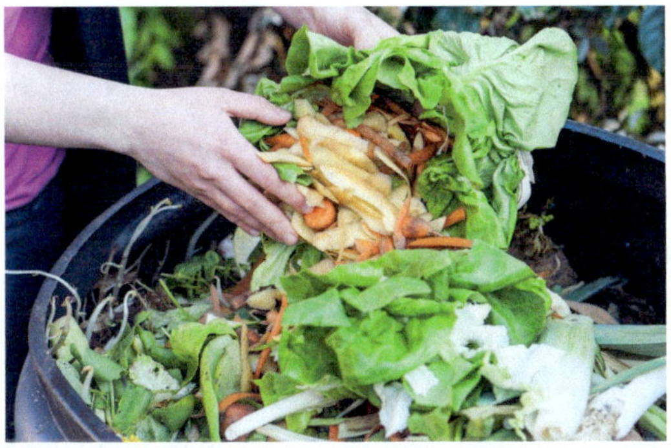

Figure 15.2. The food production sector generates a variety of waste types that significantly impact environmental sustainability.

Source: https://foodprint.org/wp-content/uploads/2018/10/food-waste-problem.jpg.

Current Statistics on Food Waste

Food loss is a fast-expanding issue that influences both economic stability and environmental balance in the food industry. Currently, almost one-third of all the food that is produced globally is lost, which amounts to approximately 1.3 billion tons annually. The wasted food not only accounts for the enormous loss of resources but also contributes to further environmental degradation as well as food insecurity. In South Africa, the issue is most acute with a loss of approximately 10.2 million tons of food, equivalent to 2.1% of national GDP annually, while a significant portion of the population is undernourished. In the US, food loss is fueling the obesity and environmental crisis, and novel community-based interventions must be taken up to address the same to have a more sustainable food system. Therefore, food waste reduction is crucial in fulfilling economic justice as well as environmental sustainability.

Environmental Impact of Food Waste

Throwing away food adds to the damage to the environment, increases climate change and leads to the loss of resources. When thrown away, organic waste rots in landfills without air, creating methane, which is more than 20 times stronger than carbon dioxide at causing global warming over twenty years. It leads to faster global warming and also means that nutrients that could improve soil fertility are lost. In addition, food waste puts more stress on water, since water is needed for farming and for handling the waste. The improper disposal of food can lead to increased reliance on plastic packaging, which further compounds environmental issues, as noted in Landrigan et al. (2023). By giving value to waste food through energy recovery processes, as indicated in Gil (2021), companies are able to utilize their potential towards sustainable biomass energy while reducing waste and minimizing the negative impacts on the environment. Therefore, addressing food waste is important for the enhancement of sustainable practices within the food industry (Figure 15.3).

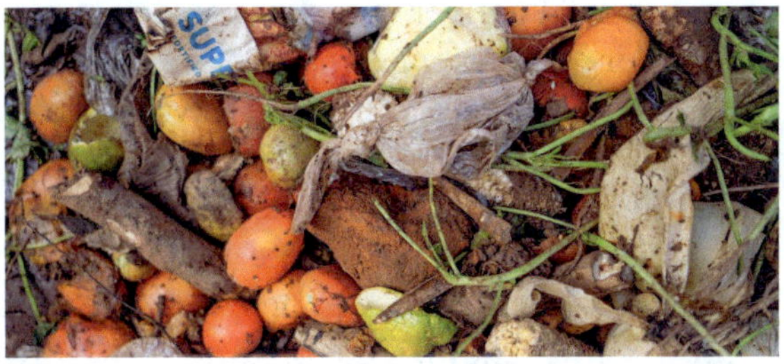

Figure 15.3. Food waste significantly contributes to environmental degradation, exacerbating climate change and resource depletion.

Source: https://global.unitednations.entermediadb.net/assets/mediadb/services/module/asset/downloads/preset/Libraries/Production%20Library/15-10-2020_FAO_Uganda.jpg/image1170x530cropped.jpg

Economic Implications of Waste in the Food Sector

The effects of food waste go past simply losing money and also impact society and the environment. Problems with food waste management cause producers to use more resources and spend more, which might be passed on to consumers. For instance, the food industry generates enormous quantities of byproducts that could be repurposed, such as the marc byproduct from winemaking, which can be converted into high-value phytopharmaceutical compounds, thereby reducing ecological footprints and fostering circular economic strategies (Bogdanof et al., 2019). Moreover, the medical sector, not traditionally attuned to food wastage, is an example of how service sectors contribute to wastage from inefficiencies in business practice and waste treatment procedures, affecting economic stability and eco-health across a number of sectors (Davies and Konisky, 2025). Improving the inefficiencies increases profits and also facilitates the use of eco-friendly products more and more needed by consumers.

Regulatory Frameworks Governing Waste Management

The governance frameworks of food waste management are increasingly shaped by the imperative for sustainability and environmental protection. Governments and institutions are promoting policy frameworks that not only aim at disposing of food waste in an efficient manner but also promote good practice across the food value chain. For instance, EU laws, such as the General Food Law, guide national measures towards heightened transparency and food safety during production, basically monitoring waste development (Barling et al., 2019). On the other hand, the inclusion of various intervention tools allows small firms to adopt green methods and enhance their operational efficiencies (Blundel et al., 2012). This comprehensive approach places heavy emphasis on having effective regulatory frameworks that not only avoid waste but also establish an enabling environment among the stakeholders in, which policy is context-driven and efficient in addressing the waste management needs of the food industry (Figure 15.4).

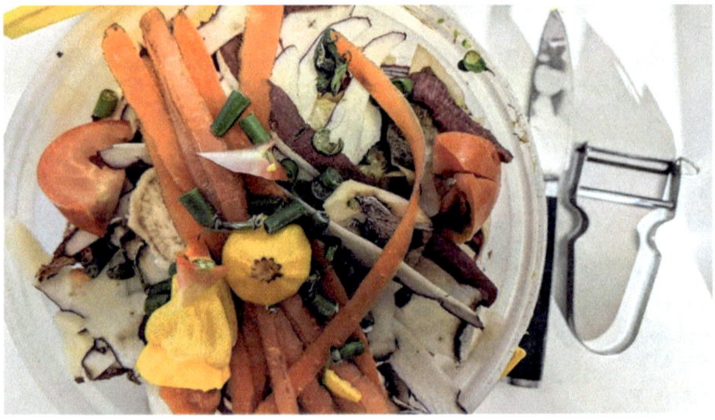

Figure 15.4. Governments and organizations are implementing structured policies that not only address the efficient handling of food waste but also promote responsible practices throughout the food value chain.

Source: https://shapiroe.com/wp-content/uploads/2024/07/benefits-of-reducing-food-waste.jpg.

15.1. Types of Waste in the Food Industry

Amongst foods, there are a number of types of waste that come under significant economic and environmental costs. Before the others is food waste itself, both unsold products and by-products generated through processing. Such waste not only represents a loss of material resources but also is a source of greenhouse gas emissions when disposed of in landfills. Additionally, waste packaging, particularly plastic, is a serious problem; plastic manufacturing globally was 335 million tons as of 2016, and the food and beverage industry has been leading the charts (Drzyzga et al., 2018). The solutions against the waste include increasing recycling activities and developing biodegradable plastics that can substitute the conventional plastic. But the diversity of managing these types of waste requires comprehensive solutions that center on sustainable methodology as well as foster industrial cooperation. Reducing the types of waste that are found in the food industry requires innovative solutions that go beyond traditional metrics of waste control (Shamseer et al., 2015).

15.1.1. Organic Waste

Organic waste plays a crucial role in food industrial waste management, which should be examined in detail. Organic waste is made up of materials that are biodegradable in nature, such as food scraps, fruit and vegetable peels, and other organic byproducts of food processing.

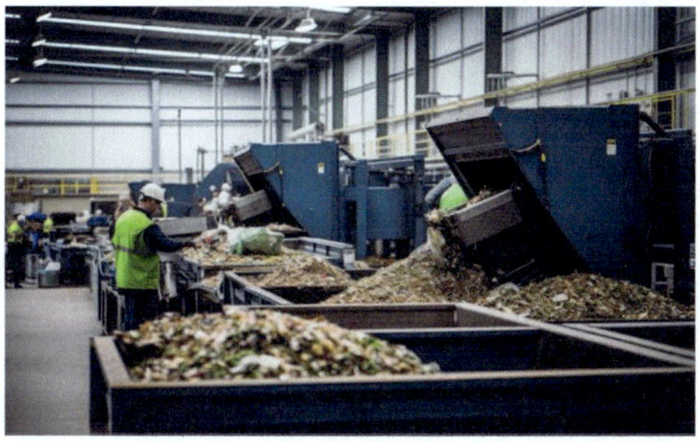

Figure 15.5. In the realm of waste management within the food industry, organic waste plays a crucial role that merits in-depth examination.

Source: https://t4.ftcdn.net/jpg/06/46/55/03/360_F_646550395_kTyeCwTLPcVcDwO1wGPzsJ97n3y8vxoi.jpg.

Proper management of organic waste not only minimizes environmental burden through reduced landfill inputs but also encourages good practices like composting that transform waste into valuable fertilizers for farming purposes. Furthermore, as shown in the literature on organic farming, organic fertilizer made from waste can enhance soil health and crop output with a minimized use of chemicals (Panday et al., 2024). However, the transition to end-to-end organic waste management is not without challenges, with most significant being implementing efficient collection, processing, and public education schemes (Landrigan et al., 2023). It is therefore essential to establish a robust organic waste management system to secure increased sustainability and loop closure within the food industry supply chain (Figure 15.5).

15.1.2. Packaging Waste

The growing problem of packaging food waste in the food sector calls for innovative solutions to packaging in order for it to be sustainable and attuned to consumers' requirements. Since packaging is also the solution to maintaining food integrity, the use of natural additives and biodegradable materials has now become a feasible option. For instance, active packaging systems may be developed based on essential oils that are derived from agro-industrial by-products in order to deliver, among other aspects, longer shelf life as well as reduce food spoilage, thereby addressing both packaging and food wastes simultaneously (Cíguez et al., 2021). Secondly, the European Union's Extended Producer Responsibility (EPR) policy will help address plastic packaging waste through recycling and recovery of the same. Implementation of eco-design concepts in the system can result in reduced packaging alternatives being achieved, finally setting up a circular economy with the least waste (Kjær et al., 2024).

15.1.3. Hazardous Waste

The toxic waste is a critical concern in the food sector, and therefore, it must be regulated very carefully so that it does not cause environmental and health hazards. It is normally created from cleaning agents, shattered glass, and other food spoilage products and can cause contamination if not disposed of properly. The decomposition of organic waste in landfills, for instance, produces harmful methane emissions, yet another driving factor of the impacts of climate change, and leachate can bring pathogens and toxic substances into the environment (Meegoda et al., 2025). Moreover, the disposal of hazardous wastes through illegal dumping has the potential to cause the proliferation of lethal microbes, thus compromising public health. Efficient practices thus need to be established in order to handle such materials, moving towards cleaner practices with waste reduction and recycling. With practices ensuring the Circular Economy, the food industry can turn toxic waste into useful resources and ultimately ensure environmental well-being and economic sustainability (Jadidi et al., 2025) (Figure 15.6).

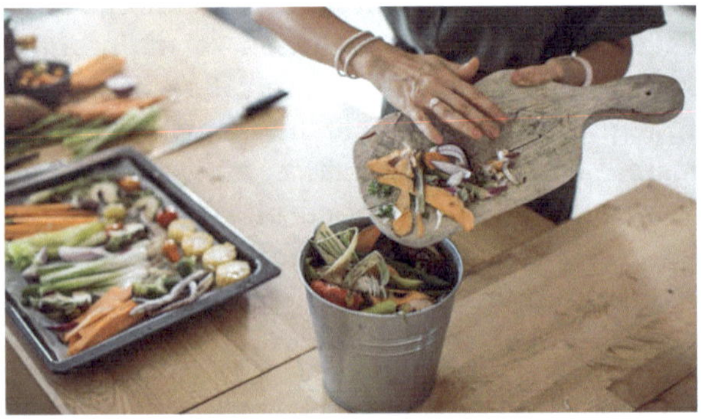

Figure 15.6. Hazardous waste presents a significant challenge within the food industry, necessitating meticulous management to mitigate environmental and health risks.

Source: https://restaurantindia.s3.ap-south-1.amazonaws.com/s3fs-public/2023-05/Sustainability_0.jpg.

15.1.4. E-Waste From Food Processing Equipment

Electronic waste (e-waste) generated by food processing equipment is a significant problem in the food industry from an environmental perspective. With the food processing industry increasingly reliant on advanced technology for efficiency and safety, the generated e-waste contributes to the industry's environmental impact. The waste also includes harmful chemicals whose elimination involves specialized procedures in order not to contaminate soil and water. Along with this, e-waste generated by food processing plant redundant equipment and electronic monitoring devices is also bringing about environmental impacts in direct and indirect ways, as explained in favor of service industry research (Davies and Konisky, 2025). The complex interaction of these effects demands rigorous waste control procedures that not only address e-waste disposal but also emphasize recycling and reducing waste generation in the first place (Davies and Konisky, 2025). Through this, existing progress in e-waste management can go a long way in preventing harmful environmental effects while transforming food processing activities into cleaner processes.

15.1.5. Wastewater and Its Treatment

Effective wastewater management is critical in the food industry since the industry is a significant water polluter through the extensive generation of organic waste during processing. Wastewater treatment is not just a regulatory requirement, but it also offers operating opportunities for resource recovery and environmental sustainability. Recent studies highlight the effectiveness of bio adsorbents, such as those from avocado peels and seeds, in the effective removal of contaminants, such as Rhodamine B dye, from wastewater, with removal efficiencies ranging from 88% to 92% under optimal conditions (Orozco et al., 2024). In addition, sustainable management practices in wastewater treatment are in harmony with larger environmental goals. By adopting forward-thinking approaches, the food industry can transform its waste crisis into a tool of sustainable resource management, thereby addressing more than just disposal and contributing towards total environmental well-being (Torrens, 2023) (Figure 15.7).

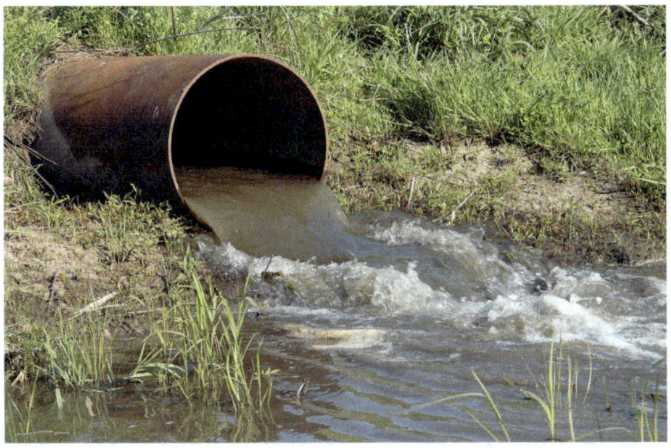

Figure 15.7. Effective wastewater management is crucial in the food industry, as this sector is a significant contributor to water pollution due to the high volume of organic waste generated during processing.

Source: https://upload.wikimedia.org/wikipedia/commons/thumb/f/fa/Discharge_pipe.jpg/1200px-Discharge_pipe.jpg

15.1.6. By-Products From Food Processing

The food processing industry generates a large amount of by-products, which, if utilized effectively, can contribute significantly to sustainable activities. As an example, grape pomace, a by-product of winemaking, is composed of skins, seeds, and stems and is a rich source of dietary fiber and polyphenols that are bioactive compounds. This waste can be used in the fortification of different food products, such as bakery, dairy, and beverages, in an effort to add nutritional value without adding more waste. In addition to this, the use of new management practices is required to reduce the environmental footprint of food processing waste. While economic progress seeks to align with environmental responsibility in the food industry, understanding the multifaceted impact of by-products, even beyond the food processing industry—can give hints into more comprehensive waste management (Davies and Konisky, 2025). Thus, utilizing by-products not only transforms what would otherwise be waste into valuable commodities but also gives zest to the visions of sustainable waste management in the food industry.

15.1.7. Spoilage and Unsold Inventory

The issue of spoilage and overstock is a significant problem within the food industry, driving the broader problem of food waste. The U.S. alone has been estimated to waste a whopping $218 billion annually on never-consumed food, in part due to overproduction and due to the inherently perishable quality of much food. Surplus stock generally comes in waste form, which not only diminishes economic efficiency but also contributes to environmental degradation. Social pressure regarding disposing of waste is compelling businesses more and more to rethink their inventory management.

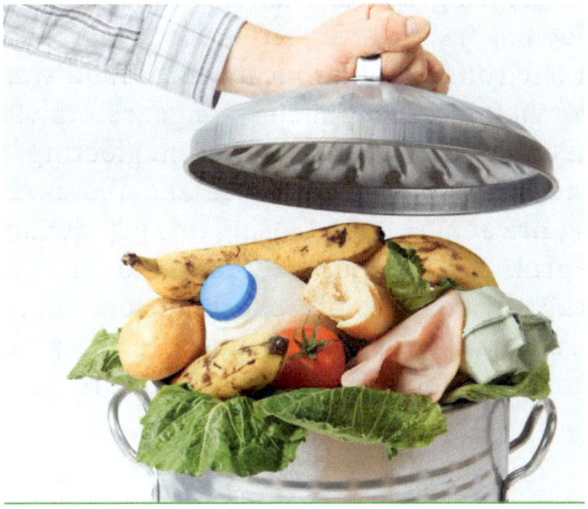

Figure 15.8. The issue of spoilage and unsold inventory represents a significant challenge within the food industry, exacerbating the broader problem of food waste.

Source: https://shapiroe.com/wp-content/uploads/2023/05/the-problem-of-food-waste.jpg.

In response to such pressures, many companies are looking for innovative solutions, such as better supply chain management and partnering with food recovery organizations, to minimize spoilage (Elia et al., 2020). Through the management of spoilage and unsold stock upfront, the food business can promote operational sustainability alongside helping toward overall environmental and social objectives (Figure 15.8).

15.1.8. Food Waste at the Consumer Level

One of the biggest issues in food industry waste management is consumer-level food waste. Billions of dollars each year in the United States alone are spent on food that does not get eaten, and it is estimated that food waste adds 1.3% to the GDP of the nation. This is a consequence of various factors that span from consumer attitudes and cultural beliefs towards disposing of food. In Canada, there has been growing concern among consumers and policymakers regarding the economic, social, and environmental implications of food waste; nevertheless, most policies are geared towards household behavior at times neglecting the broader view of food service and restaurants (Maguire et al., 2018). Closing this gap demands integral educational programs to enable a culture of responsible consumption, thereby reducing waste at source and fostering a more sustainable food management culture in our lives.

15.2. Waste Management Strategies

Sustainability in the food industry is based on sustainable waste disposal, particularly as global environmental issues worsen. Use of technology, in the form of AI-based technology, has been a game-changer way of reducing food loss in a big way. Research has indicated that hospitality businesses are employing software like Leanpath and Winnow, which calculate actual waste generation in real-time, thus providing insights for responsible consumption practices. As also argued in Clark et al. (2025), these strategies can also be adapted for home use, which indicates there is a greater likelihood of utilization. Furthermore, the practice of recycling food by-products, as reported in Wibisono et al. (2025), indicates how the sector can shift from eliminating waste to utilizing resources. This kind of trend not only benefits sustainability but is also compatible with the overall philosophy of minimizing waste across the supply chain. More cooperation among stakeholders is still required to establish robust and effective waste management systems in the food sector.

15.2.1. Waste Reduction Techniques

In the culinary world, successful waste reduction methods play an important role in maximizing sustainability and operational effectiveness. One such effective strategy is the reuse of excess ingredients, which not only reduces waste but also enables restaurants to innovate their menus. For instance, as highlighted in a recent research, small-scale ventures like Fat Ramen utilize ingredient reutilization and adapted portion size in order to align with customer demand, thereby minimizing food wastage during preparation (Mahmud et al., 2024). Second, building strong supply chain alliances can facilitate streamlined procurement and foster a cohesive approach to managing inventory. Techniques, such as flexible ordering systems, which adapt to demand fluctuations, also promote waste reduction strategies (Asian and Pacific Centre for Transfer of Technology (APCTT), UN ESCAP, 1997). Implementation of these waste reduction techniques not only benefits the environment but can also provide economic advantages, ultimately bringing the food industry to a more sustainable direction (Figure 15.9).

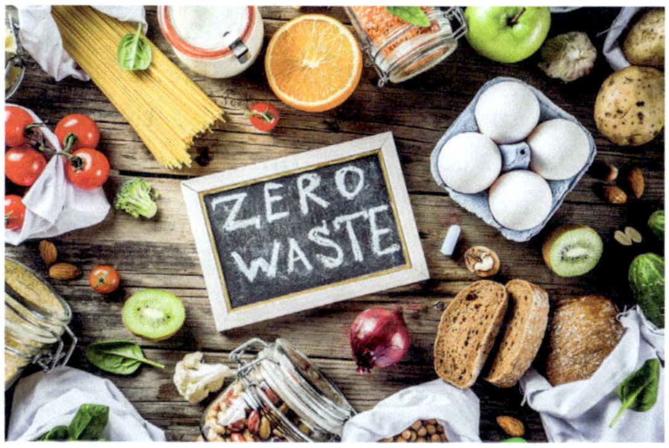

Figure 15.9. In the food industry, effective waste reduction techniques are crucial for enhancing sustainability and operational efficiency.

Source: https://hospitalityinsights.ehl.edu/hubfs/Blog-EHL-Insights/Blog-Header-EHL-Insights/AdobeStock_264542845.jpeg.

15.2.2. Recycling and Composting Initiatives

Maybe the most potent strategy for minimizing waste in the food sector is the use of recycling and composting programs. These activities, alongside excluding organic waste from landfills, also contribute significantly towards local sustainability through enhanced soil and green spaces, as presented in Frederickson et al. (2010). Besides, community composting initiatives ensure social unity as well as job and skill acquisition opportunities, affirming the variety of benefits such projects can achieve. The enormous scale of wastage of food in America, worth some $218 billion annually, reflects the necessity of embracing new waste management methods. Composting and recycling can be utilized to reduce industry operation costs while solving environmental problems simultaneously. Thus, establishing a culture of sustainability for the food industry is part of an integrated approach to waste management that addresses both economic interests and environmental interests.

15.2.3. Anaerobic Digestion for Organic Waste

The application of anaerobic digestion as a method of managing organic waste in the food sector has many environmental and economic advantages. Besides being an efficient means of waste reduction, the process also turns the waste into valuable biogas, thus the production of renewable energy. As highlighted by recent studies, the shift to anaerobic digestion can lead to substantial greenhouse gas emissions savings since findings have shown that modeled GHG emissions from current waste management practices in Myanmar range between 1500 and 1800 Gigagrams of CO_2-eq annually, while the application of improved biodegradable waste utilization could avoid 3500 to 4000 Gigagrams of CO_2-eq annually (Juchelková et al., 2018). This shift supports the broader objectives of waste reduction and resource recovery, maintaining the belief that effective waste management solutions, as set out in local Waste and Resources Strategies, can have a tangible impact on economic and environmental performance across the food sector (Limited, 2010) (Figure 15.10).

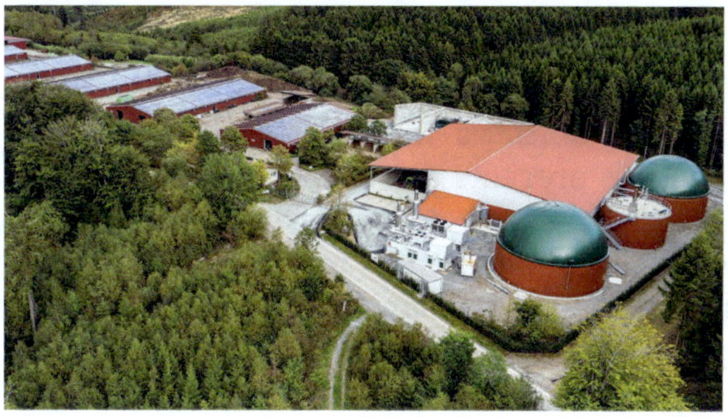

Figure 15.10. The adoption of anaerobic digestion as a method for managing organic waste within the food industry presents significant environmental and economic advantages.

Source: https://upload.wikimedia.org/wikipedia/commons/e/ee/Biogasanlage_mit_Kompostierung.jpg.

15.2.4. Use of Food Waste as Compost

The establishment of food donation programs for surplus food is a central element in averting waste in the food sector as well as helping feed the hungry and alleviating food insecurity.

By facilitating the redistribution of surplus food from farms, stores, and restaurants to charities and food banks, these programs prevent edible food from going to landfills. As quoted, approximately one out of every four calories produced is wasted, with far-reaching consequences for resource management and food security worldwide (Lipinski et al., 2013). In addition, the financial burden of food waste on the economy is astronomical; the United States alone invests $218 billion annually in food that goes uneaten. Therefore, incorporating robust food donation schemes not only prevents wastage, but also transforms surplus food into an asset that can help alleviate poverty and support vulnerable groups, thus making the food system more equitable and sustainable.

15.2.5. Technology in Waste Management

The integration of technology in waste management, particularly within the food industry, presents a revolutionary opportunity to correct the prevalent issue of food waste. Blockchain technology and the like enable greater supply chain management through greater transparency and accountability, which is crucial in the context of waste minimization across all phases of food handling and distribution. As speculated in existing literature, blockchain has the potential to greatly divide the supply chain into reasonable parts so that managers are capable of following food control and reducing waste more proactively (Kopanaki et al., 2021). In addition, the lack of sufficient policies for waste management in nations, such as Malaysia emphasizes the significance of technological advancements beyond conventional measures like landfilling and incineration (Ramlan et al., 2017). Using advanced technologies, the food industry can not only increase business efficiency but also encourage sustainable practices in harmony with global efforts to minimize food wastage (Figure 15.11).

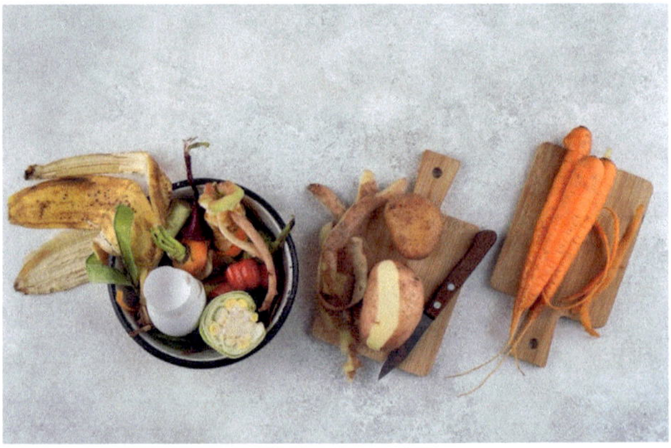

Figure 15.11. The integration of technology in waste management, particularly within the food industry, presents a transformative opportunity to address the pervasive issue of food waste.

Source: https://shapiroe.com/wp-content/uploads/2024/01/how-can-we-reduce-food-waste.jpg.

15.2.6. Employee Training and Awareness Programs

Effective employee training and sensitization are major cornerstones in waste management practices control within the food industry. Employee training on the huge financial losses arising from the wastage of food, estimated at $218 billion annually for the United States, allows organizations to instill a culture of sustainability and reduce waste.

These programs need to be accompanied by real-world know-how that enables workers to be informed of waste zones and implement best practices, such as efficient inventory control and food recycling. Besides, knowledge transfer through successful models like Hamanasi Resort, using implementation of hands-on training and participatory research, will enable the responsibility and dedication of workers (Early et al., 2011). Lastly, such training programs not only improve the environment through environmental stewardship but also meet the interests of companies in reducing waste management costs, thereby creating a win-win aspect for businesses and the environment.

15.2.7. Sustainable Packaging Solutions

The use of green packaging systems within the food industry is a major factor in encouraging waste management and minimizing environmental impacts. The utilization of compostable, biodegradable, or recyclable products by firms has the potential to limit their consumption of petroleum-based plastics as sources of pollution and squandering of resources. Recent studies targeting the circular economy indicate that innovative packaging solutions minimize waste and optimize the utilization of resources throughout the life cycle of the product (Mondello et al., 2024).

Furthermore, the negative effects of inefficient solid waste management, such as marine pollution and ground and water contamination, identify the necessity for the food sector to embrace greener practices (Ferronato et al., 2019). Moreover, the implementation of packaging innovations that are developed from the principles of the circular economy causes a shift in organizations at the system level, enforcing the tenet that management and governance must prioritize environmental sustainability. Ultimately, these practices are critical to making certain the growth of the food industry aligns with broader ecological goals (Figure 15.12).

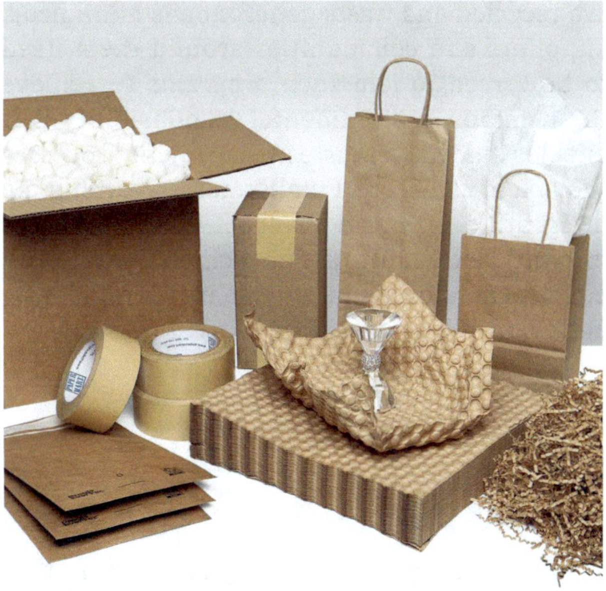

Figure 15.12. The integration of sustainable packaging solutions within the food industry is pivotal for enhancing waste management practices and minimizing environmental impact.

Source: https://blog.papermart.com/wp-content/uploads/2023/06/Eco-01-1024x1024.jpg.

15.2.8. Collaboration with Waste Management Companies

Collaboration with waste management companies is a critical element in reducing the food industry's environmental footprint. Through collaboration, food companies are able to formulate structured waste disposal and recycling strategies tailored to their own requirements, which can then reduce the environmental impact of their activities. For instance, the brewing sector has also been in mass uptake of sustainable practices, spearheaded by research inquiry for waste management strategies that promote recycling and circularity (Ravanal et al., 2024). Effective coordination not only maximizes the safe disposal of rotten food but also promotes the uptake of a circular economy in, which resources are recycled and waste generation is minimized. Suppliers and communities around them need to be forced to join such programs to achieve the common environmental responsibility that enables innovative waste management processes (Varma et al., 2024). Finally, mainstreaming the integration of waste management companies into the food industry supply chain is vital in an effort to accelerate the agenda on sustainability and establish a sustainable food industry.

15.3. Regulatory and Policy Framework

The regulatory and policy framework that governs waste management in the food industry is crucial in addressing the environmental and economic implications of food loss. As nearly 1.3 billion tons of food intended for consumption get wasted annually around the world, the significance of integrated, evidence-based rules is apparent. In particular, the Ontario Food and Organic Waste Framework exemplifies how certain policies minimize the occurrence of waste through organic waste dumping prohibition in landfills (Taylor et al., 2015). These frameworks must offer a mix of voluntary and compulsory measures that balance flexibility and transparency as emphasized by various industry actors (Taylor et al., 2015). Secondly, promoting cooperation along the entire value chain of food can enhance the effectiveness of such regulations so that food waste prevention actions are allotted the highest priority and also yield long-term ecological sustainability, and respond to timely social concerns regarding food insecurity (Taylor et al., 2015).

15.3.1. Overview of Local and National Regulations

The regulatory system of waste management in food production is controlled by an interrelated network of national and local rules intended to minimize environmental impact and promote sustainable practice. Local regulations can demand certain segregation methods, recycling mandates, and composting mandates depending on the community's needs and environmental goals. At the national level, legislation, such as the Resource

Conservation and Recovery Act (RCRA) establishes comprehensive standards for managing solid and hazardous waste, subjecting stakeholders in the food industry to responsibility for compliance with such standards. This dual-tiered approach not only allows for compliance with environmental safety but also enables public health, as seen from outcomes proving that environmental degradation is connected to rising health issues (Whitmee et al., 2015; Intergovernmental Panel on Climate Change, 2023). Strong enforcement of these policies is thus key in achieving sustainability in the food industry, as well as creating a culture of accountability for consumers and businesses (Figure 15.13).

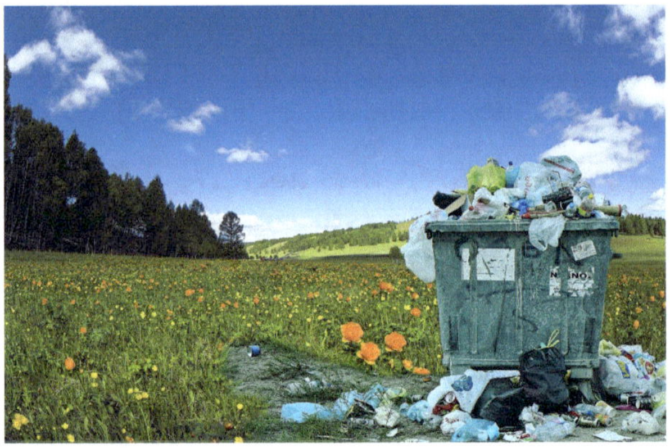

Figure 15.13. Resource Conservation and Recovery Act (RCRA).

Source: https://images.squarespace-cdn.com/content/v1/5d9f9c38a9f9dd6f0251ee7b/1619750758775-VKR32J2FXGM2XA5YBO17/pollution-3441119_1920.jpg.

15.3.2. International Guidelines on Food Waste

Global legislation on food waste plays a pivotal role in ensuring sustainable behavior within the food value chain. The legislations tend to aim at reducing wastage at every level of the food value chain, from production to consumption levels. The European Union, for instance, has an expansive framework that is responsive to food safety, sustainability, and fair trading behavior, inviting the participation of stakeholders with transparency and responsibility (Barling et al., 2019). Renewable process, such as anaerobic digestion and efficient energy management, are critical to the minimization of waste and maximization of resources (Benoit et al., 2012). Moreover, the application of food reduction processes not only contributes to the development of the global sustainability agenda but also encourages economic efficiency among producers and consumers. By harmonizing the global guidelines and local practices, the food industry will be in a position to successfully decrease wastage, lessen environmental impacts, and facilitate the circular economy, thereby stabilizing the world's food systems.

15.3.3. Role of Government in Waste Management

Effective waste management in the food industry hinges to a great extent on the role of the government, both as an authoritative regulatory institution and driver of sustainable practices. Governments can have policies that guarantee food waste reduction and recycling schemes and that stakeholders are accountable for their waste management. For instance, legislation can be enacted to issue guidelines on how agricultural and food processing residue cellulosic biomass can be used in the food industry to decrease the adverse impacts on food supplies while boosting the production of biofuels from non-food feedstocks (Ghosh, 2016). The governments can further leverage recent findings in human behavior in waste management to develop learning programs that enable recycling and establish consumer responsibility for consumption (Concari et al., 2021). Lastly, a coordinated government program can mobilize industrial and community efforts toward increased participation in sustainable waste management practices (Figure 15.14).

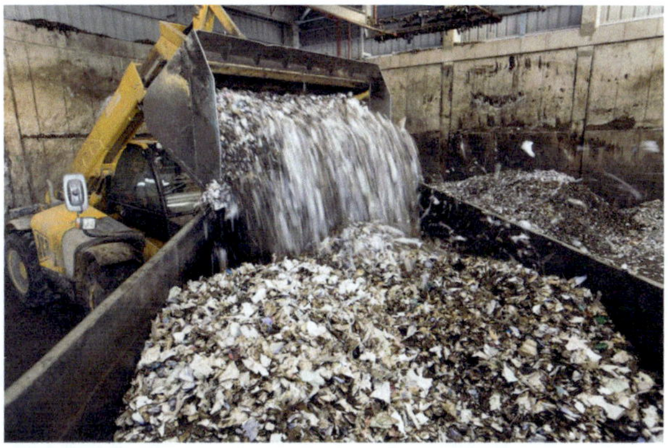

Figure 15.14. Effective waste management in the food industry hinges significantly on the role of government, which acts as a crucial regulatory body and facilitator for sustainable practices.

Source: By GST HBK - Own work, Public Domain, https://commons.wikimedia.org/w/index.php?curid=6402254

15.3.4. Incentives for Businesses to Reduce Waste

Pressure to cut waste in food production is increasingly characterized by varied incentives that seek to persuade businesses to be more sustainable. Cutting food waste, specifically, not only diminishes pressure on the environment but also reaps significant economic benefits. The U.S. alone wastes $218 billion worth of uneaten food annually, which is a cry in the wilderness to businesses to create and streamline their operations. Campaigns by groups like ReFED highlight the value of waste reduction, recovery, and recycling as major employment generation drivers and cost savers. Such techniques enhance their corporate social responsibility image to companies while exposing them to new revenue opportunities through the efficient use of resources. Therefore, the application of waste minimization strategies comes in harmony with social responsibility and cost responsibility and provides a polymorphic incentive for the food business industry.

15.3.5. Penalties for Non-Compliance

In waste management within the food industry, fines for non-compliance serve as a critical method of enforcing regulatory requirements and maintaining practice. The consequences of non-compliance in waste management can be extreme, ranging from financial fines to heightened legal consequences, such as plant shutdowns.

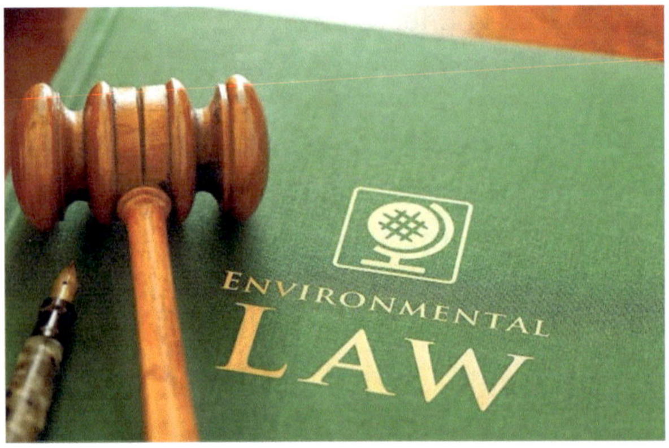

Figure 15.15. The repercussions for failing to adhere to waste management regulations can vary significantly, ranging from monetary fines to more severe legal consequences, such as facility shutdowns.

Source: https://mahabal.com/wp-content/uploads/2024/10/environmental-law.webp.

Disobedience is not just assaulting environmental integrity but is also public health, and it has made regulators impose stringent measures upon violators. However, imposition of fines is normally unpredictable, just as it is in most developing countries where funds are scarce and bribery tends to hinder strict monitoring (Dasgupta et al., 2025). Furthermore, regulatory process variation allows certain larger firms, particularly state-owned enterprises, to avoid the full force of fines, and issues of fairness and effectiveness arise (Fair Labor Association, 2012). Thus, a uniform penalty framework is essential in upholding culpability and encouraging compliance in the food industry (Figure 15.15).

15.3.6. Impact of Policies on Food Waste Reduction

The influence of policies in minimizing food waste is increasingly becoming an essential part of the solution to inefficiencies in the food industry. Actions by the government, by targeting the HoReCa (Hotels, Restaurants, and Catering) sector, play an important role in promoting sustainable practices to minimize the creation of waste.

Empirical realities indicate that effective organizational improvements can minimize food waste and associated expenditures with the support of powerful policies. For instance, Buczacki et al. (2021) emphasize stakeholder collaboration to illustrate how macro policies by governments can drive collaborative action towards the attainment of more food waste-specific Sustainable Development Goals (SDGs). Moreover, qualitative research, such as research in the Malaysian environment, discovers that collaborative work with foodservice operators and policymakers can determine the complexity of food loss and waste, thus informing more effective regulatory measures (Majid et al., 2024). In general, there is a need for collaborative policy to ensure industry-level cooperation to end towards less food wastage, eventually serving the environment and economy.

15.3.7. Stakeholder Involvement in Policy-Making

Involving stakeholders actively in policy formation is crucial in addressing the complex challenges arising from waste management for the food sector. Having a variety of stakeholders, such as local communities, government bodies, and the industry, aids in consolidating different unifications to come up with holistic waste management policies. Their contributions ensure that different perspectives are incorporated to yield effective and more sustainable policy outcomes.

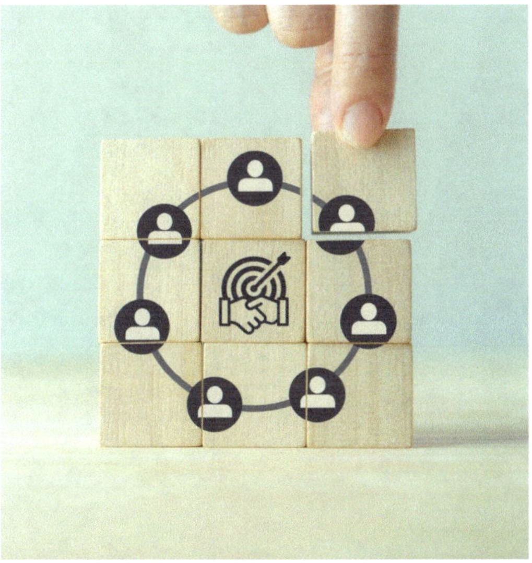

Figure 15.16. Effective stakeholder involvement in policy-making is essential for addressing the complex challenges posed by waste management in the food industry.

Source: https://aworld.org/wp-content/uploads/2024/02/shutterstock_2258443385-scaled.jpg.

For instance, as evidenced by the Intergovernmental Panel on Climate Change (2023), the interconnectedness of ecosystems and human societies underscores the importance of taking an integrated waste management practice with regard to both environmental and social impacts. Also, with the emergence of technologies like blockchain, discussed in Saberi et al. (2018), there is scope for new pathways of further transparency and traceability for supply chains, thus facilitating stakeholders to pursue sustainability goals together. Lastly, promoting the development of stakeholder involvement fosters responsibility as well as represents innovations aimed at loss minimization and overall performance maximization of food business activities (Figure 15.16).

15.3.8. Future Trends in Waste Management Legislation

With the changing face of waste management, any future regulation will certainly be more inclusive and sustainable in nature, especially in the food industry. The growing emphasis on circular economy values signals gigantic changes in the handling of food waste, with policies more centered on less landfill dependence and encouraging recycling and composting schemes. Transformation of this kind is important given that the food and drink sector is a regional economic driver, as reiterated in A Flourishing Region, underlining its contribution to the role of sustainable economic growth in regions like the East Midlands (East Midlands Development Agency, 2008). Besides, environmental management of agriculture interventions, as proposed by Tzilivakis and Lewis, accounts for a change towards robust schemes to further increase sustainable processes along the food chain (Lewis et al., 1999). Such trends suggest that future legislation will not only dictate regulatory standards but also spur innovation in waste management practices across the industry.

15.3.9. Evaluation of Existing Policies and Their Effectiveness

The policies for food industry waste management need to be carefully evaluated in order to determine their capabilities for minimizing food loss. Surprisingly, the ReFED coalition's A Roadmap to Reduce U.S. Food Waste offers integrated strategies that employ evidence-based facts in order to increase food waste reduction across all levels. The report indicates that a unified approach not only can create jobs but also resolves issues of environmental pollution and food insecurity. Besides, In California, the report Waste Not, Want Not also stresses the importance of improving the utilization of available resources, and that urban water supply can be met by reducing water wastage using effective policies and technologies. These findings collectively highlight the need for policy frameworks to be altered in order to facilitate collaboration between the stakeholders, including governments and corporations, to implement measures that combat systemic inefficiencies and capitalize on opportunities for sustainability in the food industry (Mann et al., 2003) (Figure 15.17).

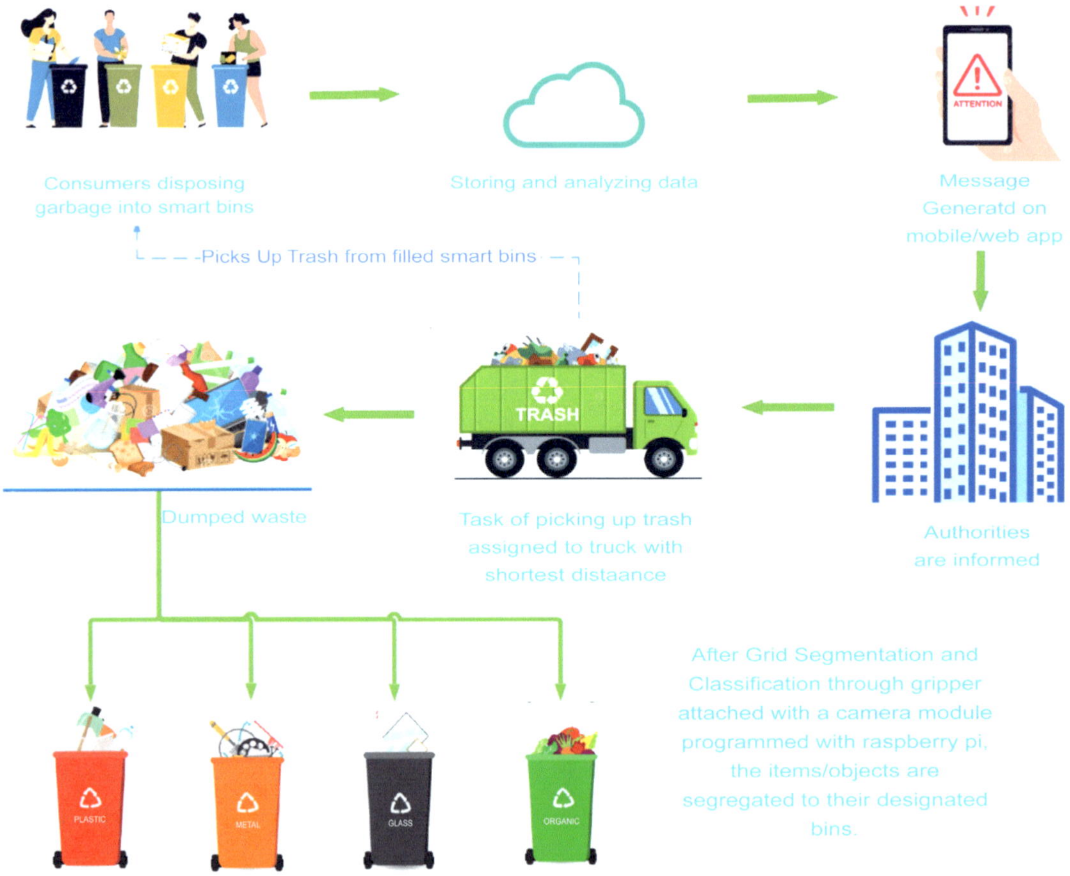

Figure 15.17. Waste management policies within the food industry require rigorous evaluation to determine their effectiveness in mitigating food waste.

Source: Cheema SM, Hannan A, Pires IM. Smart Waste Management and Classification Systems Using Cutting Edge Approach. *Sustainability*. 2022; 14(16):10226. https://doi.org/10.3390/su141610226

15.4. Economic Impact of Food Waste

The economic impact of food loss in the food industry is immense and multifaceted, with the potential for gigantic money losses and resource use inefficiencies. An estimated $1 trillion worth of food, almost one-third of food for human use, is lost each year globally (Landrigan et al., 2023). This waste not only lowers the potential market value but also encompasses the cost of wastage on waste management, such as collection, transport, and disposal. Although a few companies are beginning to adopt environmentally friendly packaging solutions in order to minimize wastage, they are often confronted by restraints that hold back the full realization of these theoretical benefits, reflecting a discrepancy between practice and theory (Molina-Besch & Pålsson, 2015). Therefore, fighting food waste in a sustainable manner can assist in reducing economic inefficiencies while enhancing resource preservation and overall societal well-being, indicating the need for systemic reform within the industry to respond to this overarching issue.

15.4.1. Cost Implications for Food Businesses

Effective waste management in the food industry has significant cost implications for organizations in terms of operational effectiveness and eventual profitability. When companies attempt to adopt sustainable practices, they are generally faced with initial investments in technologies, such as IoT and big data analytics, improving supply chain effectiveness and inventory management, as seen in Ugrinov et al. (2024). However, returns on such investments may be more than the costs in the form of reduced waste, increased brand loyalty, and cost savings in the long term. Additionally, policies of sustainability like environmental regulations and tax incentives can also alleviate costs while encouraging business managers toward judicious practice, as reported in Ngochindo et al. (2024). Last, blending these strategies not only meets regulatory needs but also builds a competitive advantage, positioning firms well in a market that increasingly values sustainability. The financial returns of waste management are, therefore, not only expenditures but strategic investments in the long-term sustainability of food businesses (Figure 15.18).

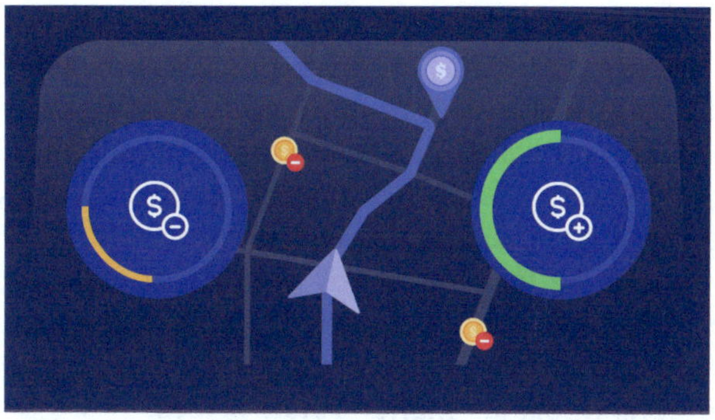

Figure 15.18. Effective waste management in the food industry carries significant cost implications for businesses, influencing both operational efficiency and long-term profitability.

Source: https://precoro.com/blog/content/images/2023/08/cost_saving1.png.

15.4.2. Economic Benefits of Waste Reduction

The cost savings from waste minimization in food processing are increasingly being considered a secret to sustainable business. By converting waste into value-added products, businesses can lower disposal and waste management expenses considerably. For instance, food waste can be a low-cost feedstock for the production of poly(3-hydroxybutyrate-co-3-hydroxyvalerate) (PHBV), a biodegradable plastic, with a possibility of 55% enhanced yield compared to traditional glucose-based processes (Wang et al., 2020). This not only minimizes the expense of waste disposal but also diminishes its effects on the environment through a reduction of dependence on landfills. Additionally, the recovery of bioactive molecules from crop residues offers potential for revenue generation in industries, such as cosmetics and nutraceuticals with the introduction of a visionary approach to harnessing resources (Dini, 2021). Overall, effective waste reduction programs not only generate sustainability but also ensure economic resilience in food production.

15.4.3. Impact on Food Prices

The intersection of food waste management in the food industry and food price is a complex and crucial issue. Unsound waste management can lead to rising production costs, thereby impacting consumers' prices. For instance, high volumes of lost foods not only cause wastage of resources but also cause transportation and processing-related costs that are passed directly to consumers as higher retail prices.

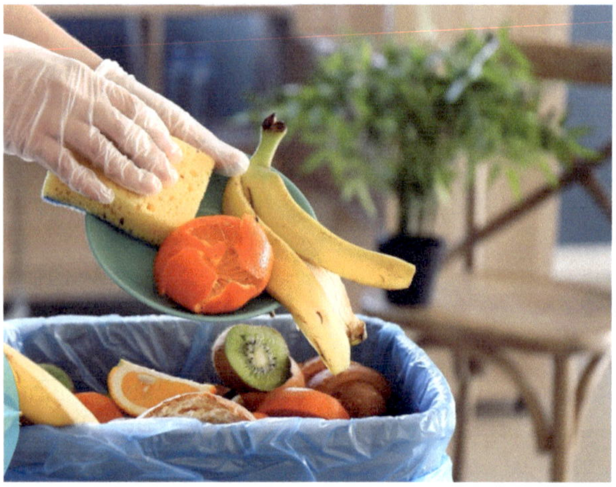

Figure 15.19. Losses of food not only contribute to resource wastage but also inflate the costs associated with transportation and processing, which are passed on to consumers through higher retail prices.

Source: https://www.retailtouchpoints.com/wp-content/uploads/2025/04/VP_Martie.png.

Moreover, the application of nitrogen fertilizers in the cultivation of crops, particularly wheat, is an area of concern in terms of sustainability. While excessive nitrogen application is essential for the provision of desirable quality, it brings about pollution and additional expenditure incurred in reversing such impacts, as cited in discussions of modern agricultural culture (Zörb et al., 2018). In contrast, investing in sustainable production and the deployment of nutritionally enhanced, water-efficient crop varieties can reverse such issues, ultimately reducing prices while enhancing food security (Dwivedi et al., 2017) (Figure 15.19).

15.4.4. Job Creation in Waste Management Sectors

The complementary partnership between job opportunities and food industry waste management is large-scale economic growth and environmental sustainability. The food industry struggles with critical problems of food loss and contamination, but sustainable waste management holds huge job potential. The initiative not only addresses the burning issues but also provides a green economy, where employees can acquire precious skills related to green strategies. As the study evidence shows, such community-level projects are also intended to enhance public and environmental health impact as well as promote economic equity. Of interest too is that non-tech industries like waste management are increasingly being viewed as a means of fostering employment generation, particularly through immigrant entrepreneurship (Jankie et al., 2013). Through this process of transformation, these communities can initiate system change that will be increasingly critical to a sustainable food system as well as a healthy workforce.

15.4.5. Investment in Sustainable Practices

In the food sector, investment in sustainability has become a decisive factor for addressing both environmental and economic objectives. With the sector experiencing challenges of depleting resources as well as regulatory pressures, integrating sustainability into its business agenda has become a top priority. For instance, though organizations are not simply compliance-oriented, they have begun to adopt innovative practices that guarantee efficiency and waste reduction.

The problem is that this is currently being made difficult by the current cost-cutting focus. As the study has explained, even as certain operators bemoan wanting to adopt sustainable programs, the larger logic of maximizing profits eclipses long-term environmental considerations, thereby preventing true strides (Dainty et al., 2014). For there to be actual transformation, stakeholders like governments need to create a platform for promotion and finance of sustainable projects that allows all the actors in the food supply chain to contribute meaningfully to waste management goals (Lavigueur et al., 2012) (Figure 15.20).

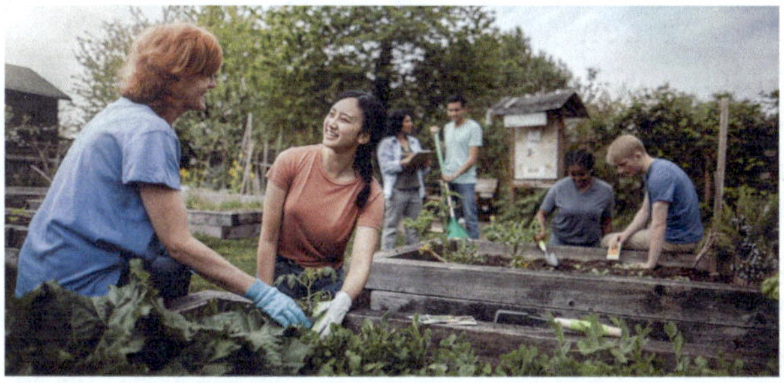

Figure 15.20. In the context of waste management in the food industry, investment in sustainable practices is increasingly recognized as a critical component for achieving both environmental and economic objectives.

Source: https://www.enel.com/content/dam/enel-com/immagini/master-azienda_2400x1160/storie_2400x1160/sostenibilita-economica-sociale-2400x1160.jpg.

15.4.6. Consumer Behavior and Its Economic Effects

You need to know the consumer behavior in order to reverse the economic impact of food waste, particularly in the food industry. The consumers are responsible for the market forces, and their purchasing choice directly affects production trends and wastage. For instance, an unbelievable $218 billion worth of wastage is devoured annually in America, which is an awe-inspiringly economic loss. This one generates a cascading effect, which gives rise to food processing, transportation, and waste cost, all of, which add up to environmental problems. Besides, as in the case of Vietnam, this change in demand for Western foods is also generating malnutrition and sustainability problems, and this takes economic cost (Do et al., 2020). Acknowledging the link between consumer behavior and such economic effects is a necessity for the development of useful waste reduction strategies that reduce food wastage while encouraging healthier and more sustainable patterns of consumption.

15.4.7. Long-Term Financial Sustainability

In waste management in the food industry, long-term financial sustainability is important in that it ensures not only the maximization of profitability but also environmental responsibility. Incorporating sustainable practices into waste management frameworks can make processes efficient and cut wasteful expenditure on waste disposal and resource consumption. For instance, research indicates that SSCM values ethical supply sourcing and supplier engagement for the purpose of lessening the negative impacts, hypothesizing that food companies can improve their reputation for sustainability while enhancing their bottom lines. Furthermore, as large companies like supermarkets hold strong negotiating muscles over supply chain practices, their endorsement of sustainability may encourage more ingrained changes throughout the industry overall (Dainty et al., 2014). Therefore, adopting long-term financial principles of sustainability will not only satisfy regulatory requirements but also strengthen market standing in the context of high competition where the environmental cause is on the increase (Figure 15.21).

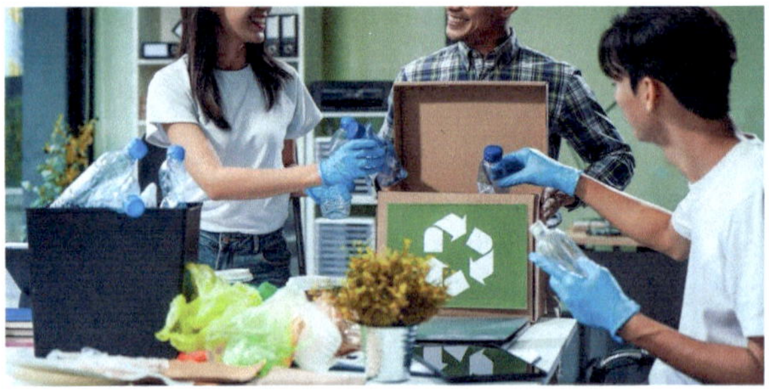

Figure 15.21. The integration of sustainable practices into waste management systems can streamline operations and reduce costs associated with waste disposal and resource consumption.

Source: https://certifiedwastesolutions.com/hubfs/shutterstock_2506586171%20%281%29.jpg.

15.4.8. Case Studies of Economic Success Through Waste Management

ood waste management does not only promote environmental sustainability but also possesses immense economic significance, as some case studies have proven. For instance, the new methods employed in food waste management have led to the recovery of useful resources, reducing operational costs and creating extra income. One good example is delivered by the results of a regional waste and resources strategies report, which identified sound examples in, which organic waste was being turned into compost and biogas, consistent with economic efficiency aims (Atkins Limited, 2010). Furthermore, institutions like Crossroads Rhode Island demonstrate how good waste management can play a role in more general social purposes. Through utilizing surplus food to share among homeless individuals, they are emulating a practice where waste reduction intersects with the public good, and both social responsibility and economic viability increase (Cooper et al., 2014). Therefore, how the food sector manages waste demonstrates its capacity for enhancing economic prosperity while meeting essential societal needs.

15.4.9. Role of Innovation in Reducing Costs

In reducing waste in food, cost-saving is driven by innovation as the key driver, enhancing the efficiency of operations as well as sustainability. Through applications of technologies, such as artificial intelligence and machine learning, food businesses are able to optimize inventory management and reduce overproduction, which impacts the bottom line directly. To ReFED, saving food waste not only alleviates environmental concerns but also offers a huge economic value since America is wasting $218 billion in one year on food that eventually gets trashed. In addition, novel trends, such as converting food waste into new products have the potential to shift hidden waste into profit streams and therefore lower disposal costs. When companies move towards these new practices, they not only save costs but also achieve more environmental goals, combining economic benefits with sustainable action. This is a double-barreled approach that emphasizes the important contribution innovation makes to reducing the cost of waste disposal.

A CLOSER LOOK

Food Security

Food security is a vital element in ensuring everyone has permanent access to sufficient, nutritious, and safe food for active and healthy living. It is founded on four pillars: availability, access, utilization, and stability. Availability entails a permanent availability of food that is reliant on agricultural yields, imports, and the supply chain. Access refers to the ability of individuals to be able to access food, depending on factors, such as income, price of food, and infrastructure. Utilization is the efficient use of food so that it is prepared, handled, and consumed in an appropriate manner concerning nutritional needs. Stability holds that food access is quite consistent in the long run and not disrupted by vagaries, such as economic vagaries or environmental changes. Food insecurity is a condition where one or more of these pillars fail, thereby leading to hunger, malnutrition, and ill health. In order to counter food security, there must be a confluence of action to build agriculture systems, eliminate poverty, increase access to food, and improve shock resilience threats to food availability.

SUMMARY

The need to discuss waste management in the food industry cannot be overemphasized, with proper measures being indispensable for environmental as well as economic viability. The analysis concludes that the waste minimization issue varies considerably across different European countries, and it results in the necessity to have specific national food waste management systems that achieve a balance between economic and technical viability to all the companies involved regardless of their waste generation capacity (Grinberga-Zalite et al., 2022). Moreover, the development of a waste minimization culture in harmony also fulfills the need for active participation of workers and employers, but primarily an educated consumer' base with a perception of the impact of their actions (Grinberga-Zalite et al., 2022). By adopting balanced waste management systems and creating awareness among everyone, the food industry itself can also contribute enormously towards minimizing wastes, thereby altering the face of a sustainable future. Dynamically flexible platforms and collective efforts will be the success mantra in curbing food wastage effectively.

In food industry waste management, there are some key problems addressed, which highlight the need for sustainability. Firstly, the amount of food waste produced underscores the need for waste minimization efforts, since, based on studies, almost one-third of the food produced worldwide ends up being wasted. This, apart from damaging the environment, also leads to food insecurity (Intergovernmental Panel on Climate Change, 2023). In addition, utilising new-generation technologies, e.g., anaerobic digestion and composting, yields efficient mechanisms of recycling organic waste to useful resources that support the circular economy (Gatta, 2022). Also not to be ruled out are consumer education and awareness, since properly informed choices can actually contribute towards lowering demand for such products that create waste. All these factors taken together imply a multi-dimensional approach towards improving waste management practice within the food sector with an emphasis on inter-stakeholder cooperation towards sustainability.

KEY TERMS FROM THIS CHAPTER

- Circular Economy
- Decomposition
- Environmental conservation
- Environmental degradation
- Grape pomace
- Health hazards
- Novel community-based interventions
- Organic waste
- Packaging food waste
- Cleaning agents
- Electronic waste (e-waste)
- Environmental damage
- Environmental sustainability
- Hazardous wastes
- Lean Thinking
- Obesity
- Overstock
- Red meat industry

REFERENCES

1. AL Jadidi, M., & AL Ghassani, G. (2025). Waste 2 wealth: Non-hazardous waste recycling approaches in oil and gas fields. *SPE Conference at Oman Petroleum & Energy Show.* https://www.semanticscholar.org/paper/47261768ffcb8b68eb55412d80f56feb77b6065b (accessed on 29 May 2025).
2. Taylor, C. M., Pollard, S. J. T., Rocks, S. A., & Angus, A. J. (2015). Better by design: business preferences for environmental regulatory reform. *The Science of the total environment, 512-513*, 287–295. https://doi.org/10.1016/j.scitotenv.2015.01.062 (accessed on 29 May 2025).
3. Arachchige, R., & Attanayake, L. (2018). Implementing an activity-based costing system: A case study based on Platform Plus Limited. https://core.ac.uk/download/187724411.pdf (accessed on 29 May 2025).
4. Asian and Pacific Centre for Transfer of Technology (APCTT), UN ESCAP. (1997). *VATIS Update: Waste Technology (Vol. 5, No. 23, Nov–Dec 1997).* https://core.ac.uk/download/641687675.pdf (accessed on 29 May 2025).
5. Atkins Limited. (2010). *Towards a Regional Resources Strategy Consultation.* A Guide to Waste Resources and Our Services. https://core.ac.uk/download/30624569.pdf (accessed on 29 May 2025).
6. Barling, D., Gresham, J., Mylona, K., Sharpe, R., et al. (2019). *Characterization Framework of Key Policy, Regulatory and Governance Dynamics and Impacts Upon European Food Value Chains: Fairer Trading Practices, Food Integrity, And Sustainability Collaborations (VALUMICS Deliverable D3.3).* https://core.ac.uk/download/287582350.pdf (accessed on 29 May 2025).
7. Batista L, Saes S, Fouto N. Sustainability of food supply chains – mapping food waste and by-product synergies. 2015. Paper presented at The 21st LRN Annual Conference and PhD Workshop 2016, United Kingdom.Benoit, L., Boustead, I., Callaghan, P., Carbon Trust, Environmental KTN, Finkbeiner, M., Hall, G. M., et al. (2012). *Energy From Waste and The Food Processing Industry.* https://core.ac.uk/download/6112944.pdf (accessed on 29 May 2025).
8. Blundel, R., Monaghan, A., & Thomas, C. (2012). *Promoting Environmentally Sustainable Enterprises: Some Policy Options.* In book: Government, SMEs and Entrepreneurship Development: Policy, Practice and Challenges (pp.171–184) Edition: 1 Chapter: Promoting environmentally sustainable enterprises: some policy options Publisher: Gower. Editors: Robert Blackburn, Michael Schaper.
9. Bogdanof, C. G., Ciupercă, R., Milea, D., Paraschiv, D., et al. (2019). Technological and ecological aspects of some wine waste recycling and their capitalization in food industry. https://core.ac.uk/download/229956318.pdf (accessed on 29 May 2025).
10. Cooper, Joel; Brookes, Joe; Lake, Darci; Fernandez, Victoria; Rosenfield, Matt; and Robinson, Arnold, "Crossroads Rhode Island: Proposed Social Enterprise Business Plan" (2014). *Business.* 8. https://docs.rwu.edu/cpc_business/8 (accessed on 29 May 2025).
11. Buczacki A, Gładysz B, Palmer E. HoReCa Food Waste and Sustainable Development Goals—A Systemic View. *Sustainability.* 2021; 13(10):5510. https://doi.org/10.3390/su13105510(accessed on 29 May 2025).

12. Carpena Rodríguez, M., Garcia-Oliveira, P., Núñez Estévez, B., Prieto Lage, M., et al. (2021). Essential oils and their application on active packaging systems: A review. https://core.ac.uk/download/484072295.pdf (accessed on 29 May 2025).
13. Clark, Q. M., Kanavikar, D. B., Clark, J., & Donnelly, P. J. (2025). Exploring the potential of AI-driven food waste management strategies used in the hospitality industry for application in household settings. *Frontiers in Artificial Intelligence, 7*. https://www.semanticscholar.org/paper/056ace0cfbd547e5a770c87670134e9f24e635b5 (accessed on 29 May 2025).
14. Concari, A., Kok, G., & Martens, P. (2021). Recycling behaviour: Mapping knowledge domain through bibliometrics and text mining. *Journal of Environmental Management, 303*, 114160. https://doi.org/10.1016/j.jenvman.2021.114160.
15. Dainty, A. J. D., Aerts, G., Ageron, B., Amaeshi, K., Bai, C., Ball, P., Baumann, H., et al. (2014). An institutional theory perspective on sustainable practices across the dairy supply chain. https://core.ac.uk/download/19595551.pdf (accessed on 29 May 2025).
16. Dasgupta, S., Huq, M., & Wheeler, D. (2025). *Bending the Rules: Discretionary Pollution Control in China*. https://core.ac.uk/download/pdf/6243306.pdf (accessed on 29 May 2025).
17. Davies, J. C., & Konisky, D. (2025). *Environmental Implications of The Foodservice and Food Retail Industries*. https://core.ac.uk/download/pdf/9307900.pdf (accessed on 29 May 2025).
18. Davies, J. C., & Lowe, A. (2025). *Environmental Implications of The Health Care Service Sector*. https://core.ac.uk/download/pdf/9307987.pdf (accessed on 29 May 2025).
19. Dikel, S., & Dikel, Ç. (2024). *A Gastronomic Approach to Industrial Aquaculture Waste Utilization*. https://core.ac.uk/download/635265907.pdf (accessed on 29 May 2025).
20. Dini, I. (2021). *Bio Discarded from Waste to Resource*. https://core.ac.uk/download/541677600.pdf (accessed on 29 May 2025).
21. Do, H., Kennedy, G., Nguyen, P. H., Nguyen, V. T., et al. (2020). *Determining Key Research Areas for Healthier Diets and Sustainable Food Systems in Viet Nam*. https://core.ac.uk/download/288633287.pdf (accessed on 29 May 2025).
22. Drzyzga, O., & Prieto, M. A. (2018). Plastic waste management, a matter for the 'community.' *Microbial Biotechnology, 12*(1), 66–68. https://doi.org/10.1111/1751-7915.13328.
23. Dwivedi, S. L., Lammerts Van Bueren, E., Ceccarelli, S., Grando, S., Upadhyaya, H. D., & Ortíz, R. (2017). Diversifying food systems in the pursuit of sustainable food production and healthy diets. *Trends in Plant Science, 22*(10), 842–856. https://doi.org/10.1016/j.tplants.2017.06.011.
24. Early, K. (2011). *Eco-Tourism Resorts: A Case Study of Best Practices at the Hamanasi Resort in Belize*. https://core.ac.uk/download/72047947.pdf (accessed on 29 May 2025).
25. East Midlands Development Agency. (2008). *East Midlands Food & Drink Sector Strategy*. https://core.ac.uk/download/30624571.pdf (accessed on 29 May 2025).
26. Elia, A. (2020). *Fashion's Destruction of Unsold Goods: Responsible Solutions for An Environmentally Conscious Future*. https://core.ac.uk/download/286697818.pdf (accessed on 29 May 2025).
27. Fair Labor Association. (2012). *Assessment Report 2012 Patagonia, China AA0000000003*. https://core.ac.uk/download/33602197.pdf (accessed on 29 May 2025).
28. Ferronato, N., & Torretta, V. (2019). Waste mismanagement in developing countries: A review

of global issues. *International Journal of Environmental Research and Public Health, 16*(6), 1060. https://doi.org/10.3390/ijerph16061060.

29. Font, X., Tapper, R., Schwartz, K., & Kornilaki, M. (2006). *Sustainable Supply Chain Management in Tourism*. https://core.ac.uk/download/29019010.pdf (accessed on 29 May 2025).
30. Frederickson, J., Slater, R., & Yoxon, M. (2010). *Unlocking the Potential of Community Composting: Full Project Report*. https://core.ac.uk/download/109365.pdf (accessed on 29 May 2025).
31. Frino, B., Verma, G., Schutz, J., Buchanan, J., Jakubauskas, M., Yu, S., & Bretherton, T. (2025). *Minimum Wages and Their Role in The Process and Incentives to Bargain*. https://core.ac.uk/download/pdf/30673958.pdf (accessed on 29 May 2025).
32. Frondel, M., Horbach, J., Rennings, K., Requate, T., et al. (2025). *Environmental Policy Tools and Firm-Level Management Practices: Empirical Evidence for Germany*. https://core.ac.uk/download/pdf/6406240.pdf (accessed on 29 May 2025).
33. Gatta, P. P. (2022). *The State of World Fisheries and Aquaculture 2022*. FAO eBooks. https://doi.org/10.4060/cc0461en.
34. Ghosh, S. K. (2016). Biomass & bio-waste supply chain sustainability for bio-energy and bio-fuel production. *Procedia Environmental Sciences, 31*, 31–39. https://doi.org/10.1016/j.proenv.2016.02.005.
35. Gil, A. (2021). Challenges on waste-to-energy for the valorization of industrial wastes: Electricity, heat and cold, bioliquids and biofuels. *Environmental Nanotechnology Monitoring & Management, 17*, 100615. https://doi.org/10.1016/j.enmm.2021.100615.
36. Gonzalez-Soria, J. (2012). *Environmental Dynamics in Animal Waste Reclamation in The Scaling Up of Livestock in Thailand*. https://core.ac.uk/download/9640100.pdf (accessed on 29 May 2025).
37. Grinberga-Zalite, G., & Zvirbule, A. (2022). *Analysis of Waste Minimization Challenges to European Food Production Enterprises*. https://core.ac.uk/download/542929982.pdf (accessed on 29 May 2025).
38. Intergovernmental Panel on Climate Change. (2023). *Climate Change 2022–Impacts, Adaptation and Vulnerability*. https://doi.org/10.1017/9781009325844.
39. Jankie, A., Chawla, C. H., Jennings, J., Lawrence, J., & Bryant, M. L. (2013). *Immigrant Entrepreneurs Creating Jobs and Strengthening the U.S. Economy in Growing Industries*. https://core.ac.uk/download/71361719.pdf (accessed on 29 May 2025).
40. JosephNg, P. S., Vasu, K. P., Phan, K. Y., Sun, J., & Wei, Z. (2024). Managing sustainable E-waste resilient infrastructure effectively with the introduction of smart bin. *Journal of Advanced Research in Applied Mechanics*. https://www.semanticscholar.org/paper/f46b3333359faeb3d8a372f71cf4cd0606591630 (accessed on 29 May 2025).
41. Juchelková, D., Raclavská, H., Sassmanová, V., Tun, M. M., et al. (2018). *Utilization of Biodegradable Wastes as A Clean Energy Source in The Developing Countries: A Case Study in Myanmar*. https://core.ac.uk/download/161968078.pdf (accessed on 29 May 2025).
42. Kjær, T., & Lybæk, R. (2024). *How Can Circular Economy Strengthen the Recycling of Plastic Packaging Wastes? Exploratory And Qualitative Case Study of The Danish Plastic Industry*. https://core.ac.uk/download/630942995.pdf (accessed on 29 May 2025).

43. Kopanaki, E., Oikonomou, M., & Stroumpoulis, A. (2021). *The Impact of Blockchain Technology on Food Waste Management in The Hospitality Industry*. https://core.ac.uk/download/493040446.pdf.

44. Landrigan, P. J., Raps, H., Cropper, M., Bald, C., Brunner, M., Canonizado, E. M., Charles, D., et al. (2023). The Minderoo-Monaco Commission on plastics and human health. *Annals of Global Health, 89*, Article 24. https://doi.org/10.5334/aogh.4056.

45. Lavigueur, A., Knutson, B., Roberts, C., Lee, K., Kneeland, K., Lee, L., Wells, L., et al. (2012). *Environmental Policy Update 2012: Development Strategies and Environmental Policy in East Africa*. https://core.ac.uk/download/75779500.pdf (accessed on 29 May 2025).

46. Lewis, K., & Tzilivakis, J. (1999). *Environmental Management for Agriculture (EMA) and Sustainable Agriculture*. https://core.ac.uk/download/29850652.pdf (accessed on 29 May 2025).

47. Lipinski, B., Hanson, C., Lomax, J., Kitinoja, L., Waite, R., & Searchinger, T. (2013). *Creating a Sustainable Food Future: Reducing Food Loss and Waste (Installment 2)*. https://core.ac.uk/download/71362194.pdf (accessed on 29 May 2025).

48. Maguire, M. A. (2018). *Wasted Potential: A Food Waste Reduction Strategy for Toronto Restaurants*. https://core.ac.uk/download/160283147.pdf (accessed on 29 May 2025).

49. Mahmud, K. T. (2024). *Reducing Food Waste Through Efficient Logistics: A Case Study*. https://core.ac.uk/download/638725929.pdf (accessed on 29 May 2025).

50. Majid, A., Arsat, A., Aliffaizi, A., Zahari, M., Salehuddin, M., Zulkifly, M., et al. (2024). Strengthening food security: A conceptual scholarly examination of the linkages between food loss and food waste. https://core.ac.uk/download/635321904.pdf (accessed on 29 May 2025).

51. Mann, A., Henges-Jeck, C., Haasz, D., Wolff, G., Cushing, K., Gleick, P. H., & Srinivasan, V. (2003). *Waste not, Want Not: The Potential for Urban Water Conservation in California*. https://core.ac.uk/download/75783416.pdf (accessed on 29 May 2025).

52. Meegoda, J. N., Chande, C., & Bakshi, I. (2025). Biodigesters for sustainable food waste management. *International Journal of Environmental Research and Public Health, 22*. https://www.semanticscholar.org/paper/2912f48593d5da4981f3bde47f9e4bb7bfd93e67 (accessed on 29 May 2025).

53. Meikle, B. (2018). *Envisioning Ontario's Food and Organic Waste Disposal Ban: A Comparative Case Analysis*. https://core.ac.uk/download/189494620.pdf (accessed on 29 May 2025).

54. Molina-Besch, K., & Pålsson, H. (2015). A supply chain perspective on green packaging development—Theory versus practice. *Packaging Technology and Science, 29*, 45–63. https://doi.org/10.1002/pts.2186.

55. Mondello, A., Salomone, R., & Mondello, G. (2024). Exploring circular economy in the cosmetic industry: Insights from a literature review. *Environmental Impact Assessment Review, 105*, 107443. https://doi.org/10.1016/j.eiar.2024.107443.

56. Ngochindo, A., Igwe, A. N., Louis, N., Eyo-Udo, E., Toromade, A. S., & Tosin, T. (2024). Policy implications and economic incentives for sustainable supply chain practices in the food and FMCG sectors. *Comprehensive Research and Reviews Journal*. https://www.semanticscholar.org/paper/34ffc7bea1e42cf762156501ca7676fbd8012870 (accessed on 29 May 2025).

57. Obioma, A., Sc, A., & Bc, A. (2024). Possible outbreak of Newcastle virus infection in the face of increasing trend of backyard poultry farm management interface in Nigeria: A public health and food security threat. *Journal of Quality in Health Care & Economics*. https://www.semanticscholar.org/paper/1f5bf89a83d1942652088d9039110c129680fff4 (accessed on 29 May 2025).

58. Orozco, S., Montiel, E., Valencia, J. E., González, R. G., Chávez Parga, M. del C., Cortés, J. A., & Rivero, M. (2024). Effective RhB dye removal using sustainable natural bio adsorbents synthesized from avocado seed and skin. *Water, Air, & Soil Pollution*. https://www.semanticscholar.org/paper/8d1537bca1a7caac988ae44bbaa824aa02cdfa8c (accessed on 29 May 2025).

59. Panday, D., Bhusal, N., Das, S., & Ghalehgolabbehbahani, A. (2024). Rooted in nature: The rise, challenges, and potential of organic farming and fertilizers in agroecosystems. *Sustainability, 16*, 1530. https://doi.org/10.3390/su16041530.

60. Ramlan, M. H., & Yaacob, S. N. A. (2017). *A Review of Food Waste Management Strategies and Policies in Malaysia's Hospitality Industry*. https://core.ac.uk/download/635281165.pdf (accessed on 29 May 2025).

61. Ravanal, M., Doussoulin, J., & Mougenot, B. (2024). Does sustainability matter in the global beer industry? Bibliometrics trends in recycling and the circular economy. *Frontiers in Sustainable Food Systems*. https://www.semanticscholar.org/paper/3d8563a09208abba7d0786a81210a3c3668ac7ed (accessed on 29 May 2025).

62. Saberi, S., Kouhizadeh, M., Sarkis, J., & Shen, L. (2018). Blockchain technology and its relationships to sustainable supply chain management. *International Journal of Production Research, 57*(7), 2117–2135. https://doi.org/10.1080/00207543.2018.1533261.

63. Shamseer, L., Moher, D., Clarke, M., Ghersi, D., Liberati, A., Petticrew, M., Shekelle, P., et al. (2015). Preferred reporting items for systematic review and meta-analysis protocols (PRISMA-P) 2015: Elaboration and explanation. *BMJ, 349*, g7647. https://doi.org/10.1136/bmj.g7647.

64. Simons, D., & Zokaei, K. (2025). *Performance Improvements Through Implementation of Lean Practices: A Study of the U.K. Red Meat Industry*. https://core.ac.uk/download/pdf/6653206.pdf (accessed on 29 May 2025).

65. Torrens, F. (2023). Natural genera, scientific classifications, life, fireworks and COVID. *Nereis. Interdisciplinary Ibero-American Journal of Methods, Modelling and Simulation*. https://www.semanticscholar.org/paper/905ff903f9734e9f09aed6aa0d9ee78c216a474e (accessed on 29 May 2025).

66. Ugrinov, S., Ćoćkalo, D., & Bakator, M. (2024). Optimization and sustainability of supply chains in the food and beverage industry. *Ekonomika*. https://www.semanticscholar.org/paper/f82dc5d023917652f7d11cb1e080854b750c924a (accessed on 29 May 2025).

67. Varma, S., Patra, P., & Shankar, R. (2024). The food industry supply chain: Synergy of environmental orientation and collaboration in implementing circularity. *Business Strategy and the Environment*. https://www.semanticscholar.org/paper/c3b3259f78d20985addfa1b14eb86a3a5a29862a (accessed on 29 May 2025).

68. Wang, K., & Zhang, R. (2020). Production of polyhydroxyalkanoates (PHA) by *Haloferax mediterranei* from food waste derived nutrients for biodegradable plastic applications. https://core.ac.uk/download/617034709.pdf (accessed on 29 May 2025).

69. Whitmee, S., Haines, A., Beyrer, C., Boltz, F., Capon, A., de Souza Dias, B. F., Ezeh, A., et al. (2015). Safeguarding human health in the Anthropocene epoch: Report of the Rockefeller Foundation–Lancet Commission on planetary health. *The Lancet, 386*(10007), 1973–2028. https://doi.org/10.1016/S0140-6736(15)60901-1.

70. Wibisono, D. A. S., Saw, C. Y., Wu, T. Y., & Chau, C. F. (2025). Advancing industrial food byproduct management: Strategies, technologies, and progress in waste reduction. *Processes*. https://www.semanticscholar.org/paper/20b1549c0435ffa5892f6e86a19b684fd505aa21 (accessed on 29 May 2025).

71. Zörb, C., Ludewig, U., & Hawkesford, M. J. (2018). Perspective on wheat yield and quality with reduced nitrogen supply. *Trends in Plant Science, 23*, 1029–1037. https://doi.org/10.1016/j.tplants.2018.08.012.

INDEX

A

abdominal discomfort 210
accountability 55, 65, 71, 72, 247
accurate subtyping methods 303
additives 28, 35, 38, 182, 190
adulterated samples 160, 163
advisory 2
aflatoxins 262
Aflatoxins 31, 32
agro-biotechnology 182, 201
agroterrorism 234
AI-driven analytics 85
airtight containers 108, 114, 117, 125
Aji Santoso International Football Academy (ASIFA) 6
Alaska 111
allergen-free food products 276, 280
allergen immunotherapy (AIT) 285
allergens 182, 185, 186, 190, 199, 200, 275, 276, 277, 278, 279, 280, 281, 283, 284, 286, 287, 288, 290, 291, 292
anaphylaxis 274, 275, 278, 279, 286, 287
animal welfare 186, 188, 204
applesauce 223
Aspergillus 262
assessment 7, 22, 26
association 2
asthma 63, 75
authenticity 160, 162, 163, 169, 171, 174, 180
automated cleaning systems 89, 91
automation 85, 104
awareness 56, 58, 64, 66, 67, 74, 78
Azarcón 220

B

bacteria 4, 5, 6, 7, 9, 28, 29, 30, 32, 44, 54
bananas 223
barley 134, 157
bathing 56
beverages 139, 157
bioaccumulate 256, 257, 258
biofilms 81, 82, 83, 85, 88, 91, 93, 95, 97, 103, 104
biological contaminants 30, 32
bisphenol A (BPA) 258
blockchain 247
body tissues 257
brand 85
brushing teeth 56

C

cadmium 216
caffeine 223
Campylobacter 1, 8, 9, 26
canning 119, 120
Canning 119
carotenoid production 166
chemical contamination 28, 37, 256, 257, 261, 265

chemical methods 160
chemical residues 210
chemicals 136, 140, 144
Chemical spills 329
chemometric analysis 161
chemometrics 137, 138, 157
chicory 134, 157
childhood allergies 274
chilling 120
chlorine compounds 89
chromatography 160, 161, 179
chronic health implications 257
Ciguatera 261, 270
Circular Economy 358, 377
citrus fruits 113
cleaning agents 357
cleaning surfaces 82, 100
cleanliness 1, 2, 5, 8, 14, 17, 82, 83, 84, 85, 88, 90, 91, 92, 93, 95, 96, 97
climate change 4
Clostridium difficile 216
Clostridium perfringens 212, 213, 216, 217, 218, 228, 229
Codex Alimentarius 212, 215
Cold chains 114
commercialization 166
Commission of the European Communities 289
communication 187, 189, 201
Community-based Outbreak Investigation and Response (COIR) 314
community health 6, 18
companies 59, 60, 69, 70
complexity 233, 234, 236, 237, 238, 239, 243, 248
compliance 55, 57, 61, 62, 65, 70, 72, 74, 76, 77, 78
conjunction 111
consumer 2, 5, 14, 15, 16
consumer attitudes 183, 195, 201
consumer awareness 182, 183, 184, 186, 187, 188, 189, 190, 191, 193, 194, 195, 200, 203, 207
consumer empowerment 182, 191
consumer knowledge 184, 186, 187, 190, 200, 203
consumer rights 184, 191
consumers 56, 58, 59, 60, 61, 63, 66, 67, 68, 69, 70, 72, 74, 77
consumption 2, 31, 32, 33, 34, 38, 134, 135, 137, 149
contaminants 27, 28, 30, 32, 34, 37, 38, 39, 40, 41, 42, 44, 47, 49
contaminated snacks 302
contamination 2, 3, 4, 6, 7, 8, 9, 10, 11, 15, 17, 18, 26
contamination pathways 29
contamination risks 107, 119, 121
COVID-19 pandemic 8, 18, 23, 26
CRISPR-based technologies 308
crop environments 209
cross-contamination 5, 7
cultural traditions 60
culture-based assays 161, 162
customs 83

D

dairy 6, 9, 10
dairy products 136, 140, 143
dangers 2, 15
danger zone 113, 114, 115, 120
data collection 302, 307
Date labeling 187
Date labels 112
decision-making 184, 186, 188, 194, 199, 201
decomposition 358
deli meats 10
deoxynivalenol 262
developing nations 1, 2
diarrhea 210, 213, 216, 217, 218, 219, 220, 221, 223, 225
digital 60
digital interfaces 186
diseases 2, 3, 4, 5, 8, 9, 10, 11, 13, 18, 19, 21, 25, 26
disinfectants 82, 85, 97
disorient food chains 325
dizziness 302
DNA barcoding 162, 163, 174, 179
DNA quality 163
dry goods 118

E

earthquakes 326, 328, 329
eco-labels 184, 194

E. coli 6, 7, 8, 9, 15, 22
ecological health 32
ecology 212
economic adulteration 136
economic security 234
economy 181, 197
ecosystems 32, 34
effluent disposal 257
Egg Macaroni 311
eggs 9
electrical property 133
electrolyte beverages 220
Electronic waste (e-waste) 358
elementary school 302, 311, 322
emerging organic groundwater contaminants (EGCs) 34
employers 57, 60
enforcement 165, 167, 168, 169, 170, 175
environmental conservation 354
environmental contamination 137
environmental damage 354
environmental degradation 354, 355, 359, 364
environmental factors 307, 312
environmental management 239
environmental pollution 257
environmental problems 2
environmental sustainability 182, 186, 205, 355, 358, 363, 370, 372
equipment 81, 82, 83, 84, 85, 86, 87, 88, 89, 90, 91, 93, 94, 95, 96, 97, 98, 99, 101
equipment maintenance 83, 90, 101
European Food Safety Authority (EFSA) 8
exclusion 210

F

fake products 163
fats 133, 135, 137, 156, 157
FIFO (First In, First Out) method 111
floods 326, 328, 329
food adulterants 160, 161, 163
Food adulteration 134, 136, 142, 145, 153, 154
Food and Agriculture Organization (FAO) 2
food attribution 234, 237, 240, 241, 242, 244
food authenticity 141
foodborne agents 302
foodborne diseases (FBDs) 29
foodborne illness 3, 8, 15, 23
foodborne illnesses 56, 57, 58, 59, 61, 62, 64, 65, 66, 67, 68, 70, 71, 72
food choices 60
food consumption 181, 184, 185, 189, 194, 200
food distribution 114, 126
food handler 55, 63, 64, 68, 74, 77
food hygiene 1, 2, 4, 5, 10, 11, 15, 17, 19, 21
food hypersensitivity 274, 279, 280, 281, 284, 287, 292, 296
Food intolerances 274, 280, 281, 282, 283
food label awareness 183
Food laboratories 163
food leftovers 82
food manufacturing 3
food piracy detection 137
food poisoning 1, 5, 17
food preparation areas 2, 5
food production 83, 84, 88, 91, 92, 98, 134, 135, 137, 145, 151, 209, 210
food production systems 184
food products 29, 31, 34, 39, 41, 42, 43, 44, 50
food proteins 278
food recovery 182
food safety 1, 2, 3, 4, 5, 6, 7, 8, 10, 11, 12, 13, 14, 15, 16, 17, 18, 19, 20, 21, 22
food safety culture 210
food safety culture (FS-culture) 58
food safety management 107
food safety protocols 82, 84, 90
food sanitation 1, 3, 7, 12, 21
food service 82, 87, 91, 93, 94, 95, 97, 99, 101
food service industry 55, 66
food services 83
food supply chains 4, 17
food system 186
food web 32, 34
Fourier transform infrared (FTIR) spectroscopy 138
Frafra potato 111, 130

fragment size 163
freezing 108, 114, 120, 125
frozen food 58, 78
fruit juices 109
fruits 138
FS-culture 58, 59, 61, 65, 69, 72
fungal growth 32
fungal infections 114
fungi 29, 30, 31, 32, 33, 36
Fusarium 262

G

Gas Chromatography (GC) 161
genetically modified (GM) food 182
genetic predisposition 276
geographical indications (GI) 181
geographical origin labels 181
geographic information systems (GIS) 307
glass 28, 38, 39, 40, 42
global food production 186
globalization 4, 325, 333
Gloves 62
gluten-free diets 186
Gluten-free pasta 186
gluten-free products 119
gluten sensitivity 274
Goldband goatfish 138
Good Hygiene Practices (GHP) 93
good manufacturing practices (GMP) 265
grape pomace 359
grooming 63

H

habitats 32
hair restraints 61
hand eczema 56, 61, 62, 79
Handwashing 61, 62, 75
Hazard Analysis Critical Control Point (HACCP) 1, 6, 13, 20
hazardous wastes 358
hazards 2, 5, 12, 20
hazelnut oil 133, 140, 142, 146
health 27, 28, 29, 30, 31, 32, 33, 34, 35, 36, 37, 38, 39, 40, 42, 43, 44, 45, 46, 49, 50, 51, 53, 54
healthcare 2, 8, 19
health checkups 63
health crises 325, 332, 335, 338
health hazards 357
health-related quality of life (HRQL) 275
health standards 60
healthy meal 60
heavy metals 28, 29, 32, 34, 36, 39, 42, 43, 44, 47, 49, 50, 53, 54
hepatitis 31
hepatitis A 238, 241
herbs 137, 139, 155
heterogeneity 305, 306, 319
high-intensity sweeteners (HIS) 139
High-Performance Liquid Chromatography (HPLC) 161
high-value oils 137
Honey 136, 155
hospital-acquired infections 212
human cognition 182
human health 255, 256, 257
humidity 215
hurricanes 328, 329
Hydration 221
hydrogen peroxide 89
hygiene 1, 2, 3, 4, 5, 6, 7, 8, 9, 10, 11, 12, 13, 14, 15, 16, 17, 18, 19, 21, 22, 23
hygiene training 59

I

illnesses 107, 108, 109, 110, 111, 112, 115, 118, 121, 123, 126, 131
immune system 223
immunoglobulin E antibodies 278
industrial emissions 280
industrial farming 29
industrial revolution 83
Industry 4.0 technologies 2, 22
industry size 84
informed decision-making 184
ingestion 1
ingredients 134, 135, 136, 139, 140, 142, 146, 149

innovations 2, 162, 166, 171
insecticides 83, 105
integrated pest management (IPM) 83
Intergovernmental Panel on Climate Changes 2
ionizing radiation 111
IoT monitoring devices 89
irritable bowel syndrome (IBS) 223

J

juvenile crayfish 32

K

knowledge 2, 6, 15, 16, 23
knowledge, attitude, and practice (KAP) 62

L

labeling 112, 119
labels 112
Laos 239, 253
law enforcement agencies 234
lax enforcement 138
lead 256, 257, 262, 263, 264, 266, 269
Lean Thinking 354
legal frameworks 82, 91
legislation 135, 149, 156
likelihood 307
liquid chromatography-high-resolution mass spectrometry (LC-HRMS) 161
Listeria monocytogenes 28, 29, 41, 82, 83, 87, 88, 89, 90, 95, 97, 100, 102, 104, 111, 112
local agencies 302
local health departments (LHDs) 223
Local health departments (LHDs) 306

M

malaise 302
management systems 55, 60, 61, 72
man-made activities 29
man-made disasters 329
manufacturers 164, 167
manufacturing 28, 29, 36
marine ecosystem 256, 258
market integration 167
meat 6, 8, 9
medical bills 84
Mediterranean diet 183
menstrual products 186
mercury 216, 256, 257
metal pieces 28
microalgae 164, 165, 166
microbial communities 81
microbial growth 32
microbial hazards 56
microbial risks 82
microbial source tracking (MST) 28
Microorganisms 81, 104, 105
Milk 136
misinformation 185, 194
mislabeling 138, 139
moisture 110, 111, 113, 117, 118
mold 31, 32
mold contamination 32
mortality data 234
Mossville 258, 259, 272
motivation 61
Mullus barbatus 138
Mullus surmuletus 138
mycotoxins 32, 33, 36, 37
Mycotoxins 260, 262, 270, 272

N

natural antiviral compounds 213
natural calamities 325
Natural disasters 328, 329
natural extracts 110
natural food toxins 210
Natural Language Processing 327
natural toxins 255, 256, 258, 259, 260, 261, 262, 263, 264, 265, 266, 267, 269
natural watercourses 32
nausea 210, 216, 219
navigation proficiency 182
near-infrared (NIR) spectroscopy 137
next-generation sequencing (NGS) 304
non-governmental organizations (NGOs) 150, 151

non-IgE-mediated allergies 277, 278
normal cell functions 242
norovirus 31
Norovirus 238, 242, 253
novel community-based interventions 355
nut-free 119
nutrients 32, 35
Nutritional awareness 186
nutritional deficiencies 135
nutritional information 275, 286
nutritional value 108, 109
Nutrition Facts Panel 198
nutrition labeling 187
Nutrition Labeling and Education Act (NLEA) 182, 189, 190
Nutrition Labeling Education Act (NLEA) 184

O

obesity 355
objective measurement 160
ochratoxin 262
Oils 137
olive oil 133, 135, 136, 140, 142, 146, 156
online food delivery apps 60
operation 86, 105
Oral rehydration solutions 220
organic food 27, 48, 182, 197
organic livestock 31
organic matter 88, 89
Organic waste 357
organizational culture 55
orrellanine (OR) poisoning 263
outbreaks 28, 29, 44, 52
overstock 359
over-the-counter (OTC) medications 221
ownership 86

P

packaging 29, 40, 45
packaging food waste 357
packaging materials 117
Pandemics 325, 329
pantry 112
parasites 28, 30, 31
parasitic pathogen amplification 213
Parkinson's disease 255, 259
pasteurization 108
pathogenic microorganisms 118
pathogens 1, 2, 3, 4, 5, 6, 7, 8, 9, 10, 11, 18, 22, 26
pathogen transmission 8, 30
patulin 109, 131
peanuts 276, 277
Penicillium 262
perishable foods 108, 112, 113, 114, 120, 125
peroxyacetic acid (PAA) 88
personal cleanliness 55
personal hygiene 55, 56, 57, 58, 59, 60, 61, 62, 63, 64, 67, 68, 69, 70, 72, 74, 78
pesticides 28, 34, 36, 37, 41, 43, 44, 48
phthalates 258
Physical adulteration 141
phytosterol profiles 135
phytosterols 133, 146
plant material 163
policymakers 11, 182, 189, 193, 234, 235, 237, 240, 241, 245, 248, 250
pollutants 29, 32, 34, 37, 38, 39, 82
polychlorinated biphenyls (PCBs) 258
polycyclic aromatic hydrocarbons (PAHs) 32
polymerase chain reaction (PCR) 151
poor sanitation 239
positive hygiene culture 58
postbiotics 109, 112, 130
post-harvest activities 215
post-harvest decay 114
pre-clean 89
probability 184
production 2, 4, 7, 8, 11, 12, 17, 20, 25
proper waste disposal 83
protected designation of origin (PDO) labeling 181
Pseudupeneus prayensis 139
psittacosis 301
public health 1, 2, 3, 4, 5, 7, 10, 11, 12, 13, 14, 15, 16, 17, 18, 19, 21, 22, 24
public health hazards 256
public health institutions 302

public health laws 82, 83, 86, 99
public trust 83
pulsed-field gel electrophoresis (PFGE) 305

Q

qualitative assessment 120
quality 1, 2, 4, 5, 7, 15, 17, 20, 24
quality of water 29
quality products 160
quantitative standards 2, 215
quaternary ammonium compounds 89

R

rapid detection systems 161, 162
rapid testing kits 162
ready-to-eat (RTE) items 10
Real-time communication 327
red meat industry 354
red mullet 138
refrigeration 108, 114, 115, 119
reheating 119, 120
reliance 60
resource allocation 210
resource recovery 358, 361
responsible 56, 58, 59, 60, 66, 68, 72
restroom 61, 62
Rhodamine B dye 358
rice 220, 221, 223
rinse 89
Risk analysis 329
roasted coffee 160

S

Safe Moisture Content (SMC) 118
salads 10
Salmonella enteritidis 109, 127
sanitary 2, 3, 6, 24
sanitation protocols 9, 11, 81, 82, 83, 85, 89, 91, 93, 95, 97
sanitize 88, 89
scientists 233, 234, 237, 240, 241, 245, 248, 250
Seafood 135, 138, 154
self-values 184
sensitization 276, 294
sensors 160
sensory analysis 160, 175
serum antibody tests 279
severe acute respiratory syndrome coronavirus 2 (SARS-CoV-2) 81
shattered glass 357
shelf life 108, 109, 110, 111, 113, 116, 119, 122, 125, 129, 130
Shiga toxin-producing Escherichia coli (STEC) 236
Shigella 10
sick 2, 3, 5, 8
single HyBeacon(®) probe assay 162
skim milk 88
skin prick testing 279
skin problems 278
soap 56, 61, 62
social vulnerability 328
societal issues 186
socio-economic factors 83
soil 29, 30, 34, 36, 38, 39, 43, 47, 48, 51, 52, 54
solid-phase extraction (SPE) 141
sous vide 120
specific origin 181
Spectroscopic methods 160
spices 136, 137, 143, 151, 157
spicy foods 223
spoilage 81, 85, 90, 97
stakeholders 4, 13, 19
staple foods 134
starch 136, 145
sterilization 119
storing 2, 5
street food handlers 59
sucrose 135
sugar 139
supply chain 3, 4
surface material 82
Surveillance systems 302
sustainability 2, 4, 12, 13, 15, 22, 26
sustainable practices 108
sustainable water management 29, 43
sweeteners 139, 157

systematic documentation 307

T

temperature 215
temperature control 107, 108, 109, 110, 111, 112, 113, 116, 117, 119, 120, 121, 122, 123, 124, 126
temperature regulation 111
terrorist attacks 329
thaw 115
The Emergency Food Assistance Program (TEFAP) 332
Thin Layer Chromatography (TLC) 161
toast 220, 221, 223
toxicants 212, 226
toxic chemicals 210
toxic contaminants 257
toxic materials 164
toxins 109
Toxoplasma gondii 31, 50
Tracking Charts 89
training 55, 58, 59, 61, 62, 64, 65, 66, 67, 68, 69, 70, 71, 72, 74, 77
transmission 59, 62, 63
transmission patterns 304
transparency 181, 182, 184, 185, 186, 188, 191, 192, 193, 197, 198, 200, 201, 203, 247
transparent labeling 184, 196
tree nuts 276, 277

U

unforeseen events 325
uniforms 61, 63, 74
United States Department of Agriculture (USDA) 245
unpasteurized milk 234
Urbanization 32
utensils 82, 88, 101

V

variant growth patterns 109
vegetables 110, 112, 118, 130, 138, 141
vibrational spectroscopy (VS) 138
vinyl gloves 62
viruses 28, 30, 31
vomiting 210, 213, 216, 219, 220, 221, 223
vulnerability 31
vulnerable population 328

W

wash 89, 94
washing hands 56, 60
waste development 356
waste management 353, 354, 356, 357, 358, 359, 360, 361, 362, 363, 364, 365, 366, 367, 369, 370, 371, 372, 374, 376, 378
wastewater 2
Wastewater treatment 358
water 29, 30, 32, 34, 36, 39, 41, 43, 48, 49, 50
water management 2
well-being 55, 56, 57, 64, 71, 72, 74
West African goatfish 139
Wheat 32, 53
wildlife health 212
wildlife mortality 212
willingness 181, 201, 203
winemaking 356, 359
World Health Organization (WHO) 2
wounds 58

Z

zoonotic diseases 31, 43
zoonotic protozoan parasite 31